AMA
AMERICAN MEDICAL ASSOCIATION

ICD-10-CM Documentation

Essential Charting Guidance to Support Medical Necessity

2021

AMA publications fund initiatives that drive improvements in patient health, practice innovation and medical education.
AMAstore.com

ICD-10-CM Documentation 2021:
Essential Charting Guidance to Support Medical Necessity

Published by DecisionHealth, a Simplify Compliance brand

100 Winners Circle, Suite 300
Brentwood, TN 37027
(855) 255-5341
www.codingbooks.com

ISBN: 978-1-64016-085-9

Item Number: OP168021

Disclaimer

No part of this publication may be reproduced, stored in a retrieval system, or transmitted, in any form or by any means, electronic, mechanical, photocopy, recording, or otherwise, without the prior written permission of the publisher. This publication is sold with the understanding that the publisher is not engaged in rendering legal, medical, accounting, or other professional service in specific situations. Although prepared for professionals, this publication should not be utilized as a substitute for professional service in specific situations. If legal or medical advice is required, the services of a professional should be sought.

Our Commitment to Accuracy

The American Medical Association (AMA) is committed to producing accurate and reliable materials. To report corrections, please call the AMA Unified Service Center at (800) 621-8335. AMA publication and product updates, errata, and addenda can be found at *amaproductupdates.org*.

To purchase additional copies, contact the AMA at 800 621-8335 or visit the AMA store at *amastore.com*. Refer to item number OP168021.

Acknowledgements

Maria Tsigas, *Product Director, Information, Print Subscription Products & Services*
Renee Dudash, *Senior Manager of Operations*
Matt Sharpe, *Senior Manager, Creative Layout*
AnnMarie Lemoine, *Team Lead, Creative Layout*
Nicole Grande, *Senior Layout Artist*
Richard Scott, *Associate Content Manager*
Lori Becks, RHIA, *Clinical Technical Editor*
Laura Evans, CPC, *Senior Content Specialist*
Susana Lambert, *Production Editor and Coordinator*

CONTENTS

INTRODUCTION

Introduction

Documentation is one of the central elements that underlie patient care, coding and billing for patient care, and an effective compliance plan. Many diseases, disorders, injuries, other conditions and even signs and symptoms require specific documentation to be compliant with the code structure and provide diagnosis coding to the highest level of specificity for accurate reporting and reimbursement. An ongoing review of documentation practices will help to determine if corrective changes are needed. The *ICD-10-CM Documentation: Essential Charting Guidance to Support Medical Necessity* is designed to address this need.

Documentation and Coding

In this book, three aspects of ICD-10-CM coding and documentation are addressed. The first relates to documentation requirements. Before actual medical record documentation can be analyzed, physicians and coders must understand the ICD-10-CM requirements for commonly reported signs, symptoms, diseases, and other medical conditions. Frequently, codes capture specific information about the condition itself. For example, strep infections of the throat and tonsils must be specifically identified as strep throat or strep tonsillitis; and for patients with strep tonsillitis, the condition must be specified as acute or acute recurrent.

Codes may also capture a disease and related conditions. For example, there are combination codes that capture the type of diabetes and specific manifestations or complications, such as Type 2 diabetes with hypoglycemia, which must also be specified as with or without coma. Some codes capture a condition and common symptoms, such as intervertebral disc disorders with radiculopathy. *ICD-10-CM Documentation: Essential Charting Guidance to Support Medical Necessity* covers many commonly reported diagnoses and reviews the necessary documentation elements so that providers and coders have a good understanding of what documentation is required based on the available codes for the condition.

The next aspect of coding and documentation that is addressed is the analysis component. Each condition covered in the book includes a bulleted list of coding and documentation elements. This list is designed to be used for actual documentation analysis. A documentation and coding example is provided with bolding of the portion of the documentation that captures the information required for ICD-10-CM code assignment. Coders will need to remember that physicians do not always document using exactly the same terminology in the code descriptor. However, that does not mean that a specific code cannot be identified. The physician may use an alternate term that describes the same condition with the necessary level of specificity. So coders will need to rely on and enhance their knowledge of medical terminology and synonymous terms. In addition, coders will need to rely on coding instructions in the Alphabetic Index and Tabular List as well as the *ICD-10-CM Official Guidelines for Coding and Reporting* to determine whether the most specific code can be assigned from the documentation provided or whether the physician will need to be queried.

The last aspect of coding and documentation addressed is documentation improvement. Several documentation checklists are provided in Appendix B for physician feedback related to specific conditions. These checklists can be used to identify any missing documentation elements required to assign the most specific code. Information contained in the checklists can be compiled for each physician and any documentation deficiencies identified. Documentation and coding checklists for conditions not addressed in this book can also be created for other conditions using the formats of the checklists provided. There are a few different formats and styles of checklists so users can determine which style works best for their practice and then create additional checklists using that format and style.

In addition to the coding and documentation checklists there are clinical documentation improvement bulleted lists for three conditions that are often lacking sufficient documentation in the inpatient setting. The information in these lists identifies common indicators of the condition so that the physician can be queried to determine if the condition should be included as a diagnosis in the medical record or can be coded to a more specific diagnosis.

Documentation and Compliance

Complete and accurate provider documentation is a continuous concern for physicians and hospitals alike. In addition to supporting quality patient care and serving as a legal document to verify the services provided, provider documentation is also needed to support correct coding initiatives, coding and documentation audits, and Medicare oversight reviews.

The Social Security Act and the Centers for Medicare & Medicaid Services (CMS) regulations require that services be medically necessary, have documentation to support the claims, and be ordered by physicians. Consistent, current and complete documentation in the treatment record is an essential component of quality patient care according to the National Committee for Quality Assurance. Specific documentation criteria are required for inpatient medical records by the Joint Commission on Accreditation of Healthcare Organizations and the federal Conditions of Participation. In addition to accreditation standards and federal regulations, medical record documentation must also comply with state licensure regulations and payer policies, as well as professional practice standards. Compliance and accurate reimbursement depend on the correct application of codes, which is based on provider documentation. In addition to the reimbursement implications, provider documentation is also used in quality improvement initiatives.

The codes reported on health insurance claims must be supported by the documentation in the medical record. Most payers require reasonable documentation that services are consistent with the insurance coverage provided. In one year, for example, the Office of Inspector General (OIG) found that 43.7 percent of errors were due to insufficient documentation, posing a significant compliance risk. Recovery Audit Contractors and Medicare Administrative Contractors reviews continue to identify numerous erroneously paid claims due to a high incidence of "insufficient documentation."

Medicare specifically requires that any services billed be supported by documentation that justifies payment. The Centers for Medicare & Medicaid Services (CMS) has implemented numerous corrective actions to reduce improper payments along with efforts to educate providers about the importance of thorough documentation to support the medical necessity of services and items. CMS review contractors identify and recover improper payments made due to insufficient documentation—the review determines that the documentation is not sufficient to support the provided service or that it was medically necessary. For example, a pilot study estimated that additional documentation would have reduced the amount of improper payments identified in 2010 by approximately $956 million.

Medical record documentation must comply with all legal/regulatory requirements applicable to Medicare claims. Documentation guidelines identify the minimal expectations of documentation by providers for payment of services to the Medicare program. Additional documentation is often required by state or local laws, professional guidelines, and the policies of a practice or facility. In general, medical record documentation that specifically justifies the medical necessity of services is necessary to support approval when those services are reviewed. Services are considered medically necessary if the documentation indicates they meet the specific requirements for medical necessity.

The key to ensuring appropriate documentation hinges on understanding how much depends on the quality and completeness of provider documentation in the medical record. Providers typically do not know the specific type of documentation needed to code various diseases and disorders accurately, so education is also a key factor. Prior to conducting provider education, it is important to know the extent and type of documentation in the medical record. Conducting a provider documentation assessment of medical records will identify key areas of risk and focus education efforts.

Documentation is central to patient care, billing for patient care, and an effective compliance plan. Accurate patient record documentation is a key component of the compliance plan, as it provides the justification necessary to support claims payment. Increased scrutiny of provider documentation by auditors has added even greater emphasis to the importance of identifying documentation deficiencies, correcting them, and ensuring proper documentation for every case. One of the key components of an effective compliance program for physician practices is the implementation of a system to audit and monitor an organization's practices.

Overview of *ICD-10-CM Documentation: Essential Charting Guidance to Support Medical Necessity*

The *ICD-10-CM Documentation: Essential Charting Guidance to Support Medical Necessity* is designed around ICD-10-CM with a documentation and coding chapter for each ICD-10-CM chapter.

Chapter Introduction

Introductory information for each chapter covers general information about the chapter. A table is provided showing the chapter coding blocks, which are the ranges of 3-character categories that cover related diagnoses within the chapter. Review of this table provides coders and physicians with information about the organization of that specific chapter.

The introduction also covers chapter level instructional notes, including includes and excludes notes. Chapter level includes notes further define or give examples of the content of the chapter. Excludes notes indicate that certain diseases, injuries or other conditions are excluded from or not coded in the chapter. There are two types of excludes notes in ICD-10-CM designated as Excludes1 and Excludes2, which are defined as follows:

- **Excludes1** – A type 1 excludes note is a pure excludes note. In general, it means "NOT CODED HERE". An Excludes1 note indicates that the code excluded should rarely be used at the same time as the code above the Excludes1 note. An Excludes1 is used when two conditions cannot occur together, such as a congenital form versus an acquired form of the same condition. There are a few exceptions when both conditions may be coded such as a sequela from a prior CVA and a new CVA or chondromalacia of the patella as well as the femur.
- **Excludes2** – A type 2 excludes note represents "NOT INCLUDED HERE". An Excludes2 note indicates that the condition excluded is not part of the condition represented by the code, but a patient may have both conditions at the same time. When an Excludes2 note appears under a code, it is acceptable to use both the code and the excluded code together, when appropriate.

Chapter Guidelines

Following the introduction, the *ICD-10-CM Official Guidelines for Coding and Reporting* for the chapter are reviewed. The chapter guidelines provide information on assigning codes from the chapter which often includes information related to documentation. Many coders think of the guidelines primarily as instructions on assignment and sequencing of codes, but there are many references to information that must be included in the documentation to allow assignment of specific codes. In addition, the coding guidelines often indicate when the physician should be queried for additional information related to the diagnosis. So, the chapter-specific guidelines are an important tool that must be used to ensure that the documentation supports assignment of a specific code.

General Documentation Requirements

For each chapter, general documentation requirements are covered. Many chapters in ICD-10-CM have documentation requirements that relate to the entire chapter or to many code categories in the chapter. Examples of the types of information covered in the general documentation requirements include:

- Site specificity, such as proximal or distal, or upper/middle/lower lobe
- Laterality (right, left, bilateral)
- Combination codes that capture:
  - Etiology and manifestation
  - Related conditions
  - Disease, injury or other medical condition and complications
  - Diseases or other medical conditions and common signs or symptoms
- Identification of the fetus affected by certain complications of pregnancy, childbirth and puerperium in multiple gestation pregnancies
- Identification of the trimester for complications occurring during pregnancy
- Increased specificity related to histologic behavior of certain neoplasms
- Episode of care (initial, subsequent, sequela) for injuries, poisoning, external causes and other conditions
- Increased specificity related to type of injury
- Use of fracture classification systems (Gustilo, Salter-Harris, Neer)
- Intraoperative and postprocedural complications
- Reclassification of codes into different categories or chapters
- Revised terminology

Chapter-Specific Documentation Requirements

In this section, code categories, subcategories, and subclassifications for some of the more frequently reported diseases, disorders, or other conditions in each ICD-10-CM chapter are reviewed. Specific documentation requirements are identified. The focus is on conditions with specific clinical documentation requirements. Although not all codes with significant documentation requirements are discussed, this section provides a representative sample of the type of documentation needed for diseases, disorders, or other conditions coded in the chapter. The section is organized alphabetically by the ICD-10-CM code category, subcategory, or subclassification depending on whether the documentation affects only a single code or an entire subcategory or category.

The condition reported by the category, subcategory, or code is discussed, followed by a bulleted list identifying the specific elements that must be captured to allow assignment of the most specific code. A scenario provides an example of the documentation required to capture the most specific code and the scenario is also coded. Coding notes are provided that discuss any guidelines, includes/excludes notes and other information that affected the code assignment for the scenario.

Quiz

A self-assessment quiz is provided at the end of the chapter. The quiz covers general and chapter specific guidelines, documentation requirements, and code assignment for the conditions discussed in the chapter. Answers and rationales are listed on the pages following the quiz in each chapter.

Appendixes

There are three appendixes. Appendix A provides checklists for common diagnoses and other conditions to be used for documentation review of current records to help identify documentation deficiencies. Appendix B provides bulleted lists that can be used for clinical documentation improvement. Appendix C provides a glossary of medical terminology encountered in the book.

Other Recommended Resources

The *ICD-10-CM Documentation: Essential Charting Guidance to Support Medical Necessity* may be used alone; however, the most benefit will be derived when the book is used with other coding resources. It is recommended that the book be used in conjunction with the most recent *ICD-10-CM Code Set* and *ICD-10-CM Official Guidelines for Coding and Reporting*. A comprehensive medical dictionary is also recommended.

Summary

Patient care, documentation, coding and compliance go hand-in-hand. It is not possible to assign the most specific and most appropriate diagnosis code without complete, detailed documentation related to the patient's disease, injury, or other reason for the encounter/visit. Documentation must also support the medical necessity of any services provided or procedures performed. Detailed, consistent, complete documentation in the medical record is one of the cornerstones of compliance. In addition, the effect of documentation on reimbursement cannot be overemphasized. Failure to support the medical necessity of the services or procedures provided or performed can result in loss of reimbursement, financial penalties, and other sanctions. Because of the specificity of ICD-10-CM codes and requirements by health plans to support the services billed, current documentation must be reviewed, documentation deficiencies identified, and a corrective action plan initiated. This book is designed to help coders, physician practices, and other health care providers understand the documentation requirements and prepare for improved documentation to support the services billed and the severity of the patient's condition.

Chapter 1
INFECTIOUS AND PARASITIC DISEASES

Introduction

Codes for infectious and parasitic diseases are located in Chapter 1. Infectious and parasitic diseases are those which are generally recognized as communicable or transmissible. Conditions covered in this chapter include scarlet fever, sepsis due to an infectious organism, meningococcal infection, and genitourinary tract infections. The table below shows the blocks within Chapter 1 Certain Infectious and Parasitic Diseases and illustrates the general layout by which these conditions are classified.

ICD-10-CM Blocks	
A00-A09	Intestinal Infectious Diseases
A15-A19	Tuberculosis
A20-A28	Certain Zoonotic Bacterial Diseases
A30-A49	Other Bacterial Diseases
A50-A64	Infections with a Predominantly Sexual Mode of Transmission
A65-A69	Other Spirochetal Diseases
A70-A74	Other Diseases Caused by Chlamydiae
A75-A79	Rickettsioses
A80-A89	Viral and Prion Infections of the Central Nervous System
A90-A99	Arthropod-Borne Viral Fevers and Viral Hemorrhagic Fevers
B00-B09	Viral Infections Characterized by Skin and Mucous Membrane Lesions
B10	Other Human Herpes Viruses
B15-B19	Viral Hepatitis
B20	Human Immunodeficiency Virus (HIV) Disease
B25-B34	Other Viral Diseases
B35-B49	Mycoses
B50-B64	Protozoal Diseases
B65-B83	Helminthiases
B85-B89	Pediculosis, Acariasis and Other Infestations
B90-B94	Sequela of Infectious and Parasitic Diseases
B95-B97	Bacterial and Viral Infectious Agents
B99	Other Infectious Diseases

Not all infectious and parasitic diseases are found in chapter 1. Localized infections are found in the respective body system chapters.

Exclusions

Reviewing the chapter level exclusions provides information on which conditions may or may not be reported together, as well as some information on infectious conditions found in other chapters.

Excludes1	Excludes2
Certain localized infections are reported with codes from body system related chapters	Carrier or suspected carrier of infectious disease (Z22.-) Infectious and parasitic diseases complicating pregnancy, childbirth, and the puerperium (O98.-) Infections and parasitic diseases specific to the perinatal period (P35-P39) Influenza and other acute respiratory infections (J00-J22)

Chapter Guidelines

Detailed official coding and reporting guidelines are provided for:

- Human immunodeficiency virus (HIV)
- Infectious agents as the cause of diseases classified to other chapters
- Infections resistant to antibiotics
- Sepsis, severe sepsis, and septic shock
- Methicillin resistant *Staphylococcus aureus* (MRSA) conditions

Human Immunodeficiency Virus (HIV) Infections

Guidelines and corresponding ICD-10-CM codes for reporting HIV infections and testing for HIV are listed on the following page.

- Code only confirmed cases. This does not require documentation of positive serology or culture for HIV. The provider's diagnostic statement that the patient is HIV positive or has an HIV-related illness is sufficient.
- Selection and sequencing of HIV codes:
  - Patient admitted for HIV-related condition. The principal diagnosis should be acquired immune deficiency syndrome (AIDS) (B20) followed by additional diagnosis codes for all reported HIV-related conditions.
  - Patient with AIDS or HIV-related disease admitted for unrelated condition. The code for the unrelated condition (such as an injury) should be the principal diagnosis followed by the code for AIDS (B20), followed by additional diagnosis codes for all HIV-related conditions that are reported.

- Newly diagnosed patient. Whether the patient is newly diagnosed or has had previous admissions/encounters for HIV conditions does not affect the sequencing decision.
- Asymptomatic HIV. The code for asymptomatic HIV infection status (Z21) is reported when the patient is asymptomatic but the physician has documented that the patient is HIV positive, known HIV, HIV test positive, or any similar terminology. These codes are not used if the physician documents that the patient has AIDS, or when the patient has any HIV-related illness or any conditions resulting from the HIV positive status. In these cases, the code for AIDS is used (B20).
- Patients with inconclusive HIV serology. Inconclusive serology without a definitive diagnosis and without any manifestations associated with HIV is assigned the code for inconclusive laboratory evidence of HIV (R75).
- Previously diagnosed HIV-related illness. Once the patient has developed an HIV-related illness, the code for AIDS (B20) is assigned on every subsequent admission/ encounter. Patients previously diagnosed with an HIV-related illness are never assigned the codes for inconclusive laboratory evidence of HIV (R75) or asymptomatic HIV infection status (Z21).
- HIV related illness in pregnancy, childbirth and the puerperium. During pregnancy, childbirth and the puerperium, a patient seen for an HIV-related illness is assigned the principal diagnosis code of O98.7-, Human immunodeficiency [HIV] disease complicating pregnancy, childbirth and the puerperium, from Chapter 15, which is sequenced first followed by the code for AIDS (B20) and then the HIV-related illness.
- A patient with asymptomatic HIV infection status during pregnancy, childbirth or the puerperium is assigned a principal diagnosis code from Chapter 15 of O98.7- followed by the code for asymptomatic HIV infection status (Z21).
- Encounter for HIV testing. A patient being seen to determine his or her HIV status is assigned code Z11.4, Encounter for screening for human immunodeficiency virus [HIV]. Additional codes should be assigned for any associated high risk behavior (e.g., Z72.5-).
- Encounter for HIV testing with signs/symptoms. The code(s) for the signs/symptoms are assigned. An additional code may be assigned if counseling for HIV is provided (Z71.7) during the encounter for the testing.
- Return encounter for HIV test results. If the results are negative, the code for HIV counseling is assigned (Z71.7). If the results are positive, use the guidelines above to select the appropriate code(s).

Infectious Agents as the Cause of Diseases Classified to Other Chapters

Certain infections, particularly localized infections, are reported with codes from the corresponding body system chapter. Many of these codes do not identify the organism, so a second code from Chapter 1 is required to identify the infecting organism. These codes are found in the following three categories:

- B95 – Streptococcus, staphylococcus, and enterococcus as the cause of diseases classified elsewhere
- B96 – Other bacterial agents as the cause of diseases classified elsewhere
- B97 – Viral agents as the cause of diseases classified elsewhere

Infections Resistant to Antibiotics

There are a growing number of pathogenic microorganisms that are resistant to some or all of the drugs previously used to treat the resulting infections. All bacterial infections documented as drug-resistant or antibiotic resistant must be identified. If a combination code is not available to capture the drug resistance, a code from category Z16 Resistance to antimicrobial drugs must be used following the infection code. Codes in category Z16 will be discussed in more detail in Chapter 20.

Sepsis, Severe Sepsis, and Septic Shock

There are significant reporting guidelines for coding conditions that are documented as urosepsis, septicemia, SIRS, sepsis, severe sepsis, and septic shock. The definitions of these terms are sometimes used interchangeably; however, it should be remembered that for coding purposes they are not considered synonymous. The current ICD-10-CM definitions and terminology usage are explained below:

- Urosepsis:
  - This term is nonspecific. There is no default code in the Alphabetic Index and it is not to be considered as synonymous with sepsis. Any provider documenting a condition as 'urosepsis' must be queried for clarification before any code can be assigned.
- Septicemia:
  - Although this term has traditionally been used to refer to a systemic disease associated with the presence of pathogenic microorganisms (bacteria, viruses, fungi, or other organisms) or their toxins in the blood, this term is not referenced in the Tabular List of ICD-10-CM. The term 'septicemia' has been replaced with the term 'sepsis.' In the Alphabetic Index, there is a cross-reference to 'sepsis' when the documentation supports a diagnosis of sepsis. An unqualified diagnosis of septicemia is reported with A41.9 Sepsis, unspecified organism, which has the alternate term septicemia, NOS.
- Systemic Inflammatory Response Syndrome (SIRS):
  - SIRS is not formerly defined in the ICD-10-CM guidelines. This term was formerly defined as the systemic response to infection, trauma, burns, or other insult to the body, such as cancer. Codes for SIRS are included in category R65. Symptoms and signs specifically associated with a systemic inflammatory response, and code descriptors containing the terminology systemic inflammatory response syndrome (SIRS) are used only for SIRS of non-infectious origin (R65.10 and R65.11). Severe sepsis is the term used in ICD-10-CM for SIRS due to an infectious process with acute organ dysfunction. For SIRS of non-infectious origin with acute organ dysfunction (R65.11), additional codes are required to identify the specific acute organ dysfunction.

- Sepsis:
  - The term sepsis is not specifically defined in the guidelines, although it is generally thought of as SIRS due to infection without acute organ dysfunction. Only one code for sepsis, appropriate to the documented underlying systemic infection, is reported such as A40.0 Sepsis due to streptococcus group A. If the causal organism is not identified, code A41.9 Sepsis, unspecified organism is assigned.
  - For sepsis due to a postprocedural infection, assign a code from T81.40-T81.43, Infection following a procedure, or a code from O86.00-O86.03, Infection of obstetric surgical wound, first to identify the site of the infection, if known. Assign an additional code for sepsis following a procedure (T81.44), or sepsis following an obstetrical procedure (O86.04) and an additional code to identify the infectious agent. If the infection follows an infusion, transfusion, therapeutic injection, or immunization, report a code from subcategory T80.2- or T88.0- first, followed by the code for the specific infection.
- Severe Sepsis:
  - Severe sepsis is not specifically defined in the ICD-10-CM guidelines. However, guidance can be found in the list of alternate descriptions under the subcategory code R65.2-. Severe sepsis includes: infection with associated acute organ dysfunction; sepsis with acute organ dysfunction; sepsis with multiple organ dysfunction; SIRS due to infectious process with acute organ dysfunction. A minimum of 2 codes are required—the code for the underlying systemic infection must be reported first, followed by the code for severe sepsis, which is further differentiated as being without septic shock (R65.20) or with septic shock (R65.21). Codes from subcategory R65.2 can never be assigned as principal diagnosis. Additional code(s) are required for identifying the associated acute organ dysfunction.
  - In cases where severe sepsis was not present on admission but developed during an encounter, the underlying systemic infection and the appropriate code from subcategory R65.2- should be assigned as secondary diagnoses.
  - When sepsis or severe sepsis as well as a localized infection, such as pneumonia or cellulitis, are both reasons for admission, the code(s) for the underlying systemic infection is assigned first and a code(s) for the localized infection is assigned secondarily. When severe sepsis is present, the appropriate R65.2- code is also assigned as a secondary diagnosis. If the localized infection is the reason for the admission, and sepsis/severe sepsis develops later, the localized infection should be assigned first followed by the appropriate sepsis/severe sepsis codes.
- Septic Shock:
  - Septic shock is circulatory failure associated with severe sepsis, and therefore represents a type of acute organ dysfunction. Two codes are required, the code for the underlying systemic infection and the code for severe sepsis with septic shock (R65.21). The code for septic shock cannot be assigned as the principal diagnosis. Additional codes for any other acute organ dysfunction should also be assigned.
  - If a postprocedural infection results in postprocedural septic shock, assign the codes previously indicated for sepsis due to a postprocedural infection followed by code T81.12- Postprocedural septic shock. Do not assign the code for severe sepsis (R65.21) with septic shock. Use additional codes for any acute organ dysfunction.

Methicillin Resistant S. Aureus (MRSA) Conditions

Staphylococcus aureus is found on the skin and in the nasal cavities of 25-30% of the US population. This is called colonization and healthy individuals with *S. aureus* colonization are called carriers. In most healthy individuals colonization causes no major problems. However, if the organisms get into the body through a cut or an open area, *S. aureus* can become a serious or even life-threatening infection. If the *S. aureus* strain is resistant to most antibiotics commonly used to treat staph infections, it is referred to as MRSA. MRSA is found on the skin of approximately 1-2% of healthy individuals. MRSA infections are much more serious and difficult to treat. Like other strains of staphylococcus, MRSA bacteria usually enter the body through a broken area in the skin, although other entry sites include the respiratory tract, surgical or other open wounds, intravenous catheters, and the urinary tract. While most MRSA infections involve only the skin and present as a boil or small bump-like blemishes, serious and often life-threatening infections also occur, including cellulitis, sepsis, and pneumonia. Patients with compromised immune systems are at a significantly greater risk of symptomatic secondary infection.

For coding purposes, *S. aureus* infections are classified as methicillin resistant, also referred to as MRSA, or methicillin susceptible, also referred to as MSSA. Coding guidelines for reporting *S. aureus* infections are as follows:

- Combination codes:
  - There are combination codes for MRSA sepsis (A41.02) and MRSA pneumonia (J15.212) and for MSSA sepsis (A41.01) and MSSA pneumonia (J15.211). A code from subcategory Z16.11 Resistance to penicillins is not reported additionally for MRSA sepsis or pneumonia because the combination code captures both the infectious organism and the drug-resistant status.
- Other MRSA infections:
  - Documentation of a current infection due to MRSA that is not covered by a combination code, such as a wound infection, stitch abscess, or urinary tract infection is reported with the code for the condition along with code B95.62, Methicillin resistant *Staphylococcus aureus* (MRSA) infection as the cause of diseases classified elsewhere to identify the drug resistant nature of the infection. A code from subcategory Z16.11 Resistance to penicillins is not reported additionally.
- MRSA or MSSA colonization:
  - An individual person may be described as being colonized or a carrier of MSSA or MRSA. Colonization means that MSSA or MRSA is present on or in the body without necessarily causing illness. A positive colonization test may be documented as "MRSA/MSSA screen positive" or "MRSA/MSSA nasal swab positive".

- Documentation of MRSA or MSSA colonization without documentation of a disease process due to MRSA or MSSA is reported with code Z22.322 Carrier or suspected carrier of MRSA or Z22.321 Carrier or suspected carrier of MSSA.
- MRSA colonization and infection:
  - For a patient documented as having both MRSA colonization and a current MRSA infection during an admission, code Z22.322 Carrier or suspected carrier of Methicillin resistant Staphylococcus aureus, and a code for the MRSA infection may both be assigned.

Zika Virus Infections

- Code only confirmed cases:
  - Only confirmed cases of zika virus as documented by the physician should be coded with A92.5 Zika virus disease or P35.4 Congenital Zika virus disease. This is in exception to the inpatient hospital guidelines. Confirmation does not require documentation of the test performed; the physician's diagnostic statement that the condition is confirmed is sufficient.
  - If the provider documents 'suspected', 'possible', or 'probable' zika, do not assign code A92.5 or P35.4. Assign a code(s) for the reason for the encounter, such as fever, rash, joint pain, or contact with and (suspected) exposure to Zika virus (Z20.821).

General Documentation Requirements

The general documentation requirements related to infectious and parasitic diseases are less problematic than for many other chapters in ICD-10-CM. The main points to consider for chapter 1 have been discussed in the chapter guidelines above: codes for localized infections found within the respective body system chapters, specified terminology such as that related to sepsis and severe sepsis, and the required use of combination codes, or an additional identifying code when a combination code is not provided.

Code-Specific Documentation Requirements

In this section, some of the more frequently reported infectious and parasitic disease codes are listed and the documentation requirements are identified. The focus is on frequently reported conditions with specific clinical documentation requirements. Even though not all codes with significant documentation requirements are discussed, this section will provide a representative sample of the type of additional documentation that is required for infectious and parasitic diseases.

Chlamydial Infection of Lower/ Other Genitourinary Sites

Chlamydia is the most frequently reported bacterial sexually transmitted disease in the United States with many more cases unreported. Many people do not know they are infected because symptoms can be mild or absent, with half of infected men and three quarters of infected women having no symptoms at all. The bacteria can cause silent damage, particularly to female reproductive organs, and infertility can result.

In ICD-10-CM, there is a combination code for the etiology of infection by Chlamydia trachomatis and the manifestation (site).

Coding and Documentation Requirements

Identify site:

- Lower genitourinary tract
  - Bladder/urethra (cystitis, urethritis)
  - Vulva/vagina (vulvovaginitis)
  - Other specified lower genitourinary tract site (cervix, other sites)
  - Unspecified lower genitourinary tract site
- Pelvis/peritoneum/other genitourinary organs
  - Female pelvis/peritoneum (female pelvic inflammatory disease)
  - Other specified site (epididymis/testis, other sites)
- Unspecified genitourinary site

ICD-10-CM Code/Documentation	
A56.00	Chlamydial infection of lower genitourinary tract, unspecified
A56.01	Chlamydial cystitis and urethritis
A56.02	Chlamydial vulvovaginitis
A56.09	Other chlamydial infection lower genitourinary tract
A56.11	Chlamydial female pelvic inflammatory disease
A56.19	Other chlamydial genitourinary infection
A56.2	Chlamydial infection of genitourinary tract, unspecified

Documentation and Coding Example

Twenty-six-year-old female presents with intermittent fever, abdominal cramps, and low back pain. She states she had UTI symptoms about a month ago with frequency and burning. Symptoms resolved with fluids and cranberry juice but sexual intercourse has been uncomfortable since then. Patient is married x 6 months, husband is her only sexual partner. Current medications include oral contraceptives. On examination, this is a well-developed, well-nourished young woman. Temperature 100.6, HR 88, RR 16, BP 100/60. PERRL, ROM and pulses intact in upper extremities. Abdomen mildly tender to palpation in all quadrants but no guarding, rebound tenderness or masses are present. Mild bilateral flank tenderness is also present. Inguinal lymph nodes are slightly enlarged but non-tender to palpation. Vulva and external genitalia normal. Speculum exam difficult to perform due to extreme discomfort. Yellowish white discharge from the endocervix. Culture obtained and sent to lab. Bimanual exam causes severe discomfort. There is moderate cervical motion tenderness, uterus is anteverted in midline and fixed in place, fallopian tubes are enlarged bilaterally and ovaries cannot be palpated due to muscle guarding. Cervical culture is positive for Chlamydia.

Diagnosis: **Chlamydial PID.**

Diagnosis Code(s)

A56.11 Chlamydial female pelvic inflammatory disease

Coding Note(s)

One combination code identifies both the chlamydial infection and the site of the infection.

Gonococcal Genitourinary Infections

Neisseria gonorrhoeae is a gram-negative bacterium responsible for sexually transmitted gonococcal infections. According to the Centers for Disease Prevention and Control (CDC), it is the second most commonly reported communicable disease. The bacteria cause purulent infection of mucous membranes through sexual contact with an infected person, or through the birth canal. In men, urethral infections cause symptoms that usually result in seeking attention timely enough to prevent sequelae in the individual, but not transmission. In women, the infection may remain asymptomatic until complications such as pelvic inflammatory disease develop. Genitourinary infections can be transmitted to the eyes and throat, and can also spread to the joints and tendons, the heart, the meninges, the abdominal cavity, and the bloodstream.

Gonococcal infections are not classified as acute or chronic. Both upper and lower genitourinary tract infections are specific to site. Codes specific for gonococcal infections of the lower genitourinary tract are divided into whether or not it occurs with periurethral and accessory gland abscess. Note that there is a single subcategory code, A54.1, for reporting gonococcal infections of the lower genitourinary tract with abscess, but multiple subclassified codes for reporting lower genitourinary infections without (A54.0-) abscess, by site. The gonococcal infections of specified sites in the lower genitourinary tract include the term "unspecified" in the descriptor. The term "unspecified" as used here means that these infections have not been specified as occurring with periurethral or accessory gland abscess of the lower genitourinary tract.

Coding and Documentation Requirements

Identify site of infection:

- Lower genitourinary tract
- Pelvis/peritoneum/other genitourinary sites

For lower genitourinary tract, identify presence/absence of complications:

- With periurethral abscess/accessory gland abscess
- Without periurethral abscess/accessory gland abscess

For lower genitourinary tract infection without periurethral or accessory gland abscess, identify site more specifically:

- Bladder/urethra (cystitis/urethritis)
- Uterine cervix (cervicitis)
- Vulva/vagina (vulvovaginitis)
- Other specified lower genitourinary tract site
- Unspecified lower genitourinary tract site

For pelvis/peritoneum/other upper genitourinary sites, identify site/condition more specifically:

- Kidney/ureter (nephritis, pyelitis, ureteritis)
- Female genitourinary system/female pelvic inflammatory disease (endometritis, salpingitis, pelviperitonitis)
- Male genitourinary system
  - Prostate (prostatitis)
  - Other male genital organs (epididymo-orchitis, seminal vesiculitis)
- Other specified site

ICD-10-CM Code/Documentation	
A54.00	Gonococcal infection of lower genitourinary tract, unspecified
A54.01	Gonococcal cystitis and urethritis, unspecified
A54.02	Gonococcal vulvovaginitis, unspecified
A54.03	Gonococcal cervicitis, unspecified
A54.09	Other gonococcal infection of lower genitourinary tract
A54.1	Gonococcal infection of lower genitourinary tract with periurethral and accessory gland abscess
A54.21	Gonococcal infection of kidney and ureter
A54.22	Gonococcal prostatitis
A54.23	Gonococcal infection of other male genital organs
A54.24	Gonococcal female pelvic inflammatory disease
A54.29	Other gonococcal genitourinary infections

Documentation and Coding Example

Nineteen-year-old male presents with **painful urination and thick white penile discharge x 1 week**. Today he noticed a swollen, painful area on underside of his penis near the scrotum. Patient has been sexually active x 3 years with multiple partners. He rarely uses a condom. On examination, this is a well- developed, well-nourished anxious appearing young man. Abdomen soft with active bowels sounds in all quadrants. Denies flank tenderness. Inguinal lymph nodes are swollen and tender to palpation. Copious white drainage noted from urethra. Culture obtained and sent to lab. Posterior penis at the junction of the scrotum has a 2 cm x 3 cm, firm, tender, erythematous swelling. Area is prepped and draped. Using an 18 g needle with syringe, 3 cc of cloudy yellow fluid is aspirated. Specimen sent to lab for gram stain and culture. **Both urethral culture and aspirate fluid are positive for *Neisseria gonorrhoeae*.** Ultrasound examination of the penis and scrotum reveal urethral distensibility and extension of the periurethral abscess into the spongiosum tissue at the bulbar urethra. The patient is admitted to the hospital and started on intravenous antibiotics. He is taken to the OR where the abscess is incised and drained. The wound is packed with antibiotic soaked saline and a dressing applied.

Diagnosis: **Cystitis, urethritis, and periurethral abscess due to gonorrhea**.

Diagnosis Code(s)

A54.1 Gonococcal infection of lower genitourinary tract with periurethral and accessory gland abscess

Coding Note(s)

The code for gonococcal cystitis and urethritis (A54.01) is not reported additionally because there is an Excludes1 note under subcategory A54.0 for gonococcal infection with periurethral abscess (A54.1), which indicates that code A54.1 is never reported with any codes in subcategory A54.0.

Herpes Simplex

Herpes simplex is caused by one of two variants of the herpes simplex virus (HSV) which are designated as HSV-1 and HSV-2. HSV-1 commonly affects the mouth, lips, and conjunctiva of the eye. When it affects the mouth and face, it is often referred to as a "fever blister" or "cold sore". HSV-2 commonly affects the genitalia. Both variants are spread by direct contact. While some individuals have no symptoms, others get blisters at the site where the virus has entered the body. The blisters may be itchy and painful. The first outbreak is typically the most severe and may be accompanied by fever, body aches, and pain and burning around the site of the outbreak. While the initial outbreak eventually resolves, the virus remains in the body and once infected most people continue to have periodic outbreaks that may be triggered by illness, stress, fatigue, hormone changes, sun exposure, or exposure to extreme heat or cold.

Herpes simplex is classified in category B00 for sites other than the genitals. Anogenital herpes infection is classified with infections with a predominantly sexual mode of transmission (A50-A64) in category A60.

Coding and Documentation Requirements

Identify HSV site/manifestation/complication:

- Anogenital
  - Female
    - » Cervicitis
    - » Vulvovaginitis
  - Male
    - » Penis
    - » Other male genital organ
  - Perianal skin/rectum
  - Other urogenital site
  - Unspecified urogenital site
  - Unspecified site, anogenital region
- Disseminated
- Eczema herpeticum
- Gingivostomatitis/pharyngotonsillitis
- Hepatitis
- Nervous system
  - Encephalitis
  - Meningitis
  - Myelitis
- Ocular (eye)
  - Conjunctivitis
  - Iridocyclitis
  - Keratitis
  - Other specified ocular disease
  - Unspecified ocular disease
- Vesicular dermatitis
  - Ear (otitis externa)
  - Face
  - Lips
- Other specified site/manifestation/complication
- Unspecified site/manifestation/complication

ICD-10-CM Code/Documentation	
A60.00	Herpesviral infection of urogenital system, unspecified
A60.01	Herpesviral infection of penis
A60.02	Herpesviral infection of other male genital organs
A60.03	Herpesviral cervicitis
A60.04	Herpesviral vulvovaginitis
A60.09	Herpesviral infection of other urogenital tract
A60.1	Herpesviral infection of perianal skin and rectum
A60.9	Anogenital herpesviral infection, unspecified
B00.0	Eczema herpeticum
B00.1	Herpesviral vesicular dermatitis
B00.2	Herpesviral gingivostomatitis and pharyngotonsillitis
B00.3	Herpesviral meningitis
B00.4	Herpesviral encephalitis
B00.50	Herpesviral ocular disease, unspecified
B00.51	Herpesviral iridocyclitis
B00.52	Herpesviral keratitis
B00.53	Herpesviral conjunctivitis
B00.59	Other herpesviral disease of eye
B00.7	Disseminated herpesviral disease
B00.81	Herpesviral hepatitis
B00.82	Herpes simplex myelitis
B00.89	Other herpesviral infection
B00.9	Herpesviral infection, unspecified

Documentation and Coding Example

Fifteen-year-old Caucasian female presents to Urgent Care Clinic with a history of fever and malaise x 3 days, severe sore throat, and painful blisters on her lips and chin when she awoke this morning. She has been on a river rafting trip with her family for the past week, camping out at night and in the sun all day. She has no chronic medical problems and no known allergies. She has been taking 400 mg of Ibuprofen 2-3 x day for the past 3 days. T 100.8, P 74, R 14, BP 100/58, O2 Sat. 99% on RA. On examination, this is a quiet, cooperative, ill appearing adolescent female. Skin is tan, mild sunburn on her shoulders and face. PERRLA, conjunctiva mildly red and moist. Nares patent with clear, thin secretions. **Lower lip is markedly swollen with clusters of fluid filled vesicles extending from the left corner to just right of midline and from the vermilion border into the oral mucosa.** There are also **scattered vesicles on the epidermis of chin and the left side of the upper lip along the vermilion border**. Oral exam is somewhat limited because the patient has trouble opening her mouth due to pain from the lesions on the lip. Additional **vesicles are noted on the gums on the lower left side and the pharynx appears red, tonsils swollen and covered with a gray exudate**. Neck is supple, cervical and supraclavicular lymph nodes can be palpated. Heart rate is regular, breath sounds are clear. Abdomen soft with active bowel sounds. Patient recalls tingling and itching of her gums and lips prior to the eruption of the rash.

Impression: **Herpes viral infection of oropharynx, gums, lips and chin**, R/O Strep/bacterial infection.

Plan: Vesicles cultured for virus. Rapid strep negative. Bacterial culture of tonsils sent to lab. Valacyclovir 1 gram BID x 10 days. Keep blisters moist using Vaseline and may use viscous lidocaine topically for pain. Continue Ibuprofen as needed. Stay out of the sun and RTC in 2 days for recheck.

Follow up visit: Afebrile. **Culture positive for HSV-1**, negative for strep. Throat is still painful and the gums, lips, and chin have fresh scattered vesicles. Old lesions appear ulcerous with gray exudate on a red base with some covered with crusts/scabs. She is prescribed Mupirocin 2% ointment for the lesions. Continue Valacyclovir. Follow up with PMD if symptoms not improving. Patient is cautioned that HSV can reoccur with stress, fatigue, sun exposure, and extreme heat and cold.

Diagnosis Code(s)

B00.1	Herpes vesicular dermatitis
B00.2	Herpesviral gingivostomatitis and pharyngotonsillitis

Coding Note(s)

Two codes are also required. There is a specific code for herpes vesicular dermatitis (B00.1) and a combination code (B00.2) that captures both the lesions on the gums (gingivostomatitis) and throat and tonsils (pharyngotonsillitis).

Intestinal Infectious Diseases

Intestinal infectious diseases may be caused by a variety of bacteria, amoebas, protozoa, and viruses. When the infection is caused by contaminated food, the condition may be referred to as food poisoning. The term "food poisoning" generally refers to any illness resulting from a foodborne pathogen that causes intestinal symptoms such as nausea, vomiting, and diarrhea. The term food poisoning groups illnesses by symptoms rather than by the pathogen that causes the illness such as a toxin, bacterium, virus, or parasite. While lay people still refer to an illness caused by food as food poisoning, public health departments recognize and classify food poisoning as either due to an infection (bacterium, virus, parasite, or other microorganism), or due to a toxin. The terms used are foodborne infection and foodborne intoxication.

This terminology change can be clearly seen in the alphabetic index. If the term "Intoxication, food" is referenced, foodborne toxins are listed but because "food intoxication" and "food poisoning" are still used interchangeably, referencing the term "Poisoning, food" in ICD-10-CM will still yield codes for foodborne illnesses caused by both toxins and infections. It is also possible to find the correct code by referencing "Enteritis, infectious", or "Infection" followed by the specific microorganism, such as Shigella.

Some of the more common causes of intestinal infectious diseases include:

- Bacterial
  - Campylobacter
  - Clostridium perfringens
  - Escherichia coli
  - Listeria
  - Salmonella
- Protozoal
  - Giardiasis [lambliasis]
- Viral
  - Adenovirus
  - Rotavirus
  - Norovirus

Bacterial Food Poisoning / Intoxication

Some of the more common bacterial causes of food poisoning are classified in category A05; however, these conditions are now referred to as foodborne intoxications. Other bacterial causes of food poisoning, food intoxication, and gastroenteritis are found throughout categories A00-A09.

Coding and Documentation Requirements

Identify bacterial cause of gastroenteritis/food poisoning/ intoxication:

- Bacillus cereus
- Botulism
- Clostridium perfringens [C. welchii]
- Staphylococcal
- Vibrio
  - Parahaemolyticus
  - Vulnificus
- Other bacteria
- Unspecified bacteria

ICD-10-CM Code/Documentation	
A05.0	Foodborne staphylococcal intoxication
A05.1	Botulism food poisoning
A05.2	Foodborne Clostridium perfringens [Clostridium welchii] intoxication
A05.8	Other specified bacterial foodborne intoxications
A05.3	Foodborne Vibrio parahaemolyticus intoxication
A05.5	Foodborne Vibrio vulnificus intoxication
A05.4	Foodborne Bacillus cereus intoxication
A05.8	Other specified bacterial foodborne intoxications
A05.9	Bacterial foodborne intoxication, unspecified

Documentation and Coding Example

History: This 28-year-old female became suddenly ill this afternoon with stomach pain and cramping, nausea, and vomiting. She states that she went out for pizza with friends and she and 2 other people also got a salad from the salad bar. The friends had planned to go out to a movie, but within an hour of eating both she and the 2 friends who had salad started to experience stomach pain and nausea. She went home and her symptoms became more severe. She now has severe stomach pain and cramps that cause her to double over in pain. She has been vomiting and now has dry heaves.

Examination: This is a young woman in acute distress. B/P 108/60, T 99.2, P 92, R 18. Abdomen is soft, tender to palpation, with hyperactive bowel sounds. ENT normal. Skin warm and dry.

Impression: **Staphylococcal food poisoning.**

Plan: Patient instructed to rest. When her stomach settles, she should begin taking ice chips and progress to clear fluids. She was given a prescription for Phenergan 25 mg to be taken every 4-6 hours as needed for nausea. She was told that the symptoms usually subside in 1-3 days and was told to return if symptoms become more severe.

Diagnosis Code(s)

A05.0 Foodborne staphylococcal intoxication

Coding Note(s)

Some foodborne pathogens causing gastrointestinal symptoms are classified as bacterial foodborne intoxications and not poisoning.

Listeriosis

Listeriosis is a disease caused by eating food contaminated with the bacterium *Listeria monocytogenes*. It is classified under other bacterial diseases and is reported by specified manifestation, such as cutaneous listeriosis (A32.0) or oculoglandular listeriosis (A32.81), or by a combination condition with the etiology and the manifestation, such as listerial sepsis (A32.7) or listerial endocarditis (A32.82).

Coding and Documentation Requirements

Identify site/manifestation:

- Cutaneous
- Endocarditis
- Meningitis
- Meningoencephalitis
- Oculoglandular
- Other form/manifestation, which includes:
  - Cerebral arteritis
- Sepsis
- Unspecified listeriosis

ICD-10-CM Code/Documentation	
A32.0	Cutaneous listeriosis
A32.11	Listerial meningitis
A32.12	Listerial meningoencephalitis
A32.7	Listerial sepsis
A32.81	Oculoglandular listeriosis
A32.82	Listerial endocarditis
A32.89	Other forms of listeriosis
A32.9	Listeriosis, unspecified

Documentation and Coding Example

This 75-year-old male presents to the ED in obvious distress with a fever of 101.6, blood pressure 70/40, pulse 120, respirations 28. He states he has not been feeling well for several days with nausea, vomiting, and tiredness. His wife states that today he has experienced periods of confusion, which she believes to be due to the fever. Due to the number of listeria cases over the past several weeks, the patient was queried about whether he has consumed any cantaloupe and he stated that he had eaten some approximately 3 weeks ago, but has not had any since.

Impression: Sepsis with septic shock likely due to listerial infection. Infectious disease consultation requested. Blood tests ordered.

Follow-up: Listerial sepsis confirmed by laboratory tests **with septic shock.**

Diagnosis Code(s)

A32.7 Listerial sepsis

R65.21 Severe sepsis with septic shock

Coding Note(s)

Septic shock is circulatory failure associated with severe sepsis, and, therefore, it represents a type of acute organ dysfunction. The code for septic shock cannot be assigned as a principal diagnosis. In ICD-10-CM, for all cases of septic shock, the code for the systemic infection should be sequenced first, followed by code R65.21. Any additional codes for other acute organ dysfunctions should also be assigned. Septic shock indicates the presence of severe sepsis. Code R65.21 Severe sepsis with septic shock, must be assigned if septic shock is documented in the medical record.

Meningococcal Infections

Meningococcal infection is a serious, potentially fatal bacterial infection caused by the bacterium *Neisseria meningitides*. It causes meningococcal meningitis, an inflammation of the membranes surrounding the brain and spinal cord; meningococcemia, the presence of *N. meningitides* in the blood; meningococcal heart disease which may affect the endocardium, myocardium, and/or pericardium; meningococcal arthritis, an infection of the joints; and may also affect other organs such as the eyes and adrenal glands. Specific documentation is required for meningococcemia as to acute or chronic nature, and for arthropathy as meningococcal arthritis or post meningococcal arthritis.

Meningococcemia

Coding and Documentation Requirements

Identify meningococcemia:

- Acute
- Chronic
- Unspecified

ICD-10-CM Code/Documentation	
A39.2	Acute meningococcemia
A39.3	Chronic meningococcemia
A39.4	Meningococcemia, unspecified

Documentation and Coding Example 1

Nineteen-year-old male college student presents with a 4-week history of intermittent fever, headaches, malaise, and joint pain. He states he has no appetite and has lost about 15 lbs. Temperature is 100.2 degrees, HR 94, RR 22, BP 92/60. This is a thin, ill-appearing young man. PERRL, conjunctiva mildly red. Oral and nasal mucous membranes are moist and slightly red. Cervical, axillary, and inguinal lymph nodes are enlarged and tender to touch. Abdomen is soft, bowel sounds present in all quadrants. Liver is palpated at 2 cm below the RCM, spleen is not palpated but patient c/o tenderness with palpation of the upper left quadrant. Smooth pinpoint petechial rash noted on back, neck, and lower extremities. Patient cannot recall if he has been immunized against meningitis. A CBC, blood cultures, and PT, PTT are obtained. Blood culture is positive for *Neisseria meningitides*.

Diagnosis: **Chronic meningococcemia**.

Diagnosis Code(s)

A39.3 Chronic meningococcemia

Coding Note(s)

The codes for meningococcemia are listed in the Alphabetic Index under three main terms: Infection, Meningococcemia, and Sepsis.

Meningococcal Arthropathy

Coding and Documentation Requirements

Identify meningococcal arthropathy:

- Current/acute meningococcal arthritis
- Post-meningococcal arthritis

ICD-10-CM Code/Documentation	
A39.83	Meningococcal arthritis
A39.84	Post-meningococcal arthritis

Documentation and Coding Example 2

Forty-four-year-old female presents with a chief complaint of right swollen, painful elbow. Patient states she was **acutely ill approximately 10 weeks ago** with fever, headache, nausea, and vomiting. She was **diagnosed with meningococcemia**, hospitalized and treated with antibiotics. She has continued to feel tired since the illness. On examination, she is afebrile, HR 80, RR 14, BP 112/70. **Fingers and wrists bilaterally are slightly red and mildly swollen. Right elbow is erythematous, diffusely tender to palpation and warm to touch**. Patient complains of pain with active and passive ROM. A patchy erythematous macular rash is also noted on both lower extremities. Small amount of purulent appearing synovial fluid is aspirated from right elbow and sent to the lab for gram stain, culture, cell count, and crystal analysis. Blood for CBC, sed rate drawn and sent to lab. **Synovial culture is positive for *Neisseria meningitides*.**

Diagnosis: **Post-meningococcal arthritis**.

Diagnosis Codes:

A39.84 Post-meningococcal arthritis

Coding Note(s)

To locate the correct code in the Alphabetic Index for chronic or post meningococcal arthritis, reference Arthritis, post meningococcal. Only the code for current, acute meningococcal arthritis is listed under Arthritis, meningococcal, or Arthritis, in (due to), meningococcus.

Scarlet Fever

Scarlet fever is caused by a bacterial infection with Streptococcus Group A. Scarlet fever is typically a complication of strep throat or less commonly a skin infection caused by Group A strep. The most common symptom is a red, rough-feeling skin rash. Scarlet fever is easily treated with antibiotics. However, serious complications can occur if it is not treated including rheumatic fever, kidney disease, ear infection, skin infection, throat abscess, pneumonia, or joint inflammation.

In ICD-10-CM, there are combination codes for scarlet fever and any complications, such as scarlet fever with myocarditis (A38.1).

Coding and Documentation Requirements

Identify scarlet fever as with or without complications:

- Scarlet fever with complications
  - Otitis media
  - Myocarditis
  - Other complications
- Scarlet fever without complications

ICD-10-CM Code/Documentation	
A38.0	Scarlet fever with otitis media
A38.1	Scarlet fever with myocarditis
A38.8	Scarlet fever with other complications
A38.9	Scarlet fever, uncomplicated

Documentation and Coding Example

Nine-year-old female presents with a sore throat, fever, general malaise, and rash. Parent states child was well until four days ago when she complained of a sore throat, headache, fever to 101 degrees and that her rash appeared yesterday. On examination, the child is in no acute distress. She is well nourished but appears slightly dehydrated. Child is cooperative and quiet throughout the examination. Mucous membranes are dry and pink, tongue is slightly swollen and very red. Throat is bright red with spotty white exudate. No nasal drainage noted. **The left ear has mild otitis media with effusion, right ear has a bulging tympanic membrane with middle ear effusion and inflammation.** Fine red rash covers neck and trunk and is especially pronounced in the axilla bilaterally. Rash is dry and sandpapery to touch, skin is peeling slightly around the neck. Child denies itching, upset stomach, vomiting, or diarrhea. **Rapid strep test (throat) positive.**

Diagnosis: **Scarlet fever, right acute otitis media, left otitis media with effusion.**

Diagnosis Code(s)

A38.0	Scarlet fever with otitis media
J02.0	Streptococcal pharyngitis

Coding Note(s)

In ICD-10-CM, there is an Excludes2 note listed under code J02.0 for Scarlet fever (A38.-). This note indicates that the condition is not part of the scarlet fever, but it is possible for a patient to have both scarlet fever and strep throat at the same time. Because both scarlet fever and strep throat are documented, both conditions are reported.

Sepsis

The term septicemia is often used for infections of the bloodstream. In ICD-10-CM, this term is not used and has been replaced with the term sepsis. When the term "septicemia" is referenced in the Alphabetic Index, there is a cross-reference to see "sepsis" when the documentation supports a diagnosis of sepsis. An unqualified diagnosis of septicemia would be reported with A41.9 Sepsis, unspecified organism, which has the alternate term 'septicemia NOS'.

Streptococcal Sepsis

Streptococcal sepsis (formerly termed septicemia) is the most common form of sepsis. Streptococcal sepsis must be identified as due to group A, group B, *S. pneumoniae*, other type, or unspecified type. Coding for streptococcal sepsis is also determined by whether the sepsis is documented as postprocedural; subsequent to immunization, infusion, transfusion, or other therapeutic injection; following an abortion or ectopic or molar pregnancy; occurring during labor; or is documented as puerperal.

Coding and Documentation Requirements

Septicemia is no longer used as coding terminology.

For streptococcal sepsis, designate agent:

- Group A
- Group B
- *S. pneumoniae*
- Other
- Unspecified

For severe sepsis, assign a code from subcategory R65.2 and specify:

- With septic shock
- Without septic shock

For severe sepsis, identify any acute organ dysfunction.

Note: A code from category A40 is reported as a secondary diagnosis to identify the specific bacterial agent for the following diagnoses:

- Postprocedural streptococcal sepsis (T81.44-)
- Streptococcal sepsis during labor (O75.3)
- Streptococcal sepsis following abortion (O03.37, O03.87)
- Streptococcal sepsis following induced termination of pregnancy (O04.87) or failed attempted termination of pregnancy (O07.37).
- Streptococcal sepsis following ectopic or molar pregnancy (O08.82)
- Streptococcal sepsis following immunization (T88.0)
- Streptococcal sepsis following infusion, transfusion or therapeutic injection (T80.2)

For puerperal sepsis:

- Do not report the codes from category A40.
- Use code O85 as the principal diagnosis and B95.0, B95.1, B95.3, B95.4 or B95.5 as appropriate to identify the organism.

ICD-10-CM Code/Documentation	
A40.0	Sepsis due to streptococcus, Group A
A40.1	Sepsis due to streptococcus, Group B
A40.3	Sepsis due to Streptococcus pneumoniae
A40.8	Other streptococcal sepsis
A40.9	Streptococcal sepsis, unspecified

Documentation and Coding Example

Twenty-two-year-old female in good health until 2 days prior to admission. She presents to ED with a 2-day history of shaking, chills, fever, and dry cough. Tonight, she feels like she cannot catch her breath and has sharp pain with inspiration on the left side. On examination, this is an acutely ill-appearing young woman. Color pale with cyanosis of the oral mucosa and nail beds. Neck veins are distended. Apical HR regular with an audible ventricular gallop. Breath sounds have course rales throughout, decreased BS in left lower lobe with dullness on percussion. Abdomen soft, non-tender with active BS. There is a well healed midline abdominal scar extending from xiphoid to pubic symphysis. Patient states she had a skiing accident at age 14 and sustained multiple rib fractures, collapsed lung and a ruptured spleen. She underwent exploratory abdominal surgery at the time and spleen was removed. Patient is placed on supplemental oxygen, 2 L/m via nasal cannula with increase in O2 saturation to 95%. Arterial blood gas drawn. IV placed and blood drawn for CBC, sed rate, CRP, cultures. Chest x-ray obtained and shows an area of consolidation in left lower lobe. Thick rust-colored sputum sample obtained after nebulizer treatment by respiratory therapy. Sample sent to lab for gram stain, culture. Patient admitted to medical floor for observation, respiratory treatment and antibiotic therapy. **Sputum and blood cultures positive for *S. pneumoniae*.**

Diagnosis: **Pneumonia due to *S. pneumoniae* complicated by sepsis.**

Diagnosis code(s)

A40.3	Sepsis due to *Streptococcus pneumoniae*
J13	Pneumonia due to *S. pneumoniae*
Z90.81	Acquired absence of spleen

Coding Note(s)

If the reason for the admission is both sepsis or severe sepsis and a localized infection, such as pneumonia or cellulitis, a code for the underlying systemic infection should be assigned first and the code for the localized infection should be assigned as a secondary diagnosis.

If the patient is admitted with a localized infection such as pneumonia, and sepsis/severe sepsis doesn't develop until after admission, the localized infection should be assigned first, followed by the appropriate sepsis/severe sepsis code(s).

Staphylococcal Sepsis

Staphylococcus, particularly *S. aureus*, is a frequent cause of infections that are usually localized, but staphylococcal infections can become systemic resulting in sepsis. In ICD-10-CM, there are four codes for staphylococcal sepsis and include sepsis due to methicillin susceptible *S. aureus,* methicillin resistant *S. aureus,* other specified staphylococcus, and unspecified staphylococcus. Coding for staphylococcal sepsis is determined by whether the sepsis is documented as postprocedural; occurring subsequent to immunization, infusion, transfusion, or other therapeutic injection; following an abortion or ectopic or molar pregnancy; occurring during labor; or is documented as puerperal.

Coding and Documentation Requirements

Septicemia is no longer used as coding terminology.

For staphylococcal sepsis, designate agent:

- Due to Methicillin resistant *S. aureus* (MRSA)
- Due to Methicillin susceptible *S. aureus* (MSSA)
- Other specified staphylococcal sepsis
- Unspecified staphylococcal sepsis

For a diagnosis of severe sepsis, assign a second code from subcategory R65.2 and specify:

- Severe sepsis with septic shock
- Severe sepsis without septic shock

Note: A code for the type of staphylococcus (A41.01, A41.02, A41.1, A41.2) is reported as a secondary diagnosis to identify the specific bacterial agent for the following diagnoses:

- Postprocedural staphylococcal sepsis (T81.44-)
- Staphylococcal sepsis during labor (O75.3)
- Staphylococcal sepsis following abortion (O03.37, O03.87)
- Staphylococcal sepsis following induced termination of pregnancy (O04.87) or failed attempted termination of pregnancy (O07.37).
- Staphylococcal sepsis following ectopic or molar pregnancy (O08.82)
- Staphylococcal sepsis following immunization (T88.0)
- Staphylococcal sepsis following infusion, transfusion or therapeutic injection (T80.2)

For puerperal sepsis:

- Do not report the codes A41.01, A41.02, A41.1, or A41.2.
- Use code O85 as the principal diagnosis and B95.61, B95.62, B95.7, or B95.8 as appropriate to identify the organism.

ICD-10-CM Code/Documentation	
A40.01	Sepsis due to Methicillin susceptible Staphylococcus aureus
A40.02	Sepsis due to Methicillin resistant Staphylococcus aureus
A41.1	Sepsis due to other specified staphylococcus
A41.2	Sepsis due to unspecified staphylococcus

Documentation and Coding Example

Fifty-eight-year-old nurse presents with a 2-day history of large, painful, erythematous **swelling on left anterior thigh**. Over the past 8 hours she has developed fever, chills, nausea, and weakness. Temp. 101.8, RR 20, HR 96, BP 88/50. Patient states that she does post-op care for surgical patients with infections. On examination, patient is an anxious, ill-appearing female. Mucous membranes are moist and pink. Skin color is pale, very warm, and dry to touch. PERRL. There is no lymph enlargement in upper body. Lungs are clear to auscultation. Heart rate regular without murmur. Abdomen soft, non-tender with decreased bowel sounds in all quadrants. Liver palpated at RCM, spleen is not palpated. Inguinal lymph nodes enlarged and very tender bilaterally. Right lower extremity unremarkable. Left lower extremity has mild edema in foot/calf and weak pedal and post tibial pulses. **A 6 cm x 4 cm erythematous area is noted on the anterior thigh approximately 10 cm above knee.** The lesion is firm, warm to touch with a soft purplish/red center. IV started in right upper extremity. Blood cultures, CBC sent to lab. Incision and drainage performed on left thigh lesion and culture sent to lab. **Blood and wound cultures both positive for methicillin resistant *Staphylococcus aureus*.**

Diagnosis: **Thigh abscess complicated by sepsis.**

Diagnosis Code(s)

A41.02	Sepsis due to methicillin resistant *S. aureus*
L02.416	Cutaneous abscess of left lower limb
B95.62	Methicillin resistant *S. aureus* as the cause of diseases classified elsewhere

Coding Note(s)

If the reason for the admission is both sepsis or severe sepsis and a localized infection, such as pneumonia or cellulitis, a code for the underlying systemic infection should be assigned first and the code(s) for the localized infection should be assigned as a secondary diagnosis. Since both the blood and the wound cultured positive for methicillin resistant Staphylococcus aureus, code B95.62 is assigned to identify the causative organism for the localized thigh abscess.

Viral Diseases of the Central Nervous System, Specified

Viruses can be spread through different mediums. Arthropods are invertebrates with an exoskeleton, jointed appendages, and a segmented body. Arthropod-borne infections are caused by viruses transmitted through invertebrates such as ticks and mosquitoes. Other invertebrates that are not arthropods, such as worms, may also transmit viruses. ICD-10-CM provides codes that distinguish arthropod-borne viral fevers and infections of the central nervous system by the vector of transmission, but there are no codes specifically designating non-arthropod borne viral illnesses. The codes for viral infections of the central nervous system are specific to site and must be specified as the brain (encephalon) (A85, A86) or meninges (A87). There are 3 codes available for reporting non-arthropod-borne viral encephalitis: enteroviral (A85.0), adenoviral (A85.1), and other specified viral encephalitis (A85.8). When the condition is not specified as encephalitis or meningitis, the code for other specified viral infections of the central nervous system not elsewhere classified (A88.8) is used. There is also a code for unspecified viral infection of central nervous system (A89).

Coding and Documentation Requirements

Specify viral type of encephalitis:

- Adenoviral
- Enteroviral
- Other viral, which may include the following descriptors:
  - Encephalitis lethargica
  - Von Economo disease
- Unspecified

Specify viral type of meningitis:

- Adenoviral
- Enteroviral, which may include:
  - coxsackievirus
  - echovirus
- Lymphocytic choriomeningitis
- Other viral
- Unspecified
- Other specified viral infection of the CNS

ICD-10-CM Code/Documentation	
A85.0	Enteroviral encephalitis
A85.1	Adenoviral encephalitis
A85.8	Other specified viral encephalitis
A70.0	Enteroviral meningitis
A87.1	Adenoviral meningitis
A87.2	Lymphocytic choriomeningitis
A87.8	Other viral meningitis
A88.8	Other specified viral infections of central nervous system

Documentation and Coding Example

Twenty-two-month-old male presents with a 4-day history of URI symptoms. Parent states he is usually very active and happy but has been irritable all day, crying inconsolably especially when touched or picked up. His URI symptoms have included fever to 102.6, nasal congestion, conjunctivitis, and cough. On examination, the patient has a maculopapular rash on the back of his head and neck. Child admitted to pediatric floor with **suspected acute viral meningitis** and placed in respiratory isolation. Neurological functioning continued to decline after admission. Symptoms included agitation, confusion, and seizures. Cross section and 3-D MRI imaging revealed **inclusion bodies** in the neurons and glial cells of the brain.

Diagnosis: **Acute inclusion body encephalitis.**

Diagnosis Code(s)

A85.8 Other specified viral encephalitis

Coding Note(s)

In the Alphabetic Index, the code is found under Encephalitis, acute, inclusion body.

Viral Diseases of Central Nervous System, Unspecified

There are two codes for unspecified viral diseases of the central nervous system, one for unspecified viral encephalitis (A86) and one for unspecified viral infection of the central nervous system when the condition is not specified as encephalitis or meningitis (A89).

Coding and Documentation Requirements

For viral infection of the CNS specify:

- Viral encephalitis/encephalomyelitis/meningoencephalitis NOS
- Viral infection of CNS, NOS

ICD-10-CM Code/Documentation	
A86	Unspecified viral encephalitis
A89	Unspecified viral infection of the central nervous system

Documentation and Coding Example

Thirty-year-old male presents with a 3-day history of flu-like symptoms, fever, headache, fatigue, muscle and joint pain, congestion and cough. Today he noticed neck stiffness and severe sensitivity to light. Patient denies exotic travel but recently spent a week skiing in Colorado. He denies falls or injuries but states he developed a large sore on this lip which he attributed to excessive sun exposure. On examination, this is an ill appearing, thin white male lying quietly with his eyes closed. Skin color is pale/pasty, skin is cool and clammy to touch. Temperature 98.2, HR 90, RR 20, BP 100/66. Unable to examine pupils due to extreme sensitivity to light. Limited anterior/posterior neck flexion due to pain with movement. Mild lymph node swelling noted in cervical area. No other lymphadenopathy appreciated. Hyperactive reflexes noted in all extremities. HR regular without murmur. Fine scattered rales noted in lungs bilaterally, clear with coughing. Abdomen soft and non-tender. Liver palpated at RCM, spleen is not palpated. Denies flank pain or difficulty with urination. Lower extremities are without edema, pulses are intact. Blood samples obtained for CBC, culture, sed rate, herpes antibody testing. Neuroimaging obtained with MRI scan of head and neck. Lumbar puncture performed and CSF sent to lab for gram stain, cell count, culture, protein, glucose, lactic acid, IgG antibodies, CRP. Patient is admitted with a diagnosis of probable viral encephalomyelitis.

Final diagnosis: **Viral encephalomyelitis.**

Diagnosis Code(s)

A86 Unspecified viral encephalitis

Coding Note(s)

In the Alphabetic Index, under Encephalomyelitis, follow the instruction "see also Encephalitis". The code is found under

Encephalitis, viral/virus. Since the specified type is not known, the code for unspecified viral encephalitis is reported.

Summary

Best practices in documentation of infectious and parasitic diseases require information on the infectious organism as well as the site of the infection. Coders will find that some aspects of coding infectious and parasitic diseases are streamlined because of many combination codes that identify both the infection and the manifestation. Some disease processes such as sepsis require an understanding of updated terminology and definitions and the detailed documentation required to code the complete clinical picture correctly. Capturing the most specific diagnosis will likely require physician training and more frequent queries of physicians to assign the proper codes.

Resources

Documentation checklists are available in Appendix A for the following condition(s):

- Sepsis, Severe Sepsis, Septic Shock, and SIRS

Clinical indicator checklists are available in Appendix B for the following condition(s):

- Sepsis, Severe Sepsis, Septic Shock, and SIRS

Chapter 1 Quiz

1. The code for a carrier or suspected carrier of an infectious disease without manifestation of acute illness is reported with a code from what chapter?
   a. Chapter 1 – Certain Infectious and Parasitic Diseases
   b. The appropriate body system chapter
   c. Chapter 21 – Factors Influencing Health Status and Contact with Health Services
   d. There are no codes for carrier or suspected carrier status
2. Which statement about localized infections is true?
   a. Localized infections reported with codes from body system chapters always identify the infectious organism
   b. The infectious organism may be reported with a code from categories B95-B97
   c. Localized infections always require an additional code for infectious organism
   d. The code for the infectious organism is always the first listed diagnosis with the site of the infection reported as a secondary code
3. Sepsis with septic shock (R65.21) is classified as a type of severe sepsis. Why?
   a. It always involves failure of multiple organ systems
   b. It is caused by kidney failure
   c. It is associated with respiratory failure
   d. It generally refers to circulatory failure associated with severe sepsis and is therefore a type of acute organ dysfunction
4. When a nasal swab is performed and documented as positive for MRSA screen but the patient has no manifestations of infection or illness, the condition is reported as:
   a. Z22.322 Carrier or suspected carrier of MRSA, for patients documented as having MRSA colonization
   b. B95.62 MRSA infection as the cause of diseases classified elsewhere
   c. A49.02 MRSA infection, unspecified site
   d. A41.02 Sepsis due to MRSA
5. Sepsis due to meningococcus is coded as:
   a. Acute meningococcemia (A39.2)
   b. Chronic meningococcemia (A39.3)
   c. Unspecified meningococcemia (A39.4)
   d. Any of the above depending on whether the condition is documented as acute, chronic, or is unspecified
6. Gonococcal infections are classified by site. Which site is considered to be part of the lower genitourinary tract in the classification of gonococcal infections?
   a. Kidney
   b. Bladder
   c. Prostate
   d. Epididymis
7. Chlamydial infection of the lower genitourinary tract has specific codes for what sites?
   a. Bladder/urethra, vulva/vagina
   b. Bladder/urethra, cervix, vulva/vagina
   c. Bladder/urethra, cervix, epididymis, testis
   d. Urethra, cervix, epididymis, testes
8. A diagnosis of listerial sepsis is reported as follows:
   a. A32.7 Listerial sepsis, R65.20 Severe sepsis without septic shock
   b. A32.7 Listerial sepsis, R65.10 SIRS of non-infectious origin without acute organ dysfunction
   c. R65.20 Severe sepsis without septic shock
   d. A32.7 Listerial sepsis
9. Documentation of severe sepsis always requires a minimum of:
   a. 1 code
   b. 2 codes
   c. 3 codes
   d. 4 codes
10. Herpes simplex virus infections are classified in which categories?
   a. A60, B00
   b. A60, B00, B10
   c. A60, B08, B10
   d. B00, B10

See next page for answers and rationales.

1. Infectious and Parasitic Diseases

Chapter 1 Answers and Rationales

1. The code for a carrier or suspected carrier of an infectious disease without manifestation of acute illness is reported with a code from what chapter?

 c. Chapter 21 – Factors Influencing Health Status and Contact with Health Services

 Rationale: *Carrier or suspected carrier status is reported with codes from category Z22 in Chapter 21.*

2. Which statement about localized infections is true?

 b. The infectious organism may be reported with a code from categories B95-B97

 Rationale: *Localized infections may or may not identify the infectious organism in the code descriptor. If the code descriptor does not identify the infectious organism, a code from category B95-B97 should be listed additionally when the specific infectious organism is documented. If the infectious organism is part of the descriptor for the localized infection, such as strep throat (J02.0), a second code from Chapter 1 is not required. The code for the infectious organism may or may not be the first listed diagnosis. Sequencing instructions differ depending on a number of factors and sequencing instructions contained in ICD-10-CM should be followed for each specific circumstance.*

3. Sepsis with septic shock (R65.21) is classified as a type of severe sepsis because:

 d. It generally refers to circulatory failure associated with severe sepsis and is therefore a type of acute organ dysfunction

 Rationale: *According to the Official ICD-10-CM Coding Guidelines – Septic shock is circulatory failure associated with severe sepsis, and, therefore, it represents a type of acute organ dysfunction. For all cases of septic shock, the code for the systemic infection should be sequenced first, followed by code R65.21. Any additional codes for other acute organ dysfunction should also be assigned.*

4. When a nasal swab is performed and documented as positive for MRSA screen but the patient has no manifestations of infection or illness, the condition is reported as:

 a. Z22.322 Carrier or suspected carrier of MRSA, for patients documented as having MRSA colonization

 Rationale: *According to the Official ICD-10-CM Coding Guidelines – A positive MRSA colonization test might be documented by the provider as "MRSA screen positive" or MRSA nasal swab positive". Assign code Z22.322 Carrier or suspected carrier of MRSA for patients documented as having MRSA colonization.*

5. Sepsis due to meningococcus is coded as:

 d. Any of the above depending on whether the condition is documented as acute, chronic, or is unspecified

 Rationale: *In the Alphabetic index under Sepsis, meningococcal, all three codes are listed. In order to select the most specific code the provider must document the sepsis as acute or chronic. If this is not documented, the code for unspecified should be used.*

6. Gonococcal infections are classified by site. Which site is considered to be part of the lower genitourinary tract in the classification of gonococcal infections?

 b. Bladder

 Rationale: *Gonococcal cystitis/urethritis is reported with code A54.01. This is classified in subcategory A54.0- Gonococcal infection of the lower genitourinary tract without periurethral or accessory gland abscess. The remaining sites are reported with codes from subcategory A54.2-.*

7. Chlamydial infection of the lower genitourinary tract has specific codes for what sites?

 a. Bladder/urethra, vulva/vagina

 Rationale: *Only the bladder (cystitis)/urethra (urethritis) and vulva/vagina (vulvovaginitis) have specific codes. The other lower genitourinary tract sites are reported with code A56.09 Other chlamydial infection lower genitourinary tract. Codes for the cervix, epididymis, testes are not classified under the lower genitourinary tract and are reported with a code from subcategory A56.1- Chlamydial infection of pelviperitoneum and other genitourinary organs.*

8. A diagnosis of listerial sepsis is reported as follows:

 d. A32.7 Listerial sepsis

 Rationale: *Documentation of listerial sepsis without documentation of severe sepsis, organ failure, or septic shock is reported with a single code A32.7.*

9. Documentation of severe sepsis always requires a minimum of:

 b. 2 codes

 Rationale: *Severe sepsis requires a minimum of two (2) codes. The underlying systemic infection is coded first, followed by a code from subcategory R65.2- Severe sepsis. In the case of a diagnosis of severe sepsis with septic shock in the absence of other documented organ failure, a sepsis code from Chapter 1 and code R65.21 for severe sepsis with septic shock would be reported. Because severe sepsis is defined as involving organ dysfunction or failure, additional codes are typically required to identify any specific organ dysfunction, so in most cases more than 2 codes would be necessary.*

10. Herpes simplex virus infections are classified in which categories?

 a. A60, B00

 Rationale: *Herpes simplex virus infections are reported with codes from category A60 for anogenital regions and with codes from category B00 for other organs, such as skin and eyes.*

Chapter 2

NEOPLASMS

Introduction

Codes for all neoplasms are located in Chapter 2. Neoplasms are classified primarily by site and then by behavior (benign, carcinoma in-situ, malignant, uncertain behavior, and unspecified). In some cases, the morphology (histologic type) is also included in the code descriptor. Some neoplasms require documentation of the histologic type for assignment of the most specific code.

Many codes require specific documentation of the site of the malignancy and laterality (right, left, bilateral), which is required for paired organs and the extremities. Other malignant neoplasms require documentation of morphology. The categories of codes with significant documentation requirements are those for lymphomas, myelomas, and leukemias. Representative examples of these documentation requirements are provided in this chapter and checklists are provided in Appendix A to help identify documentation deficiencies so that physicians and coders can confidently assign the correct ICD-10-CM codes.

The code blocks for neoplasms are displayed in the table below.

ICD-10-CM Blocks	
C00-C14	Malignant Neoplasm of Lip, Oral Cavity, and Pharynx
C15-C26	Malignant Neoplasm of Digestive Organs
C30-C39	Malignant Neoplasm of Respiratory and Intrathoracic Organs
C40-C41	Malignant Neoplasm of Bone and Articular Cartilage
C43-C44	Melanoma and Other Malignant Neoplasms of Skin
C45-C49	Malignant Neoplasms of Mesothelial and Soft Tissue
C50	Malignant Neoplasm of Breast
C51-C58	Malignant Neoplasms of Female Genital Organs
C60-C63	Malignant Neoplasms of Male Genital Organs
C64-C68	Malignant Neoplasms of Urinary Tract
C69-C72	Malignant Neoplasms of Eye, Brain, and Other Parts of Central Nervous System
C73-C75	Malignant Neoplasms of Thyroid and Other Endocrine Glands
C7A	Malignant Neuroendocrine Tumors
C7B	Secondary Neuroendocrine Tumors
C76-C80	Malignant Neoplasms of Ill-Defined, Other Secondary, and Unspecified Sites
C81-C96	Malignant Neoplasms of Lymphoid, Hematopoietic and Related Tissue
D00-D09	In Situ Neoplasms
D10-D36	Benign Neoplasms, Except Benign Neuroendocrine Tumors
D3A	Benign Neuroendocrine Tumors
D37-D48	Neoplasms of Uncertain Behavior, Polycythemia Vera and Myelodysplastic Syndromes
D49	Neoplasms of Unspecified Behavior

Glancing at the table above reveals the following:

- The In Situ Neoplasms (D00-D09) block is not specific for carcinoma in situ. It also includes codes for melanoma in situ.
- Polycythemia vera and myelodysplastic syndromes (D37-D48) are specifically identified and have their own codes instead of being in a category with other and unspecified neoplasms of uncertain behavior.
- Neuroendocrine tumors are classified based on behavior with malignant neuroendocrine (C7A) and secondary neuroendocrine tumors (C7B) in two separate code blocks and benign neuroendocrine tumors (D3A) in another code block, following other benign neoplasms.

As an additional note, mastocytosis codes are also found in separate code blocks, classified by behavior as either malignant mast cell neoplasms (C96) under the block for malignant neoplasms of lymphoid, hematopoietic, and related tissue, or mast cell neoplasms of uncertain behavior (D47) under the block for neoplasms of uncertain behavior, polycythemia vera, and myelodysplastic syndromes. Codes are provided in both categories at a more granular level for reporting further characteristic behavior as either systemic or solid neoplasm, such as cutaneous mastocytosis and other (extracutaneous) mast cell tumor of uncertain behavior, or aggressive systemic mastocytosis and mast cell sarcoma.

Chapter Guidelines

There are a number of coding notes at the chapter level related to the coding of neoplasms. The notes cover four subjects: functional activity, morphology [histology], primary malignant neoplasms overlapping site boundaries, and malignant neoplasms of ectopic tissue.

Subject	Coding Note
Functional activity	All neoplasms are classified in this chapter, whether they are functionally active or not. An additional code from Chapter 4 may be used, to identify functional activity associated with any neoplasm.
Morphology [Histology]	Chapter 2 classifies neoplasms primarily by site (topography), with broad groupings for behavior: malignant, in situ, benign, etc. The Table of Neoplasms should be used to identify the correct topography code. In a few cases, such as for malignant melanoma and certain neuroendocrine tumors, the morphology (histologic type) is included in the category and codes.

Subject	Coding Note
Primary malignant neoplasms overlapping site boundaries	A primary malignant neoplasm that overlaps two or more contiguous (next to each other) sites should be classified to the subcategory/code .8 ('overlapping lesion'), unless the combination is specifically indexed elsewhere. For multiple neoplasms of the same site that are not contiguous, such as tumors in different quadrants of the same breast, codes for each site should be assigned.
Malignant neoplasm of ectopic tissue	Malignant neoplasms of ectopic tissue are to be coded to the site mentioned, e.g., ectopic pancreatic malignant neoplasms are coded to pancreas, unspecified (C25.9).

There are no chapter level Includes or Excludes notes for neoplasms.

General Guidelines

- To assign the most specific code possible, documentation must be reviewed to determine the histologic behavior which may be benign, in-situ, malignant, or of uncertain behavior. Malignant neoplasms must be further differentiated as primary or secondary. Records containing documentation of a primary malignant neoplasm should also be reviewed for documentation of any secondary or metastatic sites.
- The Alphabetic Index and Table of Neoplasms should be referenced as follows:
  - The Neoplasm Table should be referenced first. However, if the histological type is documented, that term is referenced instead of going directly to the Neoplasm Table first in order to identify the histological behavior as benign, malignant, or uncertain behavior, and which column of the Neoplasm Table is appropriate. The Neoplasm Table is then used to identify the correct category, subcategory, or code and the Tabular List is referenced for any additional coding instructions and to verify the code selected code is correct and that a more specific site code does not exist.
  - If a specific code is listed in the Alphabetic Index for the histological type, the Neoplasm Table need not be referenced. The Tabular List is reviewed for any additional coding instructions. For example, a liver lesion that is identified as a hepatoblastoma on the pathology report has a specific code listed in the Alphabetic Index, C22.2 Hepatoblastoma, so the neoplasm table does not need to be referenced.
  - If the histological type is not referenced but the histological behavior (benign, malignant, uncertain) is documented, the Neoplasm Table is consulted to identify the correct code and the Tabular List is then reviewed for any additional coding instructions.

Coding and Sequencing Guidelines for Treatment of Neoplasms

- Treatment of the malignant neoplasm:
  - If the treatment, excluding admission/encounter solely for the administration of chemotherapy, immunotherapy, or external beam radiation therapy, is directed at the malignancy, the malignancy is the principal or first-listed diagnosis.
    - » If treatment is directed to the primary site, the code for primary malignant neoplasm is the principal or first-listed diagnosis.
    - » If the treatment is directed to the primary site and there are known metastatic sites, the code for the primary malignant neoplasm is sequenced first followed by the code(s) for the secondary (metastatic) sites.
    - » If the treatment is directed at a secondary or metastatic site only, the code for the secondary neoplasm is the principal or first-listed diagnosis.
      - o If the malignancy of the primary site is still present and has not been excised or eradicated, the code for the primary malignancy follows the code for the secondary neoplasm.
      - o If the malignancy for the primary site has been excised or eradicated, a code from category Z85 Personal history of malignant neoplasm follows the code for the secondary neoplasm.
      - o Codes from Z85.0-Z85.7 should only be assigned for a former primary malignancy site, not a secondary one. Codes from subcategory Z85.8, however, may be assigned for the former site(s) of either primary or secondary malignancies.
  - If the treatment involves surgical removal of a primary or secondary neoplasm, followed by adjunct chemotherapy, immunotherapy, or radiotherapy during the same episode of care (admission/encounter), the code for the neoplasm is assigned as the principal or first-listed diagnosis.
  - If the admission or encounter is solely for chemotherapy, immunotherapy, or external beam radiation therapy, the following codes are reported as the principal or first-listed diagnosis followed by the code for the malignancy as a secondary diagnosis.
    - » Z51.0 Encounter for antineoplastic radiation therapy
    - » Z51.11 Encounter for antineoplastic chemotherapy
    - » Z51.12 Encounter for antineoplastic immunotherapy
  - If a patient receives more than one type of antineoplastic therapy (chemotherapy, immunotherapy, and radiation therapy) during the same encounter, a code for each therapy should be assigned, in any sequence.
  - If the patient admission/encounter is for insertion/implantation of radioactive elements, such as for brachytherapy, the malignancy is the principal or first-listed diagnosis. Code Z51.0 should not be assigned. Any complications that develop, such as uncontrolled nausea and vomiting or dehydration are listed as secondary diagnoses.
- Admission/encounter to determine the extent of malignancy:
  - The primary malignancy or appropriate metastatic site is the principal or first-listed diagnosis.
  - Codes related to the administration of chemotherapy, immunotherapy, or radiotherapy provided during the same encounter are reported as secondary diagnoses.

Coding for Complications Due to Neoplasm or Treatment of Neoplasm

- Treatment of complications due to the neoplasm and complications resulting from treatment of the neoplasm:
  - Anemia associated with the malignancy
    - » If management of anemia associated with the malignancy is the only condition being treated, codes and sequencing are as follows:
    - » The appropriate code for the malignancy is sequenced as the principal or first-listed diagnosis.
    - » The appropriate code for the anemia, such as D63.0 Anemia in neoplastic disease follows the code for the malignancy.
  - Anemia associated with chemotherapy or immunotherapy
  - If the anemia resulting from the administration of chemotherapy or immunotherapy is the only condition being treated, codes and sequencing are as follows:
    - » The code for the anemia is sequenced first.
    - » The code T45.1X5 Adverse effect of antineoplastic and immunosuppressive drug follows the anemia code.
  - Anemia associated with radiotherapy
  - If the anemia resulting from the administration of radiotherapy is the only condition being treated, codes and sequencing are as follows:
    - » The code for the anemia is sequenced first.
    - » The code Y84.2 Radiological procedure and radiotherapy as the cause of abnormal reaction of the patient, or of later complication, without mention of misadventure at the time of the procedure follows the anemia code.
  - Other complications associated with chemotherapy, immunotherapy, or radiation therapy
    - » When the admission is for the purpose of radiotherapy, immunotherapy, or chemotherapy and complications develop:
    - » The code for encounter for the chemotherapy, immunotherapy, or radiation therapy is the principal or first-listed diagnosis.
    - » Code(s) for the complication(s) such as nausea, vomiting, dehydration, and adverse drug reaction follow the therapy code.
  - Dehydration due to the malignancy
  - When management of the dehydration is the reason for the encounter/admission and the only condition treated:
    - » The code for the dehydration is sequenced first.
    - » The code for the malignancy follows the dehydration code.
  - Pathologic fracture due to the malignancy
    - » If the treatment is directed at the fracture, a code from subcategory M84.5 Pathological fracture in neoplastic disease, is sequenced first followed by the code for the neoplasm.
    - » If treatment is directed at the neoplasm that has caused the pathological fracture, the neoplasm code is sequenced first followed by a code from subcategory M84.5.
  - Other complications associated with the malignancy
    - » If the encounter is only for management of the complication, the code for the complication is sequenced first followed by the code for the malignancy.
  - Complications resulting from a surgical procedure
    - » When the encounter is for treatment directed solely at the complication resulting from a surgical procedure, the code for the complication is designated as the principal or first-listed diagnosis.

Symptoms, Signs, and Abnormal Findings Associated with Neoplasms

Codes listed in Chapter 18 for symptoms, signs, and ill-defined conditions that may be associated with an existing malignancy are never listed as the principal diagnosis to replace the malignancy as the first-listed diagnosis regardless of the number of admissions/encounters for treatment the patient is receiving for a neoplasm.

Coding for Primary Malignancy Previously Excised/Eradicated

- If the primary malignancy has been previously excised or eradicated, a code from category Z85 Personal history of malignant neoplasm is reported to indicate the former site provided that:
  - No further treatment of the malignancy is being directed to that primary site
  - There is no evidence of any remaining primary malignancy at that site
- If the primary malignant neoplasm has been previously excised or eradicated but there is documentation of extension, invasion, or metastasis to another site:
  - The code for the extension or invasion site is reported as a secondary malignant neoplasm to the eradicated primary site.
  - The code for the secondary malignant neoplasm may be the principal or first-listed diagnosis followed by a code from category Z85 as a secondary code to report the former site of the primary malignancy.
  - Codes from Z85.0-Z85.7 should only be reported for a former primary malignancy site, not a secondary one. Codes from subcategory Z85.8 may report the former site(s) of either a primary or secondary malignancy.

Special Coding Guidelines for Other Coding Scenarios Involving Malignant Neoplasms

- Primary malignant neoplasms of overlapping site boundaries:
  - If a specific code is available for the overlapping site, the specific code is used. For example, malignant neoplasm of rectosigmoid junction is reported with code C19 which is specific for neoplasms of the sigmoid colon with the rectum.

  - A primary malignant neoplasm that overlaps two or more contiguous sites (sites that are adjacent or next to each other) that does not have a specific code for the overlapping sites is classified to the subcategory/code .8 for overlapping lesion.
- Malignant neoplasms of the same site or organ, such as the breast, that are not contiguous:
- Two discrete malignant lesions, such as one in the upper outer quadrant and another in the lower outer quadrant of the right breast (female) are reported with codes for each site as follows:
  - C50.411 Malignant neoplasm of upper-outer quadrant of right female breast
  - C50.511 Malignant neoplasm of lower-outer quadrant of right female breast
- Malignant neoplasm of ectopic tissue:
- The malignancy is coded to the site of the ectopic tissue. For example, malignancy of ectopic pancreatic tissue is reported with code C25.9 Malignant neoplasm, pancreas, unspecified.
- Malignant neoplasm, unspecified site:
  - If the malignancy is documented as disseminated, generalized, or advanced metastatic disease, but no specific primary or secondary sites are identified, use code C80.0 Disseminated malignant neoplasm, unspecified.
  - If the malignancy is not documented as disseminated and no specific primary site is identified, use C80.1 Malignant (primary) neoplasm, unspecified.
- Malignant neoplasm in a pregnant patient:
  - The principal or first-listed diagnosis is a code from subcategory O9A.1- Malignant neoplasm complicating pregnancy, childbirth, and the puerperium followed by the appropriate codes from Chapter 2 to identify the malignancy.
- Malignant neoplasm associated with a transplanted organ:
  - A malignancy associated with a transplanted organ is considered to be a complication of the transplant and three codes are required:
    - » The principal or first-listed diagnosis is a code from category T86.- Complications of transplanted organs and tissue.
    - » The second code is C80.2 Malignant neoplasm associated with a transplanted organ.
    - » The third code is for the specific malignancy.

Coding for Leukemia, Multiple Myeloma, and Malignant Plasma Cell Neoplasms

- The following code categories require documentation related to whether the neoplasm has not ever achieved remission, is in remission, is in relapse, or whether the patient has been disease-free for a prolonged period and is considered "cured":
  - C90 Multiple myeloma and malignant plasma cell neoplasms
  - C91 Lymphoid leukemia
  - C92 Myeloid leukemia
  - C93 Monocytic leukemia
  - C94 Other leukemias of specified cell type
  - C95 Leukemia of unspecified cell type
- Documentation must be clear as to whether a patient is in remission or has been disease-free for a long period. If the documentation is not clear, the physician should be queried.
  - If the patient is in remission, use the appropriate code from one of the categories listed above.
  - If the patient has been disease-free or in remission for a prolonged period and is considered "cured", use the code for personal history of malignant neoplasm:
    - » Z85.6 Personal history of leukemia
    - » Z85.79 Personal history of other malignant neoplasms of lymphoid, hematopoietic, and related tissues

Aftercare following neoplasm surgery, follow-up for completed malignancy treatment, and prophylactic organ removal are reported with codes from Chapter 21 Factors influencing health status and contact with health services.

General Documentation Requirements

General documentation requirements differ depending on whether the neoplasm involves a solid organ or tissue, or whether the neoplasm involves lymph and blood forming cells or tissues (lymphatic, hematopoietic, and related tissues). Some of the general documentation requirements are discussed here but greater detail will be provided in the next section for some of the more common neoplasms.

Solid Organ/Tissue Neoplasms

In order to assign the most specific code for solid organ or tissue neoplasms, documentation must include:

- Site
- Histologic behavior:
  - Benign
  - In situ
  - Malignant
    - » Primary site
    - » Secondary (metastatic) site
  - Uncertain behavior
  - Unspecified
- Histologic type:
  - Malignant neoplasms
    - » Liver and intrahepatic bile ducts
      - o Liver cell carcinoma (hepatocellular carcinoma, hepatoma)
      - o Intrahepatic bile duct (cholangiocarcinoma)
      - o Hepatoblastoma
      - o Angiosarcoma (Kupffer cell sarcoma)
      - o Other specific liver sarcomas
      - o Other specified liver carcinomas
      - o Unspecified type primary malignancy of liver
      - o Unspecified type, liver, not specified as primary or secondary

2. Neoplasms

- » Mesothelial and soft tissue
  - ◦ Mesothelioma
  - ◦ Kaposi's sarcoma
  - ◦ Merkel cell carcinoma
- » Neuroendocrine tumors
  - ◦ Malignant carcinoid tumor (primary)
  - ◦ Secondary carcinoid tumors
- » Skin
  - ◦ Malignant melanoma
  - ◦ Basal cell carcinoma
  - ◦ Squamous cell carcinoma
  - ◦ Other specified histologic type
  - ◦ Unspecified

– In situ neoplasms
- » Skin
  - ◦ Melanoma in situ
  - ◦ Carcinoma in situ

– Benign neoplasms
- » Neuroendocrine
  - ◦ Benign carcinoid tumor
  - ◦ Other benign tumor
- » Skin
  - ◦ Melanocytic nevi (atypical nevus, blue hairy pigmented nevus, nevus NOS)
  - ◦ Other benign neoplasms
- » Uterus
  - ◦ Leiomyoma
  - ◦ Other benign neoplasm
  - ◦

- Laterality, for paired organs or extremities
- Sex, for neoplasms of the breast

Neoplasms of Lymphoid, Hematopoietic, and Related Tissues

Codes for lymphomas, leukemias, multiple myeloma, and malignant plasma cell neoplasms have undergone extensive changes from previously used classification groupings for identification. Documentation requirements for these conditions will be discussed in detail in the next section, but a few of the changes related to classifying lymphomas are listed below:

- Outdated classifications of lymphoma, such as Hodgkin's paragranuloma, granuloma, and sarcoma, have been replaced with current terms and descriptors.
- Hodgkin lymphomas are classified as lymphocyte predominant or classical with classical types being subclassified into more specific types.
- Follicular lymphomas require documentation of grade.
- Other lymphomas require documentation related to cell type with descriptors, such as large cell, small cell, mixed cell, B-cell, T-cell, mantle cell, peripheral, and cutaneous, as well as other types.

Reclassification of Neoplasm Types

In the neoplasm chapter, a number of neoplasms have been reclassified from their traditional identification into updated terminology. In addition, some conditions have been reclassified as neoplasms. For example:

- Some neoplasms previously classified as uncertain histological behavior, such as myeloproliferative disease not described as chronic is now classified in category C94 Other leukemias of specified cell type.
- Some conditions such as macroglobulinemia have been reclassified as malignant immunoproliferative diseases.

Code-Specific Documentation Requirements

In this section, some of the more frequently reported neoplasm code categories, subcategories, and subclassifications are reviewed with codes listed and documentation requirements identified. The focus is on frequently reported conditions and what specific clinical documentation is required for reporting them. Even though not all codes with significant documentation requirements are discussed, this section will provide a representative sample of the type of documentation required for neoplasms. The section is organized alphabetically by the diagnostic condition named in the examples.

Benign Neoplasm of Colon, Rectum, Anal Canal

Benign neoplasms are defined as a collection of abnormal cells or an overgrowth of cells that lack the invasive properties of cancer. Often named for the tissue or cells from which they arise (lipoma/fat cells, adenoma/gland forming cells), benign neoplasms may still produce negative health effects. Benign neoplasms of the colon, rectum, or anus are of concern because some types can evolve into malignant neoplasms. One broad type of benign neoplasm commonly found in the colon, rectum, and anus is a polyp. However, there are several different types of polyps and some types are classified in the neoplasm chapter while other types are classified in the digestive system chapter. Types of polyps classified as benign neoplasms and located in the neoplasm chapter include those described as:

- Adenomatous polyp/polyposis
- Benign neoplasm
- Polyposis, benign
- Polyposis, familial

Careful review of the documentation as well as carefully following instructions in the Alphabetic Index and Tabular List is required to assign the correct code for polyps in the colon, rectum, and anus.

Specific documentation is required related to site as each section of the colon as well as the rectosigmoid junction, rectum, and anal canal is represented by a specific code. Category D12 includes adenomatous polyps, polyposis of the colon (described as adenomatous, benign, or familial), adenomatosis, and dysplasia (including high grade focal dysplasia). Also included in category D12 are polyps where the specific site in the colon has been documented. For example, a diagnosis of polyp of the sigmoid colon is reported with code D12.5 even though none of the other qualifiers (adenomatous, benign, familial) are documented. Conditions excluded from codes in category D12 are as follows:

- Benign carcinoid tumors of the appendix, large intestine, and rectum
- Benign neoplasm of colon without a more specific site designation – those described as inflammatory polyps or colon polyps (NOS)
- Benign neoplasms of the anus and anal canal – those described as located at the anal margin or limited to the anal or perianal skin

Coding and Documentation Requirements

Identify lesion type:

- Adenomatosis
- Benign neoplasm
- Dysplasia (includes high grade focal dysplasia)
- Polyposis of the colon
  - Adenomatous
  - Benign
  - Familial

Identify lesion site:

- Cecum
- Appendix
- Colon
  - Ascending
  - Transverse
  - Descending
  - Sigmoid
  - Unspecified
- Rectosigmoid junction
- Rectum
- Anus and anal canal

ICD-10-CM Code/Documentation	
D12.0	Benign neoplasm of cecum
D12.1	Benign neoplasm of appendix
D12.2	Benign neoplasm of ascending colon
D12.3	Benign neoplasm of transverse colon
D12.4	Benign neoplasm of descending colon
D12.5	Benign neoplasm of sigmoid colon
D12.6	Benign neoplasm of colon, unspecified site
D12.7	Benign neoplasm of rectosigmoid junction
D12.8	Benign neoplasm of rectum
D12.9	Benign neoplasm of anus and anal canal

Documentation and Coding Example

Fifty-seven-year-old Caucasian female presents to urgent care clinic with a 2-day history of crampy lower abdominal pain and diarrhea. Her pain has now localized to the RLQ and she has nausea and a low grade fever. Temperature 100.2, HR 88, RR 16, BP 132/78. On examination, this is an anxious but cooperative woman. Skin is warm, dry to touch with slightly decreased turgor. PERRL, TMs clear. Mucous membranes dry and pale pink, neck supple without lymphadenopathy. Heart rate regular without murmur, bruit or rub, breath sounds clear, equal bilaterally. Abdomen is non-distended, bowel sounds hyperactive throughout. Spleen is not palpable, liver can be felt at the RCM. No tenderness is appreciated in R or L UQ. LLQ has mild tenderness to deep palpation and RLQ has moderate tenderness and some guarding at McBurney's point but no rebound tenderness. Rectal exam shows good sphincter tone, moderate tenderness on both right and left sides and guaiac positive stool. Blood drawn for CBC, ESR and Chem panel. IV started for hydration. Flat plate of abdomen shows normal bowel gas pattern. CBC has a slightly elevated WBC count but no left shift. Patient treated with IV anti-emetic and hydration. She is referred to gastroenterologist for follow up. Symptoms continued and two days later patient underwent a colonoscopy without bowel prep.

Findings: Lesion consistent with **benign intestinal fibro-epithelioma** found **in the cecum near the periappendiceal tissue** with marked inflammation and bleeding. Lesion removed and sent to pathology. **Pathology report confirmed benign fibro-epithelioma**. Symptoms resolved and patient advised to return in near future for a repeat colonoscopy with bowel prep.

Diagnosis Code(s)

D12.0 Benign neoplasm cecum

Coding Note(s)

Because the histology is provided it is possible to look up the code using the histological term fibro-epithelioma. However, the Alphabetic Index does not provide a reference for fibroepithelioma or epithelioma, fibrous/fibroid. Because the documentation states that this is a benign fibro-epithelioma, it is appropriate to assign the code for benign neoplasm. The site of the fibro-epithelioma is documented as in the cecum near the periappendiceal tissue. The correct site code is the cecum, not the appendix, because the lesion is not in the appendix. The reference to the periappendiceal tissue more specifically describes the location of the lesion in the cecum.

Benign Neoplasm of Skin

Benign neoplasms are defined as a collection of abnormal cells or an overgrowth of cells that lack the invasive properties of cancer. Often named for the tissue or cells from which they arise (dermatofibroma/skin cells, adenoma/gland forming cells), benign neoplasms may still produce negative health effects. One common type of benign neoplasm of the skin is a nevus, more often referred to in lay terms as a mole.

Melanocytic nevi have been assigned a unique category (D22) with a second category (D23) for all other benign neoplasms of the skin. Melanocytic nevi include atypical nevus, blue hairy pigmented nevus, and nevus NOS.

Coding and Documentation Requirements

Identify type of benign skin neoplasm:

- Melanocytic nevi, which includes:
  - Atypical nevus

- Blue hairy pigmented nevus
- Nevus NOS

- Other benign neoplasm of skin such as:
  - Adenoma
  - Dermatofibroma
  - Hydrocystoma
  - Syringocystadenoma
  - Syringoma
  - Trichoepithelioma
  - Trichofolliculoma
  - Tricholemmoma

Identify site:

- Lip
- Eyelid/canthus
- Ear/external auricular canal
- Face
  - Other specified site
  - Unspecified site
- Scalp/neck
- Trunk
- Upper limb/shoulder
- Lower limb/hip
- Unspecified site

For paired organs/extremities, identify laterality:

- Right
- Left
- Unspecified

ICD-10-CM Code/Documentation	
D23.0	Other benign neoplasm skin of lip
D22.0	Melanocytic nevi of lip
D23.10	Other benign neoplasm of skin of unspecified eyelid, including canthus
D23.111	Other benign neoplasm of skin of right upper eyelid, including canthus
D23.112	Other benign neoplasm of skin of right lower eyelid, including canthus
D23.121	Other benign neoplasm of skin of left upper eyelid, including canthus
D23.122	Other benign neoplasm of skin of left lower eyelid, including canthus
D22.10	Melanocytic nevi of unspecified eyelid, including canthus
D22.111	Melanocytic nevi of right upper eyelid, including canthus
D22.112	Melanocytic nevi of right lower eyelid, including canthus
D22.121	Melanocytic nevi of left upper eyelid, including canthus
D22.122	Melanocytic nevi of left lower eyelid, including canthus
D23.20	Other benign neoplasm of unspecified ear and external auricular canal
D23.21	Other benign neoplasm of right ear and external auricular canal
D23.22	Other benign neoplasm of left ear and external auricular canal
D22.20	Melanocytic nevi of unspecified ear and external auricular canal
D22.21	Melanocytic nevi of right ear and external auricular canal
D22.22	Melanocytic nevi of left ear and external auricular cana
D23.30	Other benign neoplasm of skin of unspecified part of face
D23.39	Other benign neoplasm of skin of other specified part of face
D22.30	Melanocytic nevi of unspecified part of face
D22.39	Melanocytic nevi of other specified part of face
D23.4	Other benign neoplasm of skin of scalp and neck
D22.4	Melanocytic nevi of scalp and neck
D23.5	Other benign neoplasm of skin of trunk
D22.5	Melanocytic nevi of trunk
D23.60	Other benign neoplasm of skin of unspecified upper limb, including shoulder
D23.61	Other benign neoplasm of skin of right upper limb, including shoulder
D23.62	Other benign neoplasm of skin of left upper limb, including shoulder
D22.60	Melanocytic nevi of unspecified upper limb, including shoulder
D22.61	Melanocytic nevi of right upper limb, including shoulder
D22.62	Melanocytic nevi of left upper limb, including shoulder
D23.70	Other benign neoplasm of skin of unspecified lower limb, including hip
D23.71	Other benign neoplasm of skin of right lower limb, including hip
D23.72	Other benign neoplasm of skin of left lower limb, including hip
D22.70	Melanocytic nevi of unspecified lower limb, including hip
D22.71	Melanocytic nevi of right lower limb, including hip
D22.72	Melanocytic nevi of left lower limb, including hip
D23.9	Other benign neoplasm of skin, unspecified
D22.9	Melanocytic nevi, unspecified

Documentation and Coding Example

Seven-year-old female presents to ENT accompanied by her mother having failed audiometric hearing screen, left ear, administered at school. Patient has an entirely unremarkable medical history. She is seen regularly for preventative care with her last visit 8 months ago, immunizations are UTD for age. Mother states child has never had an ear infection and has never been prescribed an antibiotic. Pregnancy and birth were uncomplicated and patient passed newborn AABR prior to discharge. Mother contacted the school nurse and was told that her daughter passed a similar screening 2 years ago. On examination, this is a cooperative young lady who is able to articulate that she has no pain in either ear but does say her left ear sometimes has a "stuffy" feel about it. She denies placing any foreign body in the ear and mother states they never use Q-tips to clean ears and child does not use headphones or ear buds to listen to music. Nares patent without drainage, oral mucosa moist and pink, pharynx without swelling, lesions or drainage. Neck supple without lymphadenopathy. Right ear exam unremarkable with patent external ear canal and intact TM without fluid, redness, or bulging. Otomicroscopic exam of the left external ear canal is almost impossible due to obstruction by a dome shaped darkly pigmented hairy lesion arising from the posterior wall of the canal. Pressure or manipulation of the lesion produces no pain according to the patient. With permission of patient and her mother a second ENT opinion is immediately obtained. Both physicians agree that this lesion requires immediate attention and would best be removed under anesthesia. Parent agrees and patient is scheduled for outpatient surgical excision.

Operative note: **Left ear external auditory canal** examined with the patient under monitored anesthesia care. Using an operating microscope an elliptical incision was made around the lesion with visually clear margins. A 0.5 x 0.6 x 0.8 cm lesion was removed and sent for pathology which was reported as **melanocytic nevi with microscopically clear margins** all around. The incision was closed with non-absorbable suture and the external auditory canal packed with sterile gauze.

Follow up note: Patient seen 5 days post op. Drain and packing removed. Incision healing well. Sutures removed 10 days post op. Hearing test administered at that time is completely normal.

Diagnosis Code(s)

D22.22 Melanocytic nevi of left ear and external auricular canal

Coding Note(s)

The code is specific for a melanocytic nevus as well as site (ear and external auricular canal) and laterality (left).

Carcinoma in Situ of Cervix Uteri

An in-situ tumor is confined to the site of origin. The neoplastic (cancer) cells are usually flat lesions that proliferate in their normal habitat (skin, cervix, mammary ducts). If left untreated, in-situ tumors can invade the surrounding tissue and spread to other areas of the body, called metastasis.

Carcinoma in situ is specific to site such as endocervix or exocervix. Documentation that supports a diagnosis of carcinoma in situ includes:

- Cervical adenocarcinoma in situ
- Cervical intraepithelial glandular neoplasia
- Cervical intraepithelial neoplasia III (CIN III)
- Severe dysplasia of the uterine cervix

Coding and Documentation Requirements

Identify site of cervix:

- Endocervix
- Exocervix
- Other parts/overlapping sites of cervix
- Unspecified part of cervix

ICD-10-CM Code/Documentation	
D06.0	Carcinoma in situ of endocervix
D06.1	Carcinoma in situ of exocervix
D06.7	Carcinoma in situ of other parts of cervix
D06.9	Carcinoma in situ of cervix, unspecified

Documentation and Coding Example

Thirty-three-year-old black female presents for routine GYN exam. Patient has a 10+ year history of genital warts and abnormal pap smears, last exam and cervical cytology 18 months ago. She has been married for one year and just completed her MBA. She works at a brokerage firm, her husband is an accountant. They plan to start a family soon. Temperature 98.4, HR 66, RR 12, BP 102/60. Patient states LMP was about 1 week ago and last intercourse 2 days ago. She is not currently using any form of contraceptive. On examination, patient is a well-groomed, healthy appearing female who looks her stated age. Skin warm, dry to touch, mucous membranes moist and pink. HR regular without murmur. Breath sounds clear, equal bilaterally. Abdomen soft and non-tender, active bowel sounds throughout. External genitalia without lesions, speculum inserted easily. Cervix visualized and appears grossly normal with clear mucus present in the os. Pap test performed using cervical brush obtaining both endocervical and exocervical cell samples, cervical HPV DNA swab also obtained due to history of genital warts. Speculum removed and bimanual exam is unremarkable with anteverted, freely mobile uterus, ovaries palpable and normal in size. Patient is reminded that with her history of HPV infection and abnormal pap tests she should have a GYN exam and testing every 6-12 months.

Cervical cytology shows many abnormal cells and **HPV DNA swab is positive for HPV type 31**.

Patient returns for colposcopic exam which reveals areas of abnormal staining on left side of exocervix. Multiple biopsies obtained including endocervical curettage cell samples. Specimens to lab along with blood sample for CBC, Chem Panel, SCCA, CEA. **Biopsies reveal Ca in situ of exocervix, no malignancy found in endocervical cell samples**, blood tests are all WNL. Patient underwent LEEP procedure with good results.

Diagnosis Code(s)

D06.1 Carcinoma in situ of exocervix

R87.810 Cervical high risk human papillomavirus (HPV) DNA test positive

Coding Note(s)

HPV types 16, 18, 31, 33, 35, 39, 45, 51, 52, 56, 58, and 59 are "high-risk" sexually transmitted HPVs that may lead to the development of cervical intraepithelial neoplasia (CIN) and cervical cancer.

Follicular Lymphoma

There are many types of lymphoma which is a cancer of the lymphatic system. Lymphomas are grouped first into two general types—Hodgkin lymphoma and non-Hodgkin lymphoma. These two broad groups are then divided into more specific types. Hodgkin lymphoma is discussed in the next section. Non-Hodgkin lymphoma is discussed here.

Non-Hodgkin lymphomas are cancers of the lymphocytes, of which there are two types, T-cells and B-cells. The disease process is not fully understood, but at some point, B-cells or T-cells develop abnormalities that cause them to divide rapidly and accumulate at different sites in the body. As the number of abnormal T-cells or B-cells increases and they crowd out normal cells, symptoms of non-Hodgkin lymphoma develop which may include: enlarged lymph nodes, loss of appetite, weight loss, fever, night sweats, respiratory symptoms (cough, difficulty breathing), chest pain, and fatigue as well as other symptoms.

Non-Hodgkin lymphoma is classified based on whether the affected lymphocyte is a B-cell or T-cell. B-cell non-Hodgkin lymphomas are the most common, of which the common B-cell subtypes include: diffuse large B-cell lymphoma, follicular lymphoma, mantle cell lymphoma, and small lymphocytic lymphoma. There are also a number of subtypes of T-cell lymphoma, which include: peripheral T-cell lymphoma, anaplastic large cell lymphoma, angioimmunoblastic lymphoma, and cutaneous T-cell lymphoma. In this section, documentation and coding for follicular lymphoma, which was previously classified as nodular lymphoma, is discussed.

The older term "nodular lymphoma" has been replaced with follicular lymphoma (C82), which is subdivided into several different types with some types being further differentiated by grade. Grade refers to the amount of cell differentiation and rate of growth of the neoplastic cells. While follicular lymphomas are generally considered to be well-differentiated, low-grade, or slow-growing types, within this subclassification there are still variations in the rate of growth and the response to treatment with lower grades tending to have better long-term outcomes. The grading system used in ICD-10-CM was developed by the Revised European-American Classification of Lymphoid Neoplasms (REAL) which has also been adopted by the World Health Organization (WHO).

The REAL/WHO classification grades the follicular lymphoma based on the number of centroblasts per high-power field (hpf). The grades are as follows:

- Grade I (1) 0-5 centroblasts per hpf with a predominance of small centrocytes
- Grade II (2) 6-15 centroblasts per hpf with centrocytes present
- Grade III (3) >15 centroblasts per hpf with a decreased number or no centrocytes present

Follicular lymphoma grade 3 can be further divided into types A and B:

- Grade IIIa (3A) >15 centroblasts per hpf with centrocytes still present
- Grade IIIb (3B) >15 centroblasts per hpf presenting as solid sheets with no centrocytes present

The REAL/WHO classification also recognizes two variants of follicular lymphomas—cutaneous follicle center lymphoma and diffuse follicle center lymphoma, which have specific ICD-10-CM codes.

Grades should not be confused with stages. Stages relate to the extent of the disease - that is, whether it is localized or limited, involves multiple lymph node regions, or has metastasized to the bone marrow, extranodal sites, and/or solid organ sites. Stages are as follows:

Stage I – The disease is limited to a single region or group of lymph nodes. Less common is disease limited to a single organ outside the lymph system.

Stage II – The disease is limited to two or more groups of lymph nodes with all disease located on one side of the diaphragm (either above or below the diaphragm). A single organ near the involved lymph nodes may also be affected.

Stage III – The disease involves lymph node groups or regions both above and below the diaphragm and organs adjacent to involved lymph nodes may also be affected. If the spleen is involved, the disease is always considered to be stage III.

Stage IV – The disease has metastasized to the bone marrow, liver, or lung or to sites that are remote from the involved lymph node regions.

Knowing the stage helps with determining the correct site designations. For example, Stage I disease would never be coded as involving multiple sites. For Stage I disease, a specific code for the involved lymph node group or region would be assigned. Conversely, Stage IV would require a code for lymph nodes of multiple sites and a code for the spleen, and/or extranodal and solid organ sites.

Coding and Documentation Requirements

Specify type/grade of follicular lymphoma:

- Follicular lymphoma
  - Grade I
  - Grade II
  - Grade III, unspecified
  - Grade IIIa
  - Grade IIIb
- Diffuse follicle center lymphoma
- Cutaneous follicle center lymphoma
- Other types of follicular lymphoma
- Unspecified follicular lymphoma

Identify site (fifth character):

- Lymph nodes
  - Head/face/neck (1)
  - Intrathoracic (2)
  - Intra-abdominal (3)
  - Axilla and upper limb (4)
  - Inguinal region and lower limb (5)
  - Intrapelvic (6)
  - Multiple sites (8)
- Spleen (7)
- Extranodal/solid organ sites (9)
- Unspecified site (0)

ICD-10-CM Code/Documentation	
C82.0-	Follicular lymphoma grade I
C82.1-	Follicular lymphoma grade II
C82.2-	Follicular lymphoma grade III, unspecified
C82.3-	Follicular lymphoma grade IIIa
C82.4-	Follicular lymphoma grade IIIb
C82.5-	Diffuse follicle center lymphoma
C82.6-	Cutaneous follicle center lymphoma
C82.8-	Other types of follicular lymphoma
C82.9-	Unspecified follicular lymphoma

Note: A fifth digit/character is required to identify which lymph node regions, extranodal and/or solid organ sites are involved.

Documentation and Coding Example

PCP visit: Sixty-three-year-old Caucasian male presents for routine physical. He is recently retired from a 40-year career as a postal carrier and fills his time with travel, golf and is a volunteer crossing guard at the local elementary school. Temperature 97.9, HR 74, RR 14, BP 144/82, Wt. 168 lbs. On examination, this is a thin, muscular man who appears younger than his stated age. Skin warm and dry, he is very tan and admits to rarely using sunscreen. There are some dry, scaly patches on face and arms and patient will be referred to dermatology to have them evaluated. PERRL, neck supple without palpable lymph nodes. Mucus membranes moist and pink, teeth in good repair, oral and nasal airways patent. Breath sounds clear and equal bilaterally, heart rate regular with Grade II heart murmur present. Patient has known aortic regurgitation and is followed by cardiology with regular ultrasound. Last exam was 6 months ago and WNL. Upper extremities have good ROM and intact pulses. Abdomen soft and non-tender, spleen palpated 2 cm below LCM, liver 1 cm below RCM. Bowel sounds active in all quadrants. There is no evidence of hernia in the inguinal region but enlarged lymph nodes can be palpated bilaterally. Lower extremities are without edema and have good ROM. Rectal exam shows good sphincter tone, prostate is smooth and normal size, stool is guaiac negative. Blood collected and sent to lab for CBC, ESR, Chem Panel. Referred to general surgery for lymph node biopsy.

F/U visit with surgeon: Inguinal lymph node was removed under local anesthesia and sent to lab for pathology and immunohistochemistry, if indicated. Lymph node biopsy came back positive for **follicular lymphoma, grade I**. A CT scan with concurrent PET scan of chest, abdomen, and pelvis was ordered subsequent to the lymph node biopsy and showed **lymphadenopathy that is limited to groin and deep pelvic area**. There does not appear to be spleen or liver involvement. A bilateral bone marrow aspirate was obtained from hips and all specimens are negative for lymphoma cells. Patient returns today to discuss treatment options.

Diagnosis: **Follicular lymphoma, stage II involving inguinal and intrapelvic regions bilaterally**.

Diagnosis Code(s)

C82.05 Follicular lymphoma grade I, lymph nodes of inguinal region and lower limb

C82.06 Follicular lymphoma grade I, intrapelvic lymph nodes

Coding Note(s)

The grade is specified on the pathology report as Grade I. While the stage of the lymphoma is not included in the diagnosis codes, the fact that the follicular lymphoma is limited to the inguinal and intrapelvic lymph nodes provides information indicating that the patient is Stage II.

Hodgkin Lymphoma

The condition previously described as Hodgkin's disease is now referred to as Hodgkin lymphoma (C81). The terms paragranuloma, granuloma, and sarcoma are no longer used. Hodgkin lymphoma is a malignant neoplasm of the lymphatic system, specifically of B-cell lymphocytes. Most types of Hodgkin lymphoma are caused by a mutation in the B-cell DNA which causes these cells to divide rapidly and not die off as normal B-cells do. These mutated B-cells are called Reed-Sternberg cells. The cancerous B-cells crowd out normal cells in the lymphatic system producing the signs and symptoms characteristic of Hodgkin lymphoma which include: enlargement of lymphatic tissue (lymph nodes, spleen, and other immune tissue), fever, loss of appetite, weight loss, fatigue, and night sweats.

There are traditionally two primary types of Hodgkin lymphoma—classical Hodgkin lymphoma and nodular lymphocyte predominant Hodgkin lymphoma. Although classification of Hodgkin lymphoma has recently dropped the nomenclature of 'classical' and considers all types as a presentation of Hodgkin lymphoma, "classical" is still included as alternate terminology. This is the most common type and it is subdivided into four specific subtypes:

- Nodular sclerosis Hodgkin lymphoma
- Mixed cellularity Hodgkin lymphoma
- Lymphocyte-depleted Hodgkin lymphoma
- Lymphocyte-rich Hodgkin lymphoma

Codes are specific to site. Lymph node involvement should be specified as to which lymphatic regions are involved if the disease is limited, or the code for multiple sites should be used. There are also specific codes for spleen, extranodal and solid organ sites, and unspecified site.

Coding and Documentation Requirements

Identify Hodgkin lymphoma type:

- Nodular lymphocyte predominant
- Nodular sclerosis
- Mixed cellularity
- Lymphocyte depleted
- Lymphocyte-rich
- Other specified type
- Unspecified type

Identify site (fifth digit):

- Lymph nodes
  - Head/face/neck (1)
  - Intrathoracic (2)
  - Intra-abdominal (3)
  - Axilla and upper limb (4)
  - Inguinal region and lower limb (5)
  - Intrapelvic (6)
  - Multiple sites (8)
- Spleen (7)
- Extranodal/solid organ sites (9)
- Unspecified site (0)

ICD-10-CM Code/Documentation	
C81.0-	Nodular lymphocyte predominant Hodgkin lymphoma
C81.1-	Nodular sclerosis Hodgkin lymphoma
C81.2-	Mixed cellularity Hodgkin lymphoma
C81.3-	Lymphocyte depleted Hodgkin lymphoma
C81.4-	Lymphocyte-rich Hodgkin lymphoma
C81.7-	Other Hodgkin lymphoma
C81.9-	Hodgkin lymphoma, unspecified

Note: A fifth digit/character is required to identify which lymph node regions, extranodal and/or solid organ sites are involved.

Documentation and Coding Example

Oncology Consultation: Fifty-two-year-old Hispanic female presented to her PCP for comprehensive physical exam 2 weeks ago. She was in her usual state of good health until four months ago when she had a febrile illness lasting over a week and has been bothered by fatigue, drenching night sweats, decreased appetite, and a 15 lb. weight loss since then. She saw her OB/GYN six months ago for routine well woman exam and mammogram which were reported as normal. She takes supplemental calcium and Vitamin D but no other medications and does not smoke or drink alcohol. Patient is married, twin daughters are in high school and she works part time as an administrative assistant. On examination, this is an anxious, tired appearing female who looks her stated age. Temperature 98.8, HR 90, RR 16, BP 128/74, Wt. 125 lbs. PMH is non-contributory. Skin is warm and dry without rashes or bruising. PERRL, mucous membranes moist and pink, marked swelling of the Waldeyer ring but patient denies throat pain, TMs normal bilaterally. There is diffuse lymphadenopathy involving the anterior and posterior cervical lymph nodes, supraclavicular and axillary nodes. Cardiac sounds are muffled making it difficult to ascertain the presence of bruits, rubs, or murmurs. Breath sounds are clear bilaterally. Abdomen is soft and non-tender, spleen palpated at the LCM and liver 3 cm below the RCM. Bowel sounds active in all quadrants. There are no enlarged lymph nodes, swelling or edema present in the groin or lower extremities. Blood collected and sent to lab for CBC, ESR, Platelets, Chem Panel.

Findings on CT with concurrent PET scan of chest, abdomen, and pelvis that was ordered by her PCP are reviewed with patient and her husband. It shows a **mediastinal mass, enlarged liver and spleen, and diffuse lymphadenopathy throughout neck, chest, abdomen, and pelvis which is suggestive of lymphoma involving multiple sites.** Patient also underwent lymph node biopsy following the CT scan and **pathology report confirms lymphocyte rich classical Hodgkin lymphoma (LRCHL).**

Treatment options are presented including risks and benefits. Patient is referred to radiation oncologist for radiation therapy treatment plan and following that visit a chemotherapy regimen will be determined.

Diagnosis: **Lymphocyte rich classical Hodgkin lymphoma.**

Diagnosis Code(s)

C81.48 Lymphocyte-rich Hodgkin lymphoma, lymph nodes of multiple sites

Coding Note(s)

The patient is receiving care (consultation) directed at the malignancy so the code for the malignancy is reported. Once radiation therapy and chemotherapy have been initiated, the code for the therapy will be reported as the first-listed diagnosis whenever the encounter is for that treatment, followed by the code for the LRCHL.

Leukemia, Lymphoid

Lymphoid leukemia is a cancer of the lymphocytes, which are a type of white blood cell. Lymphoid leukemia arises from lymphoid stem cells. Normally, lymphoid stem cells differentiate into three types of mature white blood cells—B-lymphocytes, T-lymphocytes, and natural killer cells. In lymphoid leukemia, lymphoid stem cells do not differentiate and mature. Instead they become abnormal white blood cells that proliferate in both the bone marrow and blood stream crowding out normal blood cells. There are two primary types of lymphoid leukemia, acute and chronic. In the acute form, the increase in abnormal cells is rapid and the disease progresses rapidly. Acute lymphoblastic leukemia occurs most often in children, but it is also a cancer that affects adults. In chronic lymphoid leukemia, which is seen almost exclusively in adults, the abnormal cells increase in number more slowly so the disease progresses slowly.

Lymphoid leukemia is classified as acute lymphoblastic leukemia (ALL), chronic lymphocytic leukemia of B-cell type, prolymphocytic leukemia of B-cell type, hairy cell leukemia (previously classified as a malignant neoplasm of lymphoid and histiocytic tissue), adult T-cell leukemia (HTLV-1-associated), prolymphocytic leukemia of T-cell type, mature B-cell Burkitt type, or other specified type of lymphoid leukemia. Lymphoid leukemia specified as subacute does not have a specific code and is classified as "other specified type" of leukemia.

Coding and Documentation Requirements

Identify type of lymphoid leukemia:

- Acute lymphoblastic leukemia [ALL]
- Chronic lymphocytic leukemia, B cell type
- Prolymphocytic leukemia
  - B-cell type
  - T-cell type
  - Hairy cell leukemia
  - Adult T-cell lymphoma/leukemia (HTLV-1 associated), which includes:
    - » Acute variant
    - » Chronic variant
    - » Lymphomatoid variant
    - » Smouldering variant
- Mature B-cell leukemia Burkitt type
- Other specified type, which includes:

2. Neoplasms

- T-cell large granular lymphocytic leukemia associated with rheumatoid arthritis
- Unspecified lymphoid leukemia

Specify disease status:

- In remission
- In relapse
- Not having achieved remission

ICD-10-CM Code/Documentation	
C91.10	Chronic lymphocytic leukemia of B-cell type not having achieved remission
C91.11	Chronic lymphocytic leukemia of B-cell in remission
C91.12	Chronic lymphocytic leukemia of B-cell in relapse
C91.00	Acute lymphoblastic leukemia [ALL] not having achieved remission
C91.01	Acute lymphoblastic leukemia [ALL] in remission
C91.02	Acute lymphoblastic leukemia [ALL] in relapse
C91.40	Hairy cell leukemia not having achieved remission
C91.41	Hairy cell leukemia, in remission
C91.42	Hairy cell leukemia, in relapse
C91.50	Adult T-cell lymphoma/leukemia (HTLV-1 associated) not having achieved remission
C91.51	Adult T-cell lymphoma/leukemia (HTLV-1 associated) in remission
C91.52	Adult T-cell lymphoma/leukemia (HTLV-1 associated) in relapse
C91.60	Prolymphocytic leukemia of T-cell type not having achieved remission
C91.61	Prolymphocytic leukemia of T-cell type in remission
C91.62	Prolymphocytic leukemia of T-cell type in relapse
C91.30	Prolymphocytic leukemia of B-cell type not having achieved remission
C91.31	Prolymphocytic leukemia of B-cell type in remission
C91.32	Prolymphocytic leukemia of B-cell type in relapse
C91.Z0	Other (specified type) lymphoid leukemia not having achieved remission
C91.Z1	Other (specified type) lymphoid leukemia in remission
C91.Z2	Other (specified type) lymphoid leukemia in relapse
C91.A0	Mature B-cell leukemia Burkitt-type not having achieved remission
C91.A1	Mature B-cell leukemia Burkitt-type in remission
C91.A2	Mature B-cell leukemia Burkitt-type in relapse
C91.90	Lymphoid leukemia, unspecified not having achieved remission
C91.91	Lymphoid leukemia, unspecified, in remission
C91.92	Lymphoid leukemia, unspecified, in relapse

Documentation and Coding Example

Thirty-three-year-old Japanese-American female presents to ED with c/o fast heart rate, mild chest discomfort and shortness of breath x 40 minutes. Temperature 99.2, HR 138, RR 18, BP 110/70. Patient was in her usual state of good health until three weeks ago when she developed a fever, noticed scattered red pumps on torso and arms and swollen neck glands. She was traveling in Japan at the time, was evaluated at a clinic, diagnosed with a viral infection and prescribed rest, fluids and acetaminophen. Patient is a photo-journalist and travels extensively covering natural disasters for an international news organization. She admits that when on assignment, her living conditions are often substandard with poor sanitation, limited access to clean water or fresh food sources. She is up to date on all immunizations including typhoid, cholera, yellow fever, Japanese encephalitis, meningococcal, and hepatitis A and B. EKG shows sinus tachycardia, O2 saturation on RA 96% by pulse oximetry. On examination, patient is an anxious, ill appearing young women. Color pale, skin warm, dry to touch with poor turgor. Patches of erythroderma with papules and firm raised nodules noted on torso, arms, and upper legs. PERRL, mucous membranes dry, pale pink. Throat clear, TMs normal bilaterally. There is diffuse lymphadenopathy involving the anterior and posterior cervical lymph nodes, supraclavicular and axillary nodes. HR rapid but regular, peripheral pulses intact, extremities w/o edema. Breath sounds clear, equal bilaterally. Abdomen mildly distended with hypoactive bowel sounds, patient states she has been constipated for the past week. Liver palpated 1 cm below RCM, spleen palpated at LCM. Enlarged lymph nodes are palpated in groin bilaterally. Blood drawn for CBC, ESR, cardiac enzymes, chem panel. IV started for hydration. Lab tests show elevated serum calcium and LDH, decreased RBCs, and leukocytosis with abnormal lymphocytes. Infectious disease and hematology consults obtained and patient admitted to medical floor. Additional lab tests for bilirubin level, T-cell counts, HIV, hepatitis, and HTLV-1 antibodies. Results show elevated bilirubin and **positive HTLV-1 antibodies**. CT with concurrent PET scan of chest, abdomen, and pelvis reveal enlarged retroperitoneal lymph nodes. Skin biopsy and bone marrow biopsy both show consistent pattern of abnormal T-cell lymphocytes.

Diagnosis: **Adult T-cell lymphoma with leukemia**.

Diagnosis Code(s)

C91.50 Adult T-cell lymphoma/leukemia (HTLV-1 associated) not having achieved remission

B97.33 Human T-cell lymphotropic virus, type I [HTLV-I] as the cause of diseases classified elsewhere

Coding Note(s)

HTLV-1 infection is the cause of the adult T-cell lymphoma/leukemia and is reported additionally.

Leukemia, Myeloid

Myeloid leukemia is a cancer of the blood and bone marrow that arises from immature white blood cells called myeloblasts. Normally, blood stem cells arise in the bone marrow and then differentiate into myeloid and lymphoid stem cells. Myeloid stem cells further differentiate into red blood cells, platelets, and another type of immature blood cell called myeloblasts. Healthy myeloblasts then differentiate into several types of granulocytes (neutrophils, eosinophils, and basophils) which are white blood cells. In myeloid leukemia, abnormal myeloblasts do not mature normally. They divide at an accelerated rate, do not die, and eventually crowd out normal blood cells. There are many subtypes of myeloid leukemia and treatment depends on the specific subtype.

Leukemia documented as granulocytic or myelogenous is included in the category for myeloid leukemia (C92). with 10 subcategories, which include: acute myeloblastic leukemia, chronic BCR/ABL-positive myeloid leukemia, atypical chronic BCR/ABL-negative myeloid leukemia, myeloid sarcoma, acute promyelocytic leukemia, acute myelomonocytic leukemia, acute myeloid leukemia with 11q23 abnormality, acute myeloid leukemia with multilineage dysplasia, other specified types, and unspecified type.

Coding and Documentation Requirements

Specify type of myeloid leukemia:

- Acute myeloblastic leukemia, which includes:
  - Minimal differentiation
  - With Maturation
  - 1/ETO
  - MO, M1, or M2
  - With t(8;21)
  - Not otherwise specified or without a FAB classification
  - Refractory anemia with excess blasts in transformation [RAEB T]
- Chronic BCR/ABL-positive myeloid leukemia, which includes:
  - Chronic myelogenous leukemia, Philadelphia chromosome (Ph1) positive
  - Chronic myelogenous leukemia, t(9;22) (q34;q11)
  - Chronic myelogenous leukemia with crisis of blast cells
- Atypical chronic BCR/ABL-negative myeloid leukemia
- Myeloid sarcoma, which includes:
  - Chloroma
  - Granulocytic sarcoma
  - Malignant tumor of immature myeloid cells
- Acute promyelocytic leukemia, which includes:
  - AML M3
  - AML Me with t(15;17) and variants
- Acute myelomonocytic leukemia, which includes:
  - AML M4
  - AML M4 Eo with inv(16) or t(16;16)
- Acute myeloid leukemia with 11q23 abnormality, which includes:
  - Acute myeloid leukemia with variation of MLL-gene
- Acute myeloid leukemia with multilineage dysplasia
- Other specified myeloid leukemia
- Unspecified myeloid leukemia

Specify disease status:

- Not having achieved remission (failed remission)
- In remission
- In relapse

ICD-10-CM Code/Documentation	
C92.0-	Acute myeloblastic leukemia
C92.1-	Chronic myeloid leukemia, BCR/ABL positive
C92.2-	Atypical chronic myeloid leukemia, BCR/ABL negative
C92.3-	Myeloid sarcoma
C92.4-	Acute promyelocytic leukemia
C92.5-	Acute myelomonocytic leukemia
C92.6-	Acute myeloid leukemia with 11q23 abnormality
C92.A-	Acute myeloid leukemia with multilineage dysplasia
C92.Z-	Other myeloid leukemia
C92.9-	Myeloid leukemia, unspecified

Note: A fifth digit/character is required to identify the disease status as not having achieved remission (0), in remission (1), or in relapse (2).

Documentation and Coding Example

Thirty-nine-year-old nulliparous Hispanic female referred for hematology consult by her OB-GYN because of abnormal blood tests performed during routine gynecological exam. Patient is a mezzo-soprano performing as a guest artist with small opera companies in her native Argentina, the US, and Canada. Her husband is a cellist who teaches and performs locally. Upon questioning, patient does admit to unusual fatigue during and after her most recent performance and her vocal coach has noticed some loss of voice strength/quality. Temperature 98.8, HR 90, RR 12, BP 112/68, Wt. 144. On examination, patient is a well-developed, well-nourished female who looks younger than her stated age. Color is very pale, skin warm and dry with good turgor. PERRL, TMs normal, mucous membranes moist and pale with scattered petechiae noted on gums and posterior pharynx. Neck supple without lymphadenopathy. There is no lymph node enlargement in bilateral axilla. Breath sounds clear and equal bilaterally, heart rate regular without audible murmur, bruits, or rubs. Peripheral pulses present with weak quality, no edema noted in extremities, ROM intact. No joint swelling appreciated but there are areas of bruising noted around both knees and across the sacral area which patient cannot attribute to any kind of injury. Abdomen soft with active bowel sounds in all quadrants. There is mild discomfort when palpating the abdomen especially in the upper quadrants. Liver is palpated at 2 cm below RCM and spleen at 3 cm below LCM. Patient denies pain or bleeding with urination. She states her bowel movements are regular and denies pain or bleeding when passing stools. Breast and pelvic exams are deferred due to recent normal findings by her OB/GYN. Blood drawn for CBC, platelets, comprehensive metabolic panel, PT, PTT, fibrin studies. Lumbar puncture is deferred at this time due to absence of CNS symptoms. Bone marrow biopsy is performed with samples to lab for flow cytometry and cytogenetics including FISH and RT-PCR for ML-RAR alpha transcription. **Blood tests show decreased RBCs and platelets along with immature granulocytes (promyelocytes). Molecular genetic testing is significant for positive myeloperoxidase and CD33, negative human leukocyte antigen (HLA)-DR.**

2. Neoplasms

Diagnosis: **Acute promyelocytic leukemia**

Diagnosis Code(s)

C92.40 Acute promyelocytic leukemia, not having achieved remission

Coding Note(s)

ICD-10-CM provides specific codes for conditions that have been previously classified only as acute myeloid leukemia. The code identifies the type of leukemia as acute promyelocytic leukemia, which is a distinct subtype of acute myeloid leukemia that requires a different treatment regimen.

Lipoma of Skin and Subcutaneous Tissue

A lipoma is a benign (noncancerous) lesion composed of fat cells contained in a thin, fibrous capsule that is usually situated beneath the skin in the subcutaneous tissue, although it can occur at other sites. Because a lipoma is a type of abnormal tissue growth it is classified as a benign neoplasm.

New nomenclature for a lipoma is benign lipomatous neoplasm (D17). Documentation requires site specificity.

Coding and Documentation Requirements

Identify site of skin and subcutaneous tissue benign lipomatous neoplasm:

- Head/face/neck
- Trunk
- Right arm
- Left arm
- Right leg
- Left leg
- Unspecified limb
- Other sites
- Unspecified site

ICD-10-CM Code/Documentation	
D17.0	Benign lipomatous neoplasm of skin and subcutaneous tissue of head, face, and neck
D17.1	Benign lipomatous neoplasm of skin and subcutaneous tissue of trunk
D17.20	Benign lipomatous neoplasm of skin and subcutaneous tissue of unspecified limb
D17.21	Benign lipomatous neoplasm of skin and subcutaneous tissue of right arm
D17.22	Benign lipomatous neoplasm of skin and subcutaneous tissue of left arm
D17.23	Benign lipomatous neoplasm of skin and subcutaneous tissue of right leg
D17.24	Benign lipomatous neoplasm of skin and subcutaneous tissue of left leg
D17.30	Benign lipomatous neoplasm of skin and subcutaneous tissue of unspecified sites
D17.39	Benign lipomatous neoplasm of skin and subcutaneous tissue of other sites

Documentation and Coding Example

Forty-eight-year-old fair skinned female presents for annual dermatology exam. She has one area that she is concerned about at this time. On her **right forearm midway between the wrist and elbow is a 3 x 4 cm soft, slightly mobile painless lump**. Patient recalls a fall from her bicycle approximately six months ago where she sustained relatively minor scrapes and bruises on her right hip, arm, and torso. She noticed a small lump following the accident and it has continued to increase in size. Patient finds it cosmetically bothersome and would like it removed. The right forearm is prepped, draped, and the surgical site infiltrated with local anesthetic. Small incision is made in the skin directly over the lump which is dissected free from surrounding tissue and easily delivered through the incision. Appearance is consistent with a benign lipoma, specimen sent for pathology. Incision closed in layers and a sterile dressing applied. Patient instructed to return in one week for suture removal and wound check.

Follow up: Incision site is clean and healing well. Sutures removed and steri-strips applied. Pathology confirmed a **benign lipomatous neoplasm**.

Diagnosis Code(s)

D17.21 Benign lipomatous neoplasm of skin and subcutaneous tissue of right arm

Coding Note(s)

Codes for lipomas, now classified as benign lipomatous neoplasms, are specific to site. For the extremities, laterality is also a component of the code.

Malignant Melanoma of Skin

Malignant melanoma of the skin is a malignant neoplasm that originates in the melanin (brown pigment producing) cells of the skin. These cells are also called melanocytes. While melanoma is not the most common type of skin cancer, it is the most dangerous type resulting in more deaths each year than other more common types. The success of treatment depends on whether the melanoma is recognized and treated early when it is still confined to the epidermal layer, or whether it has invaded deeper layers of the dermis and underlying tissues. When the malignant melanocytes are confined to the epidermis, the condition is classified as melanoma in situ, also referred to as Stage 0 melanoma or tumor in situ (TIS). When the malignant melanocytes have invaded deeper tissues of the dermis or underlying tissues, the condition is classified as melanoma or melanocarcinoma and is classified as stage I-IV.

Documentation is required specifying whether the melanoma is in situ (D03.-) or has invaded deeper layers of the skin (C43.-). Body sites are specific and require documentation of laterality for paired body parts (eyes, ears, upper limb, lower limb).

Coding and Documentation Requirements

Identify stage or depth of lesion:

- Melanoma in situ
  - Stage 0, also referred to as classification TIS (tumor in situ), or confined to epidermal layer only

- Melanoma (melanocarcinoma)
  - Stage I – localized
    - » Stage IA – less than 1.0 mm thick, no ulceration, no lymph node involvement, no distant metastases
    - » Stage 1B – less than 1.0 mm thick with ulceration or less than 2.0 mm thick without ulceration, no lymph node involvement, no distant metastases
  - Stage II – localized
    - » Stage IIA – 1.01-2.00 mm thick with ulceration, no lymph node involvement, no distant metastases
    - » Stage IIB – 2.01-4.00 mm thick without ulceration, no lymph node involvement, no distant metastases
    - » Stage IIC – greater than 4.00 mm thick with ulceration, no lymph node involvement, no distant metastases
  - Stage III – tumor spread to regional lymph nodes or development of in transit metastases or satellites without spread to distant sites; also marked by three substages IIIA, IIIB, IIIC
  - Stage IV – tumor spread beyond regional lymph nodes with metastases to distant sites

Identify site:

- Anal skin
- Breast
- Ear/external auricular canal
  - Left
  - Right
  - Unspecified
- Eyelid, including canthus
  - Left
    - » Lower
    - » Upper
  - Right
    - » Lower
    - » Upper
  - Unspecified
- Face
  - Other parts
  - Unspecified part
- Lip
- Lower limb, including hip
  - Left
  - Right
  - Unspecified
- Neck/Scalp
- Nose
- Skin
  - Overlapping sites
  - Unspecified site
- Trunk, other parts
- Upper limb, including shoulder
  - Left
  - Right
  - Unspecified

ICD-10-CM Code/Documentation	
C43.0	Malignant melanoma of lip
C43.10	Malignant melanoma of unspecified eyelid, including canthus
C43.111	Malignant melanoma of right upper eyelid, including canthus
C43.112	Malignant Melanoma of right lower eyelid, including canthus
C43.121	Malignant melanoma of left upper eyelid, including canthus
C43.122	Malignant melanoma of left lower eyelid, including canthus
C43.20	Malignant melanoma of unspecified ear and external auricular canal
C43.21	Malignant melanoma of right ear and external auricular canal
C43.22	Malignant melanoma of left ear and external auricular canal
C43.30	Malignant melanoma of unspecified parts of face
C43.31	Malignant melanoma of nose
C43.39	Malignant melanoma of other parts of face
C43.4	Malignant melanoma of scalp and neck
C43.51	Malignant melanoma of anal skin
C43.52	Malignant melanoma of skin of breast
C43.59	Malignant melanoma of other part of trunk
C43.60	Malignant melanoma of unspecified upper limb, including shoulder
C43.61	Malignant melanoma of right upper limb, including shoulder
C43.62	Malignant melanoma of left upper limb, including shoulder
C43.70	Malignant melanoma of unspecified lower limb, including hip
C43.71	Malignant melanoma of right lower limb, including hip
C43.72	Malignant melanoma of left lower limb, including hip
C43.8	Malignant melanoma of overlapping sites of skin
C43.9	Malignant melanoma of skin, unspecified
D03.0	Melanoma in situ of lip
D03.10	Melanoma in situ of unspecified eyelid, including canthus
D03.111	Melanoma in situ of right upper eyelid, including canthus
D03.112	Melanoma in situ of right lower eyelid, including canthus
D03.121	Melanoma in situ of left upper eyelid, including canthus
D03.122	Melanoma in situ of left lower eyelid, including canthus
D03.20	Melanoma in situ of unspecified ear and external auricular canal
D03.21	Melanoma in situ of right ear and external auricular canal
D03.22	Melanoma in situ of left ear and external auricular canal
D03.30	Melanoma in situ of unspecified parts of face
D03.31	Melanoma in situ of nose
D03.39	Melanoma in situ of other parts of face
D03.4	Melanoma in situ of scalp and neck
D03.51	Melanoma in situ of anal skin
D03.52	Melanoma in situ of skin of breast
D03.59	Melanoma in situ of other part of trunk
D03.60	Melanoma in situ of unspecified upper limb, including shoulder

ICD-10-CM Code/Documentation	
D03.61	Melanoma in situ of right upper limb, including shoulder
D03.62	Melanoma in situ of left upper limb, including shoulder
D03.70	Melanoma in situ of unspecified lower limb, including hip
D03.71	Melanoma in situ of right lower limb, including hip
D03.72	Melanoma in situ of left lower limb, including hip
D03.8	Melanoma in situ of overlapping sites of skin
D03.9	Melanoma in situ of skin, unspecified

Documentation and Coding Example

Forty-five-year-old Caucasian female presents to dermatologist's office for annual skin check. Patient has fair skin, light blond hair and blue eyes. She has a **history of basal cell carcinoma removed from right upper lip one year ago** followed by 5 FU therapy to her entire face. On examination, this is a pleasant, well-developed, well-nourished woman. Well-healed scar on upper lip, facial skin is smooth with normal signs of aging. Anterior and posterior neck and trunk have scattered freckles and normal appearing moles. Upper extremities have freckling, dry skin noted at elbows and hands, fingernails are manicured with deep red nail polish. Patient is instructed to check fingernails regularly for dark spots that could indicate melanoma. Lower extremities have small cherry angiomas and freckling, toenails are also obscured with nail polish. There is a **0.5 x 1 cm scaly brown patch of skin on the dorsal aspect of right foot**. Patient states it has been itchy and she has applied an antifungal cream without relief of symptoms.

2. Neoplasms

Impression: Superficial skin lesion R/O malignancy.

Procedure: Area prepped, draped and infiltrated with local anesthetic. Three-millimeter full thickness punch biopsy obtained and sent to pathology. Puncture wound sutured with 3-0 nylon and covered with sterile dressing.

Follow up: Punch biopsy positive for melanoma in-situ.

Labs/Tests: Molecular genetic testing, LDH, lymphoscintigraphy of right lower extremity. Patient returns for wide excision of right foot lesion, lymph node excision is not indicated. Incision lines marked with surgical ink, area is prepped, draped and infiltrated with local anesthetic. Lesion excised using an elliptical incision with 1 cm clear margins on all sides. Specimen sent to pathology. Incision undermined and closed in layers. Sterile dressing applied.

Diagnosis: **Melanoma Stage 0, right dorsal foot.**

Diagnosis Code(s)

D03.71 Melanoma in situ of right lower limb, including hip

Z85.828 Personal history of other malignant neoplasm of skin

Coding Note(s)

Stage 0 melanoma is very early stage disease known as melanoma in situ. Patients with melanoma in situ are classified as TIS (tumor in situ). The tumor is limited to the top layer of the skin (epidermis) with no evidence of invasion into the dermis, surrounding tissues, lymph nodes, or distant sites. Melanoma in situ is very low risk for recurrence or metastasis.

Malignant Neoplasm of Body of Uterus

The most common type of cancer of the body of the uterus is endometrial carcinoma which develops in the glandular cells that line the uterus. Endometrial carcinoma accounts for approximately 95% of all uterine cancers. Sarcoma is another less common type of cancer of the uterus. It originates in the myometrium which is muscle tissue that comprises the middle tissue layer of the uterus.

Documentation must state whether the malignant neoplasm is in the isthmus, endometrium, myometrium, fundus, or overlapping sites as there are specific codes for these sites.

Coding and Documentation Requirements

Identify site:

- Isthmus
- Endometrium
- Myometrium
- Fundus uteri
- Overlapping sites of corpus uteri
- Unspecified site corpus uteri
- Unspecified part of uterus

ICD-10-CM Code/Documentation	
C54.0	Malignant neoplasm of isthmus uteri
C54.1	Malignant neoplasm of endometrium
C54.2	Malignant neoplasm of myometrium
C54.3	Malignant neoplasm of fundus uteri
C54.8	Malignant neoplasm of overlapping sites of corpus uteri
C54.9	Malignant neoplasm of corpus uteri, unspecified
C55	Malignant neoplasm of uterus, part unspecified

Documentation and Coding Example

Twenty-nine-year-old female presents with her thirty-year-old husband for infertility consult. Couple has been trying to conceive without success for the past 14 months. Past medical history is significant for polycystic ovarian syndrome diagnosed at age 21. Patient states her periods have always been somewhat irregular, last menstrual period was 2 weeks ago and heavier than normal. Temperature 97.8, HR 90, RR 14, BP 136/90, HT 66", WT 150 lbs. On examination, this is a pleasant somewhat nervous, well-developed, well-nourished woman. Neck is supple without lymphadenopathy. Thyroid is smooth, normal size. Breath sounds are clear equal bilateral. HR regular with a S1 S2 split sound. Peripheral pulses intact, no edema noted in extremities. Breasts are without masses. Abdomen soft, non-tender, active bowel sounds present. External genitalia normal, speculum inserted without discomfort. Normal appearing vaginal mucosa, cervix in midline, there is clear thin mucus at the cervical os. PAP smear and endometrial biopsy performed. Bimanual exam reveals a retroflexed uterus, normal in size, right and left ovaries are palpated easily and feel slightly enlarged.

Impression: **Infertility, polycystic ovarian syndrome**, R/O neoplasm.

Lab findings: **PAP smear and endometrial biopsy positive for endometrial adenocarcinoma**. Pelvic ultrasound performed shows thickening of endometrium and numerous small cysts on the surface of both ovaries.

Diagnosis: **Adenocarcinoma of the endometrium, polycystic ovarian syndrome, and infertility**.

Diagnosis Code(s)

C54.1 Malignant neoplasm of endometrium

E28.2 Polycystic ovarian syndrome

Coding Note(s)

Under N97 Female infertility, there is an Excludes1 note for female infertility associated with Stein-Leventhal syndrome (polycystic ovarian syndrome) (E28.2), so a code for infertility is not reported additionally.

Malignant Neoplasm of Breast

The codes for malignant neoplasms of the breast are used for any type of breast cancer that is described as invasive or infiltrating. When these terms are used it means that the cancer cells are no longer limited to the membrane that lines the breast duct or lobule and that the cancer has invaded deeper tissues of the breast. Invasive breast cancers may also be described as Stage I, II, III, or IV. Cancer that begins in the breast ducts is called ductal carcinoma and this is the most common type. Lobular carcinoma is another type that accounts for approximately 10% of all breast cancers. It begins in the breast lobules where milk is produced. Far less common are cancers of the connective tissues of the breast which are called sarcomas. Breast cancer is not classified by histological type, so regardless of whether the cancer is described as ductal carcinoma, lobular carcinoma, or sarcoma, the same malignant neoplasm codes are assigned.

For coding malignant neoplasms of the breast, laterality is required (right, left) and breast cancer in males is also site-specific. Cancers of the female and male breast are classified in category C50. Malignant neoplasms of the breast are classified first by site (e.g., central portion, upper-outer quadrant, lower-inner quadrant, etc.), and then by gender. Malignant neoplasms of the female breast are identified by the fifth character 1 and malignant neoplasms of the male breast are identified by fifth character 2. The sixth character specifies laterality as right (1), left (2), or unspecified (9).

Coding and Documentation Requirements

Identify gender:

- Male
- Female

Identify site for both male/female:

- Nipple/areola
- Central portion
- Upper-inner quadrant
- Lower-inner quadrant
- Upper-outer quadrant
- Lower-outer quadrant
- Axillary tail
  - Contiguous/overlapping sites
- Unspecified site

Identify laterality:

- Right
- Left

ICD-10-CM Code/Documentation	
C50.011	Malignant neoplasm of nipple and areola, right female breast
C50.012	Malignant neoplasm of nipple and areola, left female breast
C50.019	Malignant neoplasm of nipple and areola, unspecified female breast
C50.111	Malignant neoplasm of central portion of right female breast
C50.112	Malignant neoplasm of central portion of left female breast
C50.119	Malignant neoplasm of central portion of unspecified female breast
C50.211	Malignant neoplasm of upper-inner quadrant of right female breast
C50.212	Malignant neoplasm of upper-inner quadrant of left female breast
C50.219	Malignant neoplasm of upper-inner quadrant of unspecified female breast
C50.311	Malignant neoplasm of lower-inner quadrant of right female breast
C50.312	Malignant neoplasm of lower-inner quadrant of left female breast
C50.319	Malignant neoplasm of lower-inner quadrant of unspecified female breast
C50.411	Malignant neoplasm of upper-outer quadrant of right female breast
C50.412	Malignant neoplasm of upper-outer quadrant of left female breast
C50.419	Malignant neoplasm of upper-outer quadrant of unspecified female breast
C50.511	Malignant neoplasm of lower-outer quadrant of right female breast
C50.512	Malignant neoplasm of lower-outer quadrant of left female breast
C50.519	Malignant neoplasm of lower-outer quadrant of unspecified female breast
C50.611	Malignant neoplasm of axillary tail of right female breast
C50.612	Malignant neoplasm of axillary tail of left female breast
C50.619	Malignant neoplasm of axillary tail of unspecified female breast
C50.811	Malignant neoplasm of overlapping sites of right female breast
C50.812	Malignant neoplasm of overlapping sites of left female breast
C50.819	Malignant neoplasm of overlapping sites of unspecified female breast
C50.911	Malignant neoplasm of unspecified site of right female breast
C50.912	Malignant neoplasm of unspecified site of left female breast
C50.919	Malignant neoplasm of unspecified site of unspecified female breast
C50.021	Malignant neoplasm of nipple and areola, right male breast
C50.022	Malignant neoplasm of nipple and areola, left male breast
C50.029	Malignant neoplasm of nipple and areola, unspecified male breast
C50.121	Malignant neoplasm of central portion, right male breast
C50.122	Malignant neoplasm of central portion, left male breast
C50.129	Malignant neoplasm of central portion, unspecified. male breast
C50.221	Malignant neoplasm of upper-inner quadrant, right male breast
C50.222	Malignant neoplasm of upper-inner quadrant, left male breast
C50.229	Malignant neoplasm of upper-inner quadrant, unspecified male breast
C50.321	Malignant neoplasm of lower-inner quadrant, right male breast

ICD-10-CM Code/Documentation	
C50.322	Malignant neoplasm of lower-inner quadrant, left male breast
C50.329	Malignant neoplasm of lower-inner quadrant, unspecified male breast
C50.421	Malignant neoplasm of upper-outer quadrant, right male breast
C50.422	Malignant neoplasm of upper-outer quadrant, left male breast
C50.429	Malignant neoplasm of upper-outer quadrant, unspecified male breast
C50.521	Malignant neoplasm of lower-outer quadrant, right male breast
C50.522	Malignant neoplasm of lower-outer quadrant, left male breast
C50.529	Malignant neoplasm of lower-outer quadrant, unspecified male breast
C50.621	Malignant neoplasm of axillary tail, right male breast
C50.622	Malignant neoplasm of axillary tail, left male breast
C50.629	Malignant neoplasm of axillary tail, unspecified male breast
C50.821	Malignant neoplasm of overlapping sites, right male breast
C50.822	Malignant neoplasm of overlapping sites, left male breast
C50.829	Malignant neoplasm of overlapping sites, unspecified male breast
C50.921	Malignant neoplasm of unspecified site, right male breast
C50.922	Malignant neoplasm of unspecified site, left male breast
C50.929	Malignant neoplasm of unspecified site, unspecified male breast

Documentation and Coding Example

Sixty-nine-year-old Caucasian male is sent by PCP for surgery consult with a complaint of **left nipple discharge x 3 months with a palpable lump under the nipple.** There is a family history of breast cancer in his mother and maternal grandmother. Temperature 97.2, HR 76, RR 16, BP 150/80. On examination, this is a well-developed, well-nourished gentleman in no apparent distress. PERRL, TM's clear, mucus membranes moist and pink, mouth and pharynx without lesions, nares patent. Neck supple without palpable lymph nodes and there are no enlarged lymph nodes in the axilla. Right nipple and areola are unremarkable, no swelling or tenderness appreciated. **The left nipple is examined and mild swelling is appreciated in the area immediately surrounding the nipple with a 1 cm lump palpated under the nipple. The nipple and areola are slightly tender to touch. Thin, serosanguinous fluid is easily expressed from the nipple with gentle pressure**. Sample collected for laboratory analysis. Fine needle biopsy obtained from the area and sent to pathology. If biopsy positive for malignancy, will perform estrogen/ progesterone receptor status tests. Blood drawn for CBC, chem panel, ESR, molecular genetic testing for BRCA2 and Klinefelter's. Patient scheduled for mammogram, breast US, PET scan.

Diagnosis: **Nipple discharge and FN biopsy positive for infiltrating ductal carcinoma. Estrogen and progesterone receptor status are both positive. Mammography and US show lesion confined to the area of the left nipple/areola.** No areas of uptake on PET scan. Patient is scheduled for lumpectomy.

Diagnosis Code(s)

C50.022	Malignant neoplasm of nipple and areola, left male breast
Z17.0	Estrogen receptor positive status [ER+]
Z80.3	Family history of malignant neoplasm of breast

Coding Note(s)

Under C50 Malignant neoplasm of breast, there is an instruction to use an additional code to identify estrogen receptor status (Z17.0, Z17.1).

Malignant Neoplasm of Connective and Other Soft Tissue

Primary malignant neoplasms of connective and other soft tissues are classified as sarcomas and are extremely rare. There are many types of sarcomas and often the histological type is more specifically documented. Some histological types of connective tissue neoplasms are malignant fibrous histiocytoma, neurosarcoma, rhabdomyosarcoma, fibrosarcoma, hemangiopericytoma, and angiosarcoma. Gastrointestinal stromal tumors, or GIST, is another type of sarcoma that grows from the stromal cells of the digestive organs. Stromal cells are the connective tissue cells, such as fibroblasts, that support the function of the parenchymal cells of that organ.

When the histology of a neoplasm is documented, it is necessary to reference the histological type in the Alphabetic Index before proceeding to the Tabular List. Most of these histologic types refer the coder to Neoplasm, connective tissue, malignant. However, there are some exceptions. Neurosarcoma indicates that the correct code is found under Neoplasm, nerve, malignant. In the case of hemangiopericytoma, unless the documentation specifically identifies the neoplasm as malignant, the code for neoplasm, connective tissue, uncertain behavior is assigned.

Primary malignant neoplasms of connective and other soft tissue are separated into two categories. Category C47 reports primary malignant neoplasms of peripheral nerves and the autonomic nervous system. Category C49 reports primary malignant neoplasms of all other connective and soft tissues, including gastrointestinal stromal tumors. Both categories require laterality for reporting connective and soft tissue malignant neoplasms of the upper and lower limbs.

Coding and Documentation Requirements

Identify type of connective/soft tissue:

- Peripheral nerve/autonomic nervous system
- Other connective/soft tissue, which includes:
  - Blood vessel
  - Bursa
  - Cartilage
  - Fascia
  - Fat
  - Ligament, except uterine
  - Lymphatic vessel
  - Muscle
  - Synovia
  - Tendon (sheath)

Identify site:

- Abdomen
- Head/face/neck
- Lower limb, including hip
  - Left

- Right
- Unspecified

- Overlapping sites
- Pelvis
- Thorax
- Trunk, unspecified
- Unspecified site

ICD-10-CM Code/Documentation	
C47.0	Malignant neoplasm of peripheral nerves of head, face and neck
C47.10	Malignant neoplasm of peripheral nerves of unspecified upper limb, including shoulder
C47.11	Malignant neoplasm of peripheral nerves of right upper limb, including shoulder
C47.12	Malignant neoplasm of peripheral nerves of left upper limb, including shoulder
C47.20	Malignant neoplasm of peripheral nerves of unspecified lower limb, including hip
C47.21	Malignant neoplasm of peripheral nerves of right lower limb, including hip
C47.22	Malignant neoplasm of peripheral nerves of left lower limb, including hip
C47.3	Malignant neoplasm of peripheral nerves of thorax
C47.4	Malignant neoplasm of peripheral nerves of abdomen
C47.5	Malignant neoplasm of peripheral nerves of pelvis
C47.6	Malignant neoplasm of peripheral nerves of trunk, unspecified
C47.8	Malignant neoplasm of overlapping sites of peripheral nerves and autonomic nervous system
C47.9	Malignant neoplasm of peripheral nerves and autonomic system, unspecified
C49.0	Malignant neoplasm of connective and soft tissue of head, face and neck
C49.10	Malignant neoplasm of connective and soft tissue of unspecified upper limb, including shoulder
C49.11	Malignant neoplasm of connective and soft tissue of right upper limb, including shoulder
C49.12	Malignant neoplasm of connective and soft tissue of left upper limb, including shoulder
C49.20	Malignant neoplasm of connective and soft tissue of unspecified lower limb, including hip
C49.21	Malignant neoplasm of connective and soft tissue of right lower limb, including hip
C49.22	Malignant neoplasm of connective and soft tissue of left lower limb, including hip
C49.3	Malignant neoplasm of connective and soft tissue of thorax
C49.4	Malignant neoplasm of connective and soft tissue of abdomen
C49.5	Malignant neoplasm of connective and soft tissue of pelvis
C49.6	Malignant neoplasm of connective and soft tissue of trunk, unspecified
C49.8	Malignant neoplasm of overlapping sites of connective and soft tissue
C49.9	Malignant neoplasm of connective and soft tissue, unspecified
C49.A0	Gastrointestinal stromal tumor, unspecified site
C49.A1	Gastrointestinal stromal tumor of esophagus
C49.A2	Gastrointestinal stromal tumor of stomach
C49.A3	Gastrointestinal stromal tumor of small intestine
C49.A4	Gastrointestinal stromal tumor of large intestine
C49.A5	Gastrointestinal stromal tumor of rectum
C49.A9	Gastrointestinal stromal tumor of other sites

Documentation and Coding Example

Twenty-eight-year-old male presents with pain and swelling of the right upper arm, he can recall no injury or trauma to the area. Patient is right hand dominant and has a history of neurofibromatosis, type 1. Temperature 97.8, HR 62, RR 12, BP 104/66. On examination, this is a well-developed, well-nourished young man. He has at least 25 café-au-lait spots > 1cm in size on his upper body and freckling in the axilla bilaterally. Scattered pea size neurofibromas can be palpated beneath the skin on neck, torso, and both upper extremities. There are no observable skeletal deformities and his head appears to be of average size. PERRL, 4 Lisch nodules are present on right iris, 2 on left. Neck supple without lymphadenopathy. Mucous membranes are moist and pink. Weakness noted with flexion and supination of the right forearm, peripheral pulses intact. A 4 x 6 cm firm, tender mass is palpated in the right upper arm, 6 cm above the elbow along the mid-anterior area. The skin overlying the mass is of normal temperature and color. The skin on the lateral side of right forearm is cooler to touch and both sharp and dull sensation is decreased. Impression: Neurofibroma of the right brachial plexus R/O peripheral nerve sheath tumor/soft tissue sarcoma. Labs/Tests: CBC, Sed Rate, CRP, RUE x-ray (including shoulder) and ultrasound. Radiologic and US studies confirm solid mass tumor. MRI indicates tumor with pseudocapsule and perilesional edema along musculocutaneous nerve. Ultrasound guided needle biopsy performed.

Diagnosis: **Malignant peripheral nerve sheath tumor.** Further testing ordered: CT scan of chest, PET scan, bone scan to identify any metastatic disease.

Diagnosis Code(s)

C47.11 Malignant neoplasm of peripheral nerves of right upper limb, including shoulder

Q85.01 Neurofibromatosis, type 1

Coding Note(s)

Under category C49 Malignant neoplasm of other connective and soft tissue there is an Excludes2 note for malignant neoplasm of peripheral nerves and autonomic nervous system (C47.-) indicating that it is possible to have both types of malignancies at the same time. In this case the malignancy is identified as being in the nerve sheath only, so only code C47.11 is reported. If the physician had indicated that surrounding soft tissue was also involved, it would be appropriate to report a code from both categories.

Malignant Neoplasm of Liver and Intrahepatic Bile Ducts

While there are a number of different types of primary malignancies of the liver, the most common cancers found in the liver are actually secondary malignancies or metastases. These cancers originate in other cells or tissues of the body and move into the liver. Only about 2% of all cancers found in the liver are primary malignancies and of those the most common form is hepatocellular carcinoma which begins in liver cells called hepatocytes. A second type of primary malignancy of the liver begins in the bile ducts within the liver and is called intrahepatic bile duct carcinoma, which includes cholangiocarcinoma. When cancer begins in the bile ducts outside the liver it is called extrahepatic carcinoma. Angiosarcoma is a very rare type of primary liver cancer that begins in the blood vessels of the liver and includes Kupffer cell sarcoma. Hepatoblastoma is another very rare type of primary liver cancer that primarily affects children under age 3.

Codes are specific to site and morphology (histologic type). There are also codes for unspecified morphology and for liver malignancies not specified as primary or secondary.

Coding and Documentation Requirements

Identify site:

- Liver
- Intrahepatic bile ducts

Identify morphology (histologic type) for primary malignancies:

- Angiosarcoma (includes Kupffer cell sarcoma)
- Carcinoma
- Hepatocellular and hepatoma
- Intrahepatic bile duct, cholangiocarcinoma
- Hepatoblastoma
- Other sarcoma
- Other specified carcinomas
- Unspecified histologic type, primary

Identify if neoplasm is not specified as primary or secondary

ICD-10-CM Code/Documentation	
C22.0	Liver cell carcinoma (includes hepatocellular carcinoma and hepatoma)
C22.1	Intrahepatic bile duct carcinoma (includes cholangiocarcinoma)
C22.2	Hepatoblastoma
C22.3	Angiosarcoma of liver (includes Kupffer cell sarcoma)
C22.4	Other sarcomas of liver
C22.7	Other specified carcinomas of liver
C22.8	Malignant neoplasm of liver, primary, unspecified as to type
C22.9	Malignant neoplasm of liver, not specified as primary or secondary

Documentation and Coding Example

Sixty-three-year-old African-American male presents with a 2-3 month history of intermittent right upper quadrant pain, abdominal distention and a 20 lb. weight loss. He has a poor appetite and when he does eat, experiences early satiety. On examination, this is a well-groomed, thin man. Temperature 97.8, HR 80, RR 14, BP 146/88. Skin does not appear to be jaundiced but it is difficult to assess due to naturally dark pigmentation. PERRL, sclera observed to be without jaundice. Heart rate regular without murmur. Carotid arteries are without bruit. Breath sounds clear and equal bilaterally. Abdomen is soft and slightly distended, there are no abdominal varicosities observed. Bowel sounds present in all quadrants. Liver is palpated at 4 cm below the RCM, liver border is irregular. There is an audible hepatic artery bruit. Patient states he drinks alcohol socially, usually one beer or glass of wine 2-4 times a month, denies tobacco use other than an occasional cigarette in late teens/early twenties. He cannot recall ever being tested for hepatitis. Impression: R/O hepatitis, liver tumor. Labs/Tests: CBC, AFP, Hepatitis Panel. Liver ultrasound with guided needle biopsy. MRI of abdomen and PET scan.

Diagnosis: Pathology report on liver biopsy – **hepatocellular carcinoma**

Diagnosis Code(s)

C22.0 Liver cell carcinoma

Coding Note(s)

Because malignant neoplasms of the liver are classified by morphology (histologic type), it is not possible to identify the correct code using only the Neoplasm Table. Once the pathology report is available, the histologic type must be identified in the Alphabetic Index.

Malignant Neoplasm of Spinal Cord

In adults, the spinal cord extends from the foramen magnum at the base of the skull to the level of the first or second lumbar vertebrae. The terminal end of the spinal cord is referred to as the conus medullaris. Nerve roots that extend distal to the conus medullaris form the cauda equina which is a Latin term meaning horse's tail. The conus medullaris and cauda equina are the sites where the nervous system transitions from the central nervous system to the peripheral nervous system. The motor nerve roots of the cauda equina are considered part of the peripheral nervous system.

Primary malignant spinal cord and cauda equina tumors are those that originate in cells and tissue of the spinal cord and cauda equina respectively. Primary malignant neoplasms of both sites include ependymomas and astrocytomas. Ependymomas are the most common type. Most ependymomas are primary malignant neoplasms. However, some ependymomas, such as those described as myxopapillary or papillary, are classified under neoplasm, uncertain behavior. Astrocytomas are the second most common type and they are most often classified as primary malignant neoplasms, although for astrocytoma, subependymal, giant cell, the Alphabetic Index indicates that a code for neoplasm, uncertain behavior should be assigned. Schwannomas are another type of nervous system malignant neoplasm.

The site of the malignancy must be documented as the spinal cord or the cauda equina.

Coding and Documentation Requirements

Identify site:

- Spinal cord
- Cauda equina

ICD-10-CM Code/Documentation	
C72.0	Malignant neoplasm of spinal cord
C72.1	Malignant neoplasm of cauda equina

Documentation and Coding Example

Seventeen-year-old male presents to ED with severe low back pain not relieved with ice, rest, and ibuprofen. Student was in his usual state of good health until 1 day prior to admission when he had sudden onset of pain in his lower back radiating into his buttocks after a routine water polo practice at school. He was examined by the school's athletic trainer, told it was a muscle strain and advised to take 600 mg of ibuprofen q 8 hours RTC, ice for 20 minutes q 2 hours while awake and resume normal activities in 24 hours. Patient awoke this morning with a deep aching pain in lower back and sharp pain radiating through his buttocks and down both legs. He also noticed numbness in his groin and some urinary hesitancy and weakness of urine flow. Over the past 8 hours he has developed bilateral lower extremity weakness and sensory loss. Temperature 98.6, HR 100, RR 16, BP 106/66. On examination, this is an anxious appearing, well-developed, well-nourished teenager. He denies recent injury, illness, or drug use other than ibuprofen. PERRL, neck supple without lymphadenopathy. Upper extremity pulses and reflexes grossly intact. Heart rate regular, breath sounds clear and equal bilaterally. Abdomen soft with decreased bowel sounds. Bladder is distended. There is decreased anal sphincter tone on rectal exam. Patient states pain is constant, not relieved by any position change. There is decreased muscle tone and tendon reflexes in both lower extremities. Pulses are intact and there is no peripheral edema noted in lower extremities. Impression: Cauda equina syndrome, R/O tumor, infection, injury. Neurosurgical consult obtained. Labs/Tests: IV started and blood drawn for CBC, Sed Rate, CRP, PT, PTT, Metabolic Panel. Foley catheter placed and urine sent to lab for UA, culture. MRI of spine and pelvis with gadolinium contrast obtained and **reveals a 2 x 2.5 cm mass consistent with tumor, just below the dura in the posterior cauda equina**. IV dexamethasone and broad-spectrum antibiotics administered, emergency laminectomy performed, **biopsy reveals malignant neoplasm**. Tumor successfully removed.

Diagnosis: **Malignant neoplasm of cauda equina**.

Diagnosis Code(s)

C72.1 Malignant neoplasm of cauda equina

Multiple Myeloma and Immunoproliferative Neoplasms

Multiple myeloma is a cancer of the plasma cells. Plasma cells are white blood cells that make infection-fighting antibodies. As with other blood cancers, multiple myeloma results in increased numbers of abnormal plasma cells that do not progress through the normal cell life cycle. The abnormal cells do not mature and die. This causes the body to become overwhelmed by the abnormal cells resulting in an inability to make normal blood cells. Usually there are few symptoms in the early stages of the disease, but as the disease progresses four indicators are typically present. These are:

- Elevated blood calcium levels
- Renal (kidney) failure
- Anemia and anemia-related fatigue
- Bone damage caused by osteolysis with resulting bone pain and fractures

Malignant immunoproliferative diseases, previously classified as immunoproliferative neoplasms, are a group of disorders of the immune system involving abnormal proliferation of primary cells including B-cells, T-cells, Natural Killer (NK) cells, and/or excessive production of immunoglobulins (antibodies).

There are two categories for reporting these conditions—one for malignant immunoproliferative disease and certain other B-cell lymphomas (C88) and one for multiple myeloma and malignant plasma cell neoplasms (C90). Codes for multiple myeloma and plasma cell leukemia have not been expanded from their former usage, and code descriptors remain basically the same, but there are specific codes for other malignant immunoproliferative diseases, (C88); these codes are not classified by whether or not they have never achieved remission, are in remission, or are in relapse.

Coding and Documentation Requirements

Identify condition:

- Multiple myeloma
  - Not having achieved remission
  - In remission
  - In relapse
- Plasma cell leukemia
  - Not having achieved remission
  - In remission
  - In relapse
- Plasmacytoma
  - Extramedullary
    - » Not having achieved remission
    - » In remission
    - » In relapse
  - Solitary
    - » Not having achieved remission
    - » In remission
    - » In relapse
- Malignant immunoprolierative diseases and certain other B-cell lymphomas
  - Extranodal marginal zone B-cell lymphoma of mucosa-associated lymphoid tissue [MALT]
  - Heavy chain disease
  - Immunoproliferative small intestinal disease
  - Waldenström macroglobulinemia
  - Other malignant immunoproliferative diseases
  - Unspecified immunoproliferative diseases

ICD-10-CM Code/Documentation	
C88.0	Waldenström macroglobulinemia
C88.2	Heavy chain disease
C88.3	Immunoproliferative small intestinal disease
C88.4	Extranodal marginal zone B-cell lymphoma of mucosa-associated lymphoid tissue [MALT lymphoma]
C88.8	Other malignant immunoproliferative diseases
C88.9	Malignant immunoproliferative disease, unspecified

Documentation and Coding Example

Fifty-seven-year-old Caucasian male referred to ENT by PCP with complaints of nasal stuffiness, drainage, and frequent nose bleeds x 3-4 months. He has been treated with oral antihistamines (Loratidine) and inhaled nasal corticosteroid (Nasonex) for the past month without noticeable improvement. He admits to a half pack/day smoking history from ages 19-25 and to social drinking throughout life. Temperature 98.4, HR 68, RR 16, BP 132/72. On examination, patient is a well-nourished, well developed male. Neck supple without masses. TMs normal. Oral mucosa moist and pink, no tonsil or adenoid tissue appreciated, patient recalls having had a T & A in childhood for recurrent strep infections. Posterior pharynx has a cobblestone appearance consistent with chronic post nasal drip. Clear nasal drainage is present bilaterally. No air movement is appreciated through the right nares, air movement through left nares is decreased. Endoscopic exam reveals a soft, bright red mass in the right nasal cavity narrowing the opening and making it difficult to pass the scope. Left nasal cavity is also narrowed but the scope can be passed with relative ease. Biopsy of mass obtained and sent to lab. **Pathology report is positive for malignant monoclonal plasma cell histology.** Blood drawn for CBC, renal panel, serum calcium, plasma electrophoresis, and cytogenetic testing of Chromosome 13. CT of head reveals tumor engulfing the ethmoid sinus without involvement of surrounding lymph nodes.

Diagnosis: **Extramedullary plasmacytoma**. Recommended treatment: Surgical debulking/removal of the tumor followed by radiation therapy.

Diagnosis Code(s)

C90.20 Extramedullary plasmacytoma not having achieved remission

Coding Note(s)

The Alphabetic Index lists three subterms under plasmacytoma – extramedullary, medullary, and solitary. All of these codes are classified as malignant neoplasms in category C90 Multiple myeloma and malignant plasma cell neoplasms.

Myelodysplastic Syndrome Lesions

Myelodysplastic syndrome (MDS) may be referred to as preleukemia. MDS is a diverse group of blood disorders involving poorly formed or dysfunctional myeloid (stem) cells. MDS is rarely symptomatic in the early stages. As the disease progresses, symptoms may include fatigue, unusual bleeding/bruising, and petechiae rash. Severe anemia and bone marrow failure are late manifestations of the disease.

There is a category for myelodysplastic syndromes which is part of the block that contains neoplasms of uncertain behavior and polycythemia vera. There are 11 codes for reporting specific manifesting disorders of myelodysplastic syndrome.

Coding and Documentation Requirements

Identify specific myelodysplastic disorder:

- Refractory anemia
  - Documented as without ring sideroblasts
  - With ring sideroblasts
  - With excess blasts
    - » RAEB 1
    - » RAEB 2
    - » RAEB NOS
  - Unspecified type
- Refractory cytopenia
  - With multilineage dysplasia (RCMD)
  - With multilineage dysplasia and ring sideroblasts (RCMD RS)
- Myelodysplastic syndrome
  - With isolated del(5Q) chromosomal abnormality
  - Other
  - Unspecified

ICD-10-CM Code/Documentation	
D46.20	Refractory anemia with excess of blasts, unspecified
D46.21	Refractory anemia with excess of blasts 1
D46.22	Refractory anemia with excess blasts 2
D46.C	Myelodysplastic syndrome with isolated del(5q) chromosomal abnormality
D46.9	Myelodysplastic syndrome, unspecified
D46.Z	Other myelodysplastic syndromes
D46.0	Refractory anemia without ring sideroblasts, so stated
D46.1	Refractory anemia with ring sideroblasts
D46.4	Refractory anemia, unspecified
D46.A	Refractory cytopenia with multilineage dysplasia
D46.B	Refractory cytopenia with multilineage dysplasia and ring sideroblasts

Documentation and Coding Example

Seventy-two-year-old Caucasian female presents to PCP with a 2-day history of fever, cough, and malaise. Patient is widowed, retired x 20 years from the Army Nurse Corp and stays active with tennis, travel, and looking after her grandchildren. She volunteers 2 days a week at a local homeless shelter, usually assisting in the health clinic. PMH is remarkable for mitral valve prolapse but she takes no medication other than OTC vitamins and supplements. Temperature 101.4, HR 92, RR 16, BP 138/88. O2 Saturation on RA in 97%. On examination, this is a mature, athletic appearing female. Skin very warm, dry to touch with good turgor. PERRL, TMs mildly red. Mucous membranes moist and pink, posterior pharynx red, without exudate. Neck supple without lymphadenopathy. HR regular with soft, late systolic murmur consistent with MVP. Breath sounds have fine and course scattered rales bilaterally and diminished sounds in the left base. Abdomen soft, non-tender with active bowel sounds. Liver is palpated at 2 cm below RCM, spleen is palpable at LCM. Chest x-ray obtained and shows scattered infiltrates and consolidation in the LLL. Patient is UTD on Pneumonia and Flu vaccinations. Blood drawn for CBC, ESR, Chem Panel, cultures and a sputum sample is obtained and sent to lab.

Diagnosis: **Pneumonia**. Prescribed broad spectrum antibiotic and will RTC in 2 days. Follow up: Patient returns to clinic and is feeling a little better. Afebrile, but cough and fatigue continue. **CBC shows alarmingly low levels of hemoglobin, absolute**

2. Neoplasms

neutrophil count and platelets with dysplastic features present in >30% of these cells. Bone marrow biopsy is obtained which is significant for absent Auer rods and only 2% blast cells. Additional cytogenetic testing performed which is indicative of refractory cytopenia with multilineage dysplasia.

Final Impression: **Resolving bacterial pneumonia, RCMD.** Patient is referred to hematology.

Diagnosis Code(s)

J15.9	Unspecified bacterial pneumonia
D46.A	Refractory cytopenia with multilineage dysplasia

Coding Note(s)

There is a note to code first (T36-T50) if the myelodysplastic syndrome is drug induced. In this case, there is no documentation indicating that the condition is drug induced, so only the RCMD is reported.

Summary

Documentation requirements for coding neoplasms require specific information about the site of the malignancy as well as laterality (right, left, bilateral) for paired organs and extremities. Some malignant neoplasms require documentation of morphology. Some neoplasms of uncertain behavior have specific codes and some conditions that were previously classifiedas metabolic disorders, such as macroglobulinemia are now considered neoplasms. The categories for reporting neoplasms involving lymph and blood-forming cells or tissues (lymphatic, hematopoietic, and related tissues), reflect an upgrade in medical terminology and understanding of these diseases for classification purposes.

Resources

Documentation checklists are available in Appendix A for the following neoplasms:

- Melanoma/melanoma in situ
- Lymphoma – Follicular

Chapter 2 Quiz

1. Some neoplasm codes require documentation of morphology (histological type) to assign the most specific code. Which of the following does NOT represent the histological type of the neoplasm?
   a. Hepatoblastoma
   b. Basal cell carcinoma
   c. Malignant neoplasm liver
   d. Mesothelioma
2. Melanocytic nevi of the skin have specific codes in ICD-10-CM. What alternate term may be used to describe a melanocytic nevus?
   a. Nevus
   b. Benign neoplasm skin
   c. Seborrheic keratosis
   d. Melanoma in situ
3. Coding for leukemia, multiple myeloma, and malignant plasma cell neoplasms require documentation related to whether the neoplasm has never achieved remission, is in remission, is in relapse, or is considered cured. If the coder believes the patient is in remission but the documentation is not clear, what code is assigned?
   a. A code indicating the patient has never achieved remission is assigned
   b. The physician is queried and the code is assigned based on the physician's response
   c. A code for in remission is assigned
   d. The condition is not coded
4. Some types of follicular non-Hodgkin lymphoma require documentation of the grade. Grade refers to:
   a. The extent of the disease, such as the number of lymph node sites that are involved
   b. Whether the disease is localized or has metastasized
   c. The patient's prognosis
   d. The amount of cell differentiation and rate of growth of the neoplastic cells
5. Documentation of two discrete malignant lesions of the right breast of a female patient, one located in the upper outer quadrant and a second located in the upper inner quadrant would be reported as follows:
   a. C50.211, C50.221
   b. C50.621
   c. C50.111
   d. C50.211, C50.411
6. Documentation that supports a diagnosis of carcinoma in situ of the cervix includes:
   a. Adenocarcinoma of the cervix
   b. Cervical intraepithelial neoplasia III (CIN III)
   c. Severe dysplasia of the uterine cervix
   d. Both b and c
7. What term is NOT used in classification of lymphoid and myeloid leukemias?
   a. Acute
   b. Subacute
   c. Chronic
   d. All of the above
8. A malignant neoplasm documented as located in the body of the uterus is reported as follows:
   a. C54.9 Malignant neoplasm of corpus uteri, unspecified
   b. C54.8 Malignant neoplasm of overlapping sites of corpus uteri
   c. C54.3 Malignant neoplasm of fundus uteri
   d. C54.0 Malignant neoplasm of isthmus uteri
9. What specific type of connective/soft tissue has a unique malignant neoplasm category?
   a. Cartilage and ligaments
   b. Muscles and tendons
   c. Peripheral nerves and autonomic nervous system
   d. Blood vessels and lymphatic vessels
10. What condition described below would NOT be reported with a code from category D12 Benign neoplasm of colon, rectum, anus and anal canal?
   a. Benign carcinoid tumors of colon
   b. Adenomatosis of colon
   c. Hereditary polyposis
   d. All of the above

See next page for answers and rationales.

Chapter 2 Answers and Rationales

1. Some neoplasm codes require documentation of morphology (histological type) to assign the most specific code. Which of the following does NOT represent the histological type of the neoplasm?

   c. **Malignant neoplasm liver**

   Rationale: *Malignant neoplasm of the liver describes the general behavior of the neoplasm but not the morphology. Morphology provides additional information about the characteristics of the neoplasm. There are specific codes for some histological types of malignant neoplasms of the liver including hepatoblastoma, liver cell carcinoma (hepatocellular carcinoma, hepatoma), cholangiocarcinoma, hepatoblastoma, angiosarcoma (Kupffer cell sarcoma).*

2. Melanocytic nevi of the skin have specific codes in ICD-10-CM. What alternate term may be used to describe a melanocytic nevus?

   a. **Nevus**

   Rationale: *Nevus NOS is classified as a melanocytic nevus. This can be verified using the Alphabetic Index and looking under the main term nevus, skin and by reviewing the includes note under category D22 Melanocytic nevi.*

3. Coding for leukemia, multiple myeloma, and malignant plasma cell neoplasms require documentation related to whether the neoplasm has never achieved remission, is in remission, is in relapse, or is considered cured. If the coder believes the patient is in remission but the documentation is not clear, what code is assigned?

   b. **The physician is queried and the code is assigned based on the physician's response**

   Rationale: *According to coding guidelines, the documentation must be clear as to whether the patient has achieved remission. If the documentation is not clear, the physician should be queried.*

4. Some types of follicular non-Hodgkin lymphoma require documentation of the grade. Grade refers to:

   d. **The amount of cell differentiation and rate of growth of the neoplastic cells**

   Rationale: *Grade refers to the amount of cell differentiation and the rate of growth of the neoplastic cells. The grade may affect the prognosis but grade does not specifically refer to the prognosis. Stage is used to describe the extent of the disease, i.e. how many lymph node sites are involved, whether there is involvement both above and below the diaphragm, and whether the lymphoma has metastasized to the bone marrow, extranodal, or solid organ sites.*

5. Documentation of two discrete malignant lesions of the right breast of a female patient, one located in the upper outer quadrant and a second located in the upper inner quadrant would be reported as follows:

   d. **C50.211, C50.411**

   Rationale: *Discrete lesions of different sites in the same breast are reported with the specific code for each site. The code for overlapping sites of the breast is only reported for a contiguous lesion overlapping two or more sites or regions in the breast.*

6. Documentation that supports a diagnosis of carcinoma in situ of the cervix includes:

   d. **Both b and c**

   Rationale: *Using the alphabetic index, Dysplasia, cervix, severe and Neoplasia, intraepithelial, cervix, grade III both direct the coder to category D06 Carcinoma in situ of cervix uteri. While adenocarcinoma in situ would be coded as carcinoma in situ, adenocarcinoma not specified as "in situ" is coded as malignant neoplasm of the cervix.*

7. What term is NOT used in classification of lymphoid and myeloid leukemias?

   b. **Subacute**

   Rationale: *The terms acute and chronic are still used in the classification of lymphoid and myeloid leukemias; however, the term subacute is no longer used. Lymphoid leukemia described as subacute is reported with codes for other lymphoid leukemia. Myeloid leukemia described as subacute is reported with codes for atypical chronic myeloid leukemia according to the general equivalency mappings (GEMs).*

8. A malignant neoplasm documented as located in the body of the uterus is reported as follows:

   a. **C54.9 Malignant neoplasm of corpus uteri, unspecified**

   Rationale: *The term body of the uterus is nonspecific, so the malignant neoplasm would be reported with code C54.9 Malignant neoplasm of corpus uteri, unspecified. See the Neoplasm table under Uterus, body.*

9. What specific type of connective/soft tissue has a unique malignant neoplasm category?

   c. **Peripheral nerves and autonomic nervous system**

   Rationale: *Malignant neoplasms of the peripheral nerves and autonomic nervous system are reported with codes from category C47. Malignant neoplasms of all other connective and soft tissues (blood vessel, bursa, cartilage, fascia, fat, ligament lymphatic vessel, muscle, synovia, tendon) are reported with codes from category C49.*

10. What condition described below would NOT be reported with a code from category D12 Benign neoplasm of colon, rectum, anus, and anal canal?

    a. **Benign carcinoid tumors of colon**

    Rationale: *There are more specific codes for benign carcinoid tumors of the large intestine and rectum so if the documentation states that the neoplasm is a benign carcinoid tumor, a code from subcategory D3A.02- would be reported.*

Chapter 3
DISEASES OF THE BLOOD AND BLOOD-FORMING ORGANS

Introduction

Codes in Chapter 3 classify diseases of the blood and blood-forming organs as well as certain disorders involving the immune mechanism and added intraoperative and postprocedural complications of the spleen.

Diseases of the blood and blood-forming organs include disorders involving the bone marrow, lymphatic tissue, platelets, and coagulation factors. Certain disorders involving the immune mechanism such as immunodeficiency disorders (except HIV/AIDS) are also classified to Chapter 3 by the type of disease and the cause of the disease or disorder.

Significant exclusions from Chapter 3 include HIV and related conditions, which are coded to Chapter 1. Note also that Chapter 3 does not include diseases related to the circulatory system which are classified to Chapter 9.

Documentation requirements for many diseases and conditions of the blood and immune system require specific information of the disease type and the site, including laterality (right, left, bilateral). Representative examples of documentation requirements are provided in this chapter and checklists are provided in Appendix A to help identify some potential, or typical, documentation deficiencies so that physicians and coders are able to select the highest granularity code(s) for reporting.

Understanding the coding and documentation challenges for diseases of the blood and blood-forming organs begins with a look at the code blocks, which are displayed in the table below.

ICD-10-CM Blocks	
D50-D53	Nutritional Anemias
D55-D59	Hemolytic Anemias
D60-D64	Aplastic and Other Anemias and Other Bone Marrow Failure Syndromes
D65-D69	Coagulation Defects, Purpura and Other Hemorrhagic Conditions
D70-D77	Other Disorders of Blood and Blood-Forming Organs
D78	Intraoperative and Postprocedural Complications of the Spleen
D80-D89	Certain Disorders Involving the Immune Mechanism

A quick review of the table above highlights the following:

- The first codes for blood and blood-forming organ disorders relate to anemia. "Anemia" refers to a lower than normal erythrocyte count or hemoglobin level in the blood.
- Anemia codes have been grouped into blocks based on the type of anemia.
- ICD-10-CM classifies diseases of the blood and blood-forming organs by the type of disease and the cause of the disease or disorder.
- Code block D78 classifies intraoperative and postprocedural complications of the spleen.
- The last block D80-D89 classifies disorders of the immune mechanism where immunodeficiency disorders are found—not with the endocrine, nutritional, and metabolic disorders.

Exclusions

There are no Excludes1 notes, but there are a number of Excludes2 notes which are listed in the table below.

Excludes1	Excludes2
None	Autoimmune disease (systemic) NOS (M35.9)
None	Certain conditions originating in the perinatal period (P00-P96)
None	Complications of pregnancy, childbirth and the puerperium (O00-O9A)
None	Congenital malformations, deformations and chromosomal abnormalities (Q00-Q99)
None	Endocrine, nutritional and metabolic diseases (E00-E88)
None	Human immunodeficiency virus [HIV] disease (B20)
None	Injury, poisoning and certain other consequences of external causes (S00-T88)
None	Neoplasms (C00-D49)
None	Symptoms, signs and abnormal clinical and laboratory findings, not elsewhere classified (R00-R94)

Chapter Guidelines

ICD-10-CM coding guidelines include the conventions in the Alphabetic Index and Tabular, the general coding guidelines, and chapter-specific coding guidelines. There are currently no chapter-specific coding guidelines for Chapter 3 Diseases of the Blood and Blood-Forming Organs and Certain Disorders Involving the Immune Mechanism (D50-D89), which is reserved for future guideline expansion.

There are however, related guidelines found in chapter-specific guidelines for other chapters, such as anemia associated with malignancy and anemia associated with chemotherapy, immunotherapy, and radiation therapy. When managing an anemia associated with a malignancy, it is essential that the documentation clearly states whether the reason for the admission or encounter is for treatment of the malignancy or treatment of the anemia only. The same is true when an admission or encounter is for management of an anemia associated with an adverse effect of radiation therapy, or antineoplastic or immunosuppressive drugs. In addition, the documentation must clearly link the therapy as the cause of the abnormal reaction or of the later complication.

Coding and sequencing guidelines for diseases of the blood, blood-forming organs and immune mechanism, and complications due to the treatment of these diseases and conditions, are incorporated into the Alphabetic Index and the Tabular List. These coding conventions direct correct code assignment. To assign the most specific code possible, pay close attention to the coding and sequencing instructions in the Tabular List and Alphabetic Index, particularly the Excludes1 and Excludes2 notes.

According to the *ICD-10-CM Official Guidelines for Coding and Reporting*, without consistent, complete documentation in the medical record, accurate coding cannot be achieved. A joint effort between the provider and the coder is essential to achieve complete and accurate documentation, code assignment, and reporting of diagnoses and procedures.

General Documentation Requirements

General documentation requirements differ depending on the particular disease or disorder of the blood, blood-forming organs, or immune mechanism. Some of the general documentation requirements are discussed here, but greater detail for some of the more common diseases and conditions of the blood and immune system will be provided in the next section.

Documentation of the severity and/or status of the disease in terms of acute or chronic, with or without crisis, as well as the site, etiology, and any secondary disease processes, are basic medical record documentation requirements. Physician documentation of the significance of any findings or confirmation of any diagnosis found in test reports is also a basic documentation requirement. In fact, laboratory reports are not required for code assignment. It is the physician documentation that is of greatest importance.

In general, ICD-10-CM requires a certain level of granularity regarding the type and cause of the blood or immune mechanism disorder which must be documented in the medical record. For example, specificity has been added to capture diseases and disorders of the blood, blood-forming organs, and immune mechanism due to drugs, such as neutropenia due to chemotherapy or due to other drugs.

Precise documentation is also necessary to avoid confusion between disorders such as thrombocytopenia – a platelet (thrombocytes) deficiency, and thrombocythemia – a clinical syndrome involving an increase in the number of circulating platelets in the blood. It is important to make a clear distinction in the medical record documentation.

Documentation should clearly specify the cause-and-effect relationship between the medical intervention and the blood or immune mechanism disorder, such as post-transfusion purpura. Documentation should specify whether a complication occurred intraoperatively or postoperatively, as in intraoperative hemorrhage and hematoma of the spleen complicating a procedure. In order to assign the code with the highest level of granularity, the type of procedure being performed when the complication arises, whether a procedure on the spleen itself, or another procedure, is also a required part of documentation.

In addition to these general documentation requirements, there are specific diseases and disorders that require even greater detail in documentation to ensure optimal code assignment.

Anemia

Accurate code assignment of any specific type of anemia requires physician documentation—a diagnostic statement of anemia without further qualification or description is insufficient. Even when the laboratory or other diagnostic report specifies the type of anemia, physician concurrence is required before the code may be assigned. Codes cannot be assigned solely on the basis of diagnostic reports; documentation of the physician's corroboration of a diagnosis or the significance of any test results is required.

Anemia codes have expanded to include much more specific information regarding the type of anemia. Anemia is further specified by the cause, including anemia due to loss of blood, due to the ingestion of certain drugs, or due to a form of dietary deficiency.

In order to assign the most specific code for anemia, documentation must include the type and cause of the anemia:

- Deficiency anemias:
  - Nutritional anemia, further specified as:
    - Iron deficiency anemia
    - Vitamin B12 deficiency anemia
    - Folate deficiency anemia
    - Other nutritional deficiency anemias (e.g., protein, zinc)
- Hemolytic anemias:
  - Acquired
  - Enzyme disorder anemias
  - Thalassemias
  - Sickle Cell Disorders - further specified as with or without crisis
  - Other hereditary hemolytic anemias
- Aplastic anemia and other bone marrow failure syndromes, further specified as:
  - Aplastic anemia
    - Constitutional
    - Drug-induced
    - Due to other external agents
    - Idiopathic
    - Myelophthisis
    - Pancyopenia
  - Acute posthemorrhagic anemia
  - Anemia in chronic disease (neoplastic, chronic kidney, infectious)
  - Red cell aplasia
  - Sideroblastic anemia

Neutropenia

Leukocytes, or white blood cells, are key players in the body's immune system. Leukocyte diseases are classified based on whether the white blood count is elevated or low. Neutropenia for example, is an abnormally low count of neutrophils—a type of white blood cell. Neutropenia is further specified by cause, for example:

- Congenital
- Secondary to cancer chemotherapy or other drug
- Due to infection

There are many different types of neutropenic disease. Neutropenia can be chronic, genetic, idiopathic, immune, infantile, malignant, pernicious, or splenic. To ensure assignment of the most specific code, the documentation must specify the type and cause of the neutropenia:

- Chronic granulocytopenia (due to any cause)
- Congenital (primary)
- Cyclic/Periodic
- Due to infection
- Fever
- Toxic
- Secondary
  - Drug-induced
  - Due to cytoreductive cancer chemotherapy

Neutropenia is typically diagnosed based on clinical evidence such as absolute neutrophil counts below 1,000 cells/cubic millimeter. However, the condition cannot be coded based on the laboratory findings, code assignment must be based on the physician documentation of the diagnosis.

Coagulation Disorders

As with anemia, code assignment for coagulation disorders requires specific physician documentation. For example, when bleeding occurs in a patient who is being treated with Coumadin, heparin, or other anticoagulant, the physician's documentation of the hemorrhagic disorder as due to the drug, extrinsic circulating anticoagulants, or an adverse effect of the prescribed drug, is necessary for code assignment.

To assign the most specific code for coagulation defects, purpura, and other hemorrhagic conditions, documentation must include specification of the type, such as:

- Allergic purpura
- Defibrination syndrome
- Disseminated intravascular coagulation
- Hereditary factor deficiency
- Primary or secondary thrombocytopenia
- Qualitative platelet defects

Coagulation defects involve prolonged clotting time, while hypercoagulable states are characterized by an increased tendency for blood clotting. Coagulation disorders can be congenital or acquired, which must be identified in the documentation. Here again, laboratory evidence of chronic inherited coagulation disorders must be supported by the appropriate physician documentation of the diagnosis or the significance of test results.

Coagulation defects should never be reported when only a prolonged prothrombin time or other abnormal coagulation profile is documented. Similarly, prophylactic therapy with an anti-hemophilic does not, in itself, support coding of the disorder.

Chapter-Specific Documentation Requirements

In this section, code categories, subcategories, and subclassifications for some of the commonly reported diseases and conditions of the blood and immune system are reviewed and their documentation requirements identified. The focus is on frequently reported conditions with specific clinical documentation requirements. Though not all of the codes with additional documentation requirements are discussed, this section will provide a representative sample of the type of additional documentation required for Diseases of the Blood and Blood-forming Organs and Immune System. The section is organized alphabetically by topic.

Folate Deficiency Anemia

Folic acid, or folate, is essential for red blood cell formation. Folate-deficiency anemia occurs due to a lack of folate and may also be documented as nutritional megaloblastic anemia. ICD-10-CM further specifies folate-deficiency anemia by cause. The more common causes of this anemia are poor dietary folic acid intake and certain medications. Other causes that may be documented include:

- Gastrointestinal disease such as Crohn's disease or celiac disease
- Surgeries such as weight-loss surgery that remove parts of the stomach or intestine
- Pregnancy due to an increased need for folic acid
- Congenital folate malabsorption
- Hemolytic anemia, which can also cause a deficiency due to increased red blood cell destruction

As with other anemias, the documentation must clearly indicate the type of anemia as well as the cause, such as dietary, drug-induced, or surgery-related folate deficiency anemia. The documentation in the medical record should also identify when a folate deficiency is not associated with anemia.

Coding and Documentation Requirements

Identify folate-deficiency anemia type:

- Dietary folate-deficiency anemia
- Drug-induced (also identify drug)
- Other specified type
- Unspecified type

ICD-10-CM Code/Documentation	
D52.0	Dietary folate deficiency anemia
D52.1	Drug-induced folate deficiency anemia
D52.8	Other folate deficiency anemias
D52.9	Folate deficiency anemia, unspecified

Documentation and Coding Example

Discharge Summary:

Patient is a 70-year-old male with **rheumatoid arthritis treated with an anti-inflammatory (1 g Sulfasalazine) daily for two years**. He recently developed abdominal pain, diarrhea, loss of appetite, and loss of weight. Hematological studies demonstrated a hemoglobin drop and the serum level of folic acid was significantly low; the red cell folate serum level was 146 ng/ml, with a normal serum B12. Addison's disease was excluded. He was diagnosed with **drug-induced megaloblastic anemia due to folate deficiency associated with Sulfasalazine treatment** and was admitted. Bone marrow biopsy confirmed megaloblastic erythropoiesis.

The patient's hemoglobin levels promptly recovered after discontinuing the Sulfasalazine and treatment with folic acid. Signs of clinical improvement were quickly evident. The patient's daily Sulfasalazine has been replaced with Mesalazine and patient will receive low levels of oral supplementation of folate acid replacement therapy. Patient will be monitored on an ongoing, outpatient basis for high levels of homocysteine, due to the increased risks for arteriosclerosis and thromboembolism.

Diagnosis: **Drug-induced folate deficiency anemia**

Diagnosis Code(s)

D52.1	Drug-induced folate deficiency anemia
T37.0x5A	Adverse effect of sulfonamides, initial encounter
M06.9	Rheumatoid arthritis, unspecified

Coding Note(s)

The reason for the admission is the drug-induced folate deficiency anemia so that is sequenced first. An additional code is assigned to identify the drug, which requires a 7th character to identify the episode of care. This is the initial encounter for the adverse effect of the sulfonamides, so 7th character 'A' is assigned. The code for rheumatoid arthritis is also reported.

Neutropenia, Acquired

Most cases of neutropenia in adults are acquired, although the condition may be congenital. Drugs, both cytotoxic (chemotherapy) and noncytotoxic, can induce neutropenia and are the most common cause. A decrease in neutrophil count can also be caused by infection such as tuberculosis or infection with Epstein Barr virus, cytomegalovirus, and viral hepatitis. Other forms of acquired neutropenia include cases that are related to an autoimmune disorder, such as Crohn's disease, rheumatoid arthritis, and lupus.

Drug induced neutropenia, or agranulocytosis, occurs most often due to the destruction of neutrophils rather than sequestration or hypoplasia. Neutrophils are a type of white blood cell that function as the first line responders for the immune system. Normal amounts of neutrophils are absolutely essential for the body to prevent infection. Many different types of drugs can induce neutropenia, for example, neutropenia has been reported as a side effect of vancomycin therapy. Epileptic, psychiatric, and blood pressure medications, in addition to antibiotics, have also been known to induce neutropenia. In many cases of drug induced neutropenia, discontinuation of the drug results in rapid correction of the neutrophil count within 30 days.

Drug induced neutropenia typically occurs secondary to the use of cytotoxic agents, as in chemotherapy. In these cases, the clinical documentation should include the underlying neoplasm in addition to identifying the causal drug. To ensure assignment of the most specific code, the clinical documentation must clearly indicate the cause-and-effect relationship, for example:

- Neutropenia due to cytoreductive cancer chemotherapy
- Neutropenia due to other specified drug
- Neutropenia due to infection

Neutropenia is diagnosed based on clinical evidence such as absolute neutrophil counts. However, the condition cannot be coded based on the laboratory findings, rather the medical record documentation of the physician's corroboration of the diagnosis must be the basis for code assignment.

Coding and Documentation Requirements

Identify the acquired neutropenia:

- Drug-induced
  - Secondary to cancer chemotherapy
    - » Specify the drug (T45.1X5)
    - » Identify the underlying neoplasm
- Other drug-induced agranulocytosis
  - Specify the drug (T36-T50 with 5th or 6th character 5)
- Neutropenia due to infection
- Other neutropenia

Identify any associated conditions such as fever, mucositis, or exanthem.

ICD-10-CM Code/Documentation	
D70.1	Agranulocytosis secondary to cancer chemotherapy
D70.2	Other drug-induced agranulocytosis
D70.3	Neutropenia due to infection
D70.8	Other neutropenia

Documentation and Coding Example

Sixty-three-year-old female being treated with home IV vancomycin, 250mg every 12 hours, for a gram-positive infection, presented to the ED on day 14 of vancomycin therapy after experiencing **fever** and a **fine macular rash,** which progressed over the previous 3 days. Labs indicated total leukocyte and neutrophil counts, 2.3 X 109/L and 1.2X 109/L respectively and patient was admitted for treatment of **neutropenia associated with the vancomycin therapy**. Laboratory monitoring was performed and her counts rebounded promptly after discontinuation of vancomycin. Resolution of her **vancomycin-induced neutropenia** occurred within 7 days of discontinuation and patient was discharged home, in stable condition.

Diagnosis: **Vancomycin induced neutropenia and dermatitis**

Diagnosis Code(s)

D70.2	Other drug-induced agranulocytosis
T36.8X5A	Adverse effect of other systemic antibiotics, initial encounter
R50.81	Fever presenting with conditions classified elsewhere
L27.0	Generalized skin eruption due to drugs and medicaments taken internally

Coding Note(s)

Additional codes are assigned to identify the fever and the rash. The appropriate 7th character is added to the code from category T36 to identify the encounter as the initial encounter.

Pernicious Anemia/Other Vitamin B12 Deficiency Anemia

The human body uses a special protein called intrinsic factor to absorb vitamin B12. When the stomach does not make enough intrinsic factor, the intestine cannot properly absorb vitamin B12. Pernicious anemia refers specifically to vitamin B12 deficiency resulting from a lack of production of intrinsic factor in the stomach. However, other causes of vitamin B12 deficiency do exist. Pernicious anemia is also known as Biermer's anemia, Addison's anemia, Addison–Biermer anemia, or megaloblastic anemia caused by a deficiency of vitamin B12.

In the medical record documentation, Vitamin B12 deficiency anemia must be clearly differentiated from Vitamin B12 deficiency. Vitamin B12 deficiency anemia is further specified based on cause, so the documentation must clearly indicate the underlying cause.

Coding and Documentation Requirements

Identify type of vitamin B12 deficiency anemia:

- Due to intrinsic factor deficiency, which includes:
  - Addison anemia
  - Biermer anemia
  - Pernicious (congenital) anemia
  - Congenital intrinsic factor deficiency
- Due to selective vitamin B12 malabsorption with proteinuria, which includes:
  - Imerslund (Gräsbeck) syndrome
  - Megaloblastic hereditary anemia
- Transcobalamin II deficiency
- Other dietary vitamin B12 deficiency anemia (vegan anemia)
- Other specified type of vitamin B12 deficiency anemias
- Unspecified type

ICD-10-CM Code/Documentation	
D51.0	Vitamin B12 deficiency anemia due to intrinsic factor deficiency
D51.1	Vitamin B12 deficiency anemia due to selective vitamin B12 malabsorption with proteinuria
D51.2	Transcobalamin II deficiency
D51.3	Other dietary vitamin B12 deficiency anemia
D51.8	Other vitamin B12 deficiency anemias
D51.9	Vitamin B12 deficiency anemia, unspecified

Documentation and Coding Example

A 57-year-old male presents with complaints of headache, general fatigue, weakness, and shortness of breath, all of which have slowly worsened over the past nine months. Patient states he has also been experiencing periodic dizziness and loss of balance for the past one to two weeks.

No history of ear infection, upper respiratory illness, nausea/vomiting, or fever. No cardiac history or complaints. Medical history is negative for stomach or intestinal surgeries, celiac or Crohn's disease, or other digestive disorders. **Patient has been a vegan his entire adult life; he eats no meat, fish, eggs, or dairy products**. No current medications. Family history is negative for autoimmune disorders and otherwise non-contributory.

On examination, patient's skin is warm, dry, and jaundiced. Tongue appears swollen and dark red. No ulcers or leukoplakia in buccal folds or under the tongue. Conjunctiva and sclera clear, eyes negative for ptosis, exophthalmos, lesions, or asymmetry. Pulse regular rate and rhythm; no heart murmur. Lungs clear bilaterally. Abdomen rigid, rebound tenderness, and significant hepatomegaly. Normal bowel sounds. Poor reflexes and marked muscle weakness noted in extremities; patient reports periodic numbness and tingling in his hands and feet. Gait is unsteady, but no tremors or unusual movements. Mental status exam is negative for confusion and depression.

Labs ordered: CBC, serum folate and iron, reticulocyte count, homocysteine, methylmalonic acid and vitamin B12 levels, and intrinsic factor antibodies and parietal cell antibodies.

Diagnosis: **Dietary vitamin B12 deficiency anemia**

Assessment/Plan: Patient's pernicious anemia is caused by his strict vegan diet. Administered vitamin B12 injection and patient will continue with monthly B12 injections. Patient does not desire to modify his strict vegan diet in any way but agreed to take high dose vitamin B12 supplements by mouth daily. Patient will return to office next week for follow-up.

Diagnosis Code(s)

D51.3	Other dietary vitamin B12 deficiency anemia

Coding Note(s)

While there are other forms of pernicious anemia, this patient's condition arises from his vegan diet so his diagnosis is dietary vitamin B12 deficiency anemia. "Vegan anemia" is listed as an inclusion term under the code D51.3.

Primary Hypercoagulable State

Hypercoagulability involves the presence of abnormalities associated with an increased risk of thromboembolic complications and recurrent thrombosis. Primary hypercoagulable states are generally inherited abnormalities involving a defective anticoagulant mechanism, while secondary hypercoagulable states are acquired disorders in patients with underlying systemic diseases or clinical conditions known to be linked to an increased risk of thrombosis.

The documentation must fully describe the type of coagulation disorder and laboratory evidence must be supported by the appropriate physician documentation of the diagnosis or the significance of test results.

Coding and Documentation Requirements

Identify hypercoagulable state:

- Primary thrombophilia
  - Activated protein C resistance
  - Prothrombin gene mutation
  - Other primary thrombophilia, which includes:
    - » Antithrombin III deficiency
    - » Hypercoagulable state NOS
    - » Primary hypercoagulable state NEC
    - » Primary thrombophilia NEC
    - » Protein C deficiency
    - » Protein S deficiency
    - » Thrombophilia NOS
- Other thrombophilia
  - Antiphospholipid syndrome, which includes:
    - » Anticardiolipin syndrome
    - » Antiphospholipid antibody syndrome
  - Lupus anticoagulant syndrome
  - Other specified thrombophilia (secondary hypercoagulable state NOS)

ICD-10-CM Code/Documentation	
D68.51	Activated protein C resistance
D68.52	Prothrombin gene mutation
D68.59	Other primary thrombophilia
D68.61	Antiphospholipid syndrome
D68.62	Lupus anticoagulant syndrome
D68.69	Other thrombophilia

Documentation and Coding Example

Hematology Consult Note

This 40-year-old, Caucasian female patient with a history of increased prothrombin levels and familial thrombosis was admitted for treatment of a venous thromboembolism. She was subsequently discharged and referred for hematologic consultation.

The patient has no predisposing thrombotic conditions, she is a non-smoker, she is not obese, and she is not pregnant. No history of injury, prolonged bed rest, or travel. She is not using oral contraceptives and her past medical history is negative for estrogen use or heparin use, cancer, diabetes, lupus, heart failure, or renal failure. Surgical history is negative. Her family history is significant for maternal venous thrombosis.

Physical examination was negative for fever, weight loss, malar rash, or excessive rubor. Sclera and conjunctiva clear, no exophthalmos. ENT normal. Lungs clear, no rales. Pulse rhythm and rate regular, no bruits. No hepatosplenomegaly, masses, or tenderness. No joint inflammation, or signs of rheumatoid arthritis or lupus; positive pedal pulses and no pedal edema. No tremor, onycholysis, or hyperreflexia.

Workup included CBC, chemistry, and a TSH test which were within normal limits, and lipid profiles which were negative for hypercholesterolemia. **Primary hypercoagulable state was suspected because of the high incidence of this mutation in Caucasian patients with familial thrombosis.** A **hypercoagulation panel was ordered** for protein S, protein C, and antithrombin III assay; testing for Leiden factor V mutation; prothrombin mutation; total plasma homocysteine concentration; anticardiolipin, antinuclear, and antiphospholipid antibodies; lupus anticoagulant; and fibrinogen level. **Two copies of the prothrombin G20210A mutation were detected.**

Patient was counseled at length on the diagnosis and reassured that although the prothrombin G20210A mutation increases the risk of deep vein thrombosis, stroke, and fetal loss, early recognition can provide opportunities to reduce the morbidity and mortality associated with these conditions. Treatment will include oral anticoagulation therapy.

Diagnosis: **Primary thrombophilia, Prothrombin G20210A mutation**

Diagnosis Code(s)

D68.52 Prothrombin gene mutation

Coding Note(s)

Primary thrombophilia and primary hypercoagulable states are classified by type such as Prothrombin gene mutation, activated protein C resistance, Factor V Leiden mutation, Antithrombin III deficiency, Protein C deficiency, or Protein S deficiency.

Red Cell Aplasia

Red cell aplasia is a rare, chronic condition characterized by profound anemia. Acquired pure red cell aplasia (PRCA) can be secondary to underlying disorders such as diabetes, thyroiditis, or rheumatoid arthritis; however, acquired idiopathic PRCA is the most common form of the disorder in adults. Certain medications such as antiepileptic medications are also thought to cause PRCA. The condition is also associated with thymoma, infections, and renal failure. In fact, an increased incidence of PRCA in patients with chronic renal disease secondary to treatment with Epoetin therapy has been noted.

Essential documentation for red cell aplasia includes documentation of the cause—whether known or unknown (idiopathic). Documentation must clearly differentiate acquired pure red cell anemia from a similar condition, transient erythroblastopenia, and from the congenital form of the disease known as Diamond-Blackfan anemia or syndrome.

Coding and Documentation Requirements

Identify type of acquired pure red cell aplasia:

- Chronic
- Transient
- Other acquired type
- Unspecified

3. Diseases of the Blood/ Blood-Forming Organs

ICD-10-CM Code/Documentation	
D60.0	Chronic acquired pure red cell aplasia
D60.1	Transient acquired pure red cell aplasia
D60.8	Other acquired pure red cell aplasia
D60.9	Acquired pure red cell aplasia, unspecified

Documentation and Coding Example

Discharge Summary:

This 30-year-old female school teacher presented with severe anemia. On admission her hematocrit was 13.7% with a hemoglobin concentration of 4.7 g/dl and her reticulocyte counts were abnormal at 0.1%. The patient history is significant for a current parvovirus B19 outbreak at the school. PCR test positive for parvovirus B19. A direct Coombs was negative for autoimmune hemolytic anemia. CT scans were negative for thymomas. A bone marrow examination revealed severe erythroid hypoplasia. **Acute transient PRCA secondary to parvovirus B19 infection** was diagnosed and the patient was treated with transfusions. Her hematological test results rapidly improved and she was discharged from the hospital on the 9th day. At that time, her hematocrit was 33.2%, her hemoglobin concentration was 10.0 g/dl, and her peripheral reticulocyte level was 1.8%.

Discharge Diagnosis: **Acute transient pure red cell aplasia.**

Diagnosis Code(s)

D60.1 Transient acquired pure red cell aplasia

B97.6 Parvovirus as the cause of diseases classified elsewhere

Coding Note(s)

ICD-10-CM specifies pure red cell aplasia as chronic, transient, or other specified.

Sickle-Cell Disease/Trait

Sickle cell disease refers to a group of genetic disorders affecting red blood cells when an abnormal hemoglobin "S" sickle cell gene is inherited, sometimes in combination with a gene for another type of abnormal hemoglobin or beta thalassemia. Hemoglobin is the iron-containing protein that allows normal red blood cells to carry oxygen throughout the body. Hb-SS disease, also known as sickle cell anemia, is the most severe form of sickle cell disease, which occurs when two copies of the altered gene are inherited. The red blood cells become rigid and misshapen. The crescent shaped cells get stuck in small blood vessels, blocking blood flow and causing pain and damage to organs, resulting in crisis. They also die off early, resulting in chronic and severe anemia.

People may inherit one sickle cell "S" gene from one parent and another form of abnormal hemoglobin from the other parent, resulting in Hb-SC (Sickle-cell/Hb-C disease), which is milder, or Hb-SD, Hb-SE, or Hb-SO disease with varying severity. Those with one inherited sickle cell "S" gene and one beta thalassemia gene, will have either HbS-beta zero thalassemia or HbS-beta plus thalassemia. Beta thalassemia is another type of anemia that reduces the amount of hemoglobin produced. The red blood cells in sickle cell beta thalassemia will be small and pale along with some that are misshapen and sickled as well, also resulting in anemia. In sickle cell beta zero thalassemia, the blood has no normal hemoglobin. In sickle cell beta plus thalassemia, there is some normal hemoglobin but in a lower than normal amount.

Sickle cell trait occurs when a person inherits one sickle cell "S" gene and one normal, hemoglobin "A" gene. Those with sickle cell trait do not normally show any signs of sickle cell disease but can pass it on to their children.

With sickle-cell disorders, it is important that the documentation clearly distinguish between sickle-cell disease (anemia) and sickle-cell trait. When the physician documents both sickle-cell trait and sickle-cell disease, only the sickle-cell disease is coded.

Medical record documentation of sickle-cell disease should specify the type of disorder:

- Hb-SS
- Hb-SC
- Hb-SD
- Hb-SE
- Hb-SO
- Sickle-cell thalassemia
  - Sickle-cell thalassemia beta plus
  - Sickle-cell thalassemia beta zero

ICD-10-CM classifies sickle-cell disease (D57) by type as well as by type of crisis when present, as in Hb-SS or Hb-SC disease with unspecified vaso-occlusive crisis. Further specification of the type of crisis, such as acute chest syndrome, cerebral vascular involvement, splenic sequestration or other condition, should also be documented. Documentation of vaso-occlusive and aplastic episodes should describe severity, frequency, and duration.

Documentation of sickle-cell disorders typically includes appropriate hematologic evidence for sickle-cell disease, such as hemoglobin electrophoresis. However, the condition cannot be coded based solely on the laboratory findings without physician documentation of the diagnosis.

Coding and Documentation Requirements

Identify as sickle cell:

- Disease (anemia)
- Trait

For sickle-cell disease, identify type:

- Hb-SS
- Hb-SC (Hb-S/Hb-C, Sickle-cell/Hb-C)
- Other specified type which includes:
  - Hb-SD
  - Hb-SE
  - Hb-SO

Sickle-cell thalassemia which includes:

- Sickle-cell thalassemia beta zero
- Sickle-cell thalassemia beta plus

Identify sickle-cell disease as without or with crisis:

- With crisis

- Acute chest syndrome
- Cerebral vascular involvement
- Splenic sequestration
- Other specified complication
- Unspecified

• Without crisis

ICD-1Ø-CM Code/Documentation			
D57.1	Sickle-cell disease without crisis	D57.ØØ	Hb-SS disease with crisis, unspecified
D57.2Ø	Sickle-cell/Hb-C disease without crisis	D57.Ø1	Hb-SS disease with acute chest syndrome
D57.8Ø	Other sickle-cell disorders without crisis	D57.Ø2	Hb-SS disease with splenic sequestration
		D57.Ø3	Hb-SS disease with cerebral vascular involvement
		D57.Ø9	Hb-SS disease with crisis with other specified complication
D57.4Ø	Sickle-cell thalassemia without crisis	D57.211	Sickle-cell/Hb-C disease with acute chest syndrome
D57.42	Sickle-cell thalassemia beta zero without crisis	D57.212	Sickle-cell/Hb-C disease with splenic sequestration
D57.44	Sickle-cell thalassemia beta plus without crisis	D57.213	Sickle-cell/Hb-C disease with cerebral vascular involvement
		D57.218	Sickle-cell/Hb-C disease with crisis with other specified complication
		D57.219	Sickle-cell/Hb-C disease with crisis, unspecified
D57.3	Sickle-cell trait	D57.811	Other sickle-cell disorders with acute chest syndrome
		D57.812	Other sickle-cell disorders with splenic sequestration
		D57.813	Other sickle-cell disorders with cerebral vascular Involvement
		D57.818	Other sickle-cell disorders with crisis with other specified complication
		D57.819	Other sickle-cell disorders with crisis, unspecified
		D57.431	Sickle-cell thalassemia beta zero with acute chest syndrome
		D57.432	Sickle-cell thalassemia beta zero with splenic sequestration
		D57.433	Sickle-cell thalassemia beta zero with cerebral vascular involvement
		D57.438	Sickle-cell thalassemia beta zero with crisis with other specified complication
		D57.439	Sickle-cell thalassemia beta zero with crisis, unspecified

ICD-1Ø-CM Code/Documentation		
	D57.451	Sickle-cell thalassemia beta plus with acute chest syndrome
	D57.452	Sickle-cell thalassemia beta plus with splenic sequestration
	D57.453	Sickle-cell thalassemia beta plus with cerebral vascular involvement
	D57.458	Sickle-cell thalassemia beta plus with crisis with other specified complication
	D57.459	Sickle-cell thalassemia beta plus with crisis, unspecified
	D57.411	Sickle-cell thalassemia, unspecified, with acute chest syndrome
	D57.412	Sickle-cell thalassemia, unspecified, with splenic sequestration
	D57.413	Sickle-cell thalassemia, unspecified, with cerebral vascular involvement
	D57.418	Sickle-cell thalassemia, unspecified, with crisis with other specified complication
	D57.419	Sickle-cell thalassemia, unspecified, with crisis

Documentation and Coding Example

A 26-year-old African-American male presents to the ED in sickle-cell crisis. Patient is writhing in pain. He describes his pain as 15/10. Painful extremities, no fever, no chest pain, no respiratory distress.

Past Medical History: Sickle-cell disease; pneumonia. NKDA.

s significant for sickle-cell trait

Social History: Non-contributory

Physical Exam

Temp: VS: T 98.6°F, HR 11Ø, RR 2Ø, BP 135/8Ø

ENT: EOMI, PERRL, clear TM

Cardiovascular: Sinus tachycardia, normal S1/S2, no murmurs, rubs, or gallops

Lungs: CTA bilaterally

Abdomen: Soft, non-distended, diffusely tender

Extremities: No clubbing/cyanosis/edema, pain everywhere

Neuro: Grossly intact

ED Course: IV, normal saline hydration started. Morphine IV push administered, followed by morphine drip.

Patient was afebrile with no infection, consequently no labs were obtained. No x-rays were ordered. The patient's pain was adequately controlled during his stay in the ED. Discharged home on oral pain medication and will follow-up with his primary care physician on Monday.

Disposition: Home.

Diagnosis: **Sickle cell vaso-occlusive crisis**

Diagnosis Code(s)

D57.00 Hb-SS disease with crisis, unspecified

Coding Note(s)

Sickle-cell disease or Hb-SS disease, with vaso-occlusive pain is classified as Hb-SS disease with crisis and is listed as an inclusion term. No additional code is required for the vaso-occlusive pain.

Sideroblastic Anemia

Sideroblastic anemias are classified as hereditary or acquired conditions. While many anemias are mild or moderate, sideroblastic anemia is considered severe. The three main types of sideroblastic anemia are:

- Hereditary sideroblastic anemia, caused by a recessive gene linked to the X-chromosome and so is more common in men than women
- Acquired sideroblastic anemia, which is usually caused by alcohol or substance abuse, or lead poisoning
- Idiopathic sideroblastic anemia

Documentation of sideroblastic anemia must describe the type such as acquired, congenital, hereditary, primary, or secondary. In cases of acquired and secondary sideroblastic anemia, the cause (e.g., drug-induced, due to disease) should also be fully described in the medical record documentation.

Coding and Documentation Requirements

Identify the sideroblastic anemia:

- Hereditary
- Secondary, identify cause:
  - Drug-induced (specify drug)
  - Due to disease (specify disease)
- Other specified type

ICD-10-CM Code/Documentation	
D64.0	Hereditary sideroblastic anemia
D64.1	Secondary sideroblastic anemia due to disease
D64.2	Secondary sideroblastic anemia due to drugs and toxins
D64.3	Other sideroblastic anemias

Documentation and Coding Example

A 57-year-old male, **chronic alcoholic**, well-known to this ED, presents today complaining of chest pain, headache, fatigue, and difficulty in swallowing. Workup included a complete blood count, ferritin, and total iron-binding capacity. The CBC count revealed severe anemia, and a low mean corpuscular volume. Siderocytes had been noted and alcoholism is suggested as a cause. In view of these results, a bone marrow aspirate was done which showed mixed marrow cellularity and florid sideroblastic change. A diagnosis of **alcoholic acquired sideroblastic anemia** was therefore established for this patient. Patient was admitted and treated with complete blood transfusion, and vitamin B complex.

Diagnosis: **Acquired sideroblastic anemia secondary to alcohol dependence**

Diagnosis Code(s)

T51.0X1A Toxic effect of ethanol, accidental (unintentional), initial encounter

D64.2 Secondary sideroblastic anemia due to drugs and toxins

F10.20 Alcohol dependence, uncomplicated

Coding Note(s)

Under code D64.2 there are instructional notes directing the user to code first poisoning due to drug or toxin (T36-T65 with fifth or sixth character 1-4 or 6), if applicable or in the case of an adverse effect to assign an additional code when applicable to identify the causal drug (T36-T50 with fifth or sixth character 5). In this case, the sideroblastic anemia is due to a toxic effect of alcohol and so the code for the toxic effect is the first-listed diagnosis. ICD-10-CM lists four external causes for toxic effects of alcohol, which include accidental (unintentional), intentional self-harm, assault, and undetermined. When no intent is documented, the code for accidental is reported. Undetermined intent is only for use when there is specific documentation that the intent of the toxic effect cannot be determined, even though it may be suspected. An additional code is reported for alcohol dependence. Note under code F10.2 Alcohol dependence that there is an Excludes2 note for T51.0-; however, in this case the patient has both conditions, sideroblastic anemia as a toxic effect of long-term alcohol dependence, and alcohol dependence so both conditions are reported. The code for alcohol dependence uncomplicated is reported even though the patient has a blood disorder caused by his alcohol dependence because other codes for complications relate specifically to mental and behavioral disorders associated with alcohol dependence. This is the initial encounter for the toxic effect so the 7th character 'A' is reported.

Thalassemias

Thalassemia is a recessive trait inherited disease that affects the ability to produce hemoglobin and red blood cells. Individuals with thalassemia can have mild or severe anemia. There are two primary types of thalassemia—alpha thalassemia and beta thalassemia which affect the alpha and the beta hemoglobin chain genes. Both alpha and beta thalassemia are classified as major or minor. Major thalassemia occurs when an individual inherits the defective gene from both parents, while the minor form occurs when an individual inherits the defective gene from only one parent. A diagnosis of thalassemia minor means the individual is a carrier of the gene and these individuals are typically asymptomatic. Thalassemia minor may also be referred to as alpha or beta thalassemia trait. Another condition, hereditary persistence of fetal hemoglobin (HPFH), usually caused by a mutation in the beta-globin gene cluster, results in the production of fetal hemoglobin (hemoglobin F) well into adulthood. HPFH can alleviate the severity of certain types of thalassemia.

Category D56 Thalassemia includes alpha thalassemia, beta thalassemia, delta-beta thalassemia, thalassemia minor which includes alpha, beta, and delta-beta types, hereditary persistence of fetal hemoglobin (HPFH), hemoglobin E-beta thalassemia, and other and unspecified thalassemia. Sickle cell thalassemias are classified in category D57 with sickle cell disorders.

Coding and Documentation Requirements

Identify thalassemia type:

- Alpha thalassemia
- Beta thalassemia
- Delta-beta thalassemia
- Thalassemia minor, which includes:
  - Alpha thalassemia minor
  - Alpha thalassemia silent carrier
  - Alpha thalassemia trait
  - Beta thalassemia minor
  - Beta thalassemia trait
  - Delta-beta thalassemia minor
  - Delta-beta thalassemia trait
- Hemoglobin E-beta thalassemia
- Hereditary persistence of fetal hemoglobin [HPFH]
- Other thalassemias, which include:
  - Dominant thalassemia
  - Hemoglobin C thalassemia
  - Mixed thalassemia
  - Thalassemia with other hemoglobinopathy

ICD-10-CM Code/Documentation			
D56.0	Alpha thalassemia	D56.4	Hereditary persistence of fetal hemoglobin [HPFH]
D56.1	Beta thalassemia	D56.5	Hemoglobin E-beta thalassemia
D56.2	Delta-beta thalassemia	D56.8	Other thalassemias
D56.3	Thalassemia minor	D56.9	Thalassemia, unspecified

Documentation and Coding Example

A 2-year-old African-American girl was seen by her pediatrician for assessment of poor appetite and slowed growth and development. Family medical history includes a maternal aunt with thalassemia. Based on hemoglobin tests and family genetic studies that showed only one parent with alpha thalassemia trait, she was diagnosed with alpha thalassemia minor. Treatment includes daily folic acid supplements, observation, and monitoring.

Diagnosis: **Alpha thalassemia minor**

Diagnosis Code(s)

D56.3 Thalassemia minor

Coding Note(s)

Alpha thalassemia minor is classified differently from Alpha thalassemia major. Alpha thalassemia minor is classified as thalassemia minor and includes any type of thalassemia minor (alpha, beta, delta-beta) or any type documented as thalassemia trait or silent carrier. Alpha thalassemia major is coded to D56.0.

Summary

Certain information regarding the type and cause of the blood or immune mechanism disorder must be documented in the medical record before the most appropriate and specific code can be assigned. Many codes require further specific documentation of the disease type (e.g., inherited or acquired disorder).

ICD-10-CM classifies diseases of the blood and blood-forming organs and immune mechanism by the type of disease and by the cause of the disease or disorder, such as intraoperative and postprocedural complications, or drug-induced conditions. Documentation of the severity and/or status of the disease in terms of acute or chronic, with or without crisis, as well as the site, etiology, and any secondary disease process are basic documentation requirements. Physician documentation of diagnostic test findings or confirmation of any diagnosis found in test reports is also required documentation.

Understanding the coding and documentation challenges for diseases of the blood and blood-forming organs can help in identifying documentation deficiencies so that physicians and coders can correct any areas in which the necessary documentation is lacking.

Chapter 3 Quiz

1. Notable exclusions in the classification of diseases of the blood and blood-forming organs and certain disorders involving the immune mechanism contain which of the following?
   a. AIDS
   b. Human immunodeficiency virus (HIV) disease
   c. Circulatory system diseases
   d. All of the above
2. Which of the following is NOT a true statement regarding anemia code assignment?
   a. A diagnostic report specifying the type of anemia is required for the code to be assigned.
   b. Codes cannot be assigned solely on the basis of diagnostic test findings.
   c. When a laboratory report specifies the type of anemia, physician concurrence is required before the code may be assigned.
   d. The physician's documentation of corroboration of a diagnosis or the significance of any test results is required.
3. Where are guidelines related to anemia associated with a malignancy found?
   a. In the chapter-specific guidelines for Chapter 3 Diseases of the Blood and Blood-Forming Organs and Certain Disorders Involving the Immune Mechanism
   b. In the chapter-specific guidelines for Chapter 2 Neoplasms
   c. In the coding conventions
   d. In the general guidelines
4. Where are coding and sequencing instructions for diseases of the blood, blood-forming organs, and disorders of the immune mechanism found?
   a. In the Alphabetic Index
   b. In the Tabular List
   c. Guidelines are found only in the chapter-specific guidelines for each chapter
   d. Both a. and b.
5. When bleeding occurs in a patient being treated with an anticoagulant, and the documentation states the hemorrhagic disorder is an adverse effect of the prescribed anticoagulant, what is the correct primary code assignment?
   a. Drug-induced hemorrhagic disorder
   b. Hemorrhagic disorder due to intrinsic circulating anticoagulants
   c. Adverse effect of anticoagulant
   d. None of the above
6. Coagulation defects involve prolonged clotting time, while hypercoagulable states are characterized by an increased tendency for blood clotting. Which of the following is true regarding coding coagulation defects?
   a. Coagulation defects may be reported when a prolonged prothrombin time or other abnormal coagulation profile is documented.
   b. Coagulation defects may be reported when prophylactic therapy, such as an anti-hemophilic, is documented.
   c. Coagulation defects may be reported when laboratory evidence of a coagulation disorder is supported by the physician documentation.
   d. All of the above
7. What is pernicious anemia also known as?
   a. Biermer's anemia
   b. Addison's anemia
   c. Addison–Biermer anemia
   d. All of the above
8. Which of the following is true regarding documentation required for accurate coding of sickle-cell disorders?
   a. Clear distinction is needed between sickle-cell disease (anemia), and sickle-cell trait.
   b. When the physician documents both sickle-cell trait and sickle-cell disease, only the sickle-cell disease is coded.
   c. When the physician documents both sickle-cell trait and sickle-cell disease, only the sickle-cell trait is coded.
   d. Both a and b
9. How is sickle-cell disease with vaso-occlusive pain coded?
   a. With a combination code for the manifestation
   b. With a code for Hb-SS disease followed by a code for vaso-occlusive pain
   c. As Hb-SS disease with crisis
   d. All of the above
10. How is a diagnosis documented as antineoplastic chemotherapy-induced anemia coded?
    a. Anemia due to antineoplastic chemotherapy
    b. Aplastic anemia due to antineoplastic chemotherapy
    c. Drug-induced aplastic anemia
    d. All of the above

See next page for answers and rationales.

Chapter 3 Answers and Rationales

1. Notable exclusions in the classification of diseases of the blood and blood-forming organs and certain disorders involving the immune mechanism contain which of the following?

   d. All of the above

   Rationale: *There is an Excludes2 note at the beginning of Chapter 3 indicating that HIV disease (AIDS) is not reported with codes from Chapter 3. Although not specifically stated in the excludes2 list for Chapter 3, Circulatory system diseases are reported with codes from Chapter 9 Diseases of the Circulatory System.*

2. Which of the following is NOT a true statement regarding anemia code assignment?

   a. A diagnostic report specifying the type of anemia is required for the code to be assigned.

   Rationale: *According to coding guidelines, code assignment of a patient diagnosis is based on medical record documentation from the patient's provider—the physician or other qualified healthcare practitioner legally accountable for establishing the patient's diagnosis. The associated diagnosis must be documented by the patient's provider and cannot be coded based on a diagnostic report.*

3. Where are guidelines related to anemia associated with a malignancy found?

   b. In the chapter-specific guidelines for Chapter 2 Neoplasms

   Rationale: *There are no chapter-specific guidelines for Chapter 3 Diseases of the Blood and Blood-Forming Organs and Certain Disorders Involving the Immune Mechanism. However, there are detailed guidelines in the chapter-specific guidelines for Chapter 2 Neoplasms that address coding for complications associated with malignancy, including anemia associated with the malignancy, and anemia associated with treatment of the malignancy.*

4. Where are coding and sequencing instructions for diseases of the blood, blood-forming organs, and disorders of the immune mechanism found?

   d. Both a. and b.

   Rationale: *According to Section I.A of the coding guidelines, the conventions and instructions of the classification take precedence over guidelines. The conventions for ICD-10-CM are the rules for use of the classification independent of the guidelines. These conventions are incorporated within the Alphabetic Index and Tabular List as instructional notes.*

5. When bleeding occurs in a patient being treated with an anticoagulant, and the documentation states a hemorrhagic disorder due to an adverse effect of the prescribed anticoagulant, what is the correct primary code assignment?

   a. Drug-induced hemorrhagic disorder

   Rationale: *Since the disorder is documented as being caused by the prescribed anticoagulant, the condition is drug-induced, which is coded first, followed by the adverse effect to identify the drug. Note also that drug-induced hemorrhagic disorder is reported as hemorrhagic disorder due to extrinsic circulating anticoagulants, code D68.32, which includes drug-induced hemorrhagic disorder. Intrinsic circulating anticoagulants are usually autoantibodies that work against the normal clotting mechanism, neutralizing certain clotting factors and this is not a disorder caused by a prescription anticoagulant drug.*

6. Coagulation defects involve prolonged clotting time, while hypercoagulable states are characterized by an increased tendency for blood clotting. Which of the following is true regarding coding coagulation defects?

   c. Coagulation defects may be reported when laboratory evidence of a coagulation disorder is supported by the physician documentation.

   Rationale: *Code assignment of a patient diagnosis is based on medical record documentation from the physician or provider legally accountable for establishing the patient's diagnosis according to ICD-10-CM coding guidelines. The associated diagnosis must be coded based solely on the documentation by the patient's provider. If more detailed documentation is provided in a diagnostic report, the physician may be queried for affirmation of the specified diagnosis or documentation of the significance of any test results.*

7. What is pernicious anemia also known as?

   d. All of the above

   Rationale: *Inclusion terms in the Tabular List under code D51.0 Vitamin B12 deficiency anemia due to intrinsic factor deficiency, include pernicious anemia, Addison anemia, and Biermer anemia. The ICD-10-CM Index lists Addison (-Biermer) (pernicious) as a subterm entry under Anemia.*

8. Which of the following is true regarding documentation required for accurate coding of sickle-cell disorders?

   d. Both a and b

   Rationale: *Sickle-cell disease must be differentiated from sickle-cell trait. Carriers of the sickle-cell trait do not suffer from sickle-cell anemia and sickle-cell trait is not a form of the disease. Sickle-cell trait occurs when a person has one gene for sickle hemoglobin and one gene for normal hemoglobin. People who are carriers of the trait generally don't have any medical problems and have normal lives. When the patient is documented with both, only the manifesting disease is coded.*

9. How is sickle-cell disease with vaso-occlusive pain coded?

   c. As Hb-SS disease with crisis

   Rationale: *Sickle-cell disease with vaso-occlusive pain is indexed to D57.0 Hb-SS disease with crisis. In the Tabular List, under code D57.0, Hb-SS disease with vaso-occlusive pain is listed as an included condition.*

10. How is a diagnosis documented as antineoplastic chemotherapy-induced anemia coded?

    a. Anemia due to antineoplastic chemotherapy

    Rationale: *Antineoplastic chemotherapy-induced anemia is coded to D64.81 Anemia due to antineoplastic chemotherapy. Instructional notes exclude anemia in neoplastic disease (D63.0) and aplastic anemia due to antineoplastic chemotherapy (D61.1).*

Chapter 4

ENDOCRINE, NUTRITIONAL AND METABOLIC DISEASES, AND IMMUNITY DISORDERS

Introduction

Endocrine, nutritional, and metabolic disorders are contained in Chapter 4, but certain disorders involving the immune system are in Chapter 3 and are covered with diseases of the blood and blood-forming organs within that chapter.

The blocks within the endocrine, nutritional, and metabolic diseases chapter are shown below.

ICD-10-CM Blocks	
E00-E07	Disorders of Thyroid Gland
E08-E13	Diabetes Mellitus
E15-E16	Other Disorders of Glucose Regulation and Pancreatic Internal Secretion
E20-E35	Disorders of Other Endocrine Glands
E36	Intraoperative Complications of Endocrine System
E40-E46	Malnutrition
E50-E64	Other Nutritional Deficiencies
E65-E68	Overweight, Obesity and Other Hyperalimentation
E70-E88	Metabolic Disorders
E89	Postprocedural Endocrine and Metabolic Complications and Disorders, Not Elsewhere Classified

Coding Notes

There are coding instructions related to neoplasms of the endocrine glands. Neoplasms of the endocrine glands, whether functionally active or not, are classified in the neoplasm chapter. This chapter note is further expanded to include the use of an additional code from Chapter 4, when appropriate, to indicate either functional activity by neoplasms and ectopic endocrine gland tissue, or hyperfunction and hypofunction of endocrine glands associated with neoplasms and other conditions classified elsewhere.

Exclusions

There is a single Excludes1 note at the chapter level.

Excludes1	Excludes2
Transitory endocrine and metabolic disorders specific to the newborn (P70-P74)	None

Chapter Guidelines

The only chapter guidelines for endocrine, nutritional, and metabolic diseases relate to diabetes mellitus. Diabetes mellitus codes are combination codes that capture the type of diabetes, the body system affected, and the complications or manifestations affecting each body system. The three components of the combination codes are as follows:

- The type of diabetes:
  - Drug or chemical induced (E09)
  - Due to an underlying condition (E08)
  - Type 1 (E10)
  - Type 2 (E11)
  - Other specified diabetes mellitus (E13)
- The body system affected:
  - Circulatory complications
  - Hyperosmolarity
  - Kidney complications
  - Neurological complications
  - Ophthalmic complications
  - Other specified complications, which includes:
  - arthropathy
  - dermatitis
  - hyperglycemia
  - hypoglycemia
  - oral complications
  - skin ulcer
  - Unspecified complications
  - Without complications
- Specified complications/manifestations affecting that body system (See the documentation section on diabetes mellitus)

Diabetes Mellitus General Coding and Sequencing Guidelines

As many codes within a particular category as are necessary to describe all the complications of the diabetes mellitus may be assigned. Sequencing is based on the reason for the encounter. As many codes from categories E08-E13 as are necessary to completely identify all of the associated conditions that the patient has should be assigned.

Type 1 Diabetes Mellitus:

- The age of the patient is not the sole determining factor for a diagnosis of type 1 diabetes
- Type 1 diabetes typically develops before puberty and for this reason type 1 diabetes is also referred to as juvenile diabetes

Type of Diabetes Not Documented:

- If the type of diabetes mellitus is not documented in the medical record, the default is E11.- Type 2 diabetes mellitus.

Diabetes Mellitus and the Use of Insulin:

- If use of insulin is documented, but the type of diabetes mellitus is not documented:
  - Assign a code from category E11 Type 2 diabetes mellitus
  - Assign code Z79.4 Long-term (current) use of insulin to indicate that the patient uses insulin or assign code Z79.84 Long term (current) use of oral hypoglycemic drugs to indicate that the patient uses oral hypoglycemic drugs
  - If the patient is treated with both oral medications and insulin, assign only the code for long term (current) use of insulin
  - If the patient is treated with both insulin and an injectable non-insulin antidiabetic drug, assign codes Z79.4 Long-term (current) use of insulin, and Z79.899 Other long term (current) drug therapy. If the patient is treated with both oral hypoglycemics and an injectable non-insulin antidiabetic drug, assign codes Z79.84 Long-term (current) use of oral hypoglycemic drugs, and Z79.899 Other long-term (current) drug therapy
  - Do not assign code Z79.4 if insulin is given temporarily to bring a Type 2 patient's blood sugar under control during an encounter

Diabetes Mellitus in Pregnancy and Gestational Diabetes:

- For diabetes mellitus in pregnancy, see guidelines for Chapter 15 Pregnancy, Childbirth, and the Puerperium

Complications of Insulin Pump Malfunction:

- Underdose of insulin due to insulin pump failure:
  - Principal/First-listed diagnosis code—Assign a code from subcategory T85.6- Mechanical complication of other specified internal and external prosthetic devices, implants and grafts to specify the type of pump malfunction (e.g., breakdown, displacement)
  - Second code—Assign code T38.3x6- Underdosing of insulin and oral hypoglycemic [antidiabetic] drugs
  - Additional codes—Assign additional codes to identify the type of diabetes mellitus and any associated complications due to the underdosing
- Overdose of insulin due to insulin pump failure:
  - Principal/First-listed diagnosis code—Assign a code from subcategory T85.6- Mechanical complication of other specified internal and external prosthetic devices, implants and grafts to specify the type of pump malfunction (e.g., breakdown, leakage, perforation)
  - Second code—Assign code T38.3x1- Poisoning by insulin and oral hypoglycemic [antidiabetic] drugs, accidental (unintentional)

Secondary Diabetes Mellitus:

- Always caused by another condition or event (e.g., pancreatectomy, pancreatic cancer, cystic fibrosis, adverse effect of a drug, poisoning)
- Three categories, which include:
  - E08 Diabetes mellitus due to underlying condition
  - E09 Drug or chemical induced diabetes mellitus
  - E13 Other specified diabetes mellitus
- Use of insulin
  - For patients who routinely use insulin or oral hypoglycemic drugs, assign code Z79.4 Long term (current) use of insulin or Z79.84 Long term (current) use of oral hypoglycemic drugs
  - If the patient is treated with both oral medications and insulin, assign only the code for long term (current) use of insulin
  - If the patient is treated with both insulin and an injectable non-insulin antidiabetic drug, assign codes Z79.4 Long-term (current) use of insulin, and Z79.899 Other long term (current) drug therapy. If the patient is treated with both oral hypoglycemics and an injectable non-insulin antidiabetic drug, assign codes Z79.84 Long-term (current) use of oral hypoglycemic drugs, and Z79.899 Other long-term (current) drug therapy
  - Do not assign code Z79.4 for temporary use of insulin to bring a patient's blood sugar under control during an encounter
- Assigning and sequencing secondary diabetes codes and its causes
  - Sequencing of secondary diabetes codes in relation to causative codes is based on tabular instructions
    - » For E08 Diabetes mellitus due to underlying condition, the underlying condition is coded first followed by the diabetes code(s)
    - » For E09 Drug or chemical induced diabetes mellitus, the drug or chemical poisoning (T36-T65) is coded first followed by the diabetes code(s)
  - Secondary diabetes due to pancreatectomy
    - » Principal/First listed diagnosis—Assign code E89.1 Postprocedural hypoinsulinemia
    - » Assign a code from category E13 Other specified diabetes mellitus
    - » Assign an additional code from subcategory Z90.41- Acquired absence of pancreas
    - » Assign code Z79.4 to identify any current, long-term use of insulin
  - Secondary diabetes due to drugs
    - » May be caused by an adverse effect of correctly administered medications, by poisoning, or as a late effect of poisoning
    - » See guidelines in Chapter 19 Injury, poisoning, and certain other consequences of external causes and Chapter 20 External causes of morbidity for additional coding guidelines

General Documentation Requirements

There are some general documentation requirements related to coding endocrine, nutritional, and metabolic diseases. Like all body system chapters, intraoperative and postprocedural complications specifically affecting the endocrine system are listed within this body system chapter, although in two different categories, which will be discussed next. Gout is not listed here, but is classified to another body system. Both chronic types of gout and acute gout attacks are found within the musculoskeletal system chapter and must be reported by type, site, and the presence or lack of tophi.

Intraoperative and Postprocedural Complications NEC

Intraoperative and postprocedural complications are typically found in the same code block at the end of the chapter. However, for endocrine, nutritional, and metabolic diseases, these complications are handled differently. Because intraoperative complications apply only to the endocrine system, codes for intraoperative complications are found in category E36 at the end of the endocrine system section of Chapter 4. Postoperative complications apply to the endocrine system and to metabolic disorders and are found at the end of the chapter in category E89.

Intraoperative complications located in category E36 are those related to intraoperative hemorrhage and hematoma (E36.0-) and accidental puncture and laceration (E36.1-) of an endocrine system organ or structure. These codes are specific to the procedure performed which must be designated as complicating an endocrine system procedure or complicating a procedure on organs or structures in another body system. There is also a code for other specified intraoperative complications of the endocrine system (E36.8-).

Conditions in category E89 include those that relate to changes in endocrine function due to removal of part or all of the endocrine gland, or damage to the gland such as that caused by radiation therapy. Following removal or damage of an endocrine gland, hormones produced by that gland are absent or lower than normal. In some cases, these hormones must be replaced by medication. For example, in the case of hypoinsulinemia or hyperglycemia caused by removal of the pancreas, insulin must be administered. For other postprocedural conditions such as ovarian failure, replacement of the hormones is not always required. This category also reports postprocedural hemorrhage or hematoma. These codes differentiate between hemorrhage or hematoma that results from a procedure on an endocrine system organ or structure, and hemorrhage or hematoma that results from a procedure on another body system or organ.

Reclassification of Codes

Some conditions have traditionally or formerly been considered one particular type of disease or disorder, but were later determined to fit more appropriately in another group and have consequently been moved in their clinical listing. For instance, gout was formerly considered a metabolic disorder but is now classified as an inflammatory polyarthropathy along with conditions like rheumatoid arthritis, juvenile arthritis, and other crystal arthropathies in the musculoskeletal chapter. Some specific cerebral degenerative disorders were traditionally considered nervous system diseases, such as leukodystrophy and cerebral lipidoses, but are now listed as disorders of sphingolipid metabolism and other lipid storage disorders in category E75. Certain congenital conditions are also listed in category E78 Disorders of lipoprotein metabolism and other lipidemias that were formerly classified as congenital anomalies.

Combination Codes

As has already been discussed in the guidelines, diabetes mellitus codes are combination codes that include the type of diabetes, the body system affected, and the specific complication in that body system, as well as laterality, when applicable. It is not necessary to assign a code from the diabetes category and one or more codes from other chapters to identify the complications or manifestations of the diabetes, although additional codes may be used to identify the complication or manifestation with even greater clarity.

Code-Specific Documentation Requirements

In this section, the appropriate codes for the named condition are listed and their documentation requirements are identified. The focus is on frequently reported conditions with specific clinical documentation requirements, particularly those that may differ in their present reporting from formerly accepted classification. Though not all of the codes with updated documentation requirements are discussed, this section will provide a representative sample of the type of additional documentation required for coding endocrine, nutritional, and metabolic diseases. The section is organized alphabetically with related diseases or conditions grouped together.

Cushing's Syndrome

Cushing's syndrome is an endocrine disorder that occurs when the body is exposed to high levels of the hormone cortisol. This may result from excessive intake of corticosteroids (e.g., prednisone) or by an overproduction of cortisol in the adrenal glands (e.g., adrenal gland tumors). Overproduction of the hormone may also be triggered by an excess of ACTH production by the pituitary gland (e.g., pituitary tumor), or by ACTH-producing or cortisol-producing tumors in other areas of the body such as the lungs, pancreas, or thyroid.

Multiple codes are available for Cushing's syndrome that identify the specific type or cause of Cushing's syndrome (E24). Documentation must specifically state the condition as pituitary-dependent Cushing's disease, drug-induced, alcohol-induced pseudo-Cushing's syndrome, Nelson's syndrome, Ectopic ACTH syndrome, or other specified type of Cushing's syndrome for proper code assignment.

Coding and Documentation Requirements

Identify type of Cushing's syndrome:

- Alcohol-induced pseudo-Cushing's syndrome
- Drug-induced
- Ectopic ACTH syndrome
- Nelson's syndrome
- Pituitary-dependent Cushing's disease
- Other specified type of Cushing's syndrome
- Unspecified Cushing's syndrome

Use an additional code for drug-induced Cushing's syndrome, if applicable, to identify the drug (T36-T50 with fifth or sixth character 5).

ICD-10-CM Code/Documentation	
E24.0	Pituitary-dependent Cushing's disease
E24.1	Nelson's syndrome
E24.2	Drug-induced Cushing's syndrome
E24.3	Ectopic ACTH syndrome
E24.4	Alcohol-induced pseudo-Cushing's syndrome
E24.8	Other Cushing's syndrome
E24.9	Cushing's syndrome unspecified

Documentation and Coding Example

Intake Note: Forty-year-old Caucasian male admitted for inpatient detoxification from excessive alcohol use. He has always been a social drinker but began **binge drinking approximately 12 weeks ago** after the sudden death of his wife. Friends describe his moods as very erratic and he has been unable to work for the past 3 weeks. He is a chef and owns a number of high-end restaurants with a group of investors. On examination, this is an unkempt man of medium height and weight. His face has a round cushingoid appearance with supraclavicular fat pads present and a small fat pad at the base of neck/upper back. Blood is drawn for CBC, coagulation studies, comprehensive metabolic panel, serum cortisol, TSH, and toxicology screen. A urine sample is obtained for toxicology and a 24-hour urine collection for cortisol and creatinine is started. Salivary cortisol will be obtained this evening. There are numerous areas of ecchymosis in varying stages of healing, patient cannot recall exactly how or why they appeared. Patient states his last alcohol intake was about 2 hours ago. He denies use of prescription, OTC, or illegal drugs. He is oriented to the facilities and his individual program.

Progress Note: Labs are significant for elevated salivary cortisol, serum transaminase, and BGL. WBCs moderately elevated at 15,000 with no left shift to indicate acute infection, serum potassium is low. Still awaiting 24-hour urine cortisol and creatinine results. Urine and serum toxicology screen positive for ethanol only.

Diagnosis: **Episodic ethanol abuse with alcohol-induced pseudo-Cushing's syndrome.**

Plan: Ethanol detoxification and behavioral therapy. Monitor labs closely. Anticipate 30 day inpatient stay.

Diagnosis Code(s)

F10.10 Alcohol abuse, uncomplicated

E24.4 Alcohol-induced pseudo-Cushing's syndrome

Coding Note(s)

The patient is admitted for treatment of his alcohol abuse. The pseudo-Cushing's syndrome is a secondary diagnosis. Category F10 reports alcohol related disorders and there are three subcategories—F10.1 Alcohol abuse; F10.2 Alcohol dependence; and F10.9 Alcohol use, unspecified. The physician must clearly document the condition being treated. In this case, the diagnosis is alcohol abuse without any accompanying mental or behavioral complications that would be reported in a combination code. The only related complication identified is the pseudo-Cushing's syndrome, so code F10.10 is reported. There is also a code for alcohol abuse with other alcohol-induced disorders (F10.188), but codes in Chapter 5 are reported for mental and behavioral disorders, not for other physical or physiological medical conditions associated with the alcohol abuse, so code F10.188 would not be appropriate. The endocrine condition caused by the alcohol abuse is reported with a code from the endocrine chapter, E24.4. There is a note under category F10 to use additional code for blood alcohol level, if applicable. No blood alcohol level has been documented here, but if it had been provided, a code from category Y90 would also be reported.

Diabetes Mellitus

In ICD-10-CM, code categories include diabetes mellitus due to an underlying condition (E08); drug or chemical induced diabetes mellitus (E09); Type 1 diabetes mellitus (E10); Type 2 diabetes mellitus (E11); and other specified diabetes mellitus (E13). Other specified types of diabetes mellitus include diabetes due to identified genetic defects, such as defects of beta cell function or insulin action, as well as secondary diabetes due to surgery (postpancreatectomy, postprocedural). Diabetes not specified as due to an underlying cause and not specified as Type 1 or Type 2 is reported as Type 2 diabetes by default. Since these categories are available for identifying and reporting differing types of diabetes, it is important for the underlying cause of the diabetes to be documented.

Diabetes codes also capture the body system affected in the 4th character with the complication or manifestation typically identified by the 5th character. The 6th character allows for capture of multiple complications or manifestations often seen together such as diabetic retinopathy with macular degeneration. The 7th character denotes laterality, such as left eye or right eye. Each individual code does not, however, capture whether or not the diabetes is controlled or uncontrolled. Diabetes documented as uncontrolled or poorly controlled is captured by reporting an additional code for hyperglycemia. For example, Type II diabetes documented as poorly controlled as evidenced by elevated blood sugar (hyperglycemia) would be reported with code E11.65. As many diabetes codes as are necessary to report the complete clinical picture of all manifestations and complications of the diabetic patient should be reported.

The underlying condition, or drug or chemical poisoning identified as the cause of secondary diabetes is reported as the first-listed diagnosis with the secondary diabetes code listed next. Fourth character subcategories for secondary diabetes identify the body system affected by the complication, with the specific complication or manifestation identified by the fifth character. Some secondary diabetes codes capture multiple complications or manifestations with the sixth character, and some report laterality with a seventh character. This means that to capture the most specific code, providers will need to document not only the underlying cause but also clearly describe all complications and manifestations. Documenting any long-term insulin use is also required.

Capturing the correct code for diabetes mellitus requires clear and precise documentation of the underlying cause. Secondary diabetes is defined as a diabetic condition with an underlying cause other than genetics or environmental conditions and includes diabetes mellitus secondary to drugs and chemicals or due to an underlying disease, medical condition, surgical procedure, or trauma. Some of the drugs and chemical agents identified as causing secondary diabetes include:

- Anticonvulsants
- Antihypertensive drugs including diuretics and beta blockers
- Antipsychotics including lithium and some antidepressants
- Antiretroviral drugs
- Chemotherapy drugs
- Hormone supplements, including:
  - Anabolic steroids
  - Contraceptives
  - Estrogen
  - Growth hormones
  - Hormones prescribed for prostate cancer
- Immunosuppressive drugs including corticosteroids

Some of the other causes of secondary diabetes include:

- Autoimmune diseases
- Carcinoid tumors of some sites, including:
  - Gastrointestinal tract
  - Lungs
- Endocrine disorders, including:
  - Cushing's syndrome
  - Excessive levels of growth hormones
  - Hyperthyroidism
- Hemochromatosis
- Liver diseases, including:
  - Hepatitis C
  - Fatty liver disease
- Pancreatic disease or injury, including:
  - Chronic pancreatitis
  - Pancreatic cancers
  - Pancreatic damage due to malnutrition
  - Other endocrine diseases that affect pancreatic function or damage the insulin-producing beta cells
- Trauma to the pancreas

Surgical procedures may also result in secondary diabetes mellitus. Procedures most often associated with secondary diabetes include total or partial removal of the pancreas for malignant neoplasm or severe pancreatic disease, or orchiectomy performed for testicular or prostate cancer.

Coding and Documentation Requirements

Identify the type of diabetes mellitus:

- Drug or chemical induced
- Due to underlying condition
- Type 1
- Type 2
- Other specified diabetes mellitus, which includes:
  - Due to genetic defects of beta-cell function
  - Due to genetic defects in insulin action
  - Postpancreatectomy
  - Postprocedural
  - Secondary diabetes not elsewhere classified

Identify the body system affected, the manifestations or complications, and laterality, when applicable:

- Arthropathy
  - Neuropathic
  - Other arthropathy
- Circulatory complications
  - Peripheral angiopathy
    - » With gangrene
    - » Without gangrene
  - Other specified circulatory complication
- Hyperglycemia
- Hyperosmolarity
  - with coma
  - without coma
- Hypoglycemia
  - With coma
  - Without coma
- Ketoacidosis
  - With coma
  - Without coma
- Kidney complications
  - Diabetic nephropathy
  - Chronic kidney disease
  - Other diabetic kidney complication
- Neurological complications
  - Amyotrophy
  - Autonomic (poly)neuropathy
  - Mononeuropathy
  - Polyneuropathy
  - Other specified neurological complication
  - Unspecified diabetic neuropathy
- Ophthalmic complications
  - Diabetic retinopathy
    - » Mild nonproliferative
      - o With macular edema
      - o Without macular edema
    - » Moderate nonproliferative
      - o With macular edema
      - o Without macular edema
    - » Severe nonproliferative
      - o With macular edema
      - o Without macular edema
    - » Proliferative
      - o With macular edema
      - o Without macular edema
      - o With traction retinal detachment involving the macula

- With traction retinal detachment not involving the macula
- With combined traction retinal detachment and rhegmatogenous retinal detachment

» Stable proliferative

» Unspecified diabetic retinopathy

- With macular edema
- Without macular edema

– Diabetic macular edema, resolved following treatment

– Laterality

» Right eye

» Left eye

» Bilateral

» Unspecified eye

– Diabetic cataract

– Other diabetic ophthalmic complication

- Oral complications
  - Periodontal disease
  - Other oral complications
- Skin complication
  - Dermatitis
  - Foot ulcer
  - Other skin ulcer
  - Other skin complication
- Other specified complication
- Unspecified complication
- Without complications

Example 1

Type 1 Diabetes Mellitus with Ophthalmic Manifestations

ICD-10-CM Code/Documentation			
E10.311	Type 1 diabetes mellitus with unspecified diabetic retinopathy with macular edema	E10.319	Type 1 diabetes mellitus with unspecified diabetic retinopathy without macular edema
E10.321-	Type 1 diabetes mellitus with mild nonproliferative diabetic retinopathy with macular edema	E10.329-	Type 1 diabetes mellitus with mild nonproliferative diabetic retinopathy without macular edema
E10.331-	Type 1 diabetes mellitus with moderate nonproliferative diabetic retinopathy with macular edema	E10.339-	Type 1 diabetes mellitus with moderate nonproliferative diabetic retinopathy without macular edema
E10.341-	Type 1 diabetes mellitus with severe nonproliferative diabetic retinopathy with macular edema	E10.349-	Type 1 diabetes mellitus with severe nonproliferative diabetic retinopathy without macular edema

ICD-10-CM Code/Documentation			
E10.351-	Type 1 diabetes mellitus with proliferative diabetic retinopathy with macular edema	E10.359-	Type 1 diabetes mellitus with proliferative diabetic retinopathy without macular edema
E10.352-	Type 1 diabetes mellitus with proliferative diabetic retinopathy with traction retinal detachment involving the macula	E10.353-	Type 1 diabetes mellitus with proliferative diabetic retinopathy with traction retinal detachment not involving the macula
E10.354-	Type 1 diabetes mellitus with proliferative diabetic retinopathy with combined traction retinal detachment and rhegmatogenous retinal detachment	E10.355-	Type 1 diabetes mellitus with stable proliferative diabetic retinopathy
E10.36	Type 1 diabetes mellitus with diabetic cataract	E10.39	Type 1 diabetes mellitus with other diabetic ophthalmic complication
E10.37X-	Type 1 diabetes mellitus with diabetic macular edema, resolved following treatment	Note: 1 2 3 9	Subcategories E10.32-E10.35 and E10.37 require a 7th digit to denote laterality: right eye left eye bilateral unspecified eye

Documentation and Coding Example

Thirty-eight-year-old Caucasian female is seen in ophthalmology for ongoing diabetes related eye problems. Patient experienced onset of **Type I diabetes mellitus** at age seven. She has experienced rare episodes of DKA and has kept fairly tight glycemic control using an insulin pump for the past 10 years. She has no renal, hepatic, or peripheral vascular involvement, no elevated lipids or triglycerides. Last HbA1c was 6.5 %. She had stable, mild nonproliferative diabetic retinopathy for many years with no visual acuity problems; however, patient is now 6 months post-delivery of a healthy baby boy and during her pregnancy **her retinopathy advanced to moderate nonproliferative in both eyes, and she developed signs of macular edema in her right eye**. Fundoscopy exam performed today under stereopsis and high magnification reveals **stable areas of microaneurysms in left eye and no evidence of macular edema**. Exam of **right eye shows microaneurysms and retinal hemorrhage, thickening, and focal edema consistent with macular edema**. These findings are virtually unchanged from 3 months ago. Near and far visual acuity remains at 20/30 in each eye. Patient is advised that she is not a candidate for treatment at this time. She is encouraged to continue with her excellent control of BGL and reminded to see her endocrinologist regularly. She will return in 3 months for continued monitoring of her retinopathy and macular edema.

Diagnosis Code(s)

E10.3311 Type 1 diabetes mellitus with moderate non-proliferative diabetic retinopathy with macular edema, right eye

E10.3392 Type 1 diabetes mellitus with moderate non-proliferative diabetic retinopathy without macular edema, left eye

Coding Note(s)

A combination code captures the Type 1 diabetes mellitus, the body system affected (eye), and the specific complication, which in this case includes both moderate non-proliferative diabetic retinopathy and macular edema, present only in the right eye. Laterality is a component of diabetes codes with all types of diabetic retinopathy and also for cases of diabetic macular edema resolved following treatment. Since the left eye shows no signs of macular edema, the code for moderate non-proliferative diabetic retinopathy without macular edema is reported.

Example 2

Secondary Diabetes with Neurological Complications

ICD-10-CM Code/Documentation			
E08.41	Diabetes mellitus due to underlying condition with diabetic mononeuropathy	E08.40	Diabetes mellitus due to underlying condition with diabetic neuropathy, unspecified
E09.41	Drug or chemical induced diabetes mellitus with neurological complications with diabetic mononeuropathy	E09.40	Drug or chemical induced diabetes mellitus with neurological complications with diabetic neuropathy, unspecified
E13.41	Other specified diabetes mellitus with diabetic mononeuropathy	E13.40	Other specified diabetes mellitus with diabetic neuropathy, unspecified
E08.43	Diabetes mellitus due to underlying condition with diabetic autonomic (poly) neuropathy	E08.42	Diabetes mellitus due to underlying condition with diabetic polyneuropathy
E09.43	Drug or chemical induced diabetes mellitus with neurological complications with diabetic autonomic (poly)neuropathy	E09.42	Drug or chemical induced diabetes mellitus with neurological complications with diabetic polyneuropathy
E13.43	Other specified diabetes mellitus with diabetic autonomic (poly)neuropathy	E13.42	Other specified diabetes mellitus with diabetic polyneuropathy
E08.49	Diabetes mellitus due to underlying condition with other diabetic neurological complication	E08.44	Diabetes mellitus due to underlying condition with diabetic amyotrophy
E09.49	Drug or chemical induced diabetes mellitus with neurological complications with other diabetic neurological complication	E09.44	Drug or chemical induced diabetes mellitus with neurological complications with diabetic amyotrophy
E13.49	Other specified diabetes mellitus with other diabetic neurological complication	E13.44	Other specified diabetes mellitus with diabetic amyotrophy
		E08.610	Diabetes mellitus due to underlying condition with diabetic neuropathic arthropathy
		E09.610	Drug or chemical induced diabetes mellitus with diabetic neuropathic arthropathy
		E13.610	Other specified diabetes mellitus with diabetic neuropathic arthropathy

Documentation and Coding Example

Forty-four-year-old Caucasian female is seen by PMD for c/o fatigue, dizziness, and unusual sweating. Patient has a 20 + year history of excessive **alcohol use** and was diagnosed with **chronic calcifying pancreatitis 6 years ago** resulting from her excessive alcohol consumption. She developed diabetes 2 years ago as a result of the pancreatic disease. She has cut down on her consumption of alcohol but continues to drink **2-3 glasses of wine daily. Diabetes is fairly well controlled on Lantus and Novolog insulin**. She was experiencing low BG levels with Lantus at HS but less since the dose was split and she is injecting BID. WT 126 lbs., T 97.8, P 62, R 12, BP 104/50, O2 Sat 98% on RA, BGL=206. On examination, this is a thin, athletic appearing woman who looks her stated age. Skin is very tan, mucous membranes moist and pink, eyes are clear. She states she normally is able to play tennis or work out at the gym daily for 60-90 minutes. For the past month she finds she is exhausted after exercising and in the past week has become fatigued during the workout and has to stop. She has also noticed excessive perspiration even when she is not active. The dizziness occurs upon rising from bed and sometimes from sitting to standing. She denies falls. PERRLA, neck supple. HR regular. Pulses full and intact in extremities. No evidence of edema. Reflexes 2 + and muscle tone is good. Breath sounds clear, equal bilaterally. Abdomen is soft and flat, bowel sounds present in all quadrants. Supine BP 110/52, Sitting 90/50, Standing 90/52.

Impression: **Diabetes due to chronic calcifying pancreatitis with related new onset autonomic neuropathy, orthostatic hypotension, and excessive sweating.**

Plan: Increase salt in diet. Refer to cardiology for echocardiogram and treadmill to assess HR and BP during exercise. She is again counseled about her **use of alcohol including availability of inpatient treatment programs for her dependency**. She declines these services.

Note electronically sent to Cardiology and Endocrinologist. Follow up after Cardiology workup. Sooner if symptoms worsen.

Diagnosis Code(s)

K86.0	Alcohol-induced chronic pancreatitis
E08.43	Diabetes mellitus due to underlying condition with diabetic autonomic (poly)neuropathy
F10.20	Alcohol dependence, uncomplicated
R53.83	Other fatigue
I95.1	Orthostatic hypotension
R61	Generalized hyperhidrosis
Z79.4	Long term (current) use of insulin

Coding Note(s)

This patient has secondary diabetes which is due to chronic calcifying pancreatitis which has been more specifically documented as being caused by excessive alcohol use and dependence. She has developed a new manifestation of autonomic neuropathy which is due to her secondary diabetes. There is a code first note for category E08 indicating that the code for the underlying condition is listed first and the secondary diabetes code is listed as the second diagnosis.

Codes for secondary diabetes are combination codes that identify the body system affected and the type of complication, which has been identified as new onset diabetic autonomic neuropathy. The manner in which the diabetic autonomic neuropathy is manifesting could be any number of specified conditions, and since the actual neuropathic complication the patient is experiencing is not included in the code title, additional codes that further identify the specific autonomic complication(s) may also be reported.

Example 3

Diabetes with Gastroparesis

ICD-10-CM Code/Documentation	
E08.43	Diabetes mellitus due to underlying condition with diabetic autonomic (poly)neuropathy
E09.43	Drug or chemical induced diabetes mellitus with neurological complications with diabetic autonomic (poly)neuropathy
E10.43	Type 1 diabetes mellitus with diabetic autonomic (poly)neuropathy
E11.43	Type 2 diabetes mellitus with diabetic autonomic (poly)neuropathy
E13.43	Other specified diabetes mellitus with diabetic autonomic (poly)neuropathy

Note: All diabetes codes reporting diabetic autonomic (poly) neuropathy have an inclusion term listed underneath for that particular type of diabetes stating 'with diabetic gastroparesis'.

Documentation and Coding Example

Patient is a 60-year-old Hispanic female referred to GI Clinic by PMD for weight loss, bloating, and constipation. PMH is significant for **Type 2 diabetes** diagnosed 5 years ago and well controlled on Metformin 850 mg BID. Patient was not obese when she was diagnosed with diabetes. LADA was considered but she was subsequently found to have elevated C-Peptide levels and negative ICA, IAA, and GAD tests with no family history of autoimmune disorders. HT 63 inches, WT 94 lbs. T 96.7, P 88, R 14, BP 132/88, BGL=133. On examination, this is a thin, cachectic appearing woman who looks older than her stated age. Skin is sallow, eyes dull, hair is dry and thin. Patient states she has had a 15 lb. weight loss in 2 months due to early satiety and frequent indigestion. She also states her bowel movements have become less frequent, large and hard to pass. Oral mucosa dry and pink, throat without redness. Apical pulse normal. Breath sounds clear. Abdomen mildly distended. Bowel sounds hypoactive. There is no evidence of ascites. No pain or tenderness with palpation, liver at 2 cm below RCM, spleen at LCM. No hernia appreciated. Anal sphincter has good tone, the rectum is full of hard stool. Labs including cortisol, TSH and T4 ordered by PMD are normal.

Impression: **New onset gastroparesis with underlying Type 2 diabetes.**

Plan: EGD and colonoscopy to rule out obstruction or other disease process.

Procedure note: Patient had a satisfactory bowel prep and was NPO for procedure. IV started in right hand with LR infusing. Patient sedated with Versed and Fentanyl. EGD showed normal esophagus and stomach. Pyloric sphincter somewhat stiff but scope was passed into duodenum without difficulty. The duodenum has a few patchy areas of inflammation but no ulcer. The endoscope was withdrawn and with patient positioned on left side, the colonoscopy was performed without incident. There are no polyps, narrowing, or inflammation from rectum to cecum. A large hemorrhoid is present just inside the rectal sphincter.

Diagnosis: **Gastroparesis**

Plan: Start metoclopramide 10 mg QID, 30 minutes before meals and at bedtime. Citrucel daily. Patient would benefit from nutritional counseling since she is now underweight and she has not spoken to the dietician since her diabetes diagnosis 5 years ago. She also needs a referral to new endocrinologist, due to change in insurance. Follow up in GI clinic in 1 month.

Note electronically sent to PMD.

Diagnosis Code(s)

E11.43	Type 2 diabetes mellitus with diabetic autonomic (poly)neuropathy
K31.84	Gastroparesis

Coding Note(s)

Even though only a single code is technically required to report the type 2 diabetes with gastroparesis, since there is an inclusion term listed under code E11.43 that states "Type 2 diabetes mellitus with diabetic gastroparesis," this specific manifestation is not identified in the code title. Because the manner in which a diagnosis of diabetic autonomic neuropathy manifests in a person could be any number of specified conditions, it is appropriate to assign an additional code to identify the gastroparesis in this patient. This is supported by AHA Coding Clinic.

Example 4

Secondary Diabetes with Foot Ulcer

ICD-10-CM Code/Documentation	
E08.621	Diabetes mellitus due to underlying condition with foot ulcer
E09.621	Drug or chemical induced diabetes mellitus with foot ulcer
E13.621	Other specified diabetes mellitus with foot ulcer WITH: A code from L97.4- or L97.5- to designate site, laterality, and depth of non-pressure chronic ulcer

Documentation and Coding Example

Thirty-one-year-old Caucasian male is referred to the Wound Care Clinic by PMD for **left foot ulcer.** Patient has been **insulin dependent x 6 years after undergoing total pancreatectomy due to blunt force trauma of the abdomen following a bicycle accident.** He is very physically active and even on low doses of insulin he experiences frequent episodes of hypoglycemia. Patient is married with 2 young children and works for the county as a building inspector. Patient states he is an avid runner and sees a podiatrist regularly for toenail trimming and callus shaving. He states he noticed discomfort in **left great toe** 2 weeks ago but attributed it to an increase in his workouts as he trained for an event. After completing the event, he had increased pain in the toe and noticed the skin on the bottom of the toe looked red and swollen. Epson salt soaks did not relieve the inflammation or discomfort, the **skin began peeling and he noticed yellow drainage** on his soak. He was seen by PMD 2 days ago who did a culture and x-ray, ordered blood tests, and referred for wound care. HT 69 inches, WT 155 lbs., T 98.6, P 58, R 12, BP 104/64. On examination, this is a thin but muscular man who looks younger than his stated age. Both lower extremities have intact circulation, sensation, and movement. Pedal, dorsalis pedis, and posterior tibial pulses are all strong and equal. CRT 2-3 seconds. No sign of dystrophic nails or loss of hair. Both feet have thin plantar calluses at the edge of heels, ball of foot, and distal end of great toes. There is **localized cellulitis at distal end of left great toe, with a 1 x 1 cm crater on dorsal surface** that appears fairly superficial. There is a rim of hyperkeratotic tissue surrounding the crater with thick yellow exudate in the center. X-ray is reviewed and shows no bone involvement. CBC, serum glucose, glycohemoglobin, creatine, and HbA1c are all within normal limits. **Culture is positive for Staph aureus, sensitive to cephalexin.**

Impression: **Neurogenic foot ulcer limited to skin breakdown due to diabetes. Superimposed staph infection.**

Plan: Debridement, walking boot, Keflex 500 mg QID x 10 days. RTC in 1 week. Note electronically sent to PMD.

Diagnosis Code(s)

E89.1	Postprocedural hypoinsulinemia
E13.621	Other specified diabetes mellitus with foot ulcer
L97.521	Non-pressure chronic ulcer of other part of left foot limited to breakdown of skin
L03.032	Cellulitis of left toe
B95.61	Methicillin susceptible Staphylococcus aureus infection as the cause of diseases classified elsewhere
Z90.410	Acquired total absence of pancreas
S36.209S	Unspecified injury of unspecified part of pancreas, sequela
Z79.4	Long term (current) use of insulin
V19.9XXS	Pedal cyclist (driver) (passenger) injured in unspecified traffic accident, sequela

Coding Note(s)

This patient had a total pancreatectomy following a blunt trauma injury to the pancreas that resulted from a bicycle accident. Conditions such as secondary diabetes and complications of diabetes are sequela of the accident that necessitated the pancreatectomy. An injury code should be assigned with 7th character S to designate the sequela. In ICD-10-CM, an external cause code may also be assigned with 7th character S to designate the external cause of the sequela. Sequencing of secondary diabetes codes is based on Tabular List instructions and the official guidelines. Sequencing instructions in the Tabular List take precedence over sequencing instructions in the official guidelines.

In category E13 in the Tabular List, there are no instructions related to sequencing of codes. However, there are sequencing instructions in the official guidelines for secondary diabetes due to pancreatectomy. Code E89.1 is listed first to identify the postprocedural hypoinsulinemia. A code from category E13 is listed additionally along with a code from subcategory Z90.41- to identify the acquired absence of the pancreas.

The diabetes code E13.621 identifies the type of diabetes, body system affected, and the specific manifestation/complication as a foot ulcer. A second code is required to identify the specific site of the foot ulcer, and its stage. Even though the foot ulcer is not documented as chronic, it is documented as neurogenic and this type of ulcer codes to non-pressure chronic ulcer. The depth of the ulcer is described as superficial and limited to skin breakdown.

There is an Excludes2 note listed under category L97 for skin infections (L00-L08). However, since the patient has both a dorsal surface ulcer and a superimposed infection at the distal end of the same left toe, it is appropriate to assign both codes. An additional code is assigned to identify the causative agent as *Staphylococcus aureus.* In this case, the code for Methicillin susceptible *S. aureus* is used because the infection is sensitive to Cephalexin which is a cephalosporin. Cephalosporins are classified as beta lactam antibiotics and *S. aureus* infections that can be treated with beta lactam antibiotics, are classified as methicillin susceptible infections.

Example 5

Secondary Diabetes Mellitus with Kidney Complications

ICD-10-CM Code/Documentation	
E08.21	Diabetes mellitus due to underlying condition with diabetic nephropathy
E08.22	Diabetes mellitus due to underlying condition with diabetic chronic kidney disease
E08.29	Diabetes mellitus due to underlying condition with other diabetic kidney complication
E09.21	Drug or chemical induced diabetes mellitus with diabetic nephropathy
E09.22	Drug or chemical induced diabetes mellitus with diabetic chronic kidney disease
E09.29	Drug or chemical induced diabetes mellitus with other diabetic kidney complication
E13.21	Other specified diabetes mellitus with diabetic nephropathy
E13.22	Other specified diabetes mellitus with diabetic chronic kidney disease
E13.29	Other specified diabetes mellitus with other diabetic kidney complication

Documentation and Coding Example

Forty-nine-year-old Black male is referred to nephrology by PMD for new onset fatigue and loss of appetite with elevated serum creatinine, BUN, and proteinuria. PMH is significant for asthma since childhood, often requiring steroids, **HIV infection documented at age 25** and **diabetes, onset nine years ago following pentamidine administration for acute *Pneumocystis carinii* infection.** Patient is a dancer/choreographer, active in theater and performing arts. He is accompanied to the appointment today by his partner of 20 years. Current medications include Lantus **Insulin** 12 units HS, Novolog sliding scale AC and HS for BG correction and carbohydrate intake, Singulair 5 mg at HS, Advair Diskus 500/50 BID and Stribild 1 capsule q AM. HT 70 inches, WT 160 lbs., T 98.8, P 72, R 14, BP 140/90, O2 Sat on RA 97%, BG=112. On examination, this is a thin, muscular, immaculately groomed, articulate gentleman who appears relaxed, alert, and oriented. Patient states he has been able to maintain his active lifestyle until just a few weeks ago and thought his fatigue was simply due to holiday travel and entertainment. He had a regularly scheduled appointment with his PMD so he just planned to mention his symptoms at that time. He had routine labs done a week prior to that appointment and his doctor saw him emergently for abnormal findings. PMD's note and all labs are available for review at this appointment. PERRLA, cranial nerves grossly intact. Neck supple without lymphadenopathy. Mucous membranes moist and pink, nares patent, TMs clear. HR regular without bruit, rub, or murmur. Breath sounds have occasional soft expiratory wheeze. CSM intact to extremities, no edema noted. Abdomen soft and flat, BS active all quadrants. Liver is palpated 1 cm below RCM, spleen 2 cm below LCM. No hernia appreciated, testes down, circumcised penis without urethral drainage. Renal ultrasound performed. Findings consistent with Kimmelstiel-Wilson disease.

Impression: **Secondary diabetes due to pentamidine therapy status post 9 years ago with new onset Kimmelstiel-Wilson disease secondary to diabetes.**

Plan: Discuss findings with PMD/Infectious Disease including current use of Stribild which is contraindicated with creatinine >50. Repeat labs in 2 weeks with follow up appointment at that time.

Diagnosis Code(s)

E09.21	Drug or chemical induced diabetes mellitus with diabetic nephropathy
T37.3X5S	Adverse effect of other antiprotozoal drugs, sequela
B20	Human immunodeficiency virus [HIV] disease
Z79.4	Long term (current) use of insulin

Coding Note(s)

Pentamidine is an antiprotozoal drug that may cause severe fasting hypoglycemia as an adverse effect. Some patients who have experienced severe fasting hypoglycemia due to pentamidine administration later develop insulin dependent diabetes as a sequela (late effect) of pentamidine. Diabetes that develops as a sequela of a chemical or drug is coded as secondary diabetes. The secondary diabetes code is listed first as Tabular instructions under category E09 state to use additional code for adverse effect, if applicable, to identify the drug with fifth or sixth character 5. The patient has a documented previous admission for an HIV-related illness so the code for HIV disease is assigned for every encounter. Sequencing of HIV disease is dependent on the reason for the encounter. In this case, the patient is being seen in consultation for new onset kidney disease related to diabetes, so the HIV cannot be listed first.

The combination code E09.21 captures the type of diabetes and the body system affected as well as the nature of the complication. In this case, it is Kimmelstiel-Wilson disease, which is listed as an inclusion term under code E09.21.

Example 6

Type 1 Diabetes Mellitus Poorly Controlled (with Hyperglycemia)

ICD-10-CM Code/Documentation	
E10.65	Type 1 diabetes mellitus with hyperglycemia

Documentation and Coding Example

Thirteen-year-old Caucasian male is seen in Pediatric Endocrine Clinic accompanied by his mother. Patient is well known to this practice. He was diagnosed with **Type 1 diabetes** at age 7, presenting with acute DKA and a BGL of 535. He has had multiple hospitalizations for HHS and DKA in the past 5 years, largely due to **patient non-compliance** and poor follow through of mother. The family was referred to CWS 2 years ago when the patient, unsupervised by mother, gave an incorrect dose of insulin causing severe hypoglycemia and seizure. The family received counseling and support and for the most part they have been compliant with care.

Review of labs: **HbA1c elevated at 7.7 and triglycerides at 360.** Urine and serum positive for ketones. Anion gap 11. Kidney and liver function tests moderately elevated. HT 65 inches, WT 145 lbs., T 98.4, P 76, R 14, BP 110/66, O2 Sat on RA 99, **BGL=182.** On examination, this is a somewhat sullen and uncooperative adolescent male who communicates only a little better when his mother is asked to leave the room. Patient states he will be finishing the 7th grade in 2 months, his grades are passing, his main interest is skateboarding and he is largely unsupervised in his diabetes care and food preparation because his mother works all the time. PERRLA, skin is oily, he has mild acne on his forehead and chin, hair is clean and cut short. Oral mucosa moist and pink, posterior pharynx mildly red with cobblestone appearance and clear mucus drainage noted. Patient has a history of seasonal allergies treated with Zyrtec. He states he has not taken it in over a week because he ran out and forgot to tell his mother. Neck supple with no lymphadenopathy. HR regular. BS clear and equal. Abdomen soft and flat. Liver palpated at RCM, spleen is not palpated. No evidence of hernia, normal genitalia. CSM intact in both upper and lower extremities. He has areas of bruising and scabs on his right forearm and right knee that he states is from a fall while skateboarding. Patient states he is taking Lantus insulin 22 units at bedtime and Humalog with meals. He does check his BGL in the health office at school and doses for BGL and carbs with the assistance of a school nurse but admits to not always checking at other times. His morning meal is cold cereal, lunch is a sandwich or cheeseburger bought from school cafeteria and he snacks on diet soda, chips, and ice cream. Dinner is brought home by his mother usually pizza, burgers and fries, tacos, or chicken fingers. He does not have a very concrete understanding of carbohydrate counts for the foods he frequently consumes and **appears to be under dosing** much of the time. Patient and mother are counseled together regarding the need for tighter control of his diabetes and the health risks for his hyperglycemia.

Impression: **Type 1 diabetes poorly controlled with frequent episodes of hyperglycemia. Noncompliant with diet and BGL control.**

Plan: See dietician for food counseling. Patient to attend a one-week summer camp program for diabetic youth, scholarship will be arranged. Mother is given information on parent support groups. Patient will do daily AC and HS BG monitoring and keep a log. Mother will call his numbers in weekly along with insulin doses and carbohydrate calculations. RTC in 1 month. Patient will have blood drawn for CBC, comprehensive metabolic panel, cholesterol and lipids at least 2 days prior to appointment.

Diagnosis Code(s)

E10.65	Type 1 diabetes mellitus with hyperglycemia
Z91.11	Patient's noncompliance with dietary regimen
Z91.14	Patient's other noncompliance with medication regimen

Coding Note(s)

Diabetes described as poorly controlled or uncontrolled is reported with the code for the specific type of diabetes with hyperglycemia. Noncompliance is reported additionally, with codes for both dietary regimen and medication regimen. There are specific codes for noncompliance including codes for intentional and unintentional underdosing, and also other noncompliance. The physician has not stated whether the underdosing of insulin is intentional or unintentional, indicating that the patient does not appear to understand carbohydrate counts and appears to be underdosing. For this reason, the code Z91.14 Patient's other noncompliance with medication regimen is reported, which includes underdosing of medication NOS.

Lipoid Metabolism Disorders

Lipids are fats present in the body. Lipid metabolism refers to the breakdown of lipids into constituents that can be used by the body. Some genetic and medical conditions can cause dysfunction of lipid metabolism. The exact manifestations of dysfunction in lipid metabolism depend on the specific metabolic disorder. Some specific types of lipids include lipoproteins, sphingolipids, glycosaminoglycans, and glycoproteins.

Lipoprotein metabolic disorders and lipidemias are some of the most common types of lipoid metabolic disorders. Two types of lipoproteins found in the blood are cholesterol and triglycerides. Elevated levels of one form of cholesterol called low density lipoprotein (LDL), along with elevated levels of triglycerides, are strongly linked to atherosclerotic heart disease. Disorders of lipoprotein metabolism are often inherited diseases that cause elevated levels of remnant lipoproteins in the blood and deposits in body organs. These diseases include Barth syndrome, Smith-Lemli-Opitz syndrome, hyperchylomicronemia, familial hypercholesterolemia, pure hyperglyceridemia, and mixed and familial combined hyperlipidemia.

Sphingolipids are a class of lipids made of fatty acid derivatives of sphingosine (e.g., ceramides, gangliosides, sphingomyelins, and cerebrosides) occurring mainly in the brain and are a constituent of nervous tissue. Sphingolipid metabolic disorders are usually monogenetic inherited diseases resulting in enzymatic defects in lysosomal sphingolipid degradation. The defects cause an accumulation of lipids in one or more body organs. Diseases caused by sphingolipid metabolic disorders include Tay-Sachs, Sandhoff, Fabry-Anderson, Gaucher, Krabbe, and Niemann-Pick. Sphingolipid disorders may be treated with enzyme replacement therapy (ERT), cell mediated therapy (CMT) including bone marrow transplant (BMT), cell mediated cross correction, and gene therapy.

Glycosaminoglycan metabolic disorders are usually inherited genetic diseases that cause a failure in the breakdown of long chain sugar molecules causing them to accumulate and damage body organs. Diseases caused by glycosaminoglycan metabolic disorders include Hurler, Hurler-Scheie, Scheie, Morquio, and Sanfilippo. Glycosaminoglycan disorders are most often treated with enzyme replacement therapy (ERT).

Glycoprotein metabolic disorders are rare inherited genetic diseases characterized by a failure to synthesize or degrade glycoprotein molecules, causing them to accumulate in body organs and tissue.

ICD-10-CM includes multiple categories with subclassified specificity for many types of conditions— particularly those formerly known as lipidoses. Codes for conditions previously identified as disorders of lipoid metabolism are classified in the following 5 categories:

- E75 Disorders of sphingolipid metabolism and other lipid storage disorders
- E76 Disorders of glycosaminoglycan metabolism
- E77 Disorders of glycoprotein metabolism

- E78 Disorders of lipoprotein metabolism and other lipidemias
- E88 Other and unspecified metabolic disorders

Coding and Documentation Requirements

Identify the disorder:

- Defects of glycoprotein metabolism
  - Defects in glycoprotein degradation
  - Defects in post-translational modification of lysosomal enzymes
  - Other specified disorders in glycoprotein metabolism
  - Unspecified disorder of glycoprotein metabolism
- Disorders of glycosaminoglycan metabolism
  - Mucopolysaccharidosis, type I
    - » Hurler syndrome
    - » Hurler-Scheie syndrome
    - » Scheie syndrome
  - Mucopolysaccharidosis, type II
  - Other mucopolysaccharidoses
    - » Morquio A
    - » Morquio B
    - » Morquio, unspecified
    - » Sanfilippo
    - » Other specified types
    - » Unspecified type
  - Other specified disorders of glycosaminoglycan metabolism
  - Unspecified disorder of glycosaminoglycan metabolism
- Disorders of sphingolipid metabolism and other lipid storage disorders
  - Gangliosidosis
    - » GM2 type
      - o Sandhoff disease
      - o Tay-Sachs disease
      - o Other specified GM2 type
      - o Unspecified GM2 type
    - » Other and unspecified type
      - o Mucolipidosis IV
      - o Other gangliosidoses (includes GM1, GM3)
      - o Unspecified type gangliosidosis
  - Neuronal ceroid lipofuscinosis
  - Sphingolipidosis
    - » Fabry (-Anderson) disease
    - » Gaucher disease
    - » Krabbe disease
    - » Niemann-Pick disease
      - o Type A
      - o Type B
      - o Type C
      - o Type D
      - o Other specified type
      - o Unspecified type
    - » Metachromatic leukodystrophy
    - » Other specified sphingolipidosis
    - » Unspecified sphingolipidosis
  - Other specified type of lipid storage disorder
  - Unspecified lipid storage disorder
- Disorders of lipoprotein metabolism and other lipidemias
  - Lipidemia
    - » Hyperchylomicronemia
    - » Mixed hyperlipidemia
    - » Pure hypercholesterolemia
      - o Familial
      - o Unspecified
    - » Pure hyperglyceridemia
    - » Other hyperlipidemia
    - » Unspecified hyperlipidemia
  - Lipodystrophy, NEC/NOS
  - Lipomatosis, NEC/NOS
  - Lipoprotein deficiency
  - Other specified disorders of lipoprotein metabolism
    - » Lipoid dermatoarthritis
    - » Other specified type
  - Unspecified disorder of lipoprotein metabolism
  - Disorders of bile acid and cholesterol metabolism
    - » Barth syndrome
    - » Smith-Lemli-Opitz syndrome
    - » Other specified disorder
    - » Unspecified disorder

ICD-10-CM Code/Documentation			
E75.00	GM2 gangliosidosis	E78.00	Pure hypercholesterolemia, unspecified
E75.01	Sandhoff disease	E78.01	Familial hypercholesterolemia
E75.02	Tay-Sachs disease	E78.1	Pure hyperglyceridemia
E75.09	Other GM2 gangliosidosis	E78.2	Mixed hyperlipidemia
E75.10	Unspecified gangliosidosis	E78.3	Hyperchylomicronemia
E75.11	Mucolipidosis IV	E78.41	Elevated lipoprotein (a)
E75.19	Other gangliosidosis	E78.49	Other hyperlipidemia
E75.21	Fabry (-Anderson) disease	E78.5	Hyperlipidemia, unspecified
E75.22	Gaucher disease	E78.6	Lipoprotein deficiency
E75.23	Krabbe disease	E78.70	Disorder of bile acid and cholesterol metabolism, unspecified
E75.240	Niemann-Pick disease type A	E78.71	Barth syndrome
E75.241	Niemann-Pick disease type B	E78.72	Smith-Lemli-Opitz syndrome
E75.242	Niemann-Pick disease type C	E78.79	Other disorders of bile acid and cholesterol metabolism
E75.243	Niemann-Pick disease type D	E78.81	Lipoid dermatoarthritis
E75.248	Other Niemann-Pick disease	E78.89	Other lipoprotein metabolism disorders
E75.249	Niemann-Pick disease unspecified	E78.9	Disorder of lipoprotein metabolism, unspecified
E75.25	Metachromatic leukodystrophy		
E75.26	Sulfatase deficiency		
E75.29	Other sphingolipidosis		
E75.3	Sphingolipidosis, unspecified		
E75.4	Neuronal ceroid lipofuscinosis		
E75.5	Other lipid storage disorders		
E75.6	Lipid storage disorder, unspecified		

ICD-10-CM Code/Documentation			
E77.0	Defects in post-translational modification of lysosomal enzymes	E76.01	Hurler's syndrome
E77.1	Defects in glycoprotein degradation	E76.02	Hurler-Scheie syndrome
E77.8	Other disorders of glycoprotein metabolism	E76.03	Scheie's syndrome
E77.9	Disorder of glycoprotein metabolism, unspecified	E76.1	Mucopolysaccharidosis, type II
		E76.210	Morquio A mucopolysaccharidoses
		E76.211	Morquio B mucopolysaccharidoses
		E76.219	Morquio mucopolysaccharidoses, unspecified
		E76.22	Sanfilippo mucopolysaccharidoses
		E76.29	Other mucopolysaccharidoses
		E76.3	Mucopolysaccharidosis, unspecified
		E76.8	Other disorders of glucosaminoglycan metabolism
		E76.9	Glucosaminoglycan metabolism disorder, unspecified
		E88.1	Lipodystrophy, not elsewhere classified
		E88.2	Lipomatosis, not elsewhere classified

Documentation and Coding Example

Twenty-seven-year-old female presents to Infusion Clinic for her bi-monthly intravenous VPRIV infusion. She was diagnosed with **Gaucher's Disease** 6 months ago when she presented with a traumatic fracture, bone pain, and fatigue. Her Ashkenazi Jewish ancestry led to molecular genetic studies and the diagnosis of Gaucher's was made. She had severe osteopenia on DEXA scan at that time, decreased serum glucocerebrosidase, mild anemia, thrombocytopenia, and pinguecula. She was started on oral Miglustat which she was not able to tolerate and was switched to infusions. Intravenous VPRIV has stabilized her disease with no progression of osteopenia on DEXA scan performed last week, stable pinguecula lesions in both eyes per ophthalmology, RBCs and platelets back in normal range. Temperature 97.8, HR 78, RR 12, BP 122/80. Wt. 122 lbs. Ht. 64 inches. Skin without bruising or discoloration. PERRL, neck supple without lymphadenopathy. Heart rate regular, peripheral pulses full. Breath sounds clear and equal bilaterally. Abdomen soft and non-distended. Liver palpated at 2 cm below RCM, spleen is palpated at LCM. IV started in right hand and she is pre-medicated with oral diphenhydramine and acetaminophen. VPRIV is infused over 2 hours with only mild nausea reported by patient. Angiocath removed intact, gentle pressure applied with no excess bleeding noted.

Diagnosis: **Gaucher's Disease**

Plan: Patient will return in two weeks for repeat infusion. Standing lab orders are on file and she will have blood drawn prior to her infusion appointment.

Diagnosis Code(s)

E75.22 Gaucher disease

Coding Note(s)

Gaucher disease is a type of cerebral lipidoses, which is classified under sphingolipidoses. Sphingolipidoses are an inherited group of disorders of lipid metabolism that primarily affect the central nervous system. Each of the various types of sphingolipidoses is linked to a defect in specific lysosomal enzymes. The deficient enzyme in Gaucher disease is glucocerebrosidase which causes glucocerebrosides to accumulate in the red blood cells, liver, and spleen. Symptoms include hepatosplenomegaly, anemia, thrombocytopenia, bone pain, and a deformity of the femur referred to as an Erlenmeyer flask deformity. The pattern of inheritance for Gaucher disease is autosomal recessive and it affects primarily individuals of Ashkenazi Jewish descent.

Overweight and Obesity

Overweight is generally defined as excess body fat that can impair health. One measurement used to determine overweight is body mass index (BMI), which is a measurement of height and weight that is used to assess the total proportion of fat in the body. BMI is not, however, a direct measure of body fat. A BMI of 25-29.9 is considered overweight for most individuals.

Obesity and morbid obesity are large amounts of excess fat in the body often associated with profound health risks including diabetes, respiratory compromise, and cardiac disease. Obesity is a BMI of 30-39.9 or body weight at least 20% greater than normal for height. Morbid obesity is a BMI >40 or body weight 50-100% greater than normal for height.

Category E66 Overweight and obesity contains codes for overweight; obesity and morbid obesity due to excess calories; drug-induced obesity; morbid obesity with alveolar hypoventilation; other specified types of obesity; and unspecified obesity.

Coding and Documentation Requirements

Identify condition:

- Obesity
  - Drug-induced
  - Due to excess calories
    - Morbid (severe)
    - Other
  - Morbid/severe with alveolar hypoventilation
  - Other
  - Overweight

ICD-10-CM Code/Documentation	
E66.01	Morbid (severe) obesity due to excess calories
E66.09	Other obesity due to excess calories
E66.1	Drug induced obesity
E66.2	Morbid (severe) obesity with alveolar hypoventilation
E66.3	Overweight
E66.8	Other obesity
E66.9	Obesity, unspecified

Documentation and Coding Example

Thirty-three-year-old presents to pulmonology for pre-operative work-up prior to bariatric surgery. Temperature 97.6, HR 92, RR 16, BP 156/94, HT 62 inches, WT 282 lbs. **BMI 51.6.** Patient states she has been heavy all of her life, is recently engaged to be married, and they would like to have children. She hopes that bariatric surgery will allow her to lose weight and improve her health. She is chronically short of breath and was prescribed CPAP for sleep apnea a year ago but rarely uses it. On examination, this is a pleasant, well groomed, **morbidly obese** Black female. Breath sounds are clear in upper lobes and over bronchioles, muffled in middle and lower lobes. PFTs show decreased lung volume consistent with obesity. ABG drawn pH 7.3, PaCo2 52, HCO3 30, PaO2 75, O2 Sat 92%. Impression: **Chronic hypercapnic respiratory failure secondary to morbid obesity**. Patient is a good candidate for bariatric surgery and her respiratory condition should improve with weight loss. She is sent to cardiology to complete her pre-op testing.

Diagnosis Code(s)

E66.2 Morbid (severe) obesity with alveolar hypoventilation

Z68.43 Body mass index [BMI] 50.0-59.9, adult

Coding Note(s)

An Excludes1 note under E66.01 Morbid (severe) obesity due to excess calories indicates that E66.01 is not reported with E66.2 Morbid (severe) obesity with alveolar hypoventilation so only code E66.2 is reported for the obesity. The patient's BMI is reported additionally.

Thyroid Gland Disorders

Disorders of the thyroid gland are the first codes listed within the endocrine chapter. There are eight categories. Some disorders, such as congenital iodine deficiency syndrome (that was previously classified with congenital hypothyroidism and reported with a single code), are identified specifically as to type: neurological type (E00.0), myxedematous type (E00.1), and mixed type (E00.2). Congenital hypothyroidism is also differentiated as with or without goiter. Some acquired kinds of hypothyroid conditions also have specific codes, such as E02 Subclinical iodine-deficiency hypothyroidism (which was previously reported under other specified acquired hypothyroidism).

Hypothyroidism, Acquired

Hypothyroidism is a condition in which the thyroid gland does not produce adequate levels of thyroid hormones (thyroxine and/or T3). The most common form of hypothyroidism is due to iodine deficiency. Code E89.0 Postprocedural hypothyroidism captures hypothyroidism due to surgical and irradiation procedures. Other hypothyroid conditions also have specific codes, including E02 Subclinical iodine-deficiency hypothyroidism and E03.3 Postinfectious hypothyroidism.

Coding and Documentation Requirements

Identify acquired hypothyroidism:

- Due to acquired atrophy of thyroid gland
- Due to medicaments/exogenous substances
- Iodine deficiency related
  - Hypothyroidism
  - Subclinical hypothyroidism
- Postinfectious
- Postprocedural
- Other specified type of hypothyroidism
- Unspecified type

ICD-10-CM Code/Documentation	
E01.8	Other iodine deficiency related thyroid disorders and allied conditions
E02	Subclinical iodine-deficiency hypothyroidism
E03.2	Hypothyroidism due to medicaments and other exogenous substances
E03.3	Postinfectious hypothyroidism
E03.4	Atrophy of thyroid (acquired)
E03.8	Other specified hypothyroidism
E03.9	Hypothyroidism, unspecified
E89.0	Postprocedural hypothyroidism

Documentation and Coding Example

This 45-year-old female is 6 months status post radioactive iodine treatment for Graves' disease. She comes in to the clinic today because she is concerned about **symptoms that may be indicative of postablative hypothyroidism**. She has classic symptoms of hypothyroidism which include cold intolerance, lethargy, and weight gain. Thyroid function studies are performed including T4, free T4, T3, and TSH. Comparison with previous thyroid function studies show a progressive decline in the amount of T4, free T4, and T3 to lower than normal levels. During the same period there has been a progressive increase in TSH. Impression: Findings are consistent with **postablative hypothyroidism**.

Plan: Will begin thyroid hormone replacement therapy.

Diagnosis Code(s)

E89.0 Postprocedural hypothyroidism

Coding Note(s)

Postprocedural complications and disorders that are commonly associated with a specific body system are classified in the body system chapter. These codes are usually found in the code block at the end of the chapter. Postprocedural hypothyroidism is classified together with other postprocedural endocrine and metabolic complications and disorders, such as postprocedural hypoinsulinemia, postprocedural hypoparathyroidism, postprocedural hypopituitarism, and postprocedural ovarian or testicular failure.

Hypothyroidism, Congenital

Congenital hypothyroidism is a condition that is present at birth. It occurs when the thyroid gland does not develop properly in utero or when it does not function properly. The thyroid gland may be entirely absent or much smaller than normal. It may also be in an abnormal location. In some cases, newborns have a normal-sized or enlarged thyroid gland, but the thyroid gland does not produce adequate amounts of thyroid hormones.

The code for congenital hypothyroidism without goiter (E03.1) is reported when the thyroid is absent (aplasia of thyroid), smaller than normal (atrophy), or when the thyroid does not produce enough thyroid hormones and there is no documentation of goiter or enlargement of the thyroid. Congenital iodine deficiency syndrome in a fetus or newborn is a condition where there is an inadequate level of iodine in the body which is needed to produce thyroid hormones. This results in insufficient hormone production and slowed metabolic processes that can lead to brain damage and developmental delays. This condition may manifest with neurological or myxedematous symptoms, or with a combination of both (mixed type). Neurological symptoms include deafness/hearing loss, dysarthria, muscle spasticity (primarily in the lower extremities) and cognitive deficits. Characteristics of myxedematous type include large head and edema of the genitals and extremities. Characteristics of mixed type can include large head and edema of genitals and extremities as well as cognitive deficits, muscle spasticity, and hearing loss.

Coding and Documentation Requirements

Identify congenital condition:

- Congenital hypothyroidism
  - With goiter
  - Without goiter
- Congenital iodine-deficiency syndrome
  - Mixed type
  - Myxedematous type
  - Neurological type
  - Unspecified

ICD-10-CM Code/Documentation	
E00.0	Congenital iodine-deficiency syndrome, neurological type
E00.1	Congenital iodine-deficiency syndrome, myxedematous type
E00.2	Congenital iodine-deficiency syndrome, mixed type
E00.9	Congenital iodine-deficiency syndrome, unspecified
E03.0	Congenital hypothyroidism with diffuse goiter
E03.1	Congenital hypothyroidism without goiter

Documentation and Coding Example

Seven-day-old infant is referred to Pediatric Endocrine Clinic by PMD for abnormal Newborn Screening Test. This Hispanic male is the first child of a 33-year-old mother, 32-year-old father. He was delivered at 39.5 weeks via scheduled C-section for breech presentation. BW 3150 grams, length 51 cm, HC 35 cm. Parents report infant remained in the transition nursery for >12 hours due to sleepiness, poor tone, and problems maintaining body temperature but eventually joined mother and roomed in for the 4 days that she was hospitalized. BW on discharge was 2900 grams. Mother received assistance from a lactation consultant because infant was sleepy and feeding poorly. He was seen by pediatric nurse practitioner yesterday and parents reported infant still **feeding poorly** and weight was 2780 grams. During that appointment, clinic received a call from the lab indicating that the newborn screening test showed an abnormally low T4 level and TSH also out of range. Blood drawn for repeat TSH and Free T4 confirmed abnormal levels and infant is seen emergently today by pediatric endocrinologist. On exam this is a sleepy infant. Skin is dry and peeling. Head round, fontanels sunken, sutures override. Muscle tone is floppy. Generalized appearance of muscle wasting is present. PERRLA with normal red reflex. Mucous membranes moist and pink, no macroglossia. Palate intact. Weak suck. Nares patent. Ears normal in shape and location. TMs clear. Apical pulse regular. Breath sounds clear and equal. Abdomen soft and round with hypoactive bowel sounds. No evidence of hernia. Parents report green-yellow stool being passed 2-3 x day. Testis down, penis uncircumcised.

Impression: **Congenital hypothyroidism, dehydration**. Plan: Admit to Pediatric floor for hydration and initiate levothyroxine therapy. Possible technetium thyroid scan and radioactive iodine scan.

Diagnosis Code(s)

E03.1	Congenital hypothyroidism without goiter
P74.1	Dehydration of newborn
P92.9	Feeding problem of newborn, unspecified

Coding Note(s)

There are two codes for congenital hypothyroidism, one for with goiter and one for without goiter. There are also codes for congenital iodine deficiency syndrome. Congenital iodine deficiency syndrome may present in a fetus or newborn when there are inadequate levels of iodine to produce thyroid hormones. In this case, the documentation does not state that the newborn has congenital iodine deficiency syndrome nor is there any documentation of a goiter, so the code for congenital hypothyroidism without goiter is assigned.

The newborn also has feeding problems described only as "poor feeding". There are more specific codes for feeding problems in newborns, such as slow feeding, underfeeding, and difficulty feeding at breast, but because the condition is documented only as poor feeding, the code for unspecified feeding problem must be assigned. The newborn is being admitted for hydration as well as treatment of congenital hypothyroidism so the dehydration is reported additionally. Note that it is a specific code for dehydration of newborn.

Simple and Unspecified Goiter/ Nontoxic Nodular Goiter

Goiter refers to any abnormal enlargement of the thyroid gland. A simple goiter refers to diffuse enlargement of the thyroid gland that is not caused by inflammation or malignant disease. Thyroid function is usually normal with a simple goiter. A nontoxic goiter is an enlarged thyroid gland that may also be described more specifically as a uninodular or multinodular goiter. Nontoxic goiters do not affect thyroid function so thyroid function tests are normal.

Nontoxic goiters are reported with codes from three categories: E01 Iodine-deficiency related thyroid disorders and allied conditions, E03 Other hypothyroidism, and E04 Other nontoxic goiter. A simple goiter is classified as a nontoxic diffuse goiter and is included in category E04 Other nontoxic goiter along with codes for nontoxic uninodular and multinodular goiters.

Coding and Documentation Requirements

For nontoxic goiter, identify type:

- Diffuse
  - Iodine deficiency related
  - With congenital hypothyroidism
  - Other nontoxic diffuse (simple)
- Multinodular
  - Iodine deficiency related
  - Other nontoxic multinodular
- Single thyroid nodule (uninodular)
- Other specified type nontoxic goiter
- Unspecified
  - Iodine deficiency related (not described as diffuse or multinodular)
  - Unspecified nontoxic goiter (nodular, NOS)

ICD-10-CM Code/Documentation	
E04.0	Nontoxic diffuse goiter
E04.1	Nontoxic single thyroid nodule
E04.2	Nontoxic multinodular goiter
E04.8	Other specified nontoxic goiter
E04.9	Nontoxic goiter, unspecified
E01.0	Iodine-deficiency related diffuse (endemic) goiter
E01.1	Iodine-deficiency related multinodular (endemic) goiter
E01.2	Iodine-deficiency related (endemic) goiter, unspecified
E03.0	Congenital hypothyroidism with diffuse goiter

Documentation and Coding Example

Fifty-one-year-old Black female is seen for **annual physical exam**. She states she has been feeling well and has no new complaints. She continues to work full time as a pharmacist, her husband's landscaping business is doing well and her daughters are both in high school, one active in drama and the other in sports. PMH includes dysfunctional uterine bleeding treated with endometrial ablation 3 years ago, hypertension x 20 years treated with Lopressor 50 mg BID and hypothyroid treated with Synthroid 50 mcg. QD. HT 66 in. WT 168 lbs. T 97.9, P 72, R 14, BP 138/88. On examination, this is a well-developed, well-nourished female who looks her stated age. Eyes clear, PERRLA. Nares patent. Oral mucosa moist and pink. Neck supple, there is some fullness noted in the right side of the thyroid gland, patient denies cough or hoarseness, dysphagia, or problems breathing. No lymphadenopathy appreciated. Cranial nerves grossly intact. Carotid arteries are without murmur, bruit, or rub. Apical pulse regular without murmur and peripheral pulses strong and equal. Breath sounds clear and equal bilaterally. Abdomen soft, bowel sounds present in all quadrants. Liver palpated at 2 cm below RCM, spleen is not palpated. Breast and gynecological exams are deferred as patient had a mammogram and saw her GYN 6 months ago and a note is available in the chart stating exam was WNL. There are scattered skin tags across her back, consistent with location of her bra. Discussed lab work which was done prior to visit. CBC, metabolic and cholesterol/lipid panel are WNL. Her TSH is 3.38 so she will continue on present dose of Synthroid. BP appears well controlled on Lopressor. Written RX for both medications are given to patient. Discussed the need for colonoscopy now that she is over age 50 and patient states she will make an appointment. Thyroid ultrasound can be done today in radiology and patient is sent over for that procedure and will return afterward for results.

Post procedure note: Per radiologist, thyroid ultrasound shows a 1.0 x 1.5 cystic mass on right side of the thyroid. The walls are irregular with fine debris noted within the lumen of the cyst. The thyroid vasculature appears normal and no blood vessels are within the cyst.

Impression: Hemorrhagic colloid cyst. Recommend repeat ultrasound in 2-3 months.

Patient was apprised of the findings from the ultrasound and agrees with the watch and follow plan with repeat US in 2 months.

Diagnosis Code(s)

Z00.01	Encounter for general adult medical examination with abnormal findings
E04.1	Nontoxic single thyroid nodule
I10	Essential hypertension
E03.9	Hypothyroidism, unspecified

Coding Note(s)

The reason for the encounter is an annual routine general medical examination so that is the first listed diagnosis. The patient has two chronic conditions, hypertension and hypothyroidism. These conditions were evaluated and affect the patient care so they are reported additionally. A new finding is the mass on the right side of the thyroid which is evaluated by ultrasound and determined to be cystic in nature. The thyroid cyst has been more specifically described as a colloid cyst.

There are two codes for reporting general adult medical examinations, one for without abnormal findings and another for with abnormal findings. In this case, the patient has chronic conditions as well as a new abnormal finding of a cystic mass of the thyroid, so the code for examination with abnormal findings is reported. Under Cyst, thyroid, the Alphabetic Index identifies E04.1 Nontoxic single thyroid nodule as the correct code, and colloid nodule (cystic) (thyroid) is listed as an inclusion term under E04.1 in the Tabular List. Codes for essential hypertension and unspecified hypothyroidism are also reported.

Thyrotoxicosis with or without Goiter

Thyrotoxicosis is a hypermetabolic clinical condition which occurs with elevated circulating levels of the thyroid hormones, thyroxine and/or T3, in blood serum. This condition may result from destruction of thyroid gland follicles and thyrocytes associated with thyroiditis or from the excessive intake of exogenous thyroid hormones. It may also occur due to functionally active neoplasms. Symptoms of thyrotoxicosis include sudden weight loss without decrease in caloric intake, tachycardia, increased appetite, nervousness, anxiety, restlessness, irritability, tremor, sweating, changes in menstrual cycle and bowel habits, fatigue, muscle weakness, sleep disturbances, and changes in skin and hair.

Thyrotoxicosis may occur with or without enlargement of the thyroid gland (toxic goiter) and may be complicated by thyrotoxic crisis or storm. Thyroid crisis or storm is a rare but severe complication of hyperthyroidism (elevated thyroid function). The condition is often precipitated by physical illness or stress. Symptoms can include elevated body temperature and heart rate, cardiac arrhythmias, vomiting, diarrhea, dehydration, and in extreme cases, even coma and death.

Toxic goiters are classified as diffuse or nodular. For nodular goiters there are two subcategories, one for a toxic single thyroid nodule, and another for toxic multinodular goiter. If the documentation does not specify single or multiple nodules, a code for thyrotoxicosis with toxic multinodular goiter is used. There is also a subcategory for thyrotoxicosis factitia, which is elevated thyroid function caused by the voluntary or involuntary ingestion of large amounts of exogenous thyroid hormone.

Coding and Documentation Requirements

For thyrotoxicosis, identify as with or without goiter:

- With goiter
  - Diffuse (simple)
  - Nodular
    - » Uninodular (single thyroid nodule)
    - » Multinodular
  - Unspecified
- Without goiter
  - Ectopic thyroid tissue
  - Thyrotoxicosis factitia
  - Other specified origin
  - Unspecified

Identity presence or absence of thyrotoxic crisis or storm:

- With thyrotoxic crisis or storm
- Without thyrotoxic crisis or storm

ICD-10-CM Code/Documentation	
E05.00	Thyrotoxicosis with diffuse goiter without thyrotoxic crisis or storm
E05.01	Thyrotoxicosis with diffuse goiter with thyrotoxic crisis or storm
E05.10	Thyrotoxicosis with toxic single thyroid nodule without thyrotoxic crisis or storm
E05.11	Thyrotoxicosis with toxic single thyroid nodule with thyrotoxic crisis or storm
E05.20	Thyrotoxicosis with toxic multinodular goiter without thyrotoxic crisis or storm
E05.21	Thyrotoxicosis with toxic multinodular goiter with thyrotoxic crisis or storm
E05.30	Thyrotoxicosis from ectopic thyroid tissue without thyrotoxic crisis or storm
E05.31	Thyrotoxicosis from ectopic thyroid tissue with thyrotoxic crisis or storm
E05.40	Thyrotoxicosis factitia without thyrotoxic crisis or storm
E05.41	Thyrotoxicosis factitia with thyrotoxic crisis or storm
E05.80	Other thyrotoxicosis without thyrotoxic crisis or storm
E05.81	Other thyrotoxicosis with thyrotoxic crisis or storm
E05.90	Thyrotoxicosis, unspecified without thyrotoxic crisis or storm
E05.91	Thyrotoxicosis, unspecified with thyrotoxic crisis or storm

Documentation and Coding Example

Preoperative Diagnosis: Enlarged thyroid

Postoperative Diagnosis: **Hypersecretory Thyroid Malignancy with Thyrotoxicosis**

History: This 26-year-old Caucasian female has been referred by her PMD for evaluation of a diffusely enlarged thyroid with symptoms of thyrotoxicosis. Over the past few months she has experienced weight loss, restlessness, and anxiety which she attributed to the stress of a new job. During her annual examination her PMD noted a **diffusely enlarged thyroid. Thyroid function studies obtained at that time were elevated, consistent with hyperthyroidism**. She presents today for ultrasound guided needle biopsy of her thyroid.

Operative Note: The skin over the thyroid gland was cleansed and a local anesthetic was administered. Using ultrasound guidance, the biopsy needle was introduced into the thyroid and a tissue sample was obtained. Three additional sites are biopsied using the same technique. The tissue samples are prepared and sent to the laboratory for pathological exam.

Pathological Findings: The findings are consistent with **malignant neoplasm of the thyroid**.

Plan: Refer to Oncology for additional work-up and treatment of her **functionally active thyroid malignancy**, hypersecretion of thyroid hormones, and resulting thyrotoxicosis.

Diagnosis Code(s)

C73	Malignant neoplasm of thyroid gland
E05.80	Other thyrotoxicosis without thyrotoxic crisis or storm

Coding Note(s)

The malignancy is sequenced first followed by a code from the endocrine chapter to capture the thyrotoxicosis. Even though the thyroid is enlarged, the enlargement is due to a malignant neoplasm, so the condition is not classified as a goiter. Following instructions in the chapter level note related to neoplasms that are functionally active, an additional code is assigned to capture the functional activity. The chapter level note identifies the subcategory for functional activity of the thyroid due to malignancy as E05.8-. In this case the patient is experiencing thyrotoxicosis but there is no documented thyrotoxic crisis or storm, so code E05.80 is assigned.

Thyroiditis/Other Disorders of the Thyroid

Thyroiditis is an inflammation of the thyroid gland, usually accompanied by pain and swelling. Thyroiditis is classified as acute, subacute, and chronic. Autoimmune thyroiditis is classified as a chronic form of thyroiditis. Thyroiditis may also be caused by certain drugs and medicinal agents. Acute thyroiditis is a rare condition as the thyroid gland is normally resistant to microorganisms that cause infection due to the level of iodine in the tissue, the high degree of vascularity, and a good lymphatic drainage system. The condition usually follows an upper respiratory infection and a pyriform sinus fistula is frequently present. Symptoms include fever, pain, swelling, dysphagia, and dysphonia. Thyroid hormones T3, T4, and TSH levels are usually normal. Subacute thyroiditis is usually precipitated by a viral upper respiratory infection and presents with fever, malaise, and pain/swelling in the anterior neck/thyroid gland. The condition causes thyrotoxicosis due to the sudden discharge of stored thyroid hormone. Other names for this disorder include: De Quervain's thyroiditis, giant cell thyroiditis, granulomatous or subacute granulomatous thyroiditis. Chronic thyroiditis is usually caused by an autoimmune response. Hashimoto's thyroiditis is the most common form of chronic thyroiditis. Other chronic types include chronic fibrous thyroiditis, ligneous thyroiditis, and Riedel thyroiditis.

Other disorders of the thyroid include hypersecretion of calcitonin and dyshormonogenetic goiter. A thyroid cyst is classified as a nontoxic single thyroid nodule and is reported with code E04.1. Sick euthyroid syndrome is no longer considered as sign or symptom and is coded within the endocrine chapter. Acquired atrophy of the thyroid is coded in category E03 Other hypothyroidism.

Coding and Documentation Requirements

Identify thyroiditis/other thyroid disorders:

- Thyroiditis
  - Acute
  - Autoimmune
  - Chronic
    - » With transient thyrotoxicosis
    - » Other (includes fibrous, ligneous, Riedel)
  - Drug-induced
  - Subacute
  - Unspecified
- Other thyroid disorder
  - Hypersecretion of calcitonin
  - Dyshormonogenetic goiter
  - Other specified disorder (includes hemorrhage/infarction)
  - Sick euthyroid syndrome
  - Unspecified disorder

ICD-10-CM Code/Documentation	
E06.0	Acute thyroiditis
E06.1	Subacute thyroiditis
E06.2	Chronic thyroiditis with transient thyrotoxicosis
E06.3	Autoimmune thyroiditis
E06.4	Drug-induced thyroiditis
E06.5	Other chronic thyroiditis
E06.9	Thyroiditis, unspecified
E07.0	Hypersecretion of calcitonin
E07.1	Dyshormonogenetic goiter
E07.81	Sick euthyroid syndrome
E07.89	Other specified disorders of thyroid
E07.9	Disorder of thyroid, unspecified

Documentation and Coding Example

This 47-year-old white male presents for follow-up on **Riedel thyroiditis**. Initial symptoms included a thyroid mass, hypocalcemia, and hypothyroidism. Thyroid uptake scan was performed with malignancy and Grave's disease ruled out. Other systemic symptoms all pointed to chronic thyroiditis. A needle biopsy was performed and histopathological exam of thyroid tissue confirmed Riedel thyroiditis. There was no compression of the trachea and it was elected to begin treatment with corticosteroids. He has been treated for the past month with corticosteroids with some improvement of symptoms. On examination, the thyroid enlargement is stable. No complaints of difficulty swallowing or any symptoms indicating airway compression. Continue with corticosteroid therapy. Return in one month for re-evaluation, sooner if any worsening of symptoms.

Diagnosis Code(s)

E06.5 Other chronic thyroiditis

Coding Note(s)

Riedel thyroiditis is a rare type of chronic inflammatory thyroiditis in which dense fibrotic growth replaces the normal thyroid tissue and eventually extends beyond the thyroid capsule to invade surrounding neck structures. Cases of chronic fibrous types of thyroiditis are classified together as other chronic thyroiditis.

Vitamin, Mineral, and Other Nutritional Deficiencies

Vitamin and mineral deficiencies may result from inadequate intake—not getting enough of certain nutrients in the diet, or they may result from an inability of the body to break down and absorb, or utilize, the specific vitamin, mineral, or other nutrient properly. Nutritional deficiencies are classified into different code categories based on the specific vitamin, mineral, or other nutrient that is lacking, and sometimes the manifesting condition of that particular deficiency. Certain vitamin and mineral or other deficiencies, such as enzymes, that occur due to a metabolic dysfunction are not reported as a nutritional deficiency, but are reported as a metabolic disorder, sometimes by the particular known pathway or mechanism, and/or resulting condition.

Documentation must clearly differentiate between deficiencies caused by nutritional/dietary factors and those caused by metabolic disorders. For instance, a vitamin D deficiency from lack of dietary intake that results in rickets is reported under category E55 Vitamin D deficiency, with a code specific for rickets, E55.0 Rickets, active. Vitamin D deficiency resulting from an inherited defect in the receptors for vitamin D is reported with E83.32 Hereditary vitamin D-dependent rickets (type 1) (type 2). Rickets that results from an inherited resistance to vitamin D is reported with E83.31 Familial hypophosphatemia.

Dietary deficiencies of minerals and other nutrients are captured by codes in categories E50-E64. There is a category for other nutritional deficiencies (E63) that captures more generalized conditions such as essential fatty acid (EFA) deficiencies, imbalance of nutritional constituents due to food intake, as well as other specified types of nutritional deficiencies. Category E64 reports the sequelae of certain vitamin or other nutritional deficiencies. The documentation must clearly identify the mineral or other nutrient deficiency so that the most specific code can be assigned.

Coding and Documentation Requirements

Identify the dietary deficiency of the specific vitamin/mineral/nutrient element:

- Calcium
- Chromium
- Copper
- Iron
- Magnesium
- Manganese
- Molybdenum
- Selenium
- Vanadium
- Zinc
- Vitamin A
- Vitamin B
  - Niacin
  - Thiamin
  - Riboflavin
  - Pyridoxine
  - Other B group (biotin, cyanocobalamin, folic acid, pantothenic acid)
  - Vitamin C (ascorbic acid)
  - Vitamin D
  - Vitamin E
  - Vitamin K
- Other vitamins
- Multiple nutrient elements
- Other specified nutrient elements
- Unspecified nutrient element
- Other nutritional deficiencies:
- Essential fatty acid
- Imbalance of constituents of food intake
- Other specified nutritional deficiencies
- Unspecified nutritional deficiency

Identify any sequelae of nutritional deficiencies:

- Protein-calorie malnutrition
- Vitamin A deficiency
- Vitamin C deficiency
- Rickets
- Other nutritional deficiencies
- Unspecified nutritional deficiency

ICD-10-CM Code/Documentation	
E50.0	Vitamin A deficiency with conjunctival xerosis
E50.1	Vitamin A deficiency with Bitot's spot and conjunctival xerosis
E50.2	Vitamin A deficiency with corneal xerosis
E50.3	Vitamin A deficiency with corneal ulceration and xerosis
E50.4	Vitamin A deficiency with keratomalacia
E50.5	Vitamin A deficiency with night blindness
E50.6	Vitamin A deficiency with xerophthalmic scars of cornea
E50.7	Other ocular manifestations of vitamin A deficiency
E51.11	Dry beriberi
E51.12	Wet beriberi
E51.2	Wernicke's encephalopathy
E51.8	Other manifestations of thiamine deficiency
E51.9	Thiamine deficiency, unspecified
E52	Niacin deficiency [pellagra]
E53.0	Riboflavin deficiency
E53.1	Pyridoxine deficiency
E53.8	Deficiency of other specified B group vitamins
E53.9	Vitamin B deficiency, unspecified
E54	Ascorbic acid deficiency
E55.0	Rickets, active
E55.9	Vitamin D deficiency, unspecified
E56.0	Deficiency of vitamin E
E56.1	Deficiency of vitamin K
E56.8	Deficiency of other vitamins
E56.9	Vitamin deficiency, unspecified
E58	Dietary calcium deficiency
E59	Dietary selenium deficiency
E60	Dietary zinc deficiency
E61.0	Copper deficiency
E61.1	Iron deficiency
E61.2	Magnesium deficiency
E61.3	Manganese deficiency
E61.4	Chromium deficiency
E61.5	Molybdenum deficiency
E61.6	Vanadium deficiency
E61.7	Deficiency of multiple nutrient elements
E61.8	Deficiency of other specified nutrient elements
E61.9	Deficiency of nutrient element, unspecified
E63.0	Essential fatty acid [EFA] deficiency
E63.1	Imbalance of constituents of food intake
E63.8	Other specified nutritional deficiencies
E63.9	Nutritional deficiency, unspecified
E64.0	Sequelae of protein-calorie malnutrition
E64.1	Sequelae of vitamin A deficiency
E64.2	Sequelae of vitamin C deficiency
E64.3	Sequelae of rickets
E64.4	Sequelae of other nutritional deficiencies
E64.5	Sequelae of unspecific nutritional deficiency

Documentation and Coding Example

Twenty-four-year-old Caucasian female presents to PMD for routine physical and concerns about some unusual symptoms. Patient has spent the past 2 years doing post-graduate research in the Middle East on drought resistant crops. She was well until 2 months ago when her supply of vitamin and mineral supplements ran out. She has noticed a marked decrease in energy level, loss of body hair, and intermittent diarrhea. Additionally, she has a fine red rash that she states started on her face and has now spread to her hands and feet. She states she eats a strict vegan diet including unleavened bread and is not taking any supplemental products. Temperature 97.6, HR 60, RR 12, BP 110/72, Wt. 112, Ht. 65 inches. On examination, this is a thin, but healthy appearing young woman. She is deeply tanned and states she is outdoors much of the time and does use sunscreen on her face, but rarely on the rest of her body. The hair on her head is very thin and brittle in texture. Body hair is quite sparse. A fine red rash is noted on cheeks and forehead, hands and feet. PERRL, neck supple without lymphadenopathy. Thyroid gland is smooth and normal size. Mucous membranes are pale pink, moist. Cranial nerves grossly intact. HR regular without bruit, rub, murmur. Peripheral pulses full, reflexes normal. Breath sounds clear, equal bilaterally. Breast exam is benign. Abdomen soft with active BS. Liver palpated at RCM, spleen at LCM. Pelvic exam is unremarkable, a routine pap test is performed. Patient is monogamous and at low risk for STD. A quick internet search was done while patient was getting dressed and it is possible her symptoms are due to zinc deficiency. Discussed findings with patient and lab tests ordered including CBC, CRP, ESR, comprehensive metabolic panel, Zinc, D3, TSH, cholesterol and lipid panel, UA, stool for O & P. Patient is advised to start taking a vitamin-mineral supplement and referred to a nutritionist to evaluate her diet. RTC in 1 week for test results.

Follow-Up Visit: **Labs were significant for low serum zinc levels**. Patient is prescribed zinc supplements in addition to the multi-vitamin/mineral she is taking. She will see the nutritionist in 2 days and patient is given copies of all lab reports to share with her. Diarrhea has resolved and rash is fading. Overall, she is feeling more energetic. She is advised to RTC in 3 months and we will repeat labs at that time. She should return sooner if she has any concerns.

Diagnosis: **Dietary zinc deficiency**

Diagnosis Code(s)

E60 Dietary zinc deficiency

Summary

Endocrine, metabolic, and nutritional diseases require clear and precise documentation to capture the most specific code. In order to capture the most specific code for diabetes mellitus, the chapter guidelines must be studied and the Includes and Excludes notes for each diabetes mellitus category reviewed prior to code assignment. Diabetic codes with ophthalmic complication of diabetic retinopathy require specification of the type of retinopathy with or without macular edema and laterality. Obesity will require specific documentation as to cause. Cushing syndrome is reported based on its related causative inducement or type. Dysfunctions of lipid metabolism are grouped based on the type of lipid and the specific metabolic disorder.

Resources

Documentation checklists are available in Appendix A for the following condition(s):

- Diabetes Mellitus

Chapter 4 Quiz

1. What type of diabetes mellitus would NOT be classified in category E13 Other specified diabetes mellitus?
   a. Diabetes mellitus due to pancreatectomy
   b. Insulin resistant diabetes
   c. Diabetes due to genetic defects in insulin action
   d. Secondary diabetes not elsewhere classified
2. What diagnosis documented below would necessitate the assignment of code Z79.4 for long term (current) use of insulin?
   a. Use of insulin for temporary control of blood glucose in a patient with Type 2 diabetes
   b. Type 1 diabetes treated with an insulin pump
   c. Postpancreatectomy diabetes mellitus treated with daily insulin injections
   d. All of the above
3. Which condition described below would NOT be reported with a code from category E08 Diabetes mellitus due to underlying condition?
   a. Diabetes mellitus due to Cushing's syndrome
   b. Diabetes mellitus due to hyperthyroidism
   c. Diabetes mellitus juvenile type
   d. Diabetes mellitus due to liver disease
4. What is the principal or first listed code for secondary diabetes due to pancreatectomy?
   a. A code from category E13 Other specified diabetes mellitus
   b. A code from category E08 Diabetes mellitus due to underlying condition
   c. Z90.41 Acquired absence of pancreas
   d. E89.1 Postprocedural hypoinsulinemia
5. What documentation must be present to assign the proper code(s) for diabetes with ophthalmic complication of diabetic retinopathy?
   a. Type of diabetes and specific type of diabetic retinopathy
   b. Whether or not macular edema is present, or type of retinal detachment
   c. Laterality of affected eye(s)
   d. All of the above
6. What information must be clearly documented to allow assignment of the most specific code for a vitamin or mineral deficiency?
   a. Signs and symptoms that support a diagnosis of a vitamin or mineral deficiency
   b. Any suspected conditions that might cause malabsorption of the specific vitamin or mineral
   c. Laboratory results showing a lower than normal level of the vitamin or mineral in the blood
   d. The underlying cause as due to a dietary/nutritional deficiency or a metabolic disorder
7. What information is captured with codes in category E24 Cushing syndrome?
   a. Type and cause of Cushing's syndrome
   b. The duration of the condition
   c. The drug or drugs that caused the condition
   d. All of the above
8. What information is NOT needed to assign the most specific code for obesity?
   a. Cause
   b. Severity
   c. Whether or not it is complicated by alveolar hypoventilation
   d. Body mass index
9. Pure hypercholesterolemia, NOS is classified as what type of disorder?
   a. Nutritional
   b. Metabolic
   c. Endocrine
   d. Other and unspecified condition
10. The external cause of an overdose of insulin documented as due to insulin pump malfunction is always coded as:
   a. An adverse effect
   b. Poisoning, accidental
   c. Poisoning, undetermined
   d. No external cause code is assigned

See next page for answers and rationales.

Chapter 4 Answers and Rationales

1. What type of diabetes mellitus would NOT be classified in category E13 Other specified diabetes mellitus?

   b. Insulin resistant diabetes

   Rationale: *Insulin resistant diabetes is another way of describing Type 2 diabetes mellitus which is reported with a code from category E11. The other three types—postpancreatectomy diabetes, diabetes due to genetic defects in insulin action, and secondary diabetes not elsewhere classified are all reported with codes from category E13.*

2. What diagnosis documented below would necessitate the assignment of code Z79.4 for long term (current) use of insulin?

   c. Postpancreatectomy diabetes mellitus treated with daily insulin injections

   Rationale: *Since the patient requires daily insulin injections, code Z79.4 is assigned in addition to the appropriate code(s) for other specified diabetes, where postpancreatectomy diabetes mellitus is reported. An additional code is not reported for insulin use in Type 1 diabetes mellitus. An additional code is not reported for temporary use of insulin to bring blood glucose under control in patients with Type 2 diabetes mellitus.*

3. Which condition described below would NOT be reported with a code from category E08 Diabetes mellitus due to underlying condition?

   c. Diabetes mellitus juvenile type

   Rationale: *Diabetes mellitus juvenile type is reported with a code for Type 1 diabetes.*

4. What is the principal or first listed code for secondary diabetes due to pancreatectomy?

   d. E89.1 Postprocedural hypoinsulinemia

   Rationale: *According to the coding guidelines, codes are assigned as follows:*

   - Principal/First listed diagnosis - Assign code E89.1 Postprocedural hypoinsulinemia

   - Assign a code from category E13 Other specified diabetes mellitus

   - Assign an additional code from subcategory Z90.41- Acquired absence of pancreas

5. What documentation must be present to assign the proper code(s) for diabetes with ophthalmic complication of diabetic retinopathy?

   d. All of the above

   Rationale: *The type of diabetes must be known to choose the correct diabetes category. The particular type of diabetic retinopathy must be documented, such as specified type of proliferative or nonproliferative diabetic retinopathy. Whether or not macular edema is present, or the type of retinal detachment present, is also identified in the code selection, as is the laterality.*

6. What information must be clearly documented to allow assignment of the most specific code for a vitamin or mineral deficiency?

   d. The underlying cause as due to a dietary/nutritional deficiency or a metabolic disorder

   Rationale: *Vitamin and mineral deficiencies must be clearly identified as due to a dietary deficiency or due to a metabolic disorder. Dietary vitamin and mineral deficiencies are reported with codes in categories E50-E64. Metabolic disorders resulting in vitamin and mineral deficiencies are reported with codes in categories E70-E88.*

7. What information is captured with codes in category E24 Cushing syndrome?

   a. Type and cause of Cushing's syndrome

   Rationale: *Codes in category E24 identify the specific type and cause of Cushing's syndrome. The duration of the condition is not captured by the code nor is the specific drug or drugs that caused the condition when it is documented as drug-induced.*

8. What information is NOT needed to assign the most specific code for obesity?

   d. Body mass index

   Rationale: *The cause (drug-induced, due to excess calories), severity (morbid or other), and whether or not morbid obesity is complicated by alveolar hypoventilation are required to assign the most specific code. The body mass is not required, but should be reported with an additional code from category Z68 when documented.*

9. Pure hypercholesterolemia, NOS is classified as what type of disorder?

   b. Metabolic

   Rationale: *Pure hypercholesterolemia is reported with code E78.0 which is listed in code block E70-E88 Metabolic disorders. The code category E78 identifies the condition more specifically as a disorder of lipoprotein metabolism.*

10. The external cause of an overdose of insulin documented as due to insulin pump malfunction is always coded as:

    b. Poisoning, accidental

    Rationale: *According to coding guidelines, the external cause of overdose due to insulin pump malfunction is reported with code T38.3x1- Poisoning by insulin and oral hypoglycemic [antidiabetic] drugs, accidental (unintentional).*

Chapter 5
MENTAL, BEHAVIORAL, AND NEURODEVELOPMENTAL DISORDERS

Introduction

Mental disorders are described as alterations in thinking, mood, or behavior which are associated with distress and impaired functioning. Many mental disorders have an organic origin, where disease or injury causes the mental or behavioral condition.

Examples of mental and behavioral disorders include:

- Conditions caused by substance abuse
- Psychotic and delusional conditions such as schizophrenia
- Mood disorders such as depression and mania
- Developmental disorders, such as hyperactivity, and intellectual disabilities
- Behavioral and personality disorders such as those caused by stress or trauma

Codes for mental, behavioral, and neurodevelopmental disorders are located in Chapter 5. The broad categories of mental and behavioral disorders include organic origin, psychotic and non-psychotic disorders, intellectual disabilities, and personality disorders. Chapter 5 has 100 categories of disorders related to mental, behavioral and neurodevelopmental conditions. Most of these categories require detailed documentation of the disorder in order to accurately make code assignments.

Codes for mental, behavioral and neurodevelopmental disorders are arranged based upon common characteristics. A good illustration of this is the grouping of schizophrenia together with delusional disorders in code block F20-F29. The table below shows the category blocks for mental and behavioral disorders.

ICD-10-CM Blocks	
F01-F09	Mental Disorders Due to Known Physiological Disorders
F10-F19	Mental and Behavioral Disorders Due to Psychoactive Substance Use
F20-F29	Schizophrenia, Schizotypal, Delusional, and Other Non-Mood Psychotic Disorders
F30-F39	Mood [Affective] Disorders
F40-F48	Anxiety, Dissociative, Stress-related, Somatoform and Other Nonpsychotic Mental Disorders
F50-F59	Behavioral Syndromes Associated with Physiological Disturbances and Physical Factors
F60-F69	Disorders of Adult Personality and Behavior
F70-F79	Intellectual Disabilities
F80-F89	Pervasive and Specific Developmental Disorders
F90-F98	Behavioral and Emotional Disorders with Onset Usually Occurring in Childhood and Adolescence
F99	Unspecified Mental Disorder

Many codes in ICD-10-CM include sequencing instructions. For example, in coding intellectual disability, the classification instructs to code first any associated physical or developmental disorders. Therefore, all associated physical, psychiatric, or developmental disorders must be documented.

Example

ICD-10-CM Code/Documentation
Intellectual Disabilities (F70-F79) Code first any associated physical or developmental disorders

Exclusions

In addition to general chapter level notes that provide coding instructions, many chapters have chapter level exclusions. In Chapter 5 there are only Excludes2 notes which are listed below.

Excludes1	Excludes2
None	Symptoms, signs and abnormal clinical laboratory findings, not elsewhere classified (R00-R99)

Symptoms and signs related to cognition, perception, emotional state, and behavior must be clearly differentiated in the documentation from mental, behavioral, and neurodevelopmental disorders. For example, auditory hallucinations are a complication or symptom of some mental disorders, such as schizophrenia or drug psychosis. When auditory hallucinations are part of a mental disorder, the appropriate code from Chapter 5 is used rather than a symptom code. However, auditory hallucinations may have other causes and until a definitive diagnosis is made the symptom code R44.0 would be used.

Terminology in ICD-10-CM

The clinical terminology used to describe mental and behavioral disorders in ICD-10-CM reflects advances in diagnosis and treatment of mental and behavioral disorders. This includes the classification of disorders as "mixed" to define disorders that have a combination of mixed symptoms that do not fall under a simple psychiatric label. An example would be F44.7 Conversion disorder with mixed symptom presentation.

The term "disorder" is used in the classification, rather than terms such as "disease" and "illness". "Disorder" describes a clinically recognizable set of symptoms or behaviors which are, in most cases, associated with interference with personal function and distress. Behaviors that do not interfere with personal function would then not be considered as a mental disorder.

Commonly used terms "substance abuse" and "substance dependence" are classified as separate conditions, so the terms "abuse" and "dependence" can no longer be used interchangeably in clinical documentation.

Clinical Nosologies for Mental and Behavioral Disorders

A variety of clinical nosologies are used to describe mental and behavioral disorders. In the United States, psychiatrists, psychologists, physicians, and other mental health professionals use two separate classifications of diagnoses: the *Diagnostic and Statistical Manual of Mental Disorders Fifth Edition* (DSM-5) from the American Psychiatric Association (APA), and Chapter 5 of the U.S. *Clinical Modification of the International Classification of Diseases* (ICD-10-CM). Mental health professionals rely on the DSM-5 for guidance in the assessment and diagnosis process of mental disorders. The DSM-5 however is not a coding system. The table below provides an example that compares these classification systems.

DSM-V Descriptor	ICD-10-CM Code/Documentation	
Conversion Disorder (Functional Neurological Symptom Disorder)	F44.4	Conversion disorder with motor symptom or deficit
	F44.5	Conversion disorder with seizures or convulsions
	F44.6	Conversion disorder with sensory symptom or deficit
	F44.7	Conversion disorder with mixed symptom presentation

Standardization of the terms used to diagnose and describe mental, behavioral, and neurodevelopmental disorders is essential in the identification and treatment of these conditions. The APA and Centers for Disease Control and Prevention (CDC) have worked together to develop a common structure and descriptive diagnoses between the DSM-5 and the mental disorders classification in ICD-10-CM.

The DSM contains information for every official psychiatric disorder. Included with the diagnosis documentation are separate notations for psychosocial, environmental and disability determinations. Each diagnostic listing includes specific diagnostic criteria and an overview of the disorder. The overview discusses diagnostic features, subtypes, qualifiers such as sudden onset or chronic, any associated disorders, social, cultural, age and/or gender prevalence, course of the disorder, family patterns, functional consequences, differential diagnosis, and comorbidities. ICD-10-CM includes related groupings of disorders and many are similar to DSM-5; however, DSM-5 often has greater specificity. DSM-5 is not a code set but a diagnosis resource for trained clinicians. DSM-5 incorporates the ICD-10-CM codes in the manual where appropriate. The following table illustrates the similarities and differences:

Major Depressive Disorder

DSM-V Descriptor	ICD-10-CM Code/Documentation	
Mild	F23.0	Major depressive disorder, single episode, mild
	F33.0	Major depressive disorder, recurrent, mild
Moderate	F32.1	Major depressive disorder, single episode, moderate
	F33.1	Major depressive disorder, recurrent, moderate
Severe	F32.2	Major depressive disorder, single episode, severe without psychotic features
	F32.3	Major depressive disorder, single episode, severe with psychotic features
	F33.2	Major depressive disorder, recurrent severe without psychotic features
	F33.3	Major depressive disorder, recurrent, severe with psychotic symptoms
In partial remission	F32.4	Major depressive disorder, single episode, in partial remission
	F33.41	Major depressive disorder, recurrent, in partial remission
In full remission	F32.5	Major depressive disorder, single episode, in full remission
	F33.42	Major depressive disorder, recurrent, in full remission
With anxious distress; • Mild • Moderate • Moderate-severe • Severe With mixed features With melancholic features With atypical features With psychotic features With mood-congruent psychotic features With mood-incongruent psychotic features With catatonia With peripartum onset With seasonal pattern	F33.40 F33.8 F33.9	Major depressive disorder, recurrent, in remission, unspecified Other recurrent depressive disorders Major depressive disorder, recurrent, unspecified

Chapter Guidelines

Detailed guidelines are provided for coding certain conditions classified in Chapter 5 including:

- Pain disorders with related psychological factors
- Mental and behavioral disorders due to psychoactive substance use

Pain Related to Psychological Disorders

Pain disorders with related psychological factors need to be clearly distinguished in the documentation from other pain disorders.

Documentation of any psychological component to acute or chronic pain is essential for code assignment of these conditions. Specific guidelines are as follows:

- Pain exclusively related to psychological factors – Assign code F45.41 Pain disorder exclusively related to psychological factors. Do not assign a code from category G89 with code F45.41.

- Pain disorders with related psychological factors – Assign code F45.42 Pain disorder with related psychological factors, and a second code from category G89 Pain not elsewhere classified, for a documented psychological component with acute or chronic pain

Additional guidelines for coding other pain conditions are found in Chapter 6 Diseases of the Nervous System. These guidelines relate to coding of pain not elsewhere classified (G89) and those guidelines are reviewed in the nervous system chapter of this book.

Mental and Behavioral Disorders Due to Psychoactive Substance Use

Specific guidance is provided for coding psychoactive substance use, abuse, and dependence. As with all other diagnoses, the codes for psychoactive substance use, abuse, and dependence may only be assigned based on provider documentation. Coding guidelines are as follows:

- "In remission" code selection – Selection of "in remission" codes in categories F10-F19 requires the provider's clinical judgment. Codes for "in remission" are assigned only on the basis of provider documentation unless otherwise instructed by the classification.
- Mild substance use disorders in early or sustained remission are classified as substance abuse in remission, while moderate or severe substance use disorders in early or sustained remission are classified as substance dependence in remission.
- Psychoactive substance use, abuse, dependence – When documentation refers to use, abuse, or dependence of the same substance, only one code is assigned based on the following hierarchy:
  - If both use and abuse are documented, assign only the code for abuse
  - If both use and dependence are documented, assign only the code for dependence
  - If use, abuse and dependence are all documented, assign only the code for dependence
  - If both abuse and dependence are documented, assign only the code for dependence
- Psychoactive substance use, unspecified – Codes for unspecified psychoactive substance use (F10.9-, F11.9-, F12.9-, F13.9-, F14.9-, F15.9-, F16.9-, F18.9-, F19.9-) should only be assigned based on provider documentation when the psychoactive substance use meets the definition of a reportable diagnosis, and only when the psychoactive substance use is associated with a physical disorder included in chapter 5 (such as sexual dysfunction and sleep disorder), or a mental or behavioral disorder whose relationship is documented by the provider.

General Documentation Requirements

Clinical documentation for mental disorders requires such specifics as the acuity of the disease (i.e., acute or chronic), the etiology, and any associated manifestations or complications. When a patient suffers from more than one mental disorder at the same time, such as depressive illnesses with substance abuse or anxiety disorders, detailed documentation is needed for each diagnosis and treatment.

Some mental disorders have an organic origin, while others are caused by substance abuse, stress, or trauma. Mental and behavioral disorders may also result from developmental disorders or intellectual disabilities, so clearly documenting the underlying etiology of diseases is imperative.

When two conditions are linked by the terms "with" or "in" should be interpreted as meaning "associated with" or "due to" whenever it appears in a code title, Alphabetic Index, or an instructional note in the Tabular List. The classification presumes a causal relationship between the two conditions linked by these terms. These conditions should be coded as related even in the absence of provider documentation explicitly linking them, unless the documentation clearly states the conditions are unrelated, or another guideline specifically requires a documented link between two conditions.

Organic mental or behavioral disorders are caused by a physiological condition (e.g., disease or injury), so many codes in this section require documentation of the underlying disorder. Dementia is a manifestation of many diseases with the most common form of dementia being Alzheimer's disease. Documentation should clarify dementia related to other conditions and the specific type of dementia should be documented. When dementia has an associated behavioral disturbance, the behavior must also be specified. For example, Alzheimer's disease may also be associated with delirium or behavioral disturbance, so these should be documented when present and additional codes assigned.

Example

Diagnosis: Alzheimer's dementia with wandering off

ICD-10-CM Code/Documentation	
G30.9	Alzheimer's disease, unspecified
F02.81	Dementia in other diseases classified elsewhere, with behavioral disturbance
Z91.83	Wandering in diseases classified elsewhere

Note: Because Alzheimer's dementia is a manifestation diagnosis, the guidelines specify a sequencing order requiring the etiology (Alzheimer's disease) to be listed first. Codes specified as "in other diseases classified elsewhere" indicate they are a manifestation code. A more detailed discussion of coding for Alzheimer's disease will be provided in Chapter 6 – Diseases of the Nervous System.

As with most diseases, mental disorders can range from mild to severe. In some patients, mental illness is so severe it interferes with a patient's ability to function. Documenting the severity of mental illnesses such as schizophrenia, bipolar disorder, and severe forms of depression is particularly important.

Code-Specific Documentation Requirements

In this section, documentation requirements for code categories, subcategories, and subclassifications for some of the more frequently reported mental, behavioral, and neurodevelopmental disorders are discussed. Although not all codes with documentation requirements are covered, this section provides a representative sample of the documentation needed to assign codes at the highest level of specificity.

Anorexia Nervosa and Other Eating Disorders

Eating disorders are complex illnesses that can be life threatening. Anorexia nervosa is a complex eating disorder characterized by food restrictions that can lead to malnutrition and/or starvation. The disorder is grounded in a negative body self-perception called body dysmorphia and includes an irrational fear of weight gain. Bulimia nervosa is also a complex eating disorder characterized by frequent, recurrent episodes of overeating called binging followed by purging which involves forced vomiting, ingestion of laxatives and/or diuretics. The patient may also fast or exercise excessively. Individuals with this binge/purge disorder are more likely to have a normal, healthy body weight or be slightly overweight but are unhappy with their body image.

Eating disorders such as anorexia nervosa and bulimia nervosa are classified in code block F50-F59 Behavioral syndromes associated with physiological disturbances and physical factors. Category F50 contains codes for anorexia nervosa, bulimia nervosa, avoidant/restrictive food intake disorder, and other eating disorders. The codes for these conditions are described in detail and as a result, require detailed documentation.

Coding and Documentation Requirements

Specify type of eating disorder:

- Anorexia nervosa
  - Binge eating/purging type
  - Restricting type
  - Unspecified
- Avoidant/restrictive food intake disorder
- Bulimia nervosa
- Binge eating disorder
- Other type, which includes:
  - Pica
  - Psychogenic loss of appetite
- Unspecified, which includes:
  - Atypical anorexia nervosa
  - Atypical bulimia nervosa

Note: The codes for these eating disorders are not assigned when the conditions are present due to a mental disorder classified elsewhere or are of organic origin. Documentation of the etiology and any associated mental or organic illness is necessary.

Eating Disorders

ICD-10-CM Code/Documentation	
F50.00	Anorexia nervosa, unspecified
F50.01	Anorexia nervosa, restricting type
F50.02	Anorexia nervosa, binge eating/purging type
F50.2	Bulimia nervosa
F50.81	Binge eating disorder
F50.82	Avoidant/restrictive food intake disorder
F50.89	Other specified eating disorder
F50.9	Eating disorder, unspecified (includes atypical anorexia nervosa/ atypical bulimia nervosa)

Documentation and Coding Example

This 17-year-old female patient, 5'4" and 96 lbs., with a BMI of 16.5, was seen by her gynecologist after missing 3 menstrual periods in a row and becoming noticeably moody. The patient was noted to be abnormally thin and pale and her hair had thinned considerably since her last annual check-up. Pregnancy was ruled out. Electrocardiogram was negative for arrhythmia and labs ordered for anemia, to check electrolytes, and liver and kidney function, and a bone density test to check for osteoporosis. Patient was diagnosed with amenorrhea and referred for psychiatric evaluation for an eating disorder.

Patient presents today for psychiatric consultation with her mother who describes her daughter as "a picky eater" who never ate very much but who **has become "obsessive" in her dietary habits to prevent weight gain**. Mother tried cooking special dishes, in vain. States daughter exercises all the time, even when she is sick which she states is often. Her daughter's appearance and behavior have become very concerning.

The patient maintains that she is fine and is simply stressed out about school and grades, causing the moodiness. Patient denies self-induced vomiting or misuse of laxatives, diuretics, or enemas. She explains her diet is not "extreme" rather just "portion control" and avoidance of "fattening foods". Her exercise regimen is not to lose weight, but to ensure she doesn't become "fat" after being teased for being chubby in middle school.

Assessment: **Restrictive anorexia nervosa**

Plan: Cognitive-behavioral individual and group therapy and nutritional counseling. Eating disorder educational and support group information provided to patient. Full medical evaluation and treatment of any medical issues and ongoing medical monitoring will be managed by patient's primary care physician.

Diagnosis code(s)

F50.01 Anorexia nervosa, restricting type

Coding Note(s)

Anorexia nervosa is specified as restricting type, binge eating/ purging type, or unspecified. The subtype is based upon the last 3 months of eating behaviors. Restricting type indicates individuals who present with weight loss due to dieting, fasting and/or excessive exercise but without current episodes of binge eating or purging behavior. It is not unusual during the course of the disorder that the individual will fluctuate between both the restricting type and binge eating/purging type. Diagnosis is based upon the current symptoms. Atypical anorexia nervosa is not reported with a code from subcategory F50.0, but is reported instead using the unspecified code F50.9. The codes for these eating disorders are not assigned when the conditions are present due to a mental disorder classified elsewhere or are of organic origin. Documentation of the etiology and any associated mental or organic illness is necessary.

Attention Deficit Disorder

Behavioral and emotional disorders that begin in childhood and adolescence include problems related to conduct and dissocial behavior, attention deficit (hyperactivity) disorder and tic disorders.

Attention deficit disorder (ADD) is one of the most common of these childhood disorders—and it often continues through adulthood. Symptoms include difficulty staying focused and paying attention, impulsivity, and hyperactivity. Symptoms persist for a minimum of six months and interfere with the individual's functioning or development. Clinical documentation clearly differentiating attention deficit disorder from hyperkinesia, hyperkinetic syndrome or conduct/defiance disorder, and simple disturbances of activity and attention is required.

Medical science isn't sure what causes ADD, although many studies suggest that genes play a large role. In addition to genetics, researchers are studying possible environmental factors, and how brain injuries, nutrition, and the social environment might contribute to ADD. Like many other illnesses, ADD is most likely the result of a combination of factors.

There are different subtypes of attention deficit disorder:

- Predominantly hyperactive-impulsive type: The symptoms are primarily hyperactivity (excessive motor activity at inappropriate times, excessive fidgeting, tapping or talkativeness, extreme restlessness) and impulsivity (hasty actions done without forethought with the potential to harm the individual, quick decision without thought of long-term consequences or social intrusiveness), although some degree of inattention may also be present
- Predominantly inattentive type: The majority of symptoms involve inattention (wandering off task, lacking persistence, difficulty staying focused, disorganized), although some level of hyperactivity-impulsivity may still be present
- Combined type: Symptoms of both inattention and hyperactivity-impulsivity are present but neither hyperactivity nor impulsivity is predominant. Most children have the combined type of ADD.

Attention deficit hyperactive disorder that is classified as predominantly inattentive type (F90.0) can still have documented hyperactivity but the majority of symptoms must be associated with inattention. There is also a specific code for attention deficit hyperactivity disorder that is predominantly hyperactive in type (F90.1), and another for combined type (F90.2) where there is both inattention and hyperactivity but neither inattention nor hyperactivity are predominant. The term hyperkinesis is not used and hyperkinesis is either classified as other type of attention-deficit hyperactivity disorder (F90.8) or unspecified attention-deficit hyperactivity disorder (F90.9).

Coding and Documentation Requirements

Specify type of attention deficit disorder:

- Predominantly hyperactive
- Predominantly inattentive
- Combined type
- Other type
- Unspecified type

Attention-Deficit Hyperactivity Disorder

ICD-10-CM Code/Documentation	
F90.0	Attention-deficit hyperactivity disorder, predominantly inattentive type
F90.1	Attention-deficit hyperactivity disorder, predominantly hyperactive type
F90.2	Attention-deficit hyperactivity disorder, combined type
F90.8	Attention-deficit hyperactivity disorder, other type
F90.8	Attention-deficit hyperactivity disorder, unspecified type

Documentation and Coding Example

HPI: This is an adolescent male, 13, here today for recheck of his ADHD meds.

Patient was seen on referral from the school LCSW after he began to get into trouble at school **with inattention and disruptive behavior in class.** Mother stated it was a struggle to get him to complete even the simplest tasks, from chores to homework and reported he had frequent temper tantrums at home. **Patient was diagnosed with attention deficit hyperactivity disorder** and placed on 10 mg of Adderall a day. Treatment plan includes individual and family therapy focused on helping patient gain self-control and continued monitoring and assistance from the school social worker.

Since last visit, patient feels that he has been doing very well with the medicine and mother notes a "wonderful" improvement. They have two concerns—it seems like it takes a while for the medicine to kick-in in the morning and it wears off about 3pm so they have problems in the evening.

Review of Systems: He was initially having problems with his appetite which subsequently resolved. Difficulty with his appetite was early in the morning after he takes this medicine. Taking his meds with toast helped and the problem resolved. He has been eating well, sleeping okay. Review of systems is otherwise negative.

Allergies: NKA

Vitals WNL as noted. Patient is calm and well controlled in the exam room. Physical exam itself was unremarkable. No gastrointestinal distress. He is otherwise very healthy

Assessment: **Attention deficit hyperactivity disorder combined type**, doing fairly well with the Adderall.

Plan: Discussed two options with patient and mother: increase his Adderall dose by adding 5 mg in the afternoon or switch him to the extended-release Adderall, which I think has better release of the medicine for both early morning and the afternoon. We have decided at this point to change to Adderall XR 10 mg once daily. We will recheck if he is doing well, in two months. But if there are any problems, especially in the morning, then we want to see him. Mother understands and will call if there are problems. Approximately 25 minutes spent in discussion with patient and parent.

Diagnosis Code(s)

F90.2 Attention-deficit hyperactivity disorder, combined type

Coding Note(s)

Attention deficient disorders are indexed in multiple ways. For example, referencing Deficit, attention and concentration, disorder requires following multiple see notes to identify the correct code. Under Deficit, attention and concentration, disorder the first reference says to see Attention, deficit and then under Attention, deficit, with hyperactivity there is a note to see Disorder, attention-deficit hyperactivity which when referenced provides the correct codes. In addition, attention-deficient hyperactivity disorder must be clearly distinguished in the documentation from signs and symptoms related to attention and concentration. Even though codes for attention-deficit hyperactivity disorders are located in block F90-F98 with other disorders with onset usually occurring in childhood, these codes can be used regardless of the age of the patient. Attention-deficit hyperactivity disorders usually have their onset in childhood; however, they often persist into adulthood and, in some cases, may not be diagnosed until adulthood.

Mental and Behavioral Disorders Due to Psychoactive Substance Use

Alcohol-induced and drug-induced mental disorders cover a wide variety of disorders that differ in severity from intoxication to psychotic disorders and dementia. Coding of mental and behavioral disorders due to psychoactive substance use, abuse, or dependence requires the provider's clinical judgment and documentation in the medical record of the specific mental and/or behavioral disorders that are associated with the use or abuse of, or dependence on, the psychoactive substance.

Combination codes in Chapter 5 are used to report use, abuse, or dependence on psychoactive substances and the related mental and behavioral disorders due to the psychoactive substance. For mental and behavioral disorders due to a psychoactive substance, the specific substance is identified in the 3rd character of the code category; the 4th character identifies the condition as use, abuse, or dependence. The fifth character identifies any complications. Some 5-character subcategories are further expanded to describe more specifically the complication. For example, alcohol dependence withdrawal has 6th character designations that further describe the withdrawal as uncomplicated, with withdrawal delirium, with perceptual disturbance, or unspecified. Specific codes for dependence in remission are available for alcohol and all drug classes. A diagnosis of history of alcohol or drug dependence is also reported with the remission codes.

Coding and Documentation Requirements

Identify substance:

- Alcohol
- Cannabis
- Cocaine
- Hallucinogen
- Inhalant
- Nicotine
- Opioid
- Sedative/hypnotic/anxiolytic
- Stimulant related (other than cocaine)
- Other psychoactive substance

Identify type of disorder:

- Abuse
- Dependence
- Use, unspecified

For abuse, identify mental/behavioral complications (excludes nicotine):

- In remission
- Uncomplicated
- With intoxication
  - Uncomplicated
  - With intoxication delirium
  - Unspecified
- With substance-induced mood disorder
- With substance-induced psychotic disorder
  - With delusions
  - With hallucinations
  - Unspecified
- With other substance-induced disorders
  - Anxiety disorder
  - Sexual dysfunction
  - Sleep disorder
  - Other disorder
- Unspecified complication

For dependence, identify mental/behavioral complications (excludes nicotine):

- In remission
- Uncomplicated
- With intoxication
  - Uncomplicated
  - With intoxication delirium
  - Unspecified
- With persisting amnesiac disorder
- With persisting dementia
- With substance-induced mood disorder
- With substance-induced psychotic disorder
  - With delusions
  - With hallucinations
  - Unspecified
- With other substance-induced disorders
  - Anxiety disorder
  - Sexual dysfunction

  - Sleep disorder
  - Other disorder
- With withdrawal
  - Uncomplicated
  - With delirium
  - With perceptual disturbance
  - Unspecified
- Unspecified complication

For use, identify mental/behavioral complications (excludes nicotine):

- With intoxication
  - Uncomplicated
  - With intoxication delirium
  - Unspecified
- With persisting amnesiac disorder
- With persisting dementia
- With substance-induced mood disorder
- With substance-induced psychotic disorder
  - With delusions
  - With hallucinations
  - Unspecified
- With other substance-induced disorders
  - Anxiety disorder
  - Sexual dysfunction
  - Sleep disorder
  - Other disorder
- Unspecified complication

For nicotine dependence:

- Identify nicotine product:
  - Cigarettes
  - Chewing tobacco
  - Other specified product
  - Unspecified product
- Identify dependence status/complications:
  - In remission
  - Uncomplicated
  - With withdrawal
  - With other nicotine-induced disorder
  - Unspecified

Note: Use of nicotine not documented as dependence is reported with code Z72.0.

Further coding and documentation instructions for alcohol and drug related disorders with examples follow.

Alcohol-Related Disorders

Coding instructions for alcohol-related disorders requires an additional code to identify the blood alcohol level when applicable. Assignment of codes from this chapter requires documentation by the provider of a relationship between the psychoactive substance and the mental or behavioral disorder.

Unique codes distinguish between alcohol use, abuse, and dependence, so clear documentation describing that aspect of the patient's substance use is needed. Combination codes exist for alcohol use, abuse, and dependence and associated conditions such as withdrawal or delusions.

Coding and Documentation Requirements

Identify alcohol use, abuse, dependence:

- Abuse
  - In remission
  - Uncomplicated
  - With complication/other condition
- Dependence
  - In remission
  - Uncomplicated
  - With complication/other condition
- Use, unspecified (i.e., not specified as abuse or dependence)
  - With complication/other condition

Identify alcohol induced complication:

- Intoxication
  - Uncomplicated
  - Unspecified
  - With delirium
- Mood disorder
- Persisting amnestic disorder
- Persisting dementia
- Psychotic disorder
  - With delusions
  - With hallucinations
  - Unspecified
- Other disorder
  - Anxiety
  - Sexual dysfunction
  - Sleep disorder
  - Other specified disorder
- Unspecified disorder
- Withdrawal
  - Delirium
  - Perceptual disturbance
  - Uncomplicated
  - Unspecified

Identify blood alcohol level for current encounter with intoxication:

- Less than 20 mg/100 ml
- 20-39 mg/100 ml
- 40-59 mg/100 ml
- 60-79 mg/100 ml
- 80-99mg/100 ml
- 100-119 mg/100 ml
- 120-199 mg/100 ml

- 200-239 mg/100 ml
- Equal to or greater than 240 mg/100 ml

Alcohol Dependence with Withdrawal

ICD-10-CM Code/Documentation	
F10.230	Alcohol dependence with withdrawal, uncomplicated
F10.231	Alcohol dependence with withdrawal delirium
F10.232	Alcohol dependence with withdrawal with perceptual disturbance
F10.239	Alcohol dependence with withdrawal, unspecified

Documentation and Coding Example

This is a 57-year-old male, **a known alcoholic**, who was brought to the Emergency Department by his wife after witnessed convulsions. Wife reports patient was anxious and complained of nausea and insomnia. His symptoms progressively worsened to vomiting, fever, diaphoresis, and whole-body tremor and the patient became disoriented. **Onset of symptoms occurred two days ago—one day after he stopped drinking "cold turkey" following weeks of heavy binge drinking.**

No history of head injury or loss of consciousness; no history of seizures or family history of epilepsy; denies concomitant use of drugs. The patient appears confused and agitated with a marked tremor. CIWA-Ar scoring deferred; patient does not have a clear enough sensorium to provide coherent answers.

On exam the patient is diaphoretic with global confusion and marked tremor. Vital signs, as noted on intake: fever 101.6, heart rate >90bpm, and hypertension. EKG shows tachycardia.

Sclerae muddy, evidence of lacrimal gland hypertrophy. Parotid swelling. Lungs clear bilaterally; no focal consolidation or evidence of aspiration. Abdomen tender, all four quadrants; +BS. Mini-mental exam indicates altered mental status. No apparent focal neurologic deficits to indicate intracranial pathology; will consult Neuro for full neurologic evaluation.

IV benzodiazepines with a small dose of haloperidol as adjunctive therapy to treat agitation. IV fluids and electrolytes for rehydration.

Serum ethanol concentration, CBC with differential, serum chemistries including liver function tests, CT scan of the head, chest x-ray, and cerebrospinal fluid studies.

Admit patient to psychiatric unit **in alcohol withdrawal, suffering from delirium tremens.** Neurologist consult for full neurologic evaluation as indicated. Cardiology consult to rule out alcohol-induced cardiomyopathy.

Diagnosis Code(s)

F10.231 Alcohol dependence with withdrawal delirium

Coding Note(s)

Delirium tremens is indexed under Psychosis, alcoholic, delirium tremens or Psychosis, alcoholic, with delirium tremens. If the provider documents "impending" delirium tremens, this would be coded to F10.239 Alcohol dependence with withdrawal, unspecified according to the Alphabetic Index. Codes in category F10 are only used when the alcohol use, abuse, or dependence is associated with a mental or behavioral disorder, and when the provider documents a relationship between the substance use and the disorder.

In cases of psychoactive substance induced mental disorders, the documentation must identify the pattern of use (i.e., use, abuse and/or dependence of the same substance or multiple substances). Alcohol or drug use must be differentiated from nondependent abuse and from dependence. The term "alcoholism" is often used to describe both alcohol abuse and dependence on alcohol but documentation should clearly identify all aspects of the patient's alcohol use.

Other Psychoactive Substance-Induced Mental Disorders

Coding and documentation requirements for mental and behavioral disorders due to drug use are very similar to those for alcohol-induced mental disorders.

Like alcohol related mental disorders, unique codes distinguish between drug use, abuse, and dependence, so clear documentation describing that aspect of the patient's substance use is needed. There are combination codes for drug use and associated conditions such as withdrawal or delusions. Additionally, separate subcategories exist defining the type of drug such as opioid, cocaine, cannabis and sedatives.

Psychoactive Substance-Induced Psychotic Disorder with Hallucinations

ICD-10-CM Code/Documentation	
F11.951	Opioid use, unspecified, with opioid-induced psychotic disorder with hallucinations
F12.951	Cannabis use, unspecified with psychotic disorder with hallucinations
F13.951	Sedative, hypnotic or anxiolytic use, unspecified, with sedative, hypnotic, or anxiolytic- induced psychotic disorder with hallucinations
F14.951	Cocaine use, unspecified, with cocaine-induced psychotic disorder with hallucinations
F15.951	Other stimulant use, unspecified, with other stimulant-induced psychotic disorder with hallucinations
F16.951	Hallucinogen use, unspecified, with hallucinogen-induced psychotic disorder with hallucinations
F18.951	Inhalant use, unspecified with inhalant-induced psychotic disorder with hallucinations
F19.951	Other psychoactive substance use, unspecified, with other psychoactive substance-induced psychotic disorder with hallucinations

ICD-10-CM Code/Documentation	
F11.151	Opioid abuse with opioid-induced psychotic disorder with hallucinations
F12.151	Cannabis abuse with psychotic disorder with hallucinations
F13.151	Sedative, hypnotic or anxiolytic abuse, with sedative, hypnotic, or anxiolytic-induced psychotic disorder with hallucinations
F14.151	Cocaine abuse with cocaine-induced psychotic disorder with hallucinations
F15.151	Other stimulant abuse with other stimulant-induced psychotic disorder with hallucinations
F16.151	Hallucinogen abuse with hallucinogen-induced psychotic disorder with hallucinations
F18.151	Inhalant abuse with inhalant-induced psychotic disorder with hallucinations
F19.151	Other psychoactive substance abuse with other psychoactive substance-induced psychotic disorder with hallucinations
F11.251	Opioid dependence with opioid-induced psychotic disorder with hallucinations
F12.251	Cannabis dependence with psychotic disorder with hallucinations
F13.251	Sedative, hypnotic or anxiolytic dependence with sedative, hypnotic, or anxiolytic- induced psychotic disorder with hallucinations
F14.251	Cocaine dependence with cocaine-induced psychotic disorder with hallucinations
F15.251	Other stimulant dependence with other stimulant-induced psychotic disorder with hallucinations
F16.251	Hallucinogen dependence with hallucinogen-induced psychotic disorder with hallucinations
F18.251	Inhalant dependence with inhalant-induced psychotic disorder with hallucinations
F19.251	Other psychoactive substance dependence with other psychoactive substance-induced psychotic disorder with hallucinations

Documentation and Coding Example

Twenty-year-old male, brought to ED by ambulance after being found by roommate agitated and confused "in a panic" claiming he was hearing voices. Patient reported ingesting **multiple doses of his Adderall XR (20mg once daily) for approximately one week** "cramming" for finals.

Patient assessed for medical stability and level of danger. Full physical and neurologic examination performed by ED attending who administered IV hydration and propranolol to treat the patient's elevated blood pressure and pulse and also to help with the patient's anxiety and panic. Stat urine and serum toxicology screening ordered to exclude acetaminophen, tricyclic antidepressants, aspirin, and other toxins. ED attending requested this psychiatry consult in the ED.

Mental status examination is as follows: Appearance is disheveled. Patient is suspicious and paranoid, difficult to engage, with poor eye contact. Speech is decreased and rapid. Patient's perspective of time is disorganized, although he understands place and person. Thought process is guarded and paranoid with **observed evidence of auditory hallucinations**. Mood is anxious and affect is paranoid and fearful. Insight and judgment are poor; no suicidal or homicidal ideation. Patient is not in danger of harming himself or others.

Impression/Plan: **Non-dependent, episodic amphetamine abuse with psychosis, amphetamine-induced auditory hallucinations**. Patient's agitation and psychosis are likely self-limiting and removal of the amphetamines should be sufficient to medically stabilize the patient's condition. Patient has no evidence or history of liver or kidney problems so will order IV ammonium chloride 500 mg every 3 hours to acidify the urine.

Ativan injection 2 mg to 4 mg to stabilize agitation.

Admit to Psychiatric unit for inpatient substance abuse treatment and further psychiatric stabilization.

Diagnosis Code(s)

F15.151 Other stimulant abuse with stimulant-induced psychotic disorder with hallucinations

Coding Note(s)

A single combination code is all that is required to capture the substance abuse, the type of substance and the related psychotic disorder. Codes in category F15 are only used when the psychoactive substance use is associated with a mental or behavioral disorder, and when the provider documents a relationship between the psychoactive substance use and the disorder. In cases of psychoactive substance induced mental disorders, the documentation must identify the pattern of use (i.e., use, abuse and/or dependence of the same substance or multiple substances). Drug use must be differentiated from nondependent abuse and from dependence.

Summary

Best practices in documentation of mental and behavioral disorders require detailed information on the acuity and etiology of the disease, as well as any associated manifestations or complications. Organic mental or behavioral disorders caused by a physiological condition, in particular, require documentation of the underlying physiological condition and the relationship to any manifestations or complications.

Etiology/manifestation convention is used to direct coding of an underlying condition and its manifestation. The relationship between two diagnoses or a diagnosis and an associated secondary process or complication must be clearly stated in the documentation. For example, in the case of dementia due to Parkinson's disease, the underlying etiology (i.e., Parkinson's disease) must be identified as the cause of the manifestation (i.e., the dementia).

Documentation should also clarify dementia—the specific type of dementia and whether it is related to another condition should be documented. Whenever dementia has an associated behavioral disturbance, the behavior must also be specified.

Substance abuse and dependence are classified as mental disorders and as two distinct conditions that are coded differently, so clear documentation regarding patient's substance use, abuse, or dependence is essential.

Resources

Documentation checklists are available in Appendix A for the following condition(s):

- Substance Use, Abuse, Dependence
- Mood Disorders

Chapter 5 Quiz

1. Atypical anorexia nervosa is classified as:
   a. Anorexia nervosa, restricting type
   b. Anorexia nervosa, binge eating/purging type
   c. Eating disorder, unspecified
   d. Anorexia nervosa, unspecified
2. What information is not needed when documenting alcohol dependence?
   a. That the patient is in remission
   b. That the alcohol dependence is episodic or continuous
   c. That the patient has any complications related to alcohol dependence
   d. That the patient is experiencing withdrawal symptoms
3. How is history of alcohol or drug abuse classified?
   a. As "in remission"
   b. With a Z-code for personal history of alcohol/drug abuse
   c. With a supplementary code
   d. All of the above
4. Which types of mental or behavioral disorders require documentation of the underlying physiological condition and the relationship to any manifestations or complications?
   a. Organic disorders
   b. Mood disorders
   c. Psychotic disorders
   d. Nonpsychotic disorders
5. When coding disorders related to psychoactive substance use, if both abuse and dependence are documented, assign:
   a. Only the code for abuse
   b. Only the code for dependence
   c. Both abuse and dependence
   d. Only the code for substance use
6. Coding for alcohol-related disorders requires an additional code to identify what?
   a. Continuous or episodic use
   b. In remission
   c. The blood alcohol level, when applicable
   d. All of the above
7. How are substance abuse and dependence classified?
   a. As two distinct mental disorders that are coded differently
   b. As similar mental disorders that are coded the same
   c. As etiology and manifestations using combination codes
   d. As nervous system disorders
8. What statement about attention deficit hyperactivity disorder (category F90) is FALSE?
   a. Attention deficit disorder without hyperactivity is reported with codes from F90 Attention-deficit hyperactivity disorder
   b. Codes from category F90 should not be used for adults documented as having attention-deficit hyperactivity disorder
   c. Combined type involves symptoms of both inattention and hyperactivity-impulsivity
   d. Both a and c
9. The relationship between two diagnoses or a diagnosis and an associated secondary process or complication can be assumed under what circumstances?
   a. When the two diagnoses are linked by the terms "with" or "in" in the Alphabetical Index or Tabular List
   b. Only for mental and behavioral disorders
   c. For some medical conditions/disorders but not for mental and behavioral disorders
   d. A relationship can never be assumed
10. What needs to be included in the documentation of dementia?
    a. Whether it is related to other conditions
    b. The specific type of dementia
    c. Any associated behavioral disturbance
    d. All of the above

See next page for answers and rationales.

Chapter 5 Answers and Rationales

1. Atypical anorexia nervosa is classified as:

   c. **Eating disorder, unspecified**

   Rationale: *In the alphabetic index under Anorexia, nervosa, atypical, the code listed is F50.9. Correct code assignment is then verified by referencing the Tabular list where atypical anorexia nervosa is listed as an alternate term under code F50.9 Eating disorder, unspecified.*

2. What information is not needed when documenting alcohol dependence?

   b. **That the alcohol dependence is episodic or continuous**

   Rationale: *There is a specific code for alcohol dependence in remission, but there are no codes or 5th, 6th or 7th characters that capture episodic or continuous use/abuse/dependence. There are specific codes that identify alcohol use/abuse/dependence complicated by withdrawal symptoms.*

3. How is history of alcohol or drug abuse classified?

   a. **As "in remission"**

   Rationale: *According to the ICD-10-CM guidelines, codes for "in remission" in categories F10-F19 are captured by the fourth and fifth digits -.21. Using the alphabetic index, History, personal (of), alcohol dependence, identifies code F10.21 Alcohol dependence, in remission.*

4. Which types of mental or behavioral disorders require documentation of the underlying physiological condition and the relationship to any manifestations or complications?

   a. **Organic disorders**

   Rationale: *Many mental disorders have an organic origin, where disease or injury causes the mental or behavioral condition. Mental or behavioral disorders of organic origin are referred to organic disorders.*

5. When coding disorders related to psychoactive substance use, if both abuse and dependence are documented, assign:

   b. **Only the code for dependence**

   Rationale: *According to the guidelines, "when both abuse and dependence are documented, assign only the code for dependence."*

6. Coding for alcohol-related disorders requires an additional code to identify what?

   c. **The blood alcohol level, when applicable**

   Rationale: *Under code category F10 Alcohol related disorders, there is an instruction to "use additional code for blood alcohol level, if applicable (Y90.-)".*

7. How are substance abuse and dependence classified?

   a. **As two distinct mental disorders that are coded differently**

   Rationale: *There are distinct subcategories for substance abuse and dependence. The code is assigned based on physician documentation.*

8. What statement about attention deficit hyperactivity disorder (category F90) is FALSE?

   b. **Codes from category F90 should not be used for adults documented as having attention-deficit hyperactivity disorder**

   Rationale: *According to the note under block F90-F98, codes in these categories may be used regardless of the age of a patient. These disorders generally have onset within the childhood or adolescent years, but may continue throughout life or not be diagnosed until adulthood. In the Alphabetic Index, Disorder, attention deficit without hyperactivity identifies F90.0 as the appropriate code. Combined type is defined as involving symptoms of both inattention and hyperactivity-impulsivity.*

9. The relationship between two diagnoses or a diagnosis and an associated secondary process or complication can be assumed under what circumstances?

   a. **When the two diagnoses are linked by the terms "with" or "in" in the Alphabetical Index or Tabular List**

   Rationale: *When two conditions are linked by the terms "with" or "in" in a code title, Alphabetic Index, or an instructional note in the Tabular List, it should be interpreted to mean "associated with" or "due to". The classification presumes a causal relationship between the two conditions linked by these terms. These conditions should be coded as related even in the absence of provider documentation explicitly linking them, unless the documentation clearly states the conditions are unrelated, or another guidelines exists that specifically requires a documented link between the two conditions.*

10. What needs to be included in documentation of dementia?

    d. **All of the above**

    Rationale: *There are many different types and causes of dementia and the specific type or cause should be documented. Dementia may be related to other conditions and any related to conditions should also be documented. Associated behavioral disturbances are coded additionally, so any associated behavioral disturbances should also be documented.*

Chapter 6

DISEASES OF THE NERVOUS SYSTEM

Introduction

Diseases of the nervous system include disorders of the central nervous system that affect the brain and spinal cord, such as cerebral degeneration or Parkinson's disease, and diseases of the peripheral nervous system, such as polyneuropathy, myasthenia gravis, and muscular dystrophy. Some of the more commonly treated pain diagnoses are also classified as diseases of the nervous system, including: migraine and other headache syndromes, causalgia, complex regional pain syndrome I (CRPS I), neuralgia, and pain not elsewhere classified. Diseases of the nervous system are classified in Chapter 6.

Physician documentation is the basis for code assignment and the importance of proper documentation is imperative. ICD-10-CM captures a greater level of specificity than in previous systems which will require more precise clinical information documented in the medical record. Updated and standardized clinical terminology is used in ICD-10-CM to be consistent with the current standards providers use when diagnosing and treating nervous system disorders. Clinical terms such as commonly used synonyms for "intractable" migraine and more current terminology for epilepsy are found in the code descriptions.

For example, the terms "epilepsy" and "seizure disorder" describe central nervous system disorders characterized by sudden-onset seizures and muscle contractions. Seizure disorders and recurrent seizures are classified with epilepsy; however, convulsions, seizures not otherwise specified, febrile seizures, and hysterical seizures are classified as non-epileptic. So, a detailed description of the seizure is needed in order to differentiate between epilepsy and other seizures and to distinguish between seizure types.

Many nervous system conditions are manifestations of other diseases and dual coding is often required to report both the underlying condition and the manifestation. Dual coding is frequently required for infectious diseases of the central nervous system and precise documentation is needed in order to determine whether the condition is coded to the nervous system or to an infectious disease combination code.

Combination codes for common etiologies and symptoms or manifestations (e.g., dementia with Parkinsonism) are common in Chapter 6. The codes provide specific information and clinical detail. This places an even greater emphasis on the provider's documentation of the association between conditions, such as documenting the condition as "due to" a specified disease process.

Many diseases and conditions of the nervous system have additional elements which are captured in the code. For instance, providers routinely document the side of the body where disease or injury occurs (right, left, or bilateral), and laterality is included in many of the nervous system code description. Representative examples of documentation requirements are provided in this chapter and checklists are provided in Appendix A to help identify documentation deficiencies so that physicians and coders are aware of the specificity needed for proper code assignment.

There are 11 code blocks for the central and peripheral nervous system. The table below shows the category blocks for nervous system disorders.

ICD-10-CM Code Blocks	
G00-G09	Inflammatory Diseases of the Central Nervous System
G10-G14	Systemic Atrophies Primarily Affecting the Central Nervous System
G20-G26	Extrapyramidal and Movement Disorders
G30-G32	Other Degenerative Diseases of the Nervous System
G35-G37	Demyelinating Diseases of the Central Nervous System
G40-G47	Episodic and Paroxysmal Disorders
G50-G59	Nerve, Nerve Root and Plexus Disorders
G60-G65	Polyneuropathies and other Disorders of the Peripheral Nervous System
G70-G73	Diseases of Myoneural Junction and Muscle
G80-G83	Cerebral Palsy and Other Paralytic Syndromes
G89-G99	Other Disorders of the Nervous System

The organization of nervous system diseases in ICD-10-CM includes:

- Hereditary and degenerative diseases of the central nervous system subdivided into four code blocks:
  - G10-G14 Systemic Atrophies Primarily Affecting the Central Nervous System
  - G20-G26 Extrapyramidal and Movement Disorders
  - G30-G32 Other Degenerative Diseases of the Nervous System
  - G35-G37 Demyelinating Diseases of the Central Nervous System
- Pain not elsewhere classified found in category G89 of code block G89-G99 Other Disorders of the Nervous System
- Other headache syndromes classified in category G44 in code block G40-G47 Episodic and Paroxysmal Disorders which also includes epilepsy (G40), migraine (G43), transient cerebral ischemic attacks and related syndromes (G45), vascular syndromes of brain in cerebrovascular diseases (G46), and sleep disorders (G47)

- Disorders of the peripheral nervous system subdivided into three code blocks:
  - G50-G59 Nerve, Nerve Root and Plexus Disorders
  - G60-G65 Polyneuropathies and other Disorders of the Peripheral Nervous System
  - G70-G73 Diseases of Myoneural Junction and Muscle
- Intraoperative and postprocedural complications specific to the nervous system classified in Chapter 6 in code block G89-G99 Other Disorders of the Nervous System

Sleep apnea is located with diseases of the nervous system in Chapter 6. Nonspecific neuralgia and neuritis are not classified to the nervous system chapter; rather, these nonspecific diagnoses are located in the musculoskeletal chapter.

Because many underlying conditions can cause nervous system disorders, including infectious diseases, circulatory disorders, and external causes such as injury or drugs, careful review of the medical record documentation is needed in order to determine whether the condition is coded to the nervous system chapter or to another chapter.

Exclusions

There are no Excludes1 notes, but there are a number of Excludes2.

Excludes1	Excludes2
None	• Certain conditions originating in the perinatal period (P04-P96) • Certain infectious and parasitic diseases (A00-B99) • Complications of pregnancy, childbirth and the puerperium (O00-O9A) • Congenital malformations, deformations, and chromosomal abnormalities (Q00-Q99) • Endocrine, nutritional and metabolic diseases (E00-E88) • Injury, poisoning and certain other consequences of external causes (S00-T88) • Neoplasms (C00-D49) • Symptoms, signs and abnormal clinical and laboratory findings, not elsewhere classified (R00-R94)

Chapter Guidelines

Detailed guidelines are provided for coding certain conditions classified in Chapter 6 including:

- Dominant/nondominant side
- Pain not elsewhere classified

Dominant/Nondominant Side

The side of the body affected (right, left) is a component of the code for conditions that affect one side of the body. Codes such as hemiplegia and hemiparesis (G81) and monoplegia of the upper limb (G83.2), and lower limb (G83.1) or unspecified monoplegia (G83.3) also identify whether the side affected is the dominant or nondominant side. When the documentation provides laterality but fails to identify the side affected as dominant or nondominant, and the classification system does not indicate a default, ICD-10-CM provides the following guidelines:

- For ambidextrous patients, the default should be dominant
- If the left side is affected, the default is non-dominant
- If the right side is affected, the default is dominant

Pain Not Elsewhere Classified (G89)

According to the guidelines, the pain codes in category G89 Pain, not elsewhere classified, are used in conjunction with codes from other categories and chapters to provide more detail about acute or chronic pain and neoplasm-related pain. However, if the pain is not specified in the provider documentation as acute or chronic, post-thoracotomy, postprocedural, or neoplasm-related, codes from category G89 are not assigned.

Codes from category G89 are not assigned when the underlying or definitive diagnosis is known, unless the reason for the encounter is pain management rather than management of the underlying condition. When an admission or encounter is for treatment of the underlying condition, a code for the underlying condition is assigned as the principal diagnosis and no code from category G89 is assigned. For example, when a patient is admitted for spinal fusion to treat a vertebral fracture, the code for the vertebral fracture would be assigned as the principal diagnosis but no pain code is assigned.

Category G89 Codes as Principal or First-Listed Diagnosis

Guidelines for assigning pain codes as the principal or first-listed diagnosis when pain control or pain management is the reason for the admission/encounter direct the user to assign a code for the underlying cause of the pain as an additional diagnosis, if known. A case example would be a patient with nerve impingement and severe back pain seen for a spinal canal steroid injection or a patient admitted for insertion of a neurostimulator for pain control; the appropriate pain code would be assigned as the principal or first-listed diagnosis. On the other hand, if the admission or encounter is for treatment of the underlying condition and a neurostimulator is also inserted for pain control during the same episode of care, the underlying condition is the principal diagnosis and the appropriate pain code should be assigned as a secondary diagnosis.

Category G89 Codes in Conjunction with Site-Specific Pain Codes

Pain codes from category G89 may be used in conjunction with site-specific pain codes that identify the site of pain (including codes from Chapter 18) if the category G89 code provides additional diagnostic information such as describing whether the pain is acute or chronic. The sequencing of codes is dependent on the circumstances of the admission/encounter, for example:

- The category G89 code is sequenced first followed by the code identifying the specific site of pain when the encounter is for pain control or pain management
- If the encounter is for any other reason and a related definitive diagnosis has not been confirmed in the provider's documentation, the specific site of the pain is coded first, followed by the category G89 code.

Postoperative Pain

Coding of postoperative pain is driven by the provider's documentation. For post-thoracotomy and other postoperative pain that is not specified as acute or chronic, the code for the acute form is the default.

Routine or expected postoperative pain immediately after surgery is not coded, but severe or an unexpected level of postoperative pain not associated with a specific postoperative complication is assigned to the appropriate postoperative pain code in category G89. Postoperative pain associated with a specific postoperative complication (e.g., painful wire sutures) is coded to Chapter 19 Injury, Poisoning, and Certain Other Consequences of External Causes with an additional code from category G89 to identify acute or chronic pain.

Chronic Pain

Codes in category G89 differentiate between acute and chronic pain. There is no time frame defining when pain becomes chronic pain so the provider's documentation directs the use of these codes. When chronic pain is documented, it is coded to subcategory G89.2. It is important to note that central pain syndrome (G89.0) and chronic pain syndrome (G89.4) are not the same as "chronic pain," so these codes should only be used when the provider has specifically documented these conditions.

Neoplasm Related Pain

Code G89.3 is assigned when the patient's pain is documented as being related to, associated with, or due to cancer, primary or secondary malignancy, or tumor. The code for neoplasm-related pain is assigned regardless of whether the pain is documented as acute or chronic. When the reason for the admission/encounter is documented as pain control/pain management, G89.3 is assigned as the principal or first-listed code with the underlying neoplasm reported as an additional diagnosis. When the admission/encounter is for management of the neoplasm and the pain associated with the neoplasm is also documented, code G89.3 may be assigned as an additional diagnosis. It is not necessary to assign an additional code for the site of the pain.

General Documentation Requirements

General documentation requirements differ depending on the particular nervous system disease or disorder. In general, specificity of the type and cause of the nervous system disorder is required and must be documented in the medical record. Some of the general documentation requirements are discussed here, but greater detail for some of the more common diseases and conditions of the nervous system will be provided in the next section.

According to the *ICD-10-CM Official Guidelines for Coding and Reporting*, complete and accurate code assignment requires a joint effort between the provider and the coder. Without consistent, complete documentation in the medical record, accurate coding cannot be achieved. Much of the detail captured in the ICD-10-CM codes is routinely documented by providers, such as the severity or status of the disease in terms of acuity, the etiology (e.g., neoplasm-related pain), and the significance of related diagnostic findings (e.g., EEG confirms a seizure disorder). Beyond these basic medical record documentation requirements, specifically describing the site, such as the specific nerve (e.g., lesion of medial popliteal nerve, right lower limb) rather than a general anatomical site will ensure optimal code assignment for nervous system disorders.

Documentation in the patient's record should clearly specify the cause-and-effect relationship between a symptom, manifestation, or complication and a disease or a medical intervention. For example, documentation should specify whether a complication occurred intraoperatively, as in intraoperative hemorrhage, or postoperatively.

In addition to these general documentation requirements, there are specific diseases and disorders that require greater detail in documentation to ensure optimal code assignment.

Code-Specific Documentation Requirements

In this section, the ICD-10-CM code categories, subcategories, and subclassifications for some of the more commonly reported diseases and conditions of the nervous system are reviewed along with documentation requirements. Though not all of the codes with documentation requirements are discussed, this section will provide a representative sample of the type of additional documentation required for diseases of the nervous system. The section is organized alphabetically by the code category, subcategory, or subclassification, of the condition, whether or not it is coded in the Nervous System Chapter or not.

Alzheimer's Disease

Alzheimer's disease is the most common form of dementia. The progressive degeneration of nerve cells in Alzheimer's disease manifests mental changes ranging from mild memory impairment to loss of cognitive function with dementia. Accurate code assignment of Alzheimer's disease, with or without associated dementia, requires comprehensive provider documentation that clearly distinguishes Alzheimer's dementia from senile dementia, senile degeneration, or senility.

Codes include more specificity so a diagnosis of Alzheimer's disease without further description of the onset (e.g., early onset, late onset) and the type of symptoms (e.g., depression, delusions) will not support optimal code assignment. It is essential that the provider documentation clarify dementia related to other conditions. Alzheimer's disease may also be associated with delirium or behavioral disturbances, so it is equally important to document these conditions when they are present.

Coding and Documentation Requirements

Identify type/onset of Alzheimer's disease:

- Early onset
- Late onset
- Other Alzheimer's disease
- Unspecified Alzheimer's disease

Use additional code when Alzheimer's disease is associated with:

- Delirium (F05)
- Dementia with behavioral disturbance (F02.81)
- Dementia without behavioral disturbance (F02.80)

ICD-10-CM Code/Documentation	
G30.0	Alzheimer's disease with early onset
G30.1	Alzheimer's disease with late onset
G30.8	Other Alzheimer's disease
G30.9	Alzheimer's disease, unspecified

Documentation and Coding Example

A 77-year-old woman was brought for neurological evaluation by her husband because of a 6-month history of increasing memory impairment. Her husband began noticing a gradual worsening in her memory and increased difficulty finding words. He also noted a decline in social activity which he describes as "extremely out of character" for his wife. She appeared to be in a chronic state of confusion and was unable to converse in a logical or coherent manner, and her responses to questions were frequently inappropriate. Her confusion and memory problems became even more pronounced and her husband reported she was not sleeping at night.

The patient is well-groomed, alert, and friendly with no specific complaints. She worked in a secretarial position until her retirement at age 65. Her past medical history is significant for hysterectomy and although elevated blood pressure was documented on several occasions, she was never diagnosed with or medicated for HTN. All of her recent evaluations, including a CT scan, were reported as normal.

General medical and neurological exams were normal. She scored 15 out of a possible 30 on the mini mental state examination MMSE. Her speech was highly paraphasic. She couldn't remember what she had for breakfast. She was able to provide her name, but when asked about her current age, she incorrectly stated her birth month, but then became aware of this and became very angry. She was unable to give the current year, or the name of the current president.

Formal testing was conducted and she scored well below average in all cognitive domains on the Wechsler Memory scale, the Wechsler Adult Intelligence Scale, the Visuospatial Construction, and the Graphomotor Alternation Test. The results of the evaluation indicate that she meets clinical criteria for **Alzheimer's disease**. Patient was started on an empirical trial of neurotransmitters therapy, discharged home with daily home health care assistance.

Diagnosis: **Dementia in late onset Alzheimer's disease**

Diagnosis Code(s)

G30.1 Alzheimer's disease with late onset

F02.80 Dementia in other diseases classified elsewhere without behavioral disturbance

Coding Note(s)

Alzheimer's disease with dementia requires dual with the underlying condition (Alzheimer's disease) coded first followed by a code for dementia with or without behavioral disturbance. Late onset Alzheimer's disease is coded to G30.1. When Alzheimer's associated dementia is present, code F02.8- is assigned as an additional code.

Causalgia

Causalgia, also referred to as complex regional pain syndrome type II (CRPS II), is a type of neuropathic pain that occurs following a distinct nerve injury, usually to a peripheral nerve in an extremity. Symptoms include continuous burning or throbbing pain along the peripheral nerve; sensitivity to cold and/or touch; changes in skin temperature, color, and/or texture; hair and nail changes; joint stiffness and muscle spasms; and weakness and/or atrophy.

Codes for causalgia are specified by upper and lower limb and laterality. Causalgia of the upper limb is reported with codes in subcategory G56.4. Causalgia of the lower limb is reported with codes from subcategory G57.7. Fifth characters for both the upper and lower limbs identify laterality as unspecified (0), right (1), or left (2).

Coding and Documentation Requirements

Identify site:

- Upper limb
  - Right
  - Left
  - Unspecified
- Lower limb
  - Right
  - Left
  - Unspecified

ICD-10-CM Code/Documentation	
G56.40	Causalgia of unspecified upper limb (complex regional pain syndrome II)
G56.41	Causalgia of right upper limb (complex regional pain syndrome II)
G56.42	Causalgia of left upper limb (complex regional pain syndrome II)
G57.70	Causalgia of unspecified lower limb (complex regional pain syndrome II)
G57.71	Causalgia of right lower limb (complex regional pain syndrome II)
G57.72	Causalgia of left lower limb (complex regional pain syndrome II)

Documentation and Coding Example

Patient is a 12-year-old Caucasian male referred to orthopedics by his pediatrician for evaluation of right foot pain and weakness. He is non-weight bearing on right lower extremity with use of crutches. The patient is accompanied to the appointment by his father. PMH includes seasonal allergies controlled with Cetirizine. Immunizations are up to date for age. Patient sustained a displaced fracture of the right fibula approximately two months ago complicated by right peroneal nerve injury while **racing on a BMX course**. He came over a jump, **lost control of the bike and landed hard on his right leg**. No other riders were involved. The accident occurred out of town and he was initially seen in an

Urgent Care Center where X-rays showed a displaced fracture of the proximal fibular shaft with peroneal nerve compression. He underwent an ORIF with decompression of the peroneal nerve. He was placed in a hinged knee brace, given crutches to use, and told to follow up with PMD or orthopedist when he returned home. He was able to ambulate without pain initially but started noticing some weakness in his right foot two weeks after discontinuing the brace. As the weakness increased he also began to have numbness and tingling on the top of the right foot. Walking and wearing shoes now cause unbearable pain. He denies any knee pain or loss of mobility. On examination, this is an anxious appearing, well nourished, thin, adolescent male. WT 84 lbs. (37th%) HT 62 in. (86th%). Cranial nerves grossly intact. Upper extremities are normal in strength, sensation, and movement. Cervical, thoracic, and lumbar spine all normal in appearance and movement. Hips and knees in good alignment with range of motion intact. Upper leg strength normal bilaterally. Left lower extremity has normal strength, sensation, and movement. Right lower extremity feels significantly warmer to touch than left and skin color is unusually red beginning 10 cm above ankle and extending though toes. He has hyperalgesia and marked allodynia on dorsal surface of right foot when skin is lightly stroked by examiners fingers. Hyperhidrosis is not appreciated. There is no muscle wasting noted but he has marked ankle weakness and right foot drop with attempted dorsiflexion. His is able to tolerate only a few steps weight bearing and he is noted to have a slapping gait with toe drag. Comprehensive x-rays obtained of right lower extremity including AP, lateral, and oblique views of knee; AP, lateral, and mortise views of the ankle; AP and lateral views of the tibia/fibula shafts which are negative for Maisonneuve injury but show **good calcification at the site of the transverse fracture of proximal fibula**.

Impression: **S/P right fibula fracture with secondary causalgia due to common peroneal nerve injury**.

Plan: MRI to include right knee, lower leg, and foot. Consider referral to neurology for EMG and pain management.

Diagnosis Code(s)

G57.71	Causalgia of right lower limb
S82.831S	Other fracture of upper and lower end of right fibula, sequela
S84.11XS	Injury of peroneal nerve at lower leg level, right leg, sequela
V18.0XXS	Pedal cycle driver injured in noncollision transport accident in nontraffic accident, sequela

Coding Note(s)

The causalgia of the right leg is a sequela of a fracture resulting in a nerve injury of the upper end of the fibula. The causalgia is the first listed diagnosis code. Laterality is a component of the causalgia code. The code identifying the injury that resulted in the sequela is listed next. The patient had a transverse fracture of the upper end of the fibula with compression of the peroneal nerve. Both injuries are coded with 7th character S to indicate a sequela (late effect). While there are codes specific to transverse fracture of the shaft of the fibula, there is not a specific code for transverse fracture of the upper end so the code for other fracture of upper and lower end of the right fibula is reported. In this case, the use of "and" means "and/or" in the code descriptor for code S82.831S. The physician has also documented that there is good calcification at the fracture site which indicates that the fracture has healed normally. The code for the nerve injury is specific to the peroneal nerve. Laterality is also a component of both the fracture and nerve injury codes. The BMX rider was involved in a noncollision, nontraffic accident which is reported with the 7th character S to indicate that the patient is being treated for a sequela of the BMX accident.

Complex Regional Pain Syndrome I

Reflex sympathetic dystrophy (RSD) is now more commonly referred to as complex regional pain syndrome I (CRPS I). CRPS I is a type of severe, debilitating neuropathic pain that usually results from an injury, but in CRPS I there is no direct injury to the nerve itself. The precipitating injury may range from major to relatively minor trauma. It can also occur following an illness or it can occur without any known cause. Intense pain of the affected region can result even from light touch. Other symptoms related to abnormal function of the sympathetic nervous system may also be evident including abnormal circulation, temperature, and sweating. If not promptly diagnosed and treated there can be loss of function in the affected limb followed by muscle atrophy and even changes in hair and skin.

CRPS I is reported with codes from subcategory G90.5. Codes are specific to the upper or lower limbs and laterality is also a component of the codes.

Coding and Documentation Requirements

Identify the site:

- Upper limb
  - Right
  - Left
  - Bilateral
  - Unspecified side
- Lower limb
  - Right
  - Left
  - Bilateral
  - Unspecified side
- Other specified site
- Unspecified site

ICD-10-CM Code/Documentation	
G90.50	Complex regional pain syndrome I, unspecified
G90.511	Complex regional pain syndrome I of right upper limb
G90.512	Complex regional pain syndrome I of left upper limb
G90.513	Complex regional pain syndrome I of upper limb, bilateral
G90.519	Complex regional pain syndrome I of unspecified upper limb
G90.521	Complex regional pain syndrome I of right lower limb
G90.522	Complex regional pain syndrome I of left lower limb
G90.523	Complex regional pain syndrome I of lower limb, bilateral

ICD-10-CM Code/Documentation	
G90.529	Complex regional pain syndrome I of unspecified lower limb
G90.59	Complex regional pain syndrome I of other specified site

Documentation and Coding Example

Seventy-one-year-old Asian female presents to PMD with **pain and swelling in both arms**. The patient was in her usual state of good health until one month ago when she was the **victim of an attempted purse snatching** outside a local restaurant. She held onto her purse which was looped over her left forearm, elbow bent, but she felt her **shoulder wrench and elbow twist** during the altercation. She declined medical attention at the time and treated her injury conservatively with heat and Aleve. She states the **left arm pain** has progressed from mild tingling to a continuous burning sensation extending from shoulder to fingertips. The initial **bruising on her left forearm** resolved within a week but swelling around the elbow has increased and now extends into the wrist and hand. She has difficulty with movement especially elbow extension. What is most concerning to her is that **in the past week her right arm, which was not injured at the time, has developed a tingling type pain and yesterday she noticed swelling in the wrist**. Temperature 94.2 HR 84 RR 16 BP 140/82. Current medications include Aleve, Os-Cal, and a multivitamin. On examination, this is a thin, athletic appearing woman who looks significantly younger than her stated age. Cranial nerves are grossly intact. PERRLA. Eyes are clear, nares patent, mucous membranes moist and pink. Neck supple without lymphadenopathy. HR regular, without bruits or rubs, Grade II, S1 ejection murmur is present. Breath sounds clear, equal bilaterally. Abdomen soft, non-distended with active bowel sounds. Lower extremities are completely benign with intact circulation, sensation, and movement. Right upper extremity has no bruising or discoloration noted. Shoulder is freely mobile without swelling or pain. Right elbow is not swollen but gentle manipulation elicits complaint of pain and obvious stiffness in the joint. Wrist is exquisitely tender and noticeably swollen over the carpal-metacarpal joint. Sensation is normal, skin warm, dry to touch. Examination of left upper extremity is difficult due to pain. Hyperalgesia is present from just below shoulder through fingertips. Swelling is most notable in the elbow and wrist with muscle wasting in the upper arm and forearm. Skin is pale in color, cool and moist to touch.

Impression: **Complex regional pain disorder, Type I, of both upper extremities. Sequela of direct injury to muscles/tendons left upper arm. No known injury or direct cause on the right**.

Plan: Comprehensive radiographs of bilateral upper extremities to r/o fracture and bone scan of same to assess for decreased bone density. Referral made to neurologist. Patient is offered a trial of physical therapy but she declines, stating she would prefer to wait until after she has been evaluated by neurology.

Diagnosis Code(s)

G90.513 Complex regional pain syndrome I of upper limb, bilateral

S46.902S Unspecified injury of unspecified muscle, fascia and tendon at shoulder and upper arm level, left arm, sequela

Y04.8XXS Assault by other bodily force, sequela

Coding Note(s)

The code descriptor has been changed from reflex sympathetic dystrophy (RSD) to complex regional pain syndrome I (CRPS I) to reflect current terminology for the condition. Laterality is a component of the code which has been documented as bilateral. The CRPS I on the left is a sequela of the injury to the left arm so that should be coded additionally. There is no documented injury to the right arm, but CRPS I can also occur without a known cause. Sequela of injury is reported with an injury code with 7th character S. The site of the injury is documented as the muscles and tendons of the upper left arm, but the specific muscle(s)/tendon(s) are not identified and the specific type of injury is not documented so the code for unspecified injury of unspecified muscle/tendon is assigned. A code for the external cause is also assigned with 7th character S. The external cause is a pulling/wrenching injury in an attempt to snatch a purse which would be classified as an assault using bodily force. There is not a specific code for pulling/wrenching so the code for other bodily force is assigned.

Epilepsy and Recurrent Seizures

Epilepsy is a neurological condition characterized by recurrent seizures. The terms "epilepsy" and "seizure disorder" describe central nervous system disorders characterized by sudden-onset seizures and muscle contractions. Epileptic seizures may be classified as idiopathic or symptomatic. Idiopathic seizures do not have a known cause but, in some cases, there is a family history of epilepsy. Symptomatic epilepsy is due to a specific cause, such as head trauma, stroke, brain tumors, alcohol or drug withdrawal, and other conditions. Epileptic seizures can also be a manifestation of neurologic or metabolic diseases.

Different terminology may be used to describe epilepsy such as epileptic or epilepsia attack, convulsion, fit, and seizure; however, in the medical record documentation, epilepsy must be clearly differentiated from a diagnosis of seizure or convulsion which is reported with codes from the signs and symptoms chapter rather than a code for epilepsy from the nervous system chapter. This means that a clear distinction must be made between a patient who has one seizure and a patient with epilepsy. Due to legal consequences, a code of epilepsy cannot be assigned unless it is clearly diagnosed by the provider.

Accurate coding of epilepsy and recurrent seizures depends entirely on provider documentation. Current clinical terminology and codes that capture the required detail for the specific type of epilepsy and complications such as status epilepticus and intractability are found in the code options for epilepsy. In order to assign the most specific code, clinical terminology related to the different types of epilepsy must be understood. Below are definitions of the commonly used terms describing epilepsy and recurrent seizures.

Absence epileptic syndrome – A type of generalized epilepsy characterized by an alteration of consciousness of brief duration (usually less than 20 seconds) with sudden onset and termination. The alteration of consciousness may include impaired awareness and memory of ongoing events as evidenced by mental confusion, an inability to response to external stimuli, and amnesia. May also be referred to as absence petit mal seizure.

Cryptogenic epilepsy – Epilepsy that is likely due to a specific cause but the cause has not yet been identified.

Dravet syndrome – Severe form of epilepsy marked by frequent and prolonged seizures appearing in the first year

Epilepsia partialis continua – Unique type of prolonged seizure consisting of prolonged simple partial (localized) motor seizures, now more commonly referred to as Kozhevnikov's (Kojevnikoff's, Kojewnikoff's, Kojevnikov's, Kojevnikov's) epilepsy.

Epileptic spasms – Epilepsy syndrome that is clinically similar to infantile spasms, but of a broader clinical classification that captures this syndrome when onset occurs in later childhood. Note: Infantile spasms are classified to the more general code for epileptic spasms.

Focal epilepsy – Epilepsy that is localized or starts in one area of the brain (synonymous with partial epilepsy and localization related epilepsy).

Generalized epilepsy – Epilepsy that involves the entire brain at the same time.

Grand mal status – An obsolete term used to describe generalized tonic-clonic seizures.

Idiopathic epilepsy – Epilepsy with no known cause, and the person has no other signs of neurological disease.

Infantile spasms – Epilepsy syndrome of infancy and childhood also referred to as West Syndrome characterized by brief bobbing or bowing of the head followed by relaxation and a return of the head to a normal upright position. Infantile spasms are also associated with developmental regression and if not controlled can lead to mental retardation.

Juvenile myoclonic epilepsy – A type of generalized epilepsy with onset in childhood characterized by shock-like muscle contractions in a group of muscles usually in the arms or legs that result in a jerking motion and generalized tonic-clonic seizures. The patient may also experience absence seizures. May also be referred to as impulsive petit mal seizure.

Localization-related epilepsy – Epilepsy that is localized or starts in one area of the brain (synonymous with focal epilepsy and partial epilepsy).

Lennoux-Gastaut syndrome – Severe form of epilepsy usually beginning before age 4 and associated with impaired intellectual functioning, developmental delay, and behavioral disturbances. Seizure types vary but may include tonic, atonic, myoclonic, or absence seizures. The patient may experience periods of frequent seizures mixed with brief seizure-free periods. The cause is often identified with more common causes being brain malformations, perinatal asphyxia, severe head injury, central nervous system infection, and inherited degenerative or metabolic conditions. However, in about one-third of all cases no cause is identified.

Partial epilepsy – Epilepsy that is localized or starts in one area of the brain (synonymous with focal epilepsy and localization related epilepsy).

Petit mal status – An obsolete term used to describe a type of generalized epilepsy that does not involve tonic-clonic movements.

Status epilepticus – Repeated or prolonged seizures usually lasing more than 30 minutes. May be tonic-clonic (convulsive) type or nonconvulsive (absence) type.

Symptomatic epilepsy – Epilepsy due to a known cause

Tonic-clonic seizures – Seizures characterized by an increase in muscle tone and rhythmic jerking of muscles in one part or all of the body.

In addition to the specific types of epilepsy and epileptic syndromes described above, epilepsy is also classified as intractable or not intractable. Intractable seizures are those that are not responding to treatment. Terms used to describe intractable seizures include: pharmacologically resistant, pharmacoresistant, poorly controlled, refractory, or treatment resistant. Seizures that are not intractable are responding to treatment. Documentation that supports classification as not intractable would be "under control", "well-controlled", and "seizure-free."

Seizure disorders and recurrent seizures are classified with epilepsy; however, convulsions, new-onset seizure, single seizure, febrile seizure, or hysterical seizure are classified as non-epileptic. Thorough documentation of the seizure is needed in order to differentiate between epilepsy and other seizures and to distinguish seizure types.

For some specific types of epilepsy, a distinction is made between idiopathic and symptomatic epilepsy. Localization related epilepsy must be documented as idiopathic (G40.0) or symptomatic (G40.1, G40.2). In addition, generalized epilepsy is specifically described as idiopathic (G40.3). There is also a specific subcategory for epileptic seizure related to external causes such as alcohol, drugs, hormonal changes, sleep deprivation, or stress. In addition, all types of epilepsy must be documented as intractable or not intractable and as with status epilepticus or without status epilepticus. Documentation should also clearly differentiate epilepsy and recurrent seizures from the following conditions which are reported elsewhere:

- Conversion disorder with seizures (F44.5)
- Convulsions NOS (R56.9)
- Hippocampal sclerosis (G93.81)
- Mesial temporal sclerosis (G93.81)
- Post traumatic seizures (R56.1)
- Seizure (convulsive) NOS (R56.9)
- Seizure of newborn (P90)
- Temporal sclerosis (G93.81)
- Todd's paralysis (G83.8)

Coding and Documentation Requirements

Identify type of epilepsy or recurrent seizures:

- Absence epileptic syndrome
- Due to external causes
- Generalized
  - Idiopathic
  - Other generalized type
- Juvenile myoclonic epilepsy (also known as impulsive petit mal)
- Localization-related (focal) (partial)
  - Idiopathic (with seizures of localized onset)
  - Symptomatic
    - » With complex partial seizures
    - » With simple partial seizures

- Other epilepsy and recurrent seizures
  - Dravet syndrome
  - Epileptic spasms
  - Lennox-Gastaut syndrome
  - Other epilepsy
  - Other seizures
- Unspecified epilepsy

Identify response to treatment:

- With intractable epilepsy, which includes:
  - Pharmacoresistant or pharmacologically resistant
  - Poorly controlled
  - Treatment resistant
  - Refractory (medically)
- Without intractable epilepsy

Identify as with/without status epilepticus:

- With status epilepticus
- Without status epilepticus

ICD-10-CM Code/Documentation	
G40.001	Localization-related (focal) (partial) idiopathic epilepsy and epileptic syndromes with seizures of localized onset, not intractable, with status epilepticus
G40.009	Localization-related (focal) (partial) idiopathic epilepsy and epileptic syndromes with seizures of localized onset, not intractable, without status epilepticus
G40.011	Localization-related (focal) (partial) idiopathic epilepsy and epileptic syndromes with seizures of localized onset, intractable, with status epilepticus
G40.019	Localization-related (focal) (partial) idiopathic epilepsy and epileptic syndromes with seizures of localized onset, intractable, without status epilepticus
G40.101	Localization-related (focal) (partial) symptomatic epilepsy and epileptic syndromes with simple partial seizures, not intractable, with status epilepticus
G40.109	Localization-related (focal) (partial) symptomatic epilepsy and epileptic syndromes with simple partial seizures, not intractable, without status epilepticus
G40.111	Localization-related (focal) (partial) symptomatic epilepsy and epileptic syndromes with simple partial seizures, intractable, with status epilepticus
G40.119	Localization-related (focal) (partial) symptomatic epilepsy and epileptic syndromes with simple partial seizures, intractable, without status epilepticus
G40.201	Localization-related (focal) (partial) symptomatic epilepsy and epileptic syndromes with complex partial seizures, not intractable, with status epilepticus
G40.209	Localization-related (focal) (partial) symptomatic epilepsy and epileptic syndromes with complex partial seizures, not intractable, without status epilepticus
G40.211	Localization-related (focal) (partial) symptomatic epilepsy and epileptic syndromes with complex partial seizures, intractable, with status epilepticus
G40.219	Localization-related (focal) (partial) symptomatic epilepsy and epileptic syndromes with complex partial seizures, intractable, without status epilepticus
G40.301	Generalized idiopathic epilepsy and epileptic syndromes, not intractable, with status epilepticus
G40.309	Generalized idiopathic epilepsy and epileptic syndromes, not intractable, without status epilepticus
G40.311	Generalized idiopathic epilepsy and epileptic syndromes, intractable, with status epilepticus
G40.319	Generalized idiopathic epilepsy and epileptic syndromes, intractable, without status epilepticus
G40.A01	Absence epileptic syndrome, not intractable, with status epilepticus
G40.A09	Absence epileptic syndrome, not intractable, without status epilepticus
G40.A11	Absence epileptic syndrome, intractable, with status epilepticus
G40.A19	Absence epileptic syndrome, intractable, without status epilepticus
G40.B01	Juvenile myoclonic epilepsy, not intractable, with status epilepticus
G40.B09	Juvenile myoclonic epilepsy, not intractable, without status epilepticus
G40.B11	Juvenile myoclonic epilepsy, intractable, with status epilepticus
G40.B19	Juvenile myoclonic epilepsy, intractable, without status epilepticus
G40.401	Other generalized epilepsy and epileptic syndromes, not intractable, with status epilepticus
G40.409	Other generalized epilepsy and epileptic syndromes, not intractable, without status epilepticus
G40.411	Other generalized epilepsy and epileptic syndromes, intractable, with status epilepticus
G40.419	Other generalized epilepsy and epileptic syndromes, intractable, without status epilepticus
G40.42	Cyclin-Dependent Kinase-Like 5 Deficiency Disorder
G40.501	Epileptic seizures related to external causes, not intractable, with status epilepticus
G40.509	Epileptic seizures related to external causes, not intractable, without status epilepticus
G40.801	Other epilepsy, not intractable, with status epilepticus
G40.802	Other epilepsy, not intractable, without status epilepticus
G40.803	Other epilepsy, intractable, with status epilepticus
G40.804	Other epilepsy, intractable, without status epilepticus
G40.811	Lennox-Gastaut syndrome, not intractable, with status epilepticus
G40.812	Lennox-Gastaut syndrome, not intractable, without status epilepticus
G40.813	Lennox-Gastaut syndrome, intractable, with status epilepticus
G40.814	Lennox-Gastaut syndrome, intractable, without status epilepticus
G40.821	Epileptic spasms, not intractable, with status epilepticus
G40.822	Epileptic spasms, not intractable, without status epilepticus
G40.823	Epileptic spasms, intractable, with status epilepticus
G40.824	Epileptic spasms, intractable, without status epilepticus
G40.833	Dravet syndrome, intractable, with status epilepticus
G40.834	Dravet syndrome, intractable, without status epilepticus
G40.89	Other seizures
G40.901	Epilepsy, unspecified, not intractable, with status epilepticus
G40.909	Epilepsy, unspecified, not intractable, without status epilepticus

ICD-10-CM Code/Documentation	
G40.911	Epilepsy, unspecified, intractable, with status epilepticus
G40.919	Epilepsy, unspecified, intractable, without status epilepticus

Documentation and Coding Example

A previously healthy 9-year-old boy was admitted to the hospital from the Emergency Department following several episodes of vomiting over several days and then episodes of jerking movements of the left side of the body, predominantly the left leg, accompanied by an altered mental status. While in the ED, he had repeated episodes of generalized seizures and remained in status epilepticus despite treatment with intravenous pyridoxine (two doses, 100 mg each) and consequently was admitted.

He had been born at term and his developmental milestones were normal. There was no family history of seizures or mental retardation. The diagnostic workup done on admission was negative and included serum pyruvate, serum amino acids, blood lead, copper, and mercury levels, Epstein Barr virus IgG, herpes simplex virus, polymerase chain reaction and encephalitis panel, leptospira, mycoplasma, and rabies titers. The CSF protein and glucose were normal.

Initial scalp EEG recording showed frequent centrotemporal EEG spikes. Continuous scalp EEG monitoring showed multiple electroclinical seizures beginning in the right central region and spreading to both hemispheres. MRI demonstrated abnormally thickened cortex in the high right parietal lobe. Patient was treated with pentobarbital infusion and the clinical manifestations disappeared.

Diagnosis: **Refractory focal seizures, status epilepticus**.

Diagnosis Code(s)

G40.011 Localization-related (focal) (partial) idiopathic epilepsy and epileptic syndromes with seizures of localized onset, intractable, with status epilepticus

Coding Note(s)

Refractory is listed as a synonym for intractable. ICD-10-CM lists benign childhood epilepsy with centrotemporal EEG spikes under subcategory G40.0.

Extrapyramidal Disease and Movement Disorders

There are two systems of neural pathways that affect movement – the pyramidal system which is the direct activation pathway and the extrapyramidal system which is the indirect activation pathway. The pyramidal system is responsible for voluntary movement of the head, neck, and limbs. The extrapyramidal system is a second motor pathway that is responsible for control of movements. The extrapyramidal system modifies neural impulses that originate in the cerebral cortex and is responsible for selective activation and suppression of movements, initiation of movements, rate and force of movements, and coordination. Damage to the extrapyramidal system results in movement disorders.

Code block G20-G26 Extrapyramidal and Movement Disorders contains codes for reporting these conditions.

Many movement disorders present with similar extrapyramidal symptoms, such as akathisia, dyskinesias, and dystonias. These disorders often resemble Parkinson's disease, so it is important that the medical record documentation clearly describes extrapyramidal and movement disorders.

Specific and complete documentation is necessary to avoid confusion between disorders and ensure the most accurate code assignment. Tremors, for example, are commonly associated with Parkinson's disease, but essential tremor is the most common type of tremor and the two conditions differ. In addition, people with essential tremor sometimes develop other neurological signs and symptoms —such as an unsteady gait. Medical record documentation by the provider that clearly describes extrapyramidal and movement disorders is essential. Documentation should include characteristics of the specific disorder. The following list includes other types of extrapyramidal and movement disorders, such as tremor:

- Chorea
- Essential tremor
- Familial tremor
- Drug-induced movement disorder (identify drug):
  - Akathisia
  - Chorea
  - Tics
  - Tremor
  - Other
  - Unspecified
- Intention/other tremor
- Myoclonus, which includes:
  - Drug-induced myoclonus (identify drug)
  - Palatal myoclonus
- Other specified extrapyramidal and movement disorders
  - Benign shuddering attacks
  - Restless legs syndrome
  - Stiff man syndrome
- Tics of organic origin
- Unspecified movement disorder

The table below shows of the range of codes in the categories for extrapyramidal diseases and movement disorders. Four coding examples follow the table.

ICD-10-CM Category		ICD-10-CM Code/Documentation	
G20	Parkinson's Disease		
G21	Secondary parkinsonism	G21.0	Malignant neurologic syndrome
		G21.11	Neuroleptic induced parkinsonism
		G21.19	Other drug induced secondary parkinsonism
		G21.2	Secondary parkinsonism due to other external agents
		G21.3	Postencephalitic parkinsonism
		G21.4	Vascular parkinsonism
		G21.8	Other secondary parkinsonism
		G21.9	Secondary parkinsonism, unspecified

ICD-1Ø-CM Category		ICD-1Ø-CM Code/Documentation	
G23	Other degenerative diseases of basal ganglia	G23.Ø	Hallervorden-Spatz disease
		G23.1	Progressive supranuclear ophthalmoplegia [Steele-Richardson-Olszewski]
		G23.2	Striatonigral degeneration
		G23.8	Other specified degenerative diseases of basal ganglia
		G23.9	Degenerative diseases of basal ganglia, unspecified
G24	Dystonia	G24.Ø1	Drug-induced subacute dystonia
		G24.Ø2	Drug induced acute dystonia
		G24.Ø9	Other drug induced dystonia
		G24.1	Genetic torsion dystonia
		G24.2	Idiopathic nonfamilial dystonia
		G24.3	Spasmodic torticollis
		G24.4	Idiopathic orofacial dystonia
		G24.5	Blepharospasm
		G24.8	Other dystonia
		G24.9	Dystonia, unspecified
G25	Other extrapyramidal and movement disorders	G25.Ø	Essential tremor
		G25.1	Drug-induced tremor
		G25.2	Other specified forms of tremor
		G25.3	Myoclonus
		G25.4	Drug-induced chorea
		G25.5	Other chorea
		G25.61	Drug induced tics
		G25.69	Other tics of organic origin
		G25.7Ø	Drug induced movement disorder, unspecified
		G25.71	Drug induced akathisia
		G25.79	Other drug induced movement disorders
		G25.81	Restless legs syndrome
		G25.82	Stiff-man syndrome
		G25.83	Benign shuddering attacks
		G25.89	Other specified extrapyramidal and movement disorders
		G25.9	Extrapyramidal and movement disorder unspecified
G26	Extrapyramidal and movement disorders in diseases classified elsewhere		

Example 1

Secondary Parkinsonism

Parkinson's disease is a common debilitating disease affecting one out of every 1ØØ people over the age of 6Ø. The symptoms of Parkinson's disease include tremors, rigidity, and akinesia. The term "parkinsonism" refers to any condition that involves the types of movement changes seen in Parkinson's disease. Coding of secondary parkinsonism requires a clear understanding of the difference between Parkinson's disease and secondary parkinsonism. Parkinson's disease, also referred to as idiopathic parkinsonism, primary Parkinson's disease or primary parkinsonism, is not due to or caused by another underlying condition or external agent such as a drug. In contrast, secondary parkinsonism is always caused by an underlying condition or external agent, such as chemical or environmental toxins, drugs, encephalitis, cerebrovascular disease, or another physiological condition.

In the medical record documentation, secondary parkinsonism must be clearly differentiated from primary Parkinson's disease and the documentation must indicate the underlying cause of secondary parkinsonism. Parkinson's disease and secondary parkinsonism may also be associated with mental disorders such as dementia, depression, delirium, or behavioral disturbance. For Parkinson's disease, an additional code should be used to identify any dementia, either with (FØ2.81) or without behavioral disturbance (FØ2.8Ø). To ensure assignment of the most specific code, the documentation must specify the cause of secondary parkinsonism and indicate when the condition is associated with dementia, depression, delirium, or a behavioral disturbance.

Parkinson's disease and secondary parkinsonism codes are found under Extrapyramidal and movement disorders, categories G2Ø-G21.

Coding and Documentation Requirements

Identify the cause of secondary parkinsonism:

- Drug-induced
  - Malignant neuroleptic syndrome
  - Neuroleptic induced parkinsonism
  - Other drug induced secondary parkinsonism
- Due to other external agents
- Postencephalitic
- Vascular
- Other specified cause
- Unspecified cause

For drug or external agent induced secondary parkinsonism, use an additional code to identify the substance.

ICD-1Ø-CM Code/Documentation	
G21.Ø	Malignant neuroleptic syndrome
G21.11	Neuroleptic induced parkinsonism
G21.19	Other drug induced secondary Parkinsonism
G21.2	Secondary parkinsonism due to other external agents
G21.3	Postencephalitic parkinsonism
G21.4	Vascular parkinsonism
G21.8	Other secondary parkinsonism
G21.9	Secondary parkinsonism, unspecified

Documentation and Coding Example

Follow-up visit for evaluation of **parkinsonism due to adverse effect of metoclopramide**.

History and Physical: This otherwise healthy 55-year-old man was given **metoclopramide** to treat symptomatic gastroesophageal reflux. Six months later he developed severe parkinsonism exhibiting tremors, limited movements, rigidity, and postural instability. He was started on L-dopa because his primary care physician did not realize the parkinsonism was drug-induced, and the metoclopramide was continued. The patient was referred to me six months ago for evaluation of parkinsonism after one year of taking both drugs. At that time, it was recognized that **the parkinsonism was drug-induced**. The metoclopramide was stopped and the patient has been slowly withdrawn from the L-dopa over the past six-months. On exam today, the patient's parkinsonism has resolved completely.

Diagnosis: **Drug-induced secondary parkinsonism** has resolved completely

Plan: Patient is to return to the care of his primary care physician.

Diagnosis Code(s)

G21.19 Other drug induced secondary parkinsonism

T45.0X5D Adverse effect of antiallergic and antiemetic drugs, subsequent encounter

Coding Note(s)

An additional code is used to identify the drug responsible for the adverse effect.

Metoclopramide is not classified as a neuroleptic drug, so the code for other drug induced secondary parkinsonism is assigned. An additional code is assigned for the adverse effect. The drug responsible for the adverse effect is identified with a code from categories T36-T50 with fifth or sixth character of 5. Adverse effect codes in ICD-10-CM include a seventh character to indicate the episode of care (e.g., initial encounter, subsequent encounter, or sequela). This is a follow-up encounter so 7th character D is assigned for subsequent encounter.

Example 2

Other Degenerative Diseases of Basal Ganglia

Included in the extrapyramidal and movement disorders category block are other degenerative diseases of the basal ganglia. Degenerative diseases are characterized by progressive neuron degeneration. The basal ganglia are nerve cells located within the brain involved in the initiation of voluntary movement. Damage to the basal ganglia causes muscle stiffness or spasticity and tremors. Because the deficits are primarily in motor function, the extrapyramidal system and basal ganglia have been associated with movement disorders.

Many different degenerative diseases affect the brain and produce similar symptoms, so specific documentation is necessary to avoid confusion between disorders. For example, progressive supranuclear palsy is sometimes mistaken for Parkinson's disease, because both conditions are associated with stiffness, frequent falls, slurred speech, difficulty swallowing, and decreased spontaneous movement. Provider documentation in the medical record must clearly distinguish degenerative diseases of the basal ganglia from other degenerative diseases of the brain that are characterized by motor, cognitive, and psychiatric manifestations. To ensure assignment of the most specific code for degenerative diseases of the basal ganglia, provider documentation should describe:

- Etiology
- Location (e.g., the brainstem, basal ganglia, cerebellum)
- Clinical features
- Course of the disease

Coding and Documentation Requirements

Identify the type of basal ganglia degenerative disease:

- Hallervorden-Spatz disease
- Progressive supranuclear ophthalmoplegia [Steele-Richardson-Olszewski]
- Striatonigral degeneration
- Other specified basal ganglia degenerative disease, which includes:
  - Calcification of basal ganglia
- Unspecified basal ganglia degenerative disease

ICD-10-CM Code/Documentation	
G23.0	Hallervorden-Spatz disease
G23.1	Progressive supranuclear ophthalmoplegia [Steele-Richardson-Olszewski]
G23.2	Striatonigral degeneration
G23.8	Other specified degenerative diseases of basal ganglia
G23.9	Degenerative disease of basal ganglia, unspecified

Documentation and Coding Example

Follow-up Visit History: A 63-year-old male with a year-long history of headaches, dizziness, and progressive unsteadiness and stiffening of the left side of his body presented after experiencing several falls. There was no evidence of encephalitis or of previous ingestion of neuroleptic drugs, and no family history of Parkinson's. MRI scans of the brain ruled out stroke or hydrocephalus. On examination, there was akinesia and rigidity of all limbs, more pronounced on the left, and no tremor. Deep tendon reflexes were brisk, the plantar flexor sensation was intact. Command and pursuit eye movements were grossly impaired in all directions but Doll's eye movements were normal. Optokinetic nystagmus was markedly reduced in lateral gaze to either side and absent in the vertical plane, as was convergence, but the pupillary reactions were normal. There was no ptosis, nystagmus, oculomasticatory myorhythmia, or myoclonus. A diagnosis of **progressive supranuclear palsy** was considered based on the association of a supranuclear ophthalmoplegia and Parkinsonism, and the neuro-ophthalmic findings were consistent with a diagnosis of supranuclear ophthalmoplegia. He was started on trimethoprim 160 mg with sulfamethoxazole 800 mg twice daily and levodopa 100 mg with carbidopa 10 mg four times a day. There was rapid improvement in his eye movements with minimal residual restriction in upward gaze and gradual improvement in his other symptoms by day seven.

Diagnosis: **Progressive supranuclear ophthalmoplegia** responding well to current drug regimen.

Diagnosis Code(s)

G23.1 Progressive supranuclear ophthalmoplegia [Steele-Richardson-Olszewski]

Coding Note(s)

Progressive supranuclear ophthalmoplegia has a distinct code (G23.1).

Example 3

Tremor

There are three codes that describe specific types of tremors, G25.0 Essential tremor, G25.1 Drug-induced tremor, and G25.2 Other specified forms of tremor which includes intention tremor. It should be noted that a diagnosis of tremor that is not more specifically described in the documentation is reported with a symptom code, R25.1 Tremor unspecified. These codes are also found under the extrapyramidal and other movement disorders category.

Coding and Documentation Requirements

Identify the form of tremor:

- Drug-induced
- Essential/Familial
- Other specified form (includes intention tremor)

ICD-10-CM Code/Documentation	
G25.0	Essential tremor
G25.1	Drug-induced tremor
G25.2	Other specified forms of tremor

Documentation and Coding Example

Patient is a 64-year-old Caucasian female referred to Neurology by PMD for worsening tremor in her hands and head. PMH is significant for tremor that started in her hands at least twenty years ago and progressed slowly to arms and head/neck. Patient reports that most members of her family have the problem in varying degrees. She states that her symptoms have not interfered with ADLs or exercise. Her husband is a retired architect. She has not been employed outside the home in more than 40 years. The couple moved about 1 year ago from a relatively moist/cool coastal town to a warm/dry inland area to be closer to their children/grandchildren, and it was after the move that she noticed her tremor worsening. She states she spends 4-5 months of the year in England with family, and symptoms were less severe while she was there, but exacerbated upon her return home. This is a pleasant, impeccably groomed, thin but muscular woman who looks younger than her stated age. Her head nods continuously in yes/yes pattern, her voice quality is somewhat soft but she is easily understood, arm tremor is noted when she extends her right arm for a handshake, but not when her hands are resting in her lap. She states the tremor does seem to worsen when she is anxious or acutely ill. Her general health is good. She had laser surgery for acute glaucoma 10 years ago, uses Pilocarpine 2% eye gtts daily. Last eye exam was 6 weeks ago. She currently takes multivitamin and calcium supplements, but no other medications. On examination, WT 136 lbs., HT 67 inches, T 98.4, P 70, R 14, BP 130/78. PERRLA, eyes clear without redness or excessive tearing. TMs normal. Cranial nerves grossly intact. Upper extremities are negative for muscle atrophy, fasciculation, weakness, or tenderness. There is no drift, rigidity, or resistance. Reflexes are 2+, tone 4/5. Normal sensation to pin prick, temperature, and vibration. Lower extremities are the same with 3+ reflexes and 5/5 tone. Appendicular coordination normal, gait grossly normal. She has some stiffness in her left hip with a barely discernable limp which she states is residual injury from being struck by a car while walking across a street 13 years ago. Her tremor is limited to a gentle yes/yes nod of the head when upright and abates when she reclines and her head/neck is supported on a pillow. Her hand/arm tremor is characterized by a gentle, rhythmic shaking movement with all voluntary movement. It is quite pronounced when arms are extended out from the midline either forward or to the sides. She is able to hold a cup of water, bring it up to her mouth and drink using one hand but prefers to use both, especially with hot beverages to avoid spilling and possible burns. Pencil grip is normal and writing is legible but she performs the task slowly. She states she prefers to use a keyboard/computer. Using the small keyboard on her phone is laborious and she will voice activate most frequently called numbers and no longer does text messaging.

Impression: **Benign essential tremor** possibly exacerbated by move to warm climate. Discussed medication options including benefits and side effects and she agrees to a trial of propranolol. She is given samples of Inderal 40 mg to take BID and will return to clinic in 2 weeks for follow-up.

Diagnosis Code(s)

G25.0 Essential tremor

Coding Note(s)

There is a specific code for essential tremor, also referred to as benign essential tremor or familial tremor. Essential tremor is classified with other extrapyramidal and movement disorders in category G25.

Example 4

Restless Leg Syndrome (RLS)

Restless leg syndrome (RLS) is characterized by an irresistible need to move the legs due to uncomfortable sensations in them, such as creeping, crawling, tingling, or bubbling. However, movement does relieve the discomfort. Restless leg syndrome usually manifests at night or when sitting for long periods of time. The sensations are most often felt in the lower leg between the knee and ankle but can also be located in the upper leg or arms. RLS occurs most often in middle age or older adults and stress can exacerbate the condition.

Coding and Documentation Requirements

None.

ICD-10-CM Code/Documentation	
G25.81	Restless leg syndrome

Documentation and Coding Example

A 45-year-old woman presents to the office complaining of insomnia. She states she has had trouble falling asleep for many years, but the problem is worsening. In bed she feels an unbearable discomfort in the legs. She has also noticed this urge on long car rides. The problem is worse at night. She initially described the leg sensations as a "tingling" in her bones radiating from the ankles to the thighs, accompanied by the irresistible need to move her legs. Her symptoms improve when she gets up and walks around. The tingling sensation is now more like electrical shocks accompanied with involuntary, symmetrical limb jerks with restlessness occurring earlier (at 7 pm) and chronic insomnia.

Assessment/Plan: **Restless legs syndrome**. Start with small doses of pramipexole twice daily - 0.09 mg. at 6 pm and 0.18 mg at 10 pm.

Diagnosis Code(s)

G25.81 Restless legs syndrome

Coding Note(s)

There is a distinct code to report restless legs syndrome. The syndrome includes the characteristic symptoms which are not separately reported. There is no laterality requirement for this code.

Hemiplegia and Hemiparesis

The terms hemiplegia and hemiparesis are often used interchangeably, but the two conditions are not the same. Hemiplegia is paralysis of one side of the body while hemiparesis is weakness on one side of the body. Hemiparesis is less severe than hemiplegia and both are a common side effect of stroke or cerebrovascular accident. Hemiplegia and hemiparesis must be clearly differentiated in the medical record documentation. Disability in these cases is determined by the underlying diagnosis, whether the paralysis is temporary or permanent, the extent of paralysis (monoplegia, hemiplegia, paraplegia, quadriplegia), and the body parts affected.

Hemiplegia and hemiparesis are frequently sequelae of cerebrovascular disease; however, cervical spinal cord diseases, peripheral nervous system diseases, and other conditions may manifest as hemiplegia. Precise, detailed provider documentation in the medical record is key to correct code assignment.

These conditions are reported with codes in category G81. There is a note indicating that codes in these categories are used only when hemiplegia or hemiparesis is documented without further specification, or is documented as old or longstanding of unspecified cause. The hemiplegia and hemiparesis codes may also be used in multiple coding scenarios to identify the specified types of hemiplegia resulting from any cause.

In hemiplegia and hemiparesis cases, the documentation needs to identify whether the dominant or nondominant side is affected. If the affected side is documented but not specified as dominant or nondominant, Code selection for a specified side without documentation of which side is dominant is reported as follows:

- If the left side is affected, the default is non-dominant
- If the right side is affected, the default is dominant
- In ambidextrous patients, the default is dominant

It should be noted that hemiplegia documented as congenital or infantile, or due to sequela of a cerebrovascular accident or disease is not reported with codes from these categories. Congenital hemiplegia is used to describe hemiplegia demonstrated at birth while infantile hemiplegia refers to hemiplegia that develops in infancy or within the first few years of life. Congenital or infantile hemiplegia is reported with a code from category G80. Hemiplegia and hemiparesis due to sequelae of cerebrovascular disease is reported with codes from subcategories I69.05, I69.15, I69.25, I69.35, I69.85, and I69.95.

To assign the most specific code for hemiplegia or hemiparesis, the correct category must first be identified. Documentation should be reviewed for the following descriptors:

- Congenital or infantile
- Due to late effect of cerebrovascular accident
- Not otherwise specified

For hemiplegia or hemiparesis of long-standing duration, or not specified as to cause, or to report hemiplegia or hemiparesis in a multiple coding scenario, the type of hemiplegia or hemiparesis must be identified along with the side which should be specified as dominant or nondominant.

Coding and Documentation Requirements

Identify the type of hemiplegia or hemiparesis:

- Flaccid
- Spastic
- Unspecified

Identify the side affected:

- Right
  - Dominant side
  - Nondominant side
- Left
  - Dominant side
  - Nondominant side
- Unspecified side

ICD-10-CM Code/Documentation	
G81.00	Flaccid hemiplegia affecting unspecified side
G81.01	Flaccid hemiplegia affecting right dominant side
G81.02	Flaccid hemiplegia affecting left dominant side
G81.03	Flaccid hemiplegia affecting right nondominant side
G81.04	Flaccid hemiplegia affecting left nondominant side
G81.10	Spastic hemiplegia affecting unspecified side
G81.11	Spastic hemiplegia affecting right dominant side
G81.12	Spastic hemiplegia affecting left dominant side

ICD-10-CM Code/Documentation	
G81.13	Spastic hemiplegia affecting right nondominant side
G81.14	Spastic hemiplegia affecting left nondominant side
G81.90	Hemiplegia, unspecified affecting unspecified side
G81.91	Hemiplegia, unspecified affecting right dominant side
G81.92	Hemiplegia, unspecified affecting left dominant side
G81.93	Hemiplegia, unspecified affecting right nondominant side
G81.94	Hemiplegia, unspecified affecting left nondominant side

Documentation and Coding Example

Patient is a 78-year-old, **right-handed female with longstanding flaccid hemiplegia of unspecified cause affecting her left side**. On admission to the SNF, the patient is experiencing a largely flaccid hemiplegia with Chedoke-McMaster Staging scores on the left side of 1/7 in the hand and arm, 1/7 in the leg and 1/7 in the foot, and 1/7 for posture. There were no sensory problems noted. The patient uses a manual wheelchair with a lap tray for mobility. She was able to complete a 2-person pivot transfer despite problems with her balance. She requires set-up assistance with her meals and one person to assist her with dressing, grooming, and bathing. Due to her poor recovery prognosis, the plan of care will focus on minimizing contractures and palliation of pain. Ensure the flaccid arm is continuously supported when the patient is sitting or transferring—use lap tray or arm sling. Very gentle range of motion exercises with physiotherapy.

Diagnosis: **Left-sided flaccid hemiplegia**

Diagnosis Code(s)

G81.04 Flaccid hemiplegia affecting left nondominant side

Coding Note(s)

This case is coded as flaccid hemiplegia of the nondominant side because the documentation describes the patient as right-handed, so the right side is the dominant side.

Migraine

Migraine is a common neurological disorder that often manifests as a headache. Usually unilateral and pulsating in nature, the headache results from abnormal brain activity along nerve pathways and brain chemical (neurotransmitter) changes. These affect blood flow in the brain and surrounding tissue and may trigger an "aura" or warning sign (visual, sensory, language, motor) before the onset of pain. Migraine headache is frequently accompanied by autonomic nervous system symptoms (nausea, vomiting, and sensitivity to light and/or sound). Triggers can include caffeine withdrawal, stress, lack of sleep. The various types of migraines are reported with codes in category G43. All migraines must be documented as intractable or not intractable. Terms that describe intractable migraine include: pharmacoresistant or pharmacologically resistant, treatment resistant, refractory, and poorly controlled. All migraines except cyclical vomiting (G43.A-), ophthalmoplegic (G43.B-), periodic headache syndromes child/adult (G43.C-) and abdominal migraines (G43.D-) must be documented as with or without status migrainosus. Status migrainosus refers to a migraine that has lasted more than 72 hours.

Coding and Documentation Requirements

Identify migraine type:

- Abdominal
- Chronic without aura
- Cyclical vomiting
- Hemiplegic
- Menstrual
- Ophthalmoplegic
- Periodic headache syndromes child/adult
- Persistent aura
  - With cerebral infarction
  - Without cerebral infarction
- With aura
- Without aura
- Other migraine
- Unspecified

Identify presence/absence of intractability:

- Intractable
- Not intractable

Identify presence/absence of status migrainosus:

- With status migrainosus
- Without status migrainosus

Note – Status migrainosus is not required for migraines documented as abdominal, cyclical vomiting, ophthalmoplegic, or periodic head syndromes in child/adult.

Chronic Migraine without Aura

ICD-10-CM Code/Documentation	
G43.709	Chronic migraine without aura, not intractable, without status migrainosus
G43.719	Chronic migraine without aura, intractable, without status migrainosus
G43.701	Chronic migraine without aura, not intractable, with status migrainosus
G43.711	Chronic migraine without aura, intractable, with status migrainosus

Documentation and Coding Example

Presenting Complaint: Thirty-two-year-old Caucasian female is referred to Pain Management Clinic by her PMD for evaluation and treatment of **chronic migraine headache**.

History: PMH is significant for onset of migraines at age 13-14, typically associated with menstruation for 4-5 years and then becoming more frequent and unpredictable. Patient states her headaches are significantly worse in winter and summer since moving to the NE from Hawaii five years ago. She was initially treated with rizatriptan and ibuprofen for periodic pain management and when headaches became more frequent she was started on daily propranolol. She experienced symptomatic hypotension on propanolol and was switched to amitriptyline which worked well for a few years with headache days numbering 4-5 per month. Gradually her headache days increased and she was switched to topiramate daily, with dose now at 50 mg BID and Treximet taken as needed on acute pain days. She reports **15-20 pain days per month** on these medications for the past 6 months. Headaches are negative for aura, usually bilateral in the supraorbital and/or temporal area with a pulsating quality. She typically experiences photophobia and nausea without vomiting. Patient is married with a 2-year-old son and works part time as a middle school guidance counselor.

Physical Examination: Temperature 97.9 HR 74 RR 14 BP 102/60 WT 122.5 lbs. On examination, this is a pleasant, well-nourished but tired appearing young woman who looks her stated age. At this time, she is experiencing a pulsating headache of moderate intensity, location bilateral with focal area temporal on the right and temporal-supraorbital on the left. She awoke with pain this morning and it has been ongoing for the past 3 days. She denies photophobia or nausea. She has taken topiramate as prescribed but has not taken Treximet in over a week because she ran out. Cranial nerves grossly intact. Both upper and lower extremities have normal strength, movement, and sensation. PERRLA, eyes negative for conjunctival injection and excess tearing. There is no evidence of ptosis or eyelid edema. No lymphadenopathy present. Oral mucosa normal, throat benign. Nares patent without rhinorrhea or congestion. HR regular without bruits, rubs, or murmur. Breath sounds clear, equal bilaterally. Abdomen soft and non-distended, bowel sounds present all quadrants. Liver is palpated at RCM, spleen is not palpated.

Impression: **Intractable chronic migraine headache syndrome not responsive to drug therapy**. Patient is a good candidate for OnabotulinumtoxinA (Botox) therapy. The procedure was explained to patient, questions answered and informed consent obtained.

Procedure Note: Skin over treatment area prepped with alcohol. Vacuum dried powdered Botox 200 units was reconstituted with 4 ml preservative free 0.9% sodium chloride per manufacturers specification. Using a 30-gauge 0.5 inch needle, a total of 155 units (0.1 ml=5 units) of Botox was injected at 31 points including corrugator muscle (10 units/2 sites), procerus muscle (5 units/1 site), frontalis muscle (20 units/4 sites), temporalis muscle (40 units/8 sites), occipitalis muscle (30 units/6 sites), cervical paraspinal muscle group (20 units/4 sites), and trapezius muscle (30 units/6 sites). Patient tolerated the procedure well. She has some mild ptosis noted in left eyelid but it does not obstruct vision.

Plan: Patient is advised to continue current medications as prescribed and that she may experience headache, tenderness at injection site, and mild muscle weakness in the next few days. She should call if she develops any other symptoms or problems. Return to clinic in 5 days for recheck.

Diagnosis Code(s)

G43.719 Chronic migraine without aura, intractable, without status migrainosus

Coding Note(s)

Use of the code for intractable migraine requires documentation that the migraine has not responded to treatment. In this case the patient has been referred to pain medicine because of intractable migraine and that is the stated diagnosis of the pain medicine specialist. The physician has also documented a diagnosis of chronic migraine. Chronic migraine is typically defined as 15 or more headache days per month. The documentation indicates that the patient experiences 15-20 headache days per month which further supports the diagnosis of chronic migraine. Status migrainosus refers to a migraine that has lasted for more than 72 hours. There is no documentation to support status migrainosus so the code for without status migrainosus is assigned.

Migraine Variant

Migraine variant refers to a migraine that manifests in a form other than head pain. Migraine variants may be characterized by episodes of atypical sensory, motor, or visual aura, confusion, dysarthria, focal neurologic deficits, and other constitutional symptoms, with or without a headache. The provider documentation in the medical record must include enough detail to differentiate migraine variants from other migraines and other headache disorders.

The diagnosis of migraine variant is determined by the provider's documentation. Typically, there is a history of paroxysmal signs and symptoms with or without cephalgia and without other disorders that may contribute to the symptoms. Many patients have a family history of migraine.

In the medical record documentation, migraine variants must be clearly differentiated from other headache disorders such as trigeminal autonomic cephalgias (cluster headaches), stabbing headache, thunderclap headaches, hypnic headaches and hemicrania continua, and headache syndromes associated with physical activity (e.g., exertional headaches). Chronic migraine and status migrainosus are not considered migraine variants.

Coding and Documentation Requirements

Identify migraine variant:

- Abdominal migraine
- Cyclical vomiting
- Ophthalmoplegic migraine
- Periodic headache syndromes in child/adult
- Other migraine

Identify response to treatment:

- Intractable
- Not intractable

For migraine variants classified under other migraine, identify any status migrainosus:

- With status migrainosus
- Without status migrainosus

ICD-10-CM Code/Documentation	
G43.A0	Cyclical vomiting, in migraine, not intractable
G43.A1	Cyclical vomiting, in migraine, intractable
G43.B0	Ophthalmoplegic migraine, not intractable
G43.B1	Ophthalmoplegic migraine, intractable

ICD-10-CM Code/Documentation	
G43.C0	Periodic headache syndromes in child or adult, not intractable
G43.C1	Periodic headache syndromes in child or adult, intractable
G43.D0	Abdominal migraine, not intractable
G43.D1	Abdominal migraine, intractable
G43.801	Other migraine, not intractable, with status migrainosus
G43.809	Other migraine, not intractable, without status migrainosus
G43.811	Other migraine, intractable, with status migrainosus
G43.819	Other migraine, intractable, without status migrainosus

Documentation and Coding Example

A 7-year-old girl presented with complete right oculomotor palsy. She complained the previous day of a headache in the orbital region, severe and throbbing in nature. She was given children's Tylenol and went to bed early. She awakened the following morning with complete ptosis of the right upper lid, periorbital pain, and blurred vision. On examination, the right pupil was 6 mm and slightly reactive to light. The neurologic examination and skull x-rays were normal; diagnostic workup including the glucose tolerance test was all negative. MRI and magnetic resonance angiography ruled out aneurysm, tumor, and sphenoid sinus mucocele. Intermittent angle-closure glaucoma with mydriasis was also excluded on gonioscopy. She experienced near complete resolution of her symptoms following treatment with NSAIDs.

Diagnosis: **Ophthalmoplegic migraine**

Diagnosis Code(s)

G43.B0 Ophthalmoplegic migraine, not intractable

Coding Note(s)

Ophthalmoplegic migraine is specified as intractable (with refractory migraine) or not intractable (without refractory migraine). The documentation does not mention intractable migraine or refractory migraine. An intractable or refractory migraine is any migraine that is impossible to manage or resistant to usual therapies.

Other Headache Syndromes

A complaint of headache is a common reason for seeking medical care. Headaches have many causes and while most headaches are benign, a headache may also be a symptom of another underlying disease such as cerebral hemorrhage. A diagnosis of headache that is not further qualified as a specific type, such as tension or migraine, is reported with a symptom code. Other headache syndromes is a broad category that includes many specific headache types with the exception of migraine which has its own category. Below are characteristics of the various types of headaches classified under other headache syndromes.

Cluster headache – Headache characterized by a cyclical pattern of intense, usually unilateral pain with a rapid onset. They are vascular in origin, caused by the sudden dilatation of one or more blood vessels around the trigeminal nerve. The pain often centers behind or around the eye (retro-orbital, orbital, supraorbital) or in the temporal area and has a boring/drilling quality. The pain may be accompanied by one (or more) cranial autonomic nervous system symptoms. Cluster headaches are benign, but can be quite disabling. Individuals may have a genetic predisposition for this type of headache Disorders of the hypothalamus, smoking, and traumatic brain injury may also be causative factors. Cluster headaches are subclassified as episodic or chronic. Episodic cluster headaches typically occur at least once per day, often at the same time of day for several weeks. The headaches are followed by weeks, months, or years that are completely pain free. Chronic cluster headaches may have "high" or "low" cycles in the frequency or intensity of pain but no real remission.

Drug induced headache (medication overuse headache, analgesic rebound headache) – A serious and disabling condition that can occur when medication is taken daily for tension, migraine, or other acute or chronic headache or other pain. As the medication wears off, the pain returns and more medication is needed. This creates a cycle of pain, medicating to relieve the pain, and more intense pain. The condition is more common in women, typically between the ages of 30-40, but it can occur at any age. Pain is often described as a constant dull ache that is worse in the morning and after exercise. Medications associated with this rebound headache phenomena include: acetaminophen, ibuprofen, naproxen, aspirin, codeine, hydrocodone, tramadol, and ergotamine. Triptans (sumatriptan) used for vascular headaches can also induce these headaches. To stop the pain cycle, medication must be discontinued, preferably abruptly and entirely, but slow withdrawal may be necessary in certain situations. This often results in withdrawal symptoms including headache, anxiety, insomnia, and gastrointestinal upset (nausea, vomiting). Withdrawal symptoms can last as long as 12 weeks but typically subside in 7-10 days. Non-steroidal anti-inflammatory drugs (ibuprofen, naproxen) may be given to help relieve rebound headache phenomena when these drugs have not been used previously by the patient to treat the primary headache.

Hemicrania continua – A chronic, persistent, primary headache that often varies in severity as it cycles over a 24 period. It is most often unilateral in location and does not change sides. The incidence is somewhat higher in women with age of onset in early adulthood. There can be migrainous qualities including: pulsating/throbbing pain, nausea and vomiting, photophobia (light sensitivity), and phonophobia (noise sensitivity) along with autonomic nervous system symptoms. The most striking definitive characteristic of hemicrania continua is that it responds almost immediately to treatment with the drug indomethacin.

New daily persistent headache (NDPH) – A distinct, primary headache syndrome with symptoms that can mimic chronic migraine and tension-type headaches. The onset of NDPH is typically abrupt and reaches peak intensity within 3 days. Most individuals can recall the exact day/time of onset of the headache. In some instances, the pain will follow an infection or flu-like illness, surgery, or stressful life event. Autoimmune and/or inflammatory conditions and hypermobility of the cervical spine may also be contributing factors. The pain can be self-limiting (pain ends after a few months) or unrelenting (pain lasts for years) and is often unresponsive to standard therapy.

Paroxysmal hemicranias – Rare type of headache, more common in women, that usually begins during adulthood. The pain is similar to cluster headaches, but is distinguished by greater frequency and shorter duration of the individual episodes, presence of one or more cranial autonomic nervous system symptoms, and a favorable response to the drug indomethacin. Pain is unilateral (always on the same side) and severe, with a throbbing/boring quality behind or around the eye (retro-orbital, orbital, supraorbital) and/or in the temporal area. There can be localized dull pain or soreness in these areas between episodes of acute pain. Occasionally pain may radiate to the ipsilateral (same side) shoulder, arm, or neck. One or more cranial autonomic nervous system symptoms usually accompanies the pain, such as lacrimation (eye tearing), conjunctival injection (eye redness), nasal congestion, rhinorrhea (runny nose), miosis (constricted pupil), ptosis (eyelid drooping), or eyelid edema (swelling). Cause is not known and there is no familial tendency. Paroxysmal hemicranias are subclassified as episodic or chronic. Episodic paroxysmal hemicranias are less severe and less frequent. In some individuals, this non-chronic phase will be a "pass though" to chronic paroxysmal hemicranias. Chronic paroxysmal hemicranias, also referred to as Sjaastad syndrome, is more common than episodic paroxysmal hemicranias and is characterized by more severe and more frequent episodes.

Post-traumatic headache – Headache that occurs following a closed head injury or trauma to the neck area. It is a fairly common and self-limiting condition and may have characteristics of both tension and migrainous pain. The headache rarely occurs in isolation and accompanying symptoms can include: cervical (neck) pain, cognitive, behavioral, and/or somatic problems. Individuals with chronic pain disorders (other than headache), pre-existing headaches, and affective disorders are at greater risk for developing both acute and chronic post traumatic headache. The cycle of pain can be difficult to interrupt once it has been established and overuse of analgesics frequently results in rebound phenomena. This can lead to co-morbid psychiatric disorders, post-traumatic stress disorder, insomnia, substance abuse, and depression. Acute post-traumatic headache (APTH) can begin immediately or anytime in the 2 months following injury. Acute post-traumatic headache becomes chronic post- traumatic headache when the pain continues for longer than 2 months following injury.

Primary thunderclap headache – Relatively uncommon type of headache characterized by a dramatic, sudden, severe onset of pain anywhere in the head or neck area that peaks within 60 seconds and begins to fade in 1 hour. Residual pain/discomfort may be present for up to 10 days. The sympathetic nervous system is believed to be involved and nausea and vomiting may occur with the pain; however, the headache usually cannot be attributed to any specific disorder. Thunderclap headache may signal a potentially life-threatening condition including: subarachnoid hemorrhage, cerebral venous sinus thrombosis, and cervical artery (carotid, vertebral artery) dissection.

Short-lasting unilateral neuralgiform headache with conjunctival injection and tearing (SUNCT) – A rare type of primary headache belonging to a group referred to as trigeminal autonomic cephalagia (TAC). This headache is triggered by the cranial autonomic nervous system at the trigeminal (5th cranial) nerve. Pain is usually described as moderate to severe with a burning, piercing, or stabbing quality. It is unilateral, centered in or around the eye (retro-orbital, orbital, supraorbital) and/or the temporal area. It is characterized by bursts of pain, lasting from a few seconds to 5-6 minutes and can occur up to 200 times per day (most commonly 5-6 times per hour). Cranial autonomic nervous system symptoms that accompany the pain include eye tearing (lacrimation) and conjunctival injection (eye redness). Nasal congestion, runny nose (rhinorrhea), constricted pupil (miosis), eyelid drooping (ptosis), or swelling (edema) may also occur. Men are affected more often than women with onset most commonly occurring after age 50. Pain may radiate to the teeth, neck, and around the ears. It is more common during daytime hours and can occur at regular or irregular intervals without a distinct refractory period.

Tension-type headache (muscle contraction headache, stress headache) – Characterized by pain that encircles the head without a throbbing or pulsating quality. Nausea/vomiting, disruption in normal activities, photophobia (light sensitivity) and phonophobia (sound sensitivity) are not normally associated with the condition. Onset is typically gradual, often in the middle of the day and pain can be exacerbated by fatigue, poor posture, emotions, and mental stress (including depression). This headache is more common in women and no familial tendency has been identified. Tension or stress headaches are the most common type of headaches among adults. The terms tension headache and tension-type headache are considered synonymous. Tension-type headache is subclassified as episodic or chronic. Episodic and chronic tension-type headaches are differentiated from each other by the frequency with which the headache occurs with episodic being defined as greater than 10 but less than 15 headache days per month and chronic being defined as more than 15 days per month. Episodic tension headaches occur randomly and are often the result of temporary stress, anxiety, or fatigue.

Vascular headache – A broad or generalized term that includes cluster headache, migraine headache, and toxic (fever, chemical) headache. For coding purposes, headaches described as vascular but without more specific information as to type are reported with the code for vascular headache not elsewhere classified. Vascular headaches all involve changes in blood flow or in the vascular (blood vessel) system of the brain which trigger head pain and other neurological symptoms. These symptoms can include nausea and vomiting, vertigo (dizziness), photophobia (light sensitivity), phonophobia (noise sensitivity), visual disturbances, numbness and tingling (in any area of the body), problems with speech, and muscle weakness.

Other headache syndromes are reported with codes from category G44 and include: cluster headaches, vascular headache not elsewhere classified, tension-type headaches, post-traumatic headaches, drug-induced headaches as well as others. Response to treatment is a component of many codes in category G44. Cluster headache, paroxysmal hemicranias, short lasting unilateral neuralgiform headache with conjunctival injection and tearing (SUNCT), other trigeminal autonomic cephalgias (TAC), tension-type headache, post-traumatic headache, and drug-induced headache must be specified as intractable or not intractable. Intractable refers to headache syndromes that are not responding to treatment. Terms that describe intractable migraine include: pharmacoresistant or pharmacologically resistant, treatment resistant, refractory, and poorly controlled. Not intractable describes a headache that is responsive to and well controlled with treatment. In addition, vascular headache not elsewhere classified is also classified in the nervous system chapter with other headache syndromes and is reported with code G44.1.

Differentiation between the various types of headache can be difficult and patients often experience overlapping types of headache, so clearly documenting the type or types of headache the patient is experiencing is crucial to accurate diagnosis and appropriate treatment. This documentation is also needed for coding headache disorders.

Coding and Documentation Requirements

Identify the specific headache syndrome:

- Cluster headache syndrome
  - Chronic
  - Episodic
  - Unspecified
- Complicated headache syndromes
  - Hemicrania continua
  - New daily persistent headache (NDPH)
  - Primary thunderclap headache
  - Other complicated headache syndrome
- Drug induced headache, not elsewhere classified
- Other headache syndromes
  - Headache associated with sexual activity
  - Hypnic headache
  - Primary cough headache
  - Primary exertional headache
  - Primary stabbing headache
  - Other specified headache syndrome
- Other trigeminal autonomic cephalgias (TAC)
- Paroxysmal hemicranias
  - Chronic
  - Episodic
- Post-traumatic headache
  - Acute
  - Chronic
  - Unspecified
- Short lasting unilateral neuralgiform headache with conjunctival injection and tearing (SUNCT)
- Tension type headache
  - Chronic
  - Episodic
  - Unspecified
- Vascular headache, not elsewhere classified

Identify response to treatment for the following types: cluster, paroxysmal hemicranias, SUNCT, other TAC, tension-type, post-traumatic, and drug-induced:

- Intractable
- Not intractable

Cluster Headache Syndrome

ICD-10-CM Code/Documentation	
G44.001	Cluster headache syndrome, unspecified, intractable
G44.009	Cluster headache syndrome, unspecified, not intractable
G44.011	Episodic cluster headache, intractable
G44.019	Episodic cluster headache, not intractable
G44.021	Chronic cluster headache, intractable
G44.029	Chronic cluster headache, not intractable

Documentation and Coding Example

Thirty-seven-year-old Black male is referred to Pain Management Clinic by PCP for treatment of headaches. Patient is an attorney, working in a private, four-person firm focused on family law. He is in a committed relationship with his partner of 6 years and they are expecting a baby girl with a surrogate in 2 months. PMH is significant for being struck in the left temple/eye area by a baseball ten months ago during a recreational game with friends. He had no loss of consciousness or visual changes, but significant pain and swelling of the face and eye. He was evaluated in the ED, where ophthalmology exam, x-rays, and a CT scan showed no eye damage, facial/skull fracture, or intracranial bleeding. The first headache occurred 2 months after this injury and woke him from sleep with intense stabbing pain in the left eye, accompanied by tearing and eye redness. The pain subsided in about 15 minutes only to reoccur twice in the next few hours. He was seen emergently by his ophthalmologist and the exam was entirely benign. The headaches continued, usually awakening him from sleep with a stabbing sensation in his left eye that lasted 30-60 minutes. When the acute pain abated he often had residual aching in the periorbital area and stabbing pain again within a few hours. His PCP advised taking ibuprofen which was not helpful, prescribed Toradol which was also not helpful and finally Percodan which patient states caused nausea and hallucinations. Patient has researched alternative treatment options and has tried acupuncture, melatonin, and removing foods containing tyramine and MSG from his diet. He estimates headache days were 1-3 per week at the beginning, gradually decreasing until he had a 6-week period that was pain free. The headaches began again one week ago and patient requested a referral to pain specialist. On examination, this is a soft spoken, slightly built young black male who looks his stated age. HT 69 inches, WT 150 lbs. T 96.8, P 58, R 14, BP 138/88. PERRLA, left eye has increased lacrimation, conjunctival injection and mild ptosis of the upper lid. Both nares are patent and the left naris has thin, clear mucus drainage. Oral mucosa moist and pink. Neck supple, without masses. Cranial nerves grossly intact. Upper extremities have brisk reflexes and good tone. Muscles are without atrophy, weakness, rigidity or tenderness. Heart rate regular, without bruit, murmur or rub. Breath sounds clear and equal bilaterally. Abdomen soft and non-tender with active bowel sounds in all quadrants. No evidence of hernia, normal male genitalia. Lower extremities have normal reflexes and good tone, no muscle atrophy, weakness, rigidity, or tenderness appreciated. Gait is normal. EKG is obtained and shows NSR. Impression: **Episodic cluster headache, poorly controlled with current medications.**

Consider a trial of verapamil for headache prophylaxis and sumatriptan nasal spray for acute headache.

Patient is commended for his diligence in seeking alternative treatment options and is assured that the pain management team will listen and work closely with him to ensure that his headaches are managed in a way that allows him to fully participate in and enjoy life. Treatment options discussed and patient agrees to try verapamil 40 mg PO BID for 2 weeks and RTC for re-evaluation. He declines sumatriptan nasal spray at this time. He is however interested in oxygen therapy and we will discuss that at his next visit.

Diagnosis Code(s)

G44.011 Episodic cluster headache, intractable

Coding Note(s)

Codes require identification of the headache syndrome as intractable or not intractable. These terms describe the response to treatment. Intractable indicates that the episodic cluster headache is not responding to current treatment. This is documented using the term 'poorly controlled' which, according to coding notes, is a term that is considered the equivalent of intractable.

Tension-Type Headaches

ICD-10-CM Code/Documentation	
G44.201	Tension-type headache, unspecified, intractable
G44.209	Tension-type headache, unspecified, not intractable
G44.211	Episodic tension-type headache, intractable
G44.219	Episodic tension-type headache, not intractable
G44.221	Chronic tension-type headache, intractable
G44.229	Chronic tension-type headache, not intractable

Documentation and Coding Example

HPI: This 36-year-old female complains of **headaches several times per week for several months, usually at the end of the day**. The headaches are reportedly worse after increased time at the computer. The pain starts at the base of the neck and moves up to her forehead. The patient has tried regulating eating and sleeping, drinking more water and decreasing caffeine intake, without relief. OTC headache medications have provided "little to no" relief. The only thing that helps is to lie down and close her eyes.

On examination, her neck muscles are very tight and tender. There are multiple trigger points in the sub-occipital muscles and in the sternocleidomastoid on the right. Pressure on the sub-occipital trigger points reproduces the headache. Range of motion is decreased in neck flexion and right rotation. Other testing for nerve, muscle, and joint involvement was negative and the temporomandibular joint (TMJ) is not contributory.

Assessment/Plan: **Classic tension headache**. Poor posture and fatigue causes excess tension in the posterior neck muscles, especially the sub-occipital muscle group. Treatment to include massage therapy to release the muscle tension and patient education on proper posture and ergonomics.

Diagnosis Code(s)

G44.209 Tension-type headache, unspecified, not intractable

Coding Note(s)

Under the main term Headache, the Alphabetical Index lists tension (-type) as a subterm. Tension headache NOS is listed as an inclusion term in the Tabular for tension-type headache. All types of tension headache are classified in Chapter 6 Diseases of the Nervous System, under other headache syndromes, in the subcategory G44.2. This subcategory includes: tension headache, tension-type headache, episodic tension-type headache, and chronic tension-type headache. Psychological factors affecting physical conditions (F54) has an Excludes2 note listing tension-type headache (G44.2). Headache frequency and the type and severity of symptoms should be described in the clinical documentation. Detailed documentation of the etiology and any associated mental or organic illness also is necessary. Documentation of tension headache should also describe the response to treatment.

Monoplegia of Lower/Upper Limb

Monoplegia is also known as paralysis of one limb or monoplegia disorder. Sensory loss is typically more prominent in the distal segments of the limbs. It is important that the provider clearly document the etiology or underlying cause as there are many possible causes and the underlying cause can affect code assignment. Examples of causes include:

- Cerebral palsy
- Stroke
- Brain tumor
- Multiple sclerosis
- Motor neuron disease
- Nerve trauma, impingement, or inflammation
- Mononeuritis multiplex

Like hemiplegia and hemiparesis, monoplegia of a limb is frequently due to sequela of cerebrovascular disease, cervical spinal cord diseases, or peripheral nervous system diseases. The specific type of monoplegia should be clearly described in the provider documentation. For example, congenital monoplegia (demonstrated at birth) and infantile monoplegia (develops within the first few years of life) are classified to other categories, as is monoplegia due to late effect (sequela) of cerebrovascular disease/accident. Clear, complete provider documentation in the medical record of the type and cause of the monoplegia is essential for correct code assignment.

Monoplegia is classified in the category for other paralytic syndromes. Monoplegia is also classified by whether the upper (G83.2) or limb lower (G83.1) is affected; the side of the body affected; and whether the side affected is dominant or nondominant.

There is a note indicating that codes in these categories are used only when the paralytic syndrome, in this case monoplegia, is documented without further specification, or is documented as old or longstanding of unspecified cause. The monoplegia codes may also be used in multiple coding scenarios to identify the specified types of monoplegia resulting from any cause.

For monoplegia cases, the documentation needs to identify whether the dominant or nondominant side is affected. If the affected side is documented but not specified as dominant or nondominant, Code selection for a specified side without documentation of which side is dominant is reported the same as hemiplegia:

- If the left side is affected, the default is non-dominant
- If the right side is affected, the default is dominant
- In ambidextrous patients, the default is dominant

Coding and Documentation Requirements

Identify the affected limb:

- Lower
- Upper
- Unspecified

Identify the side affected:

- Right
  - Dominant side
  - Nondominant side
- Left
  - Dominant side
  - Nondominant side
- Unspecified side

Monoplegia of Lower Limb

ICD-10-CM Code/Documentation	
G83.10	Monoplegia of lower limb affecting unspecified side
G83.11	Monoplegia of lower limb affecting right dominant side
G83.12	Monoplegia of lower limb affecting left dominant side
G83.13	Monoplegia of lower limb affecting right nondominant side
G83.14	Monoplegia of lower limb affecting left nondominant side

Documentation and Coding Example

A 46-year-old male patient presented with complaints of neck pain, numbing sensation, and right leg weakness. The physical examination showed monoplegia of right leg, with intact sensory function. The other extremities had no neurologic deficits. MR imaging showed spinal cord compression and high signal intensity of spinal cord at C6-7. Therefore, the cause of monoplegia of the leg was thought to be the spinal cord ischemia.

Diagnosis: **Monoplegia, right leg, due to spinal cord ischemia.**

Diagnosis Code(s)

G95.11 Acute infarction of spinal cord (embolic) (nonembolic)

G83.11 Monoplegia of lower limb affecting right dominant side

Coding Note(s)

In this case, the affected side is documented but not specified as dominant or nondominant. ICD-10-CM code selection hierarchy states that if the right side is affected, the default is dominant. It should also be noted that this is a multiple coding scenario, requiring a code for the spinal cord ischemia, which is listed first, and a second code identifying the monoplegia.

Monoplegia of Upper Limb

ICD-10-CM Code/Documentation	
G83.20	Monoplegia of upper limb affecting unspecified side
G83.21	Monoplegia of upper limb affecting right dominant side
G83.22	Monoplegia of upper limb affecting left dominant side
G83.23	Monoplegia of upper limb affecting right nondominant side
G83.24	Monoplegia of upper limb affecting left nondominant side

Documentation and Coding Example

A 75-year-old female presented to the emergency department with sudden onset right upper limb weakness and altered sensation. The patient was previously well with an unremarkable medical history. On examination, she was apyrexial, normotensive and normoglycemic with a GCS of 15/15. Neurological examination revealed right upper limb hypotonia and power of 0/5 in all hand and wrist muscle groups, 2/5 power in biceps and triceps, and 3/5 power in the shoulder girdle. Hypoesthesia was noted throughout the right upper limb. The remainder of the neurological examination did not reveal any other deficits. Baseline labs were normal. On brain MRI, mild ischemic change was noted throughout the cerebral white matter in the absence of infarcts within the basal ganglia, brainstem or cerebellum and cerebral venography was not suggestive of a recent thrombosis. Collectively the imaging studies were indicative of an acute parenchymal event with evidence of previous superficial bleeds. Following little improvement in right arm function after neuro-rehabilitation, the patient was discharged home.

Diagnosis: **Spontaneous right arm monoplegia secondary to probable cerebral amyloid angiopathy**.

Diagnosis Code(s)

G83.21 Monoplegia of upper limb affecting right dominant side

Coding Note(s)

Here again, the affected side is documented but not specified as dominant or nondominant. According to the code selection hierarchy in ICD-10-CM, the right side is affected so the default is dominant. ICD-10-CM Coding and Reporting Guidelines for Outpatient Services direct the user not to code diagnoses documented as "probable," "suspected," "questionable," "rule out," "working diagnosis," or other similar terms indicating uncertainty; therefore, no code is assigned for "probable cerebral amyloid angiopathy".

Summary

ICD-10-CM classifies diseases of the nervous system by the type and cause of the disease or disorder, such as intraoperative and postprocedural complications, congenital conditions, infectious diseases, neoplasms, or traumatic injury. Documentation of the severity and/or status of the disease in terms of acute or chronic, as well as the site, etiology, and any secondary disease process are basic documentation requirements. Physician documentation of diagnostic test findings or confirmation of any diagnosis found in diagnostic test reports is also required documentation.

Nervous system coding requires a significant level of specificity, which makes the provider's medical 0record documentation particularly important. Precise clinical information will need to be documented in the medical record to accurately report the codes.

Resources

Documentation checklists are available in Appendix A for

- Headache syndromes
- Migraine
- Seizures

Chapter 6 Quiz

1. CRPS II is
   a. severe neuropathic pain that may be a result of an illness or injury with intense pain to light touch, abnormal circulation, temperature and sweating
   b. usually occurs at night with an irresistible urge to move the legs due to unusual sensations such as tingling, creeping and crawling
   c. a type of neuropathic pain the occurs following a peripheral nerve injury resulting in burning or throbbing pain along the nerve, sensitivity to cold and touch, changes in skin color, temperature, texture, hair and nails
   d. Disease or damage to peripheral nerves resulting in impaired sensation, movement, gland or organ dysfunction.
2. How are seizure disorders and recurrent seizures classified?
   a. Seizure disorders and recurrent seizures are classified with epilepsy
   b. Seizure disorders and recurrent seizures are classified as non-epileptic
   c. Seizure disorders and recurrent seizures are classified as signs and symptoms
   d. None of the above
3. Which of the following is an alternate term for "intractable" migraine?
   a. Pharmacoresistant
   b. Refractory (medically)
   c. Poorly controlled
   d. All of the above
4. Where are coding and sequencing guidelines for diseases of the nervous system and complications due to the treatment of the diseases and conditions of the nervous system found?
   a. In the ICD-10-CM Official Guidelines for Coding and Reporting chapter specific guidelines for Chapter 6
   b. In the Alphabetic Index and the Tabular List and the chapter specific guidelines for Chapter 6
   c. In other chapter specific guidelines in the ICD-10-CM Official Guidelines for Coding and Reporting
   d. All of the above
5. What is the correct code assignment for an encounter for treatment of a condition causing pain?
   a. A code for the underlying condition is assigned as the principal diagnosis and a code from category G89 is assigned as an additional diagnosis.
   b. A code from category G89 is assigned as the principal diagnosis and no code is assigned for the underlying condition.
   c. A code for the underlying condition is assigned as the principal diagnosis and no code from category G89 is assigned.
   d. A code from category G89 is assigned as the principal diagnosis and a code for the underlying condition is assigned as an additional diagnosis.
6. Which of the following documentation is required for accurate coding of epilepsy?
   a. With or without intractable epilepsy
   b. Type of epilepsy
   c. With or without status epilepticus
   d. All of the above
7. When an admission is for treatment of an underlying condition and a neurostimulator is also inserted for pain control during the same episode of care, what is the correct code assignment?
   a. The underlying condition is the principal diagnosis and the appropriate pain code should be assigned as a secondary diagnosis.
   b. A code for the underlying condition is assigned as the principal diagnosis and no pain code is assigned as an additional diagnosis.
   c. A pain code is assigned as the principal diagnosis and a code for the underlying condition is assigned as an additional diagnosis.
   d. A code for insertion of a neurostimulator for pain control is assigned as the principal diagnosis and a pain code is assigned as an additional diagnosis.
8. Alzheimer's disease with dementia requires dual coding. What is the proper sequencing for Alzheimer's disease with dementia?
   a. The dementia is coded first with or without behavioral disturbance followed by a code for the underlying condition (Alzheimer's disease).
   b. Only the Alzheimer's disease is coded
   c. The Alzheimer's disease is coded first followed by a code for dementia with or without behavioral disturbance.
   d. The Alzheimer's disease is coded with an additional code for any behavioral disturbance.
9. In patients with hemiplegia, if the affected side is documented but not specified as dominant or nondominant, how is this coded?
   a. When the left side is affected, the default is non-dominant
   b. When the right side is affected, the default is dominant
   c. When the patient is ambidextrous, the default is dominant
   d. All of the above
10. What is the correct coding of a diagnosis documented as post-thoracotomy pain without further specification as acute or chronic?
    a. A code from Chapter 19 Injury, poisoning, and certain other consequences of external causes, is assigned
    b. Post-thoracotomy pain is routine postoperative pain and is not coded
    c. The code for acute post-thoracotomy pain is the default
    d. The code for chronic post-thoracotomy pain is the default

See next page for answers and rationales.

Chapter 6 Answers and Rationales

1. CRPS II is

   c. **a type of neuropathic pain the occurs following a peripheral nerve injury resulting in burning or throbbing pain along the nerve, sensitivity to cold and touch, changes in skin color, temperature, texture, hair and nails**

   Rationale: *CRPS II or chronic regional pain syndrome is pain as a result of a direct injury to a nerve vs RSD or CRPS I do not have to have a direct injury to a nerve. B is the definition for restless leg syndrome and d is the definition for neuropathy. For both CRPS I and CRPS II documentation of upper or lower extremity as well as laterality is required.*

2. How are seizure disorders and recurrent seizures classified?

   a. **Seizure disorders and recurrent seizures are classified with epilepsy**

   Rationale: *The Index entry for seizure disorder directs the user to see Epilepsy. Both Seizure disorder and recurrent seizures are indexed to G40.909 Epilepsy, unspecified.*

3. Which of the following is an alternate term for "intractable" migraine?

   d. **All of the above**

   Rationale: *According to the instructional note under category G40, the following terms are to be considered equivalent to intractable: pharmacoresistant (pharmacologically resistant), treatment resistant, refractory (medically), and poorly controlled.*

4. Where are coding and sequencing guidelines for diseases of the nervous system and complications due to the treatment of the diseases and conditions of the nervous system found?

   b. **In the Alphabetic Index and the Tabular List and the chapter specific guidelines for Chapter 6**

   Rationale: *the conventions and instructions of the classification along with the general and chapter-specific coding guidelines govern the selection and sequencing of ICD-10-CM codes. According to Section I.A of the ICD-10-CM coding guidelines, the conventions are the general rules for use of the classification independent of the guidelines. These conventions are incorporated within the Alphabetic Index and Tabular List of the ICD-10-CM as instructional notes.*

5. What is the correct code assignment for an encounter for treatment of a condition causing pain?

   c. **A code for the underlying condition is assigned as the principal diagnosis and no code from category G89 is assigned.**

   Rationale: *According to the chapter specific coding guidelines for Chapter 6 of ICD-10-CM, when an admission or encounter is for a procedure aimed at treating the underlying condition, a code for the underlying condition should be assigned as the principal diagnosis and no code from category G89 should be assigned.*

6. Which of the following documentation is required for accurate coding of epilepsy?

   d. **All of the above**

   Rationale: *Epilepsy is classified by the specific type and then as intractable or not intractable, and with or without status epilepticus. A note in lists the terms pharmacoresistant, pharmacologically resistant, poorly controlled, refractory, or treatment resistant as synonyms for intractable.*

7. When an admission is for treatment of an underlying condition and a neurostimulator is also inserted for pain control during the same episode of care, what is the correct code assignment?

   a. **The underlying condition is the principal diagnosis and the appropriate pain code should be assigned as a secondary diagnosis.**

   Rationale: *Section I.B.1.a of the ICD-10-CM coding guidelines provides specific direction on coding Category G89 codes as principal diagnosis or the first-listed code. According to these guidelines, when a patient is admitted for a procedure aimed at treating the underlying condition and a neurostimulator is inserted for pain control during the same admission/encounter, a code for the underlying condition should be assigned as the principal diagnosis and the appropriate pain code should be assigned as a secondary diagnosis.*

8. What is the proper sequencing for Alzheimer's disease with dementia?

   c. **The Alzheimer's disease is coded first followed by a code for dementia with or without behavioral disturbance.**

   Rationale: *An instructional note at category G30 directs the coder to use an additional code to identify delirium, dementia with or without behavioral disturbance.*

9. In patients with hemiplegia, if the affected side is documented but not specified as dominant or nondominant?

   d. **All of the above**

   Rationale: *Section I.C.6.a of the ICD-10-CM coding guidelines provides specific direction for cases where the affected side is documented, but not specified as dominant or nondominant. According to these guidelines, the default code is dominant for ambidextrous patients, nondominant when the left side is affected and dominant when the right side is affected.*

10. What is the correct coding of a diagnosis documented as post-thoracotomy pain without further specification as acute or chronic?

    c. **The code for acute post-thoracotomy pain is the default**

    Rationale: *According to Section I.C.6.b.3 of the ICD-10-CM coding guidelines, the default is the code for the acute form for post-thoracotomy pain when not specified as acute or chronic.*

Chapter 7

DISEASES OF THE EYE AND ADNEXA (HØØ-H59)

Introduction

The codes for diseases of the eye are located in Chapter 7 Diseases of the Eye and Adnexa (H00-H59).

The chapter begins with instructions to assign an external cause code following the code for the eye condition to identify the cause of the eye condition when applicable. Along with codes for diseases of the eye, are also codes for diseases and conditions affecting the adnexa, or the structures surrounding the eye, such as the tear (lacrimal) ducts and glands, the extraocular muscles, and the eyelids.

Coding diseases of the eye and adnexa can be difficult due to the complex anatomic structures of the ocular system. Provider documentation specifying the affected site is required in detail as body sites very specific and require documentation of laterality for paired body parts and of upper versus lower sites as in right upper eyelid or right lower eyelid.

Documentation of the evaluation and treatment of eye disorders can be difficult to understand because ophthalmology has a distinctive language. Most ophthalmic terminology such as amblyopia, glaucoma, chalazion, and pterygium are derived from Greek and Latin words. For example, ophthalmologic medical record documentation often indicates "O.S." and "O.D." O.S. is an abbreviation for "oculus sinister," Latin for "left eye" and O.D. is an abbreviation for "oculus dexter," Latin for "right eye".

To help understand the coding and documentation requirements for diseases of the eye and adnexa the code blocks in ICD-10-CM are displayed in the following table.

ICD-1Ø-CM Blocks	
HØØ-HØ5	Disorders of eyelid, lacrimal system and orbit
H1Ø-H11	Disorders of conjunctiva
H15-H22	Disorders of sclera, cornea, iris and ciliary body
H25-H28	Disorders of lens
H3Ø-H36	Disorders of choroid and retina
H4Ø-H42	Glaucoma
H43-H44	Disorders of vitreous body and globe
H46-H47	Disorders of optic nerve and visual pathways
H49-H52	Disorders of ocular muscles, binocular movement, accommodation and refraction
H53-H54	Visual disturbances and blindness
H55-H57	Other disorders of eye and adnexa
H59	Intraoperative and postprocedural complications and disorders of eye and adnexa, not elsewhere classified

There is also a code block to classify all intraoperative and post procedural complications of treatment for eye and adnexal disorders.

Exclusions

There are no Excludes1 notes, but there are a number of Excludes2 notes, which are listed in the table below.

Excludes1	Excludes2
None	Certain conditions originating in the perinatal period (PØ4-P96) Certain infectious and parasitic diseases (AØØ-B99) Complications of pregnancy, childbirth and the puerperium (OØØ-O9A) Congenital malformations, deformations, and chromosomal abnormalities (QØØ-Q99) Diabetes mellitus related eye conditions (EØ8.3-, EØ9.3-, E1Ø.3-, E11.3-, E13.3-) Endocrine, nutritional and metabolic diseases (EØØ-E88) Injury (trauma) of eye and orbit (SØ5.-) Injury, poisoning and certain other consequences of external causes (SØØ-T88) Neoplasms (CØØ-D49) Symptoms, signs and abnormal clinical and laboratory findings, not elsewhere classified (RØØ-R94) Syphilis related eye disorders (A5Ø.Ø1, A5Ø.3-, A51.43, A52.71)

As can be seen in the exclusions table, several diseases coded to other chapters have associated eye manifestations, such as eye disorders associated with infectious diseases (Chapter 1) and diabetes (Chapter 4). ICD-10-CM contains many combination codes for conditions and common symptoms or manifestations. Most notably, there are combination codes for diabetes mellitus with eye conditions (E08.3-, E09.3-, E10.3-, E11.3-, E13.3-) such as diabetic retinopathy.

Besides diabetes related conditions and eye disorders associated with infectious and parasitic diseases, other disorders of the eye and adnexa are classified in different chapters, such as conditions associated with a neoplastic process, conditions originating in the perinatal period (P04-P96), complications of pregnancy, childbirth and the puerperium (O00-O9A) and congenital malformations, deformations, and chromosomal abnormalities (Q00-Q99). Conditions resulting from injury or trauma to the eye and orbit (S05.-) are classified in Chapter 19 - Injury, Poisoning and Certain Other Consequences of External Causes (S00-T88).

Chapter Guidelines

Coding and sequencing guidelines for diseases of the eye and adnexa and complications due to the treatment of these conditions are found in the coding conventions, the general coding guidelines, and the chapter-specific coding guidelines. Close attention to the instructions in the Tabular List and Alphabetic Index is also needed in order to assign the most specific code possible.

There are specific guidelines addressing assignment of glaucoma codes. For example, when a patient is admitted with glaucoma and the stage evolves during the admission, coding guidelines direct the user to assign the code for the highest stage documented. Another example involves assignment of the code for "indeterminate" stage glaucoma; guidelines state that code assignment is based on the clinical documentation. Glaucoma codes are combination codes and the seventh character "4" is assigned for glaucoma cases whose stage cannot be clinically determined. Coding guidelines caution the user not to confuse the indeterminate stage with unspecified stage which is assigned only when there is no documentation regarding the stage of the glaucoma.

Codes identify the type of glaucoma, the affected eye, and the glaucoma stage in a single combination code. Laterality is a component for choosing codes. There are guidelines for coding bilateral glaucoma:

- For bilateral glaucoma where both eyes are documented as the same type and stage, and there is a code for bilateral provided, a single code for the type of glaucoma, bilateral, is reported with the seventh character identifying the stage.
- For bilateral glaucoma where both eyes are documented as the same type and stage, and the classification does not provide a code for bilateral glaucoma (e.g. H40.10, H40.20), report only one code for the type of glaucoma with the appropriate seventh character for stage.

Different types or stages

- When each eye is documented as having a different type or stage in bilateral glaucoma, assign the appropriate code for each eye when laterality is distinguished
- When each eye is documented as having a different type or stage in bilateral glaucoma, and laterality is not distinguished, assign one code for each type of glaucoma present with the appropriate seventh digit
- When each eye is documented as having the same type but different stage in bilateral glaucoma, and laterality is not distinguished, assign a code for the type of glaucoma with the appropriate seventh digit for each eye

General Documentation Requirements

Documentation requirements depend on the particular disease or disorder affecting the eye or the surrounding adnexa. Some of the general documentation requirements are discussed here, but greater detail for some of the more common diseases of the eye and adnexa will be provided in the next section.

In general, basic medical record documentation requirements include the severity or status of the disease (e.g., acute or chronic), as well as the site, etiology, and any secondary disease process. The provider's confirmation of any diagnosis found in laboratory or other diagnostic test reports must be documented for code assignment. Provider documentation should clearly specify any cause-and-effect relationship between medical treatment and an eye disorder. Documentation in the medical record should specify whether a complication occurred intraoperatively or postoperatively, such as intraoperative versus postoperative hemorrhage.

ICD-10-CM has included specificity regarding the type and cause of eye disorders which must be documented in the medical record. Many codes also require more specific documentation of the site such as upper or lower eyelid and laterality (right, left, bilateral).

In addition to these general documentation requirements, there are specific diseases and disorders that require greater detail in documentation to ensure optimal code assignment.

Code-Specific Documentation Requirements

In this section code categories, subcategories, and subclassifications for some of the more frequently reported diseases of the eye and adnexa are reviewed. The focus is on conditions with additional and more specific clinical documentation requirements. Although not all codes with significant documentation requirements are discussed, this section will provide a representative sample of the type of additional documentation needed for diseases of the eye and adnexa. The section is organized by the code category, subcategory, or subclassification depending on whether the documentation affects only a single code or an entire subcategory or category.

Conjunctivitis

Conjunctivitis is inflammation of the conjunctiva, which is the thin, clear membrane lining the inner surface of the eyelid and the outer surface of the eye. Inflammation may be caused by bacteria, viruses, allergens, or chemicals. Chronic allergic conjunctivitis is a prolonged allergic reaction to an allergen.

Giant papillary conjunctivitis is one of the most common complications of wearing contact lenses and has its own specific code. In giant papillary conjunctivitis, the inner surface of the eyelids becomes irritated and inflamed, and large bumps or papillae occur on the underside of the eyelid. The inflammation of the palpebral conjunctiva in giant papillary conjunctivitis results from repeated contact with and irritation of the conjunctiva, or as an allergic reaction to protein deposits on the surface of the contact lens.

Giant papillary conjunctivitis is not a true allergic reaction but rather is usually associated with hypersensitivity reactions. Hay fever or other associated allergies may play a role in the onset and the severity of the signs and symptoms, so provider documentation of any associated allergy is essential for accurate code assignment. As with other allergic diseases, a chronic condition can also develop and may be associated with an increased risk for the development of cataracts and glaucoma. Clear, complete documentation of the patient's condition is needed in order to assign the most accurate diagnosis code.

The signs and symptoms of giant papillary conjunctivitis include discomfort and a reduced tolerance to contact lens wear, conjunctival redness and edema, itching, mucous discharge, photophobia, and may include blurred vision. A diagnosis of giant papillary conjunctivitis can usually be confirmed using slit lamp biomicroscopy after ruling out other possible causes with similar presentation, such as seasonal and perennial allergic conjunctivitis or chlamydial conjunctivitis. Other types of chronic conjunctivitis must be differentiated in the medical record documentation as well, such as chronic follicular conjunctivitis, vernal conjunctivitis, parasitic conjunctivitis, or other chronic allergic conjunctivitis.

There is a separate code used to report other chronic allergic conjunctivitis (H10.45) when there is not a more specific code for the documented type of chronic conjunctivitis.

ICD-10-CM Coding and Documentation Requirements

Identify type:

- Chronic giant papillary conjunctivitis
- Other specified chronic allergic conjunctivitis

For chronic giant papillary conjunctivitis identify laterality:

- Right eye
- Left eye
- Bilateral
- Unspecified

ICD-10-CM Code/Documentation	
H10.411	Chronic giant papillary conjunctivitis, right eye
H10.412	Chronic giant papillary conjunctivitis, left eye
H10.413	Chronic giant papillary conjunctivitis, bilateral
H10.419	Chronic giant papillary conjunctivitis, unspecified

Documentation and Coding Example

Patient is a 19-year-old Caucasian female who presents to ophthalmologist with a 2-year history of itchy, burning, irritated eyes. Patient has worn contact lenses for five years and started to notice problems after one year of lens wear. She reported her symptoms numerous times to her optometrist and was told she had "dry eyes" and to use wetting drops. She saw a new optometrist 4 months ago who thought her problems were allergy related and prescribed Pataday eye drops and changed her to a daily wear contact lens. Patient attends college in another state and would not be able to follow up with her new optometrist so she was advised to see an eye doctor near her school if her symptoms did not improve in 2-3 months. Patient states she has used the Pataday drops daily and also uses Blink brand lubrication drops during the day and Sustane brand at night. She is unable to tolerate contact lenses for more than 2-3 hours and has rarely worn them in the past 3 months. On examination, this is an attractive, articulate young woman who has applied light makeup to enhance her face and eyes. She does admit to not being fastidious about removing her makeup every night. She states she does have seasonal allergies treated with Claritin and she takes vitamins and Chinese herbs prescribed by her acupuncturist. On examination, there is no evidence of blepharitis, conjunctival redness or inflammation. Corneas of both eyes are mildly pitted. Inverting the lid to look at the inner surface of her eyelids is extremely painful but even a quick look confirms that the surface is rough and red with raised papillae on **both the upper and lower lids bilaterally**. She is prescribed Lotemax Eye drops BID x 6 weeks and is to add Restasis eye drops BID beginning 2 weeks after starting the Lotemax. Patient is advised to refrain from contact lens use as much as possible. RTC in 3 months. She is advised to return sooner if her symptoms worsen or have not improved in 3-4 weeks.

Diagnosis: **Chronic giant papillary conjunctivitis secondary to contact lens use.**

ICD-10-CM Diagnosis Code(s)

H10.413 Chronic giant papillary conjunctivitis, bilateral

Coding Note(s)

There are several subcategory codes for different types of chronic conjunctivitis, in addition to the codes for chronic giant papillary conjunctivitis that also identify the affected eye.

Cataract

A senile cataract, now more commonly referred to as age-related cataract, is a disorder of the lens of the eye characterized by gradual, progressive thickening of the lens which becomes cloudy and eventually leads to vision impairment. Other forms of cataract exist including those that affect infants and children, those caused by trauma, drug-induced cataracts, and cataracts caused by underlying disease of the eye so careful review of the medical record documentation is required to ensure that the most appropriate code is selected.

The term age-related cataract has replaced senile cataract, and age-related cataracts are classified in category H25 and the condition is further differentiated by other characteristics of the cataract. For example, there are specific codes for the most common types of senile cataracts which include nuclear cataract, cortical cataract, and posterior subcapsular cataract as well as for less common types. As with all paired organs, cataract codes include laterality and must be specified as right, left, or bilateral. Additionally, there have been some terminology changes. For example, the term hypermature cataract has been replaced with the term morgagnian-type cataract which is classified in subcategory H25.2. Furthermore, some conditions that previously had a specific code are now reported using code H25.89 Other age-related cataract. For example, there is no longer a specific code for total or mature cataract, so in the absence of other more specific documentation code H25.89 is assigned.

Coding and Documentation Requirements

Identify type of age-related cataract:

- Combined forms
- Incipient
  - Anterior subcapsular polar
  - Cortical
  - Posterior subcapsular polar
  - Other incipient type
- Morgagnian type
- Nuclear
- Other specified type
- Unspecified type

Identify laterality:

- Right

- Left
- Bilateral
- Unspecified

ICD-10-CM Code/Documentation	
H25.011	Cortical age-related cataract, right eye
H25.012	Cortical age-related cataract, left eye
H25.013	Cortical age-related cataract, bilateral
H25.019	Cortical age-related cataract, unspecified
H25.031	Anterior subcapsular polar age-related cataract, right eye
H25.032	Anterior subcapsular polar age-related cataract, left eye
H25.033	Anterior subcapsular polar age-related cataract, bilateral
H25.039	Anterior subcapsular polar age-related cataract, unspecified
H25.041	Posterior subcapsular polar age-related cataract, right eye
H25.042	Posterior subcapsular polar age-related cataract, left eye
H25.043	Posterior subcapsular polar age-related cataract, bilateral
H25.049	Posterior subcapsular polar age-related cataract, unspecified

Documentation and Coding Example

Seventy-three-year-old Caucasian female presents for eye exam after noticing some loss of sharpness in her distance vision. She states the change in distance vision is mild but she is concerned about it. She does not drive or watch TV, but she does knit and read and these activities have not been impaired. On examination, this is a very petite, athletic appearing septuagenarian. She states she always keeps her skin covered and wears a brimmed hat while out of doors but has never worn sunglasses. Conjunctiva are clear, without redness or excess tearing. PERRLA. Cranial nerves are grossly intact, eye muscle movement is normal. There are no areas of scotoma. Color vision intact. Autorefraction of distance vision showed 20/40 OD and 20/50 OS. Acuity tested manually confirms these results and with refraction she is easily corrected to 20/15 OU. Near vision is excellent without evidence of astigmatism. Proparacaine eye gtts instilled and tonometry shows OD pressure of 13 mm Hg and OS pressure of 15 mm Hg. Mydriacyl 1% gtts instilled and slit lamp exam shows normal optic nerve and macula OU and **nuclear cataracts bilaterally**. The cataract OD is a LOC III NO2/NC2 and the cataract OS is slightly more opaque at a LOC III NO3/NC3.

Impression: **Bilateral nuclear cataracts in early stages.**

Plan: Dispense glasses to correct myopia. She is advised to wear sunglasses when out of doors. Follow up in 3 months. If changes are minimal she can be followed at 6-month intervals. Her diet was reviewed and she eats ample fresh fruits and vegetables, no processed foods, and healthy fats and protein sources. She is advised she can take a supplemental multivitamin/mineral if she wishes and that she should look for one that contains Lutein, Zeaxanthin and Omega-3 FA.

ICD-10-CM Diagnosis Code(s)

H25.13	Age-related nuclear cataract, bilateral
H52.13	Myopia, bilateral

Coding Note(s)

The outdated terminology of 'nuclear sclerosis' has been updated in ICD-10-CM, where the same condition is now classified as 'age-related nuclear cataract.' ICD-10-CM also captures laterality with specific codes for left, right, and bilateral cataracts.

Choroidal Degeneration/Dystrophies

The choroid is a tissue layer made up of blood vessels and connective tissue located between the sclera and retina. It supplies nutrients to the inner parts of the eye. Choroidal degeneration refers to disorders that present with progressive loss of cellular or tissue function resulting in structural changes in the choroid. Choroidal degeneration can occur as part of age-related macular degeneration. Provider documentation of any associated disease process is needed for optimal code assignment.

Careful review of the documentation is necessary when coding choroidal degeneration, atrophy, or dystrophy. Atrophy refers to the anatomic changes from the loss of cells and tissue due to cell death, and dystrophy refers to acquired cell or tissue degeneration as a result of a genetic defect or mutation. Previously there was a specific code for dystrophies primarily involving Bruch's membrane of the eye and specific codes for choroidal degeneration (sclerosis) unspecified, senile atrophy of the choroid, diffuse secondary atrophy of the choroid, and angioid streaks of the choroid. There is no longer a specific code for dystrophies involving Bruch's membrane. This condition is reported with the same codes as those for unspecified choroidal degeneration (H31.10-), age-related choroidal atrophy (H31.11-), or diffuse secondary atrophy of the choroid (H31.12-) depending on the physician's documentation.

Angioid streaks of choroid are no longer classified with codes for choroidal degenerations. This condition has been moved to subcategory H35.3 Degeneration of macula and posterior pole and is reported with code H35.33 Angioid streaks of macula. Laterality is not a component of the classification of angioid streaks of the macula so there is only a single code to report this condition.

It should also be noted that disease terminology has been updated to reflect current medical knowledge. For example, senile choroidal atrophy is the same as age-related choroidal atrophy. The Alphabetic Index entry for Atrophy, choroid, senile will direct the coder to age-related choroidal atrophy.

Coding and Documentation Requirements

Identify condition:

- Choroidal degeneration (sclerosis) or atrophy
  - Age-related choroidal atrophy
  - Diffuse secondary atrophy of choroid
  - Unspecified choroidal degeneration
- Angioid streaks of macula (choroid)

Identify laterality for choroidal degeneration/atrophy:

- Right eye
- Left eye
- Bilateral
- Unspecified

ICD-10-CM Code/Documentation					
Choroidal					
Degeneration unspecified		Age-related atrophy		Diffuse secondary atrophy	
H31.101	right eye	H31.111	right eye	H31.121	right eye
H31.102	left eye	H31.112	left eye	H31.122	left eye
H31.103	bilateral	H31.113	bilateral	H31.123	bilateral
H31.109	unspecified	H31.119	unspecified	H31.129	unspecified

Documentation and Coding Example

Seventy-nine-year-old Caucasian female presents to Ophthalmology clinic with her caregiver for continued monitoring of eye disease. Patient is well known to this practice, having been treated for **senile degenerative choroidal atrophy and retinal neovascularization in both eyes** for many years. She is a well-respected artist and a valued philanthropist in the community. She walks into the examination room on the arm of her caregiver but once settled into the chair she appears quite at ease and in control of her surroundings. Visual field acuity is significant for loss centrally in both eyes but she has fairly wide peripheral fields bilaterally. Intraocular pressure is normal in both eyes. She has been previously treated with intravitreal injections of Avastin and that seems to have controlled **neovascularization in her retinas**. Today we perform rapid sequence fluorescein angiography and optical coherence tomography. Both tests show hyperfluorescence dye leakage from retinal neovascularization but her disease appears stable at the present time. RTC in 3 months for recheck.

Diagnosis: **Bilateral age-related degenerative choroidal atrophy and retinal neovascularization.**

ICD-10-CM Diagnosis Code(s)

H31.113 Age-related choroidal atrophy, bilateral

H35.053 Retinal neovascularization, unspecified, bilateral

Coding Note(s)

In the Alphabetic Index, under the main term Atrophy, and subterms choroid and senile, the coder is referred to code H31.11- Age-related choroidal atrophy. An additional code is reported for retinal neovascularization because it is not an inherent part of the disease process for age-related choroidal atrophy.

Glaucoma

Glaucoma is a group of eye disorders characterized by elevated intraocular pressure that can cause optic nerve damage. There are a number of different types of glaucoma. The most common is a chronic condition called open angle glaucoma that develops painlessly over time. Another type, acute angle closure glaucoma, is a painful condition that develops quickly and must be treated emergently if vision is to be spared in one or both eyes. Congenital glaucoma is a type that is present at birth and usually results from abnormal eye development. Secondary glaucoma is caused by another condition such as trauma, eye disease, systemic illness, or as a side effect of medications, such as corticosteroids.

There is a great deal of variability in the care and resource utilization among glaucoma patients, so diagnosis codes that reflect disease severity allow for better management and treatment outcomes. Increased specificity of glaucoma codes was integrated to identify the stages of glaucoma. Codes reflect staging of glaucoma into mild, moderate, and severe disease based on the provider's documentation of the visual field in the patient's worse eye. There are also codes for indeterminate stage glaucoma and unspecified glaucoma stage. In order to code the patient's condition to the highest level of specificity, both the specific type and stage of glaucoma must be documented.

Glaucoma codes are located in two categories. Category H40 Glaucoma is specific to type, laterality, and stage. A 7th character is appended to capture the stage. The available 7th characters for reporting the stage are as follows:

0 – Stage unspecified

1 – Mild stage

2 – Moderate stage

3 – Severe stage

4 – Indeterminate stage

Three-character category code H42 is used for Glaucoma in diseases classified elsewhere, has no additional qualifiers, and is reported secondary to the underlying condition, such as amyloidosis, aniridia, Lowe's syndrome, Rieger's anomaly, or other specified metabolic disorder.

ICD-10-CM Coding and Documentation Requirements

Identify type:

- Glaucoma in diseases classified elsewhere
  - Code first underlying condition such as:
    - » amyloidosis (E85.-)
    - » aniridia (Q13.1)
    - » glaucoma (in) diabetes mellitus (E08.39, E09.39, E10.39, E11.39, E13.39)
    - » Lowe's syndrome (E72.03)
    - » Rieger's anomaly (Q13.81)
    - » specified metabolic disorder (E70-E88)
- Glaucoma suspect
  - Anatomical narrow angle (primary angle closure suspect)
  - Open angle with borderline findings
    - » High risk
    - » Low risk
      - ◦ Ocular hypertension
      - ◦ Preglaucoma
      - ◦ Primary angle closure without glaucoma damage
      - ◦ Steroid responder
- Open-angle glaucoma
  - Capsular glaucoma with pseudoexfoliation of lens
  - Chronic simple glaucoma
  - Low-tension glaucoma
  - Pigmentary glaucoma
  - Primary open-angle glaucoma
  - Residual stage of open-angle glaucoma
  - Unspecified open angle glaucoma

- Primary angle-closure glaucoma
  - Acute angle-closure glaucoma (attack) (crisis)
  - Chronic (primary) angle-closure glaucoma
  - Intermittent angle-closure glaucoma
  - Residual stage of angle-closure glaucoma
  - Unspecified
- Secondary glaucoma (due to)
  - Drugs
  - Eye inflammation
  - Eye trauma
  - Other eye disorders
- Other specified type of glaucoma
  - Aqueous misdirection (malignant glaucoma)
  - Hypersecretion glaucoma
  - With increased episcleral venous pressure
  - Other specified type
- Unspecified type

Identify laterality:

- Right eye
- Left eye
- Bilateral
- Unspecified

Identify stage using the appropriate 7th character:

0 – Stage unspecified

1 – Mild stage

2 – Moderate stage

3 – Severe stage

4 – Indeterminate stage

Note: Stage is not required for conditions listed under glaucoma suspect, residual stage, acute or intermittent angle-closure glaucoma, other specified types of glaucoma (aqueous misdirection, hypersecretion, glaucoma with increased episcleral venous pressure), unspecified glaucoma, or glaucoma in diseases classified elsewhere.

Use an additional code for adverse effect, if applicable, to identify the drug (T36-T50 with fifth or sixth character 5) in cases of glaucoma secondary to drugs.

Code also the underlying condition for glaucoma secondary to eye trauma, eye inflammation, and other eye disorders.

ICD-10-CM Code/Documentation	
A 7th character is required to identify the stage on the glaucoma codes listed below:	
H40.111	Primary open-angle glaucoma, right eye
H40.112	Primary open-angle glaucoma, left eye
H40.113	Primary open-angle glaucoma, bilateral
H40.119	Primary open-angle glaucoma, unspecified
H40.211	Acute angle-closure glaucoma, right eye
H40.212	Acute angle-closure glaucoma, left eye
H40.213	Acute angle-closure glaucoma, bilateral
H40.219	Acute angle-closure glaucoma, unspecified

Documentation and Coding Example

Patient is a 45-year-old African-American male who presents to the office today for ongoing care of glaucoma. This gentleman was diagnosed two years ago with **angle-closure glaucoma bilaterally**. Eye pressure was initially difficult to control and his **left eye progressed fairly rapidly to moderate disease. Clinically, the stage of disease in his right eye was difficult to determine, however both eyes appeared to be stabilized** at his exam six months ago using Cosopt eye drops bilaterally BID. Patient states he is having no side effects from the medication. On examination, his visual field perception is unchanged in both eyes with only minimal visual loss in the outer periphery of the right but circumferential in the left. Visual acuity is also unchanged on the right at 20/100 but slightly improved on the left at 20/200. His current glasses prescription for distance and reading is working fine for him. Right eye pressure is 22 mmHG, left is 23 mmHG. Slit lamp exam shows no unusual tissue growth and smooth conjunctiva and corneas bilaterally. Gonioscopy exam shows adequate fluid drainage in both eyes. Scanning laser polarimetry and optical coherence tomography is performed and compared to previous studies. Disease is stable at this time. Treatment options discussed with patient. He is not experiencing any side effects from the medication and he has good insurance coverage so it is not a financial burden to obtain the prescriptions each month. Patient has some anxiety about surgery on his eyes and as long as the medication is working, he prefers not to do any other type of treatment at this time. RTC in 6 months, sooner if symptoms arise.

Diagnosis: **Bilateral chronic angle-closure glaucoma.**

ICD-10-CM Diagnosis Code(s)

H40.2222 Chronic angle-closure glaucoma, left eye, moderate stage

H40.2214 Chronic angle-closure glaucoma, right eye, indeterminate stage

Coding Note(s)

When a patient has bilateral glaucoma and each eye is documented as having a different type or stage, and the classification distinguishes laterality, assign the appropriate code for each eye rather than the code for bilateral glaucoma. The seventh code character "2" is assigned to identify moderate stage glaucoma in the left eye and the seventh character "4" is assigned to the glaucoma code for the right eye because the stage cannot be clinically determined. The seventh character "4" is used for glaucomas whose stage cannot be clinically determined, and should not be confused with the seventh character "0", unspecified, which should be assigned when there is no documentation regarding the stage of the glaucoma.

Pterygium

A pterygium is a benign growth or thickening of the conjunctiva that grows onto the cornea. As it grows, the pterygium may become red and irritated and may cause visual disturbances. Pterygium is typically associated with ultraviolet light exposure but chronic conjunctival inflammation can cause localized amyloidosis.

There are a number of specific types of pterygiums identified in ICD-10-CM including a subcategory for amyloid pterygium (H11.01) which previously was reported with an unspecified code. Amyloid is a protein that gets deposited in the body organs and tissues where it may accumulate as in amyloid deposits on the conjunctiva.

ICD-10-CM Coding and Documentation Requirements

Identify type:

- Amyloid pterygium
  - Central pterygium
  - Double pterygium
  - Peripheral pterygium
    - » Progressive
    - » Stationary
  - Recurrent
- Unspecified pterygium

Identify laterality:

- Right eye
- Left eye
- Bilateral
- Unspecified

ICD-10-CM Code/Documentation	
H11.001	Unspecified pterygium of right eye
H11.002	Unspecified pterygium of left eye
H11.003	Unspecified pterygium of eye, bilateral
H11.009	Unspecified pterygium of eye, unspecified
H11.011	Amyloid pterygium of right eye
H11.012	Amyloid pterygium of left eye
H11.013	Amyloid pterygium of eye, bilateral
H11.019	Amyloid pterygium of eye, unspecified
H11.021	Central pterygium of right eye
H11.022	Central pterygium of left eye
H11.023	Central pterygium of eye, bilateral
H11.029	Central pterygium of unspecified eye
H11.031	Double pterygium of right eye
H11.032	Double pterygium of left eye
H11.033	Double pterygium of eye, bilateral
H11.039	Double pterygium of unspecified eye
H11.041	Peripheral pterygium, stationary, of right eye
H11.042	Peripheral pterygium, stationary, of left eye
H11.043	Peripheral pterygium, stationary, of eye, bilateral
H11.049	Peripheral pterygium, stationary, of unspecified eye
H11.051	Peripheral pterygium, progressive, of right eye
H11.052	Peripheral pterygium, progressive, of left eye
H11.053	Peripheral pterygium, progressive, of eye, bilateral
H11.059	Peripheral pterygium, progressive, of unspecified eye
H11.061	Recurrent pterygium of right eye
H11.062	Recurrent pterygium of left eye
H11.063	Recurrent pterygium of eye, bilateral
H11.069	Recurrent pterygium of unspecified eye

Documentation and Coding Example

This 34-year-old Caucasian male is self-referred to Ophthalmology with concerns about excessive tearing and patchy white growths in his eyes with occasional blurred vision in the left eye. Patient teaches physical education at the local high school and is an avid outdoorsman. He snowboards in winter, plays golf at least 9 months of the year, enjoys water sports on the local lake in the summer. He always wears sunglasses and/or a hat outside. He denies eye pain other than mild irritation relieved by OTC eye drops. On examination, visual acuity is 20/20, near and far. The eyes bilaterally have mild redness of the conjunctiva with no evidence of blepharitis. A small white patch is noted in the **upper inner edge of the right cornea** and a larger patch in the **lower outer edge of the left cornea.** Slit lamp exam confirms that they are located right on the edge of the cornea, slightly raised and contain a network of small blood vessels. **The characteristics are typical of amyloid pterygium.** Lesion on right eye is approximately 3mm x 4 mm and left eye measures 7mm x 9 mm. Corneal topography and photography is performed to document size and shape. Patient is counseled that these are usually benign growths but it would be wise to remove the lesion on the left because it is starting to affect vision. Patient is in agreement with that plan and is referred for surgical consultation.

Diagnosis:

Amyloid pterygium, right eye, 3mm x 4 mm.

Amyloid pterygium left eye, 7mm x 9 mm.

ICD-10-CM Diagnosis Code(s)

H11.013 Amyloid pterygium of eye, bilateral

Coding Note(s)

ICD-10-CM includes specific subcategories for the different types of pterygium, including amyloid pterygium. These codes further specify the affected eye as right, left, or bilateral.

Summary

Best practices in documentation of disorders of the eye and adnexa require more detailed information on the diagnosis and treatment of these conditions. In addition to general documentation requirements such as the severity or status of the disease, the affected site, the etiology, and any secondary disease process, there are specific diseases and disorders that require greater detail in medical record documentation to ensure optimal code assignment.

ICD-10-CM includes specificity regarding the type and the cause of eye disorders which must be documented in the medical record. Many codes require specific documentation of the site including right, left, or bilateral and upper or lower eyelid.

Understanding new, updated, and more specific coding terminology will be needed in addition to more detailed documentation of the patient's condition. Some aspects of coding diseases of the eye and adnexa are improved in ICD-10-CM with the addition of a number of combination codes that identify both the disorder and the common manifestation.

Resources

Documentation checklists are available in Appendix A for the following condition(s):

- Cataract
- Conjunctivitis
- Glaucoma

Chapter 7 Quiz

1. Where are the combination codes for diabetes mellitus with eye conditions classified in ICD-10-CM?
   a. Chapter 1 - Certain infectious and parasitic diseases (A00-B99)
   b. Chapter 4 - Endocrine, nutritional and metabolic diseases (E00-E89)
   c. Chapter 7 - Diseases of the Eye and Adnexa (H00-H59)
   d. Chapter 18 - Symptoms, signs and abnormal clinical and laboratory findings, not elsewhere classified (R00-R99)
2. Which of the following disorders of the eye and adnexa are NOT classified in ICD-10-CM Chapter 7 Diseases of the Eye and Adnexa (H00-H59)?
   a. Conditions associated with a neoplastic process
   b. Complications of pregnancy, childbirth and the puerperium
   c. Conditions resulting from injury or trauma to the eye and orbit
   d. All of the above
3. Which of the following statements is true regarding coding of glaucoma?
   a. Dual codes are required to report the type and stage of glaucoma
   b. A combination code can be used to report the type and stage of glaucoma
   c. Laterality needs to be documented in the medical record
   d. Both B and D
4. How is a diagnosis of senile choroidal atrophy classified in?
   a. Age-related choroidal atrophy
   b. Choroidal degeneration or sclerosis
   c. Diffuse secondary atrophy of choroid
   d. All of the above
5. How are postprocedural complications of eye and adnexa classified?
   a. In Chapter 19 Injury, poisoning and certain other consequences of external causes (S00-T88)
   b. In Chapter 20 External causes of morbidity (V00-Y99)
   c. In Chapter 21 Factors influencing health status and contact with health services
   d. In Chapter 7 in a separate code block at the end of the chapter
6. The physician documents the patient's diagnosis as bilateral glaucoma but there is no documentation regarding determination of the stage of the glaucoma. What 7th character glaucoma stage is assigned in this case?
   a. 0
   b. 1
   c. 4
   d. None, the provider must be queried for documentation of the glaucoma stage
7. The physician documents bilateral glaucoma and documents each eye as having a different type or stage. How is this coded?
   a. One code is assigned for each type of glaucoma but only the 7th character for the highest glaucoma stage is assigned.
   b. The code for each eye is assigned for each type of glaucoma with the appropriate 7th character for the stage.
   c. The code for bilateral glaucoma is assigned with the 7th character for the highest glaucoma stage
   d. The code for bilateral glaucoma is assigned twice with the 7th character for Residual stage glaucoma
8. How is glaucoma associated with ocular trauma coded?
   a. With a code from Chapter 7 Diseases of the eye and adnexa (H00-H59)
   b. With a code from Chapter 19 Injury, poisoning and certain other consequences of external causes (S00-T88)
   c. With a code from Chapter 20 External causes of morbidity (V00-Y99)
   d. With a code from Chapter 21 Factors influencing health status and contact with health services
9. A patient was admitted with moderate stage glaucoma but during the admission, the stage progresses to severe glaucoma. What is the principal diagnosis?
   a. The code for the stage documented on discharge
   b. The code for the stage documented on admission
   c. The code for the highest glaucoma stage is documented
   d. The code for the indeterminate stage
10. The physician has documented that the patient has bilateral choroidal degeneration due to Bruch's membrane dystrophy. How is this coded?
   a. There are no codes for choroidal degeneration due to Bruch's membrane dystrophy so the physician must be queried.
   b. With code H31.8 Other specified disorders of the choroid
   c. With code H31.103 Choroidal degeneration, unspecified, bilateral
   d. With code H31.123 Diffuse secondary atrophy of choroid, bilateral

See next page for answers and rationales.

Chapter 7 Answers and Rationales

1. Where are the combination codes for diabetes mellitus with eye conditions classified in ICD-10-CM?

   b. **Chapter 4 - Endocrine, nutritional and metabolic diseases (E00-E89)**

   Rationale: *According to the Excludes2 note at the beginning of Chapter 7 of ICD-10-CM, diabetes mellitus related eye conditions are coded to E08.3-, E09.3-,* E10.3-, E11.3-, and E13.3-, classified in Chapter 4.

2. Which of the following disorders of the eye and adnexa are NOT classified in ICD-10-CM Chapter 7 Diseases of the Eye and Adnexa (H00-H59)?

   d. **All of the above**

   Rationale: *All of the listed conditions are included in the list of excluded conditions at the beginning of Chapter 7.*

3. Which of the following statements is true regarding coding of glaucoma?

   d. **Both B and D**

   Rationale: *ICD-10-CM Tabular List includes combination codes that identify the type, stage and laterality of glaucoma. The ICD-10-CM guidelines for coding glaucoma provide additional direction.*

4. How is a diagnosis of senile choroidal atrophy classified?

   a. **Age-related choroidal atrophy**

   Rationale: *The Index entry for atrophy of the choroid, senile directs the coder to age-related choroidal atrophy.*

5. How are postprocedural complications of eye and adnexa classified?

   d. **In Chapter 7 in a separate code block at the end of the chapter**

   Rationale: *ICD-10-CM has a separate code block at the end of Chapter 7 (H59) to classify all intraoperative and postprocedural complications from treatment of eye and adnexa disorders together.*

6. The physician documents the patient's diagnosis as bilateral glaucoma but there is no documentation regarding determination of the stage of the glaucoma. What 7th character glaucoma stage is assigned in this case?

   a. **0**

   Rationale: *The glaucoma codes in the Tabular List of ICD-10-CM include an instructional note directing the user to assign one of the listed 7th characters to the code to designate the stage of glaucoma. According to the ICD-10-CM Official Guidelines for Coding and Reporting Section I.C.7.a.5 the seventh character "0", unspecified, should be assigned when there is no documentation regarding the stage of the glaucoma.*

7. The physician documents bilateral glaucoma and documents each eye as having a different type or stage. How is this coded?

   b. **The code for each eye is assigned for each type of glaucoma with the appropriate 7th character for the stage.**

   Rationale: *According to the ICD-10-CM Official Guidelines for Coding and Reporting Section I.C.7.a.3, assign a code for the type of glaucoma for each eye with the seventh character for the specific glaucoma stage documented for each eye.*

8. How is glaucoma associated with ocular trauma coded?

   a. **With a code from Chapter 7 Diseases of the eye and adnexa (H00-H59)**

   Rationale: *In ICD-10-CM, glaucoma secondary to eye trauma is coded to H40.30-H40.33 based on the affected eye(s) with a 7th character of 0-4 to identify the glaucoma stage. An additional code is assigned also to identify the underlying condition.*

9. A patient was admitted with moderate stage glaucoma but during the admission, the stage progresses to severe glaucoma. What is the principal diagnosis?

   c. **The code for the highest glaucoma stage is documented**

   Rationale: *According to Section I.C.7.a.4 of the ICD-10-CM Official Guidelines for Coding and Reporting, when a patient is admitted with glaucoma and the stage evolves during the admission, assign the code for highest stage documented.*

10. The physician has documented that the patient has bilateral choroidal degeneration due to Bruch's membrane dystrophy. How is this coded?

    c. **With code H31.103 Choroidal degeneration, unspecified, bilateral**

    Rationale: *There is no entry in the alphabetic index for Dystrophy, Bruch's membrane. However, the physician has specified that the patient has choroidal degeneration due to Bruch's dystrophy. Searching the Alphabetic Index under the entry Degeneration, Bruch's membrane, the instruction is given to see degeneration, choroid and when that term is located, the code provided is H31.10-. The 6th character 3 is added to identify the condition as bilateral.*

Chapter 8

DISEASES OF THE EAR AND MASTOID PROCESS (H6Ø-H95)

Introduction

Codes for diseases of the ear and mastoid process were previously classified with diseases of the nervous system and diseases of the eye and adnexa. In ICD-10-CM however, there is a separate chapters for each of these significantly different disease groups. The codes for diseases of the ear and mastoid process are located in their own chapter in ICD-10-CM: Chapter 8 Diseases of the Ear and Mastoid Process (H60-H95).

Chapter 8 in ICD-10-CM classifies diseases and conditions of the ear and mastoid process by site, starting with diseases of the external ear, followed by diseases of the middle ear and mastoid, and then diseases of the inner ear. Coding diseases of the ear can be challenging due to the complex anatomic structures of the auditory system and this arrangement makes it easier to identify the different types of conditions that occur.

Chapter 8 begins with instructions to assign an external cause code to identify the cause of any condition. There is specificity captured at the fourth, fifth and sixth character levels. Body sites in general, are very specific in ICD-10-CM. Diseases of the ear, in particular, require more specific documentation, such as the laterality of the affected ear or bilateral ears.

One important documentation requirement involves the codes for otitis externa—detail is needed regarding the specific cause. For example, conditions are differentiated with codes for acute noninfective otitis externa such as actinic, chemical, contact, eczematoid, and reactive.

Understanding the coding and documentation requirements for diseases of the ear and mastoid process begins with a familiarity of the code blocks, which are displayed in the following table.

ICD-1Ø-CM Blocks	
H6Ø-H62	Diseases of external ear
H65-H75	Diseases of middle ear and mastoid
H8Ø-H83	Diseases of inner ear
H9Ø-H94	Other disorders of ear
H95	Intraoperative and postprocedural complications and disorders of ear and mastoid process, not elsewhere classified

The table above highlights the following:

- Diseases have been arranged anatomically by types of conditions affecting the external ear, middle ear and mastoid, and inner ear
- There is a code block at the end of the chapter to classify intraoperative and postprocedural complications of treatment together by specific body system rather than scattered throughout the chapter.

Exclusions

For chapter 8, there are only Excludes2 notes:

Excludes1	Excludes2
None	Certain conditions originating in the perinatal period (PØ4-P96) Certain infectious and parasitic diseases (AØØ-B99) Complications of pregnancy, childbirth and the puerperium (OØØ-O9A) Congenital malformations, deformations and chromosomal abnormalities (QØØ-Q99) Endocrine, nutritional and metabolic diseases (EØØ-E88) Injury, poisoning and certain other consequences of external causes (SØØ-T88) Neoplasms (CØØ-D49) Symptoms, signs and abnormal clinical and laboratory findings, not elsewhere classified (RØØ-R94)

Several diseases with associated ear manifestations are classified in other chapters such as disorders associated with infectious and parasitic diseases, neoplasms, and endocrine, nutritional and metabolic diseases. Conditions due to injury, congenital malformations, or complications of pregnancy are also classified in other chapters. Notable exclusions from this chapter include otitis media in influenza (J09.X9, J10.83, J11.83), measles (B05.3), scarlet fever (A38.0), and tuberculosis (A18.6).

Classification of Codes into Code Categories

Codes for postoperative complications such as post-procedural stenosis of the right external ear canal are grouped together in a separate code block at the end of the chapter and a distinction made between intraoperative complications and postprocedural disorders. ICD-10-CM expands the use of combination codes—the use of a single code to classify two diagnoses, or a diagnosis with an associated secondary process, or a diagnosis with an associated complication. But caution is needed when coding certain conditions for which combination codes exist, such as otitis media in diseases classified elsewhere. Measles complicated by otitis media (B05.3), scarlet fever with otitis media (A38.0), tuberculosis of the inner or middle ear or tuberculous otitis media (A18.6), and otitis media in influenza (J09.X9, J10.83, and J11.83), are not coded with the otitis media codes classified in Chapter 8.

Chapter Guidelines

The coding guidelines include the coding conventions, the general coding guidelines and the chapter-specific coding guidelines. No specific coding guidelines were developed for Chapter 8 and consequently remains reserved for future guideline expansion.

General coding guidelines for laterality are particularly relevant to diseases of the ear and mastoid process. When the patient has a bilateral condition and each side is treated during separate encounters, assign the bilateral code for the encounter treating the first side (as the condition exists on both sides) and for the second encounter whenever treatment on the first side did not completely resolve the condition. For the second encounter after one side has been treated, and the condition no longer exists on that side, assign the appropriate unilateral code for the side where the condition still exists.

Coding and sequencing guidelines for ear diseases are incorporated into the Alphabetic Index and the Tabular List. To assign the most specific code possible, pay close attention to the coding and sequencing instructions in the Tabular List and Alphabetic Index, particularly the Excludes1 and Excludes2 notes.

General Documentation Requirements

Documentation requirements depend on the particular disease or disorder affecting the ear or the mastoid. Some of the new general documentation requirements are discussed here, but greater detail for some of the more common diseases of the ear and mastoid process will be provided in the next section.

General medical record documentation requirements include identifying the acuity of the disease as either acute or chronic, specifying the site, the etiology, and any secondary disease process. A high degree of specificity is required regarding the type and cause of ear disorders which must be documented in the medical record. Most codes also require documentation of the site as right, left, or bilateral for paired organs such as the ears. Documentation in the medical record should clearly specify any cause-and-effect relationship between medical treatment and an ear disorder and specify whether the complication occurred intraoperatively or postoperatively.

In addition to these general documentation requirements, there are specific diseases and disorders that require greater detail in documentation to ensure optimal code assignment.

Code-Specific Documentation Requirements

In this section, code categories, subcategories and subclassifications for some of the more frequently reported diseases of the ear and mastoid process are reviewed. The corresponding codes are listed and the documentation requirements identified. The focus is on conditions with additional and more specific clinical documentation requirements. Although not all codes with significant documentation requirements are discussed, this section will provide a representative sample of the type of additional documentation needed for diseases of the ear and mastoid process. The section is organized numerically by the ICD-10-CM code category, subcategory, or subclassification depending on whether the documentation affects only a single code or an entire subcategory or category.

Acoustic Nerve Disorders

Acoustic nerve disorders are caused by lesions or other dysfunction of the cochlea and acoustic nerve, rather than a problem of conduction. The eighth cranial nerve (the acoustic nerve) controls hearing, balance and head position. The acoustic nerve is known by several names including the auditory nerve, the vestibulocochlear nerve, the cochlear nerve and the vestibular nerve. The causes of acoustic neuritis are varied and include toxins, medications, injuries, tumors, infections, and other conditions that may damage the nerve.

In ICD-10-CM, codes for disorders of the acoustic nerve are found in category H93 Other disorders of ear, not elsewhere classified and in category H94 Other disorders of ear in diseases classified elsewhere. While the subcategory H93.3 Other disorders of the acoustic nerve does not provide codes for specific conditions, the subcategory H94.0 is specific to acoustic neuritis in infectious and parasitic diseases classified elsewhere.

ICD-10-CM Coding and Documentation Requirements

Identify type:

- Disorder of acoustic nerve
- Acoustic neuritis in infectious and parasitic diseases classified elsewhere

Identify laterality:

- Right acoustic nerve
- Left acoustic nerve
- Bilateral acoustic nerves
- Unspecified

For acoustic neuritis in infectious and parasitic diseases classified elsewhere, code first underlying disease, such as:

- Parasitic disease (B65-B89)

ICD-10-CM Code/Documentation	
Disorders of acoustic nerve	
H93.3X1	Right
H93.3X2	Left
H93.3X3	Bilateral
H93.3X9	Unspecified
Acoustic neuritis in infectious and parasitic diseases classified elsewhere	
H94.00	Unspecified
H94.01	Right ear
H94.02	Left
H94.03	Bilateral

Documentation and Coding Example

Fifty-two-year-old Asian male returns for follow-up of dizziness and unsteady gait. Patient was in his usual state of good health 3 months ago when he developed a sudden onset of severe vertigo, nausea and vomiting. He thought it was a viral illness and self-treated with rest and fluids. The nausea and vomiting abated after 2 days but he continued to feel dizzy. He first presented to the clinic about 1 week after the onset of symptoms and was noted to have nystagmus in addition to an unsteady gait. His symptoms improved when lying down, intensified when sitting or standing. He was prescribed Meclizine initially and later used Scopolamine patches. He was seen 3 weeks later with continued symptoms and had an MRI to r/o tumor or stroke. MRI was negative and symptoms slowly began to improve. T 97.4, P 58, R 12, BP 136/80. On examination, this is a thin but muscular gentleman who looks younger that his stated age. Overall, he feels like he is almost back to normal. He states he still has some unsteadiness with balance when he gets fatigued but his gait is normal. He has had only 3-4 episodes of very mild vertigo in the past month that did not require medication.

Impression: **Acoustic neuritis bilaterally, resolving.**

Plan: RTC if symptoms worsen.

Diagnosis: **Bilateral acoustic neuritis.**

Diagnosis Code(s)

H93.3X3 Disorders of bilateral acoustic nerves

Coding Note(s)

The ICD-10-CM Index entries for Neuritis, acoustic (nerve) and Neuritis, auditory (nerve) direct the coder to subcategory H93.3. These codes also specify the affected ear(s).

Hearing Loss: Conductive, Sensorineural, and Mixed

Coding hearing loss is dependent upon the documentation of the type and laterality of the hearing loss. Classification of the different types of hearing loss is based on which part of the hearing pathway is affected. In central hearing loss, the auditory nerve itself is damaged, or the nerves or nuclei of the central nervous system, either in the pathways to the brain or in the brain are damaged or impaired. Conductive hearing loss is hearing loss affecting transmission of sound through the external ear canal and middle ear to the inner ear. Sensorineural hearing loss, on the other hand, involves damage to the inner ear, the acoustic nerve, or both. When a patient experiences both conductive and sensorineural hearing impairment, it is called mixed hearing loss.

Understanding the related terminology is crucial to accurate code assignment. Sensorineural hearing loss, for example, is sometimes referred to as nerve deafness, but more common synonyms are cochlear or inner-ear hearing loss. Other names for this type of hearing loss are retrocochlear, sensory or neural hearing loss. The Index entry in ICD-10-CM for loss of hearing without further specification directs the coder to H90.5 which lists central, neural, perceptive, sensorineural, and sensory hearing loss not otherwise specified, as included conditions.

The characteristics of hearing loss captured in ICD-10-CM relate to type, conductive, sensorineural, and mixed; whether the hearing loss is in one or both ears; and when only one ear is affected the codes identify the right or left ear and when a code for unilateral is assigned these codes further specify that there is unrestricted hearing on the contralateral side.

ICD-10-CM Coding and Documentation Requirements

Identify type:

- Conductive hearing loss
- Sensorineural hearing loss
- Mixed conductive and sensorineural hearing loss

Identify laterality/extent of hearing loss:

- Bilateral
- Unilateral, left ear, with unrestricted hearing on the contralateral side
- Unilateral, right ear, with unrestricted hearing on the contralateral side
- Unspecified

ICD-10-CM Code/Documentation	
H90.2	Conductive hearing loss, unspecified
H90.0	Conductive hearing loss, bilateral
H90.11	Conductive hearing loss, unilateral, right ear, with unrestricted hearing on the contralateral side
H90.12	Conductive hearing loss, unilateral, left ear, with unrestricted hearing on the contralateral side
H90.3	Sensorineural hearing loss, bilateral
H90.41	Sensorineural hearing loss, unilateral, right ear, with unrestricted hearing on the contralateral side
H90.42	Sensorineural hearing loss, unilateral, left ear, with unrestricted hearing on the contralateral side
H90.5	Unspecified sensorineural hearing loss
H90.8	Mixed conductive and sensorineural hearing loss, unspecified
H90.71	Mixed conductive and sensorineural hearing loss, unilateral, right ear, with unrestricted hearing on the contralateral side
H90.72	Mixed conductive and sensorineural hearing loss, unilateral, left ear, with unrestricted hearing on the contralateral side
H90.6	Mixed conductive and sensorineural hearing loss, bilateral

Documentation and Coding Example

Patient is a delightful 2-year-old girl with **moderate sensorineural hearing loss in her right ear identified as a newborn**. She was fitted with a CROS hearing aid at age 3 months. Speech is developing well and she continues to work with a SLP provided by an Early Start program. The therapist presently comes 2 times a week to her home. She is here today for routine monitoring of ENT status and her hearing aid. On examination, this is an active, engaging young child who does not want to take part in the examination. Hearing aid is removed and tested for function. Otoscopic exam of ear is difficult but she does finally settle down in her mother's lap and allows a very quick view into her ears. The external auditory canals look clean and are without lesions. TMs are clear.

Impression: **Stable sensorineural hearing loss right ear, normal hearing left ear.**

Plan: Continue use of CROS hearing aid and SLP services. RTC in 6 months, sooner if problems arise. This note is electronically transmitted to her pediatrician.

Diagnosis: **Sensorineural hearing loss, right ear; normal hearing left ear.**

Diagnosis Code(s)

H90.41 Sensorineural hearing loss, unilateral, right ear, with unrestricted hearing on the contralateral side

Z97.4 Presence of external hearing aid

Coding Note(s)

The patient's sensorineural hearing loss is limited to the right ear with normal hearing in the opposite ear. ICD-10-CM codes identify the specific aspects of the patient's diagnosis in one code. An additional health status code, Z97.4 Presence of external hearing-aid, from Chapter 21 may be assigned to denote the presence of the patient's hearing aid.

Otitis Externa

Otitis externa is an inflammation of the outer ear and ear canal. Inflammation can be acute or chronic. Acute otitis externa is usually associated with a bacterial or fungal infection and symptoms include rapid onset of pain, feeling of pressure or fullness in the ear, and difficulty hearing. Chronic otitis externa is most often caused by dermatitis (eczema) and presents with itching, feeling of pressure or fullness in the ear, and difficulty hearing. Chronic otitis media is generally defined as a condition that lasts more than 4 months or that recurs with more than 4 episodes in 1 year.

There are many causes of otitis externa so it is important that the provider documentation indicate the cause. Bacterial infection (e.g., Staphylococcus aureus) is one of the most common causes of acute otitis externa. If an allergen or irritant comes in contact with the ears, allergic reactions can also cause otitis externa. The use of chemicals for the ears, or from hair spray or dye, can irritate the ear and cause otitis externa as well. Swimmer's ear is inflammation, irritation, or infection of the outer ear and ear canal. In some cases, swimmer's ear may be associated with middle ear infection (otitis media) or upper respiratory infections such as colds. Provider documentation of any associated or underlying infection is also needed for accurate code assignment.

Codes for otitis externa in ICD-10-CM are more specific than historical division of infective or other. For example, these codes require documentation of the affected site as right, left, or bilateral. ICD-10-CM also contains specificity regarding the type and cause of the otitis externa or other external ear disorder, which must be documented in the medical record.

ICD-10-CM Coding and Documentation Requirements

Identify type of otitis externa:

- Abscess of external ear
- Acute noninfective otitis externa
  - Acute actinic otitis externa
  - Acute chemical otitis externa
  - Acute contact otitis externa
  - Acute eczematoid otitis externa
  - Acute reactive otitis externa
  - Other noninfective acute otitis externa
  - Unspecified noninfective acute otitis externa
- Cellulitis of external ear
- Cholesteatoma of external ear
- Chronic otitis externa, unspecified
- Disorders of external ear in diseases classified elsewhere
  - Otitis externa
  - Other disorders
- Malignant otitis externa
- Other infective otitis externa
  - Diffuse otitis externa
  - Hemorrhagic otitis externa
  - Swimmer's ear
  - Other specified infective otitis externa
- Other otitis externa
- Unspecified otitis externa

Identify laterality:

- Left ear
- Right ear
- Bilateral
- Unspecified

For disorders of external ear in diseases classified elsewhere (H62), code first the underlying disease.

Diseases of the external ear are discussed below. Review the blocks of codes to become familiar with the categories.

ICD-10-CM Code/Documentation	
H60.0	Abscess
H60.1	Cellulitis
H60.2	Malignant otitis externa
H60.31	Diffuse infective otitis externa
H60.32	Hemorrhagic otitis externa
H60.33	Swimmer's ear
H60.39	Other infective otitis externa
H60.4	Cholesteatoma of external ear
H60.50	Unspecified acute noninfective otitis externa
H60.51	Acute actinic otitis externa
H60.52	Acute chemical otitis externa
H60.54	Acute eczematoid otitis externa
H60.55	Acute reactive otitis externa
H60.59	Other noninfective acute otitis externa
H60.6	Unspecified chronic otitis externa
H60.8	Other otitis externa
H60.9	Unspecified otitis externa

Documentation and Coding Example

Twelve-year-old Caucasian female presents to ENT with c/o ear pain and decreased hearing. PMH is significant for asthma, well controlled on Singulair, Advair and occasional Xopenex for acute symptoms. Patient swims competitively and is in the pool for practice or events 6-7 days a week. She has had external ear inflammation in the past but it is usually well controlled with OTC ear drops. Patient is afebrile. There is **mild tragal tenderness on the right ear and erythema, swelling of the right external auditory canal. Yellow purulent drainage is present in the canal**; however, TM is clear. **Left ear has no tragal tenderness** but the external auditory canal has a **dry, flaky, eczema like appearance consistent with swimmer's ear.** Enlarged periauricular lymph nodes are present only on the right with no cervical lymphadenopathy appreciated. She is prescribed Ciprodex 1 drop in each ear BID x 10 days. RTC in 2 weeks for recheck.

Diagnosis: **Bilateral swimmer's otitis externa**

8. Diseases of the Ear and Mastoid Process

Diagnosis Code(s)

H60.333 Swimmer's ear, bilateral

Coding Note(s)

Swimmer's ear is indexed in ICD-10-CM to code H60.33- with the fourth code character identifying the affected ear or ears, in this case bilateral.

Other Chronic Nonsuppurative Otitis Media

Otitis media is an ear infection that occurs in the middle ear typically between the eardrum and the inner ear, including the Eustachian tube. Otitis media is quite common during childhood. Among the common types of otitis media are acute otitis media, usually associated with an underlying URI and otitis media with effusion which is also known as secretory otitis media or serous OM. Chronic suppurative otitis media involves a perforation in the eardrum with a bacterial infection inside the middle ear. Coding otitis media requires documentation of whether the otitis media is acute or chronic, nonsuppurative, or suppurative.

The category for nonsuppurative otitis media (H65) provides instructional notes, including:

- Use additional code for any associated perforated tympanic membrane (H72.-)
- Use additional code, if applicable, to identify:
  - Exposure to environmental tobacco smoke (Z77.22)
  - Exposure to tobacco smoke in the perinatal period (P96.81)
  - History of tobacco use (Z87.891)
  - Infectious agent (B95-B97)
  - Occupational exposure to environmental tobacco smoke (Z57.31)
  - Tobacco dependence (F17.-)
  - Tobacco use (Z72.0)

ICD-10-CM Coding and Documentation Requirements

Identify type of otitis media:

- Chronic allergic otitis media
- Other chronic nonsuppurative otitis media, which includes:
  - Chronic exudative otitis media
  - Chronic nonsuppurative otitis media, NOS
  - Chronic otitis media with effusion (nonpurulent)
  - Chronic seromucinous otitis media

Identify laterality:

- Right ear
- Left ear
- Bilateral
- Unspecified

ICD-10-CM Code/Documentation	
H65.411	Chronic allergic otitis media, right ear
H65.412	Chronic allergic otitis media, left ear
H65.413	Chronic allergic otitis media, bilateral
H65.419	Chronic allergic otitis media, unspecified
H65.491	Other chronic nonsuppurative otitis media, right ear
H65.492	Other chronic nonsuppurative otitis media, left ear
H65.493	Other chronic nonsuppurative otitis media, bilateral
H65.499	Other chronic nonsuppurative otitis media, unspecified

Documentation and Coding Example

Seven-year-old Caucasian male presents to ENT for audiogram and examination after he failed a hearing screen at school. Patient is well known to us having been referred at the age of 18 months for recurring ear infections. He was treated with myringotomy tubes because of delayed speech. He had excellent results and speech improved dramatically. The right tube fell out at age 5, left tube 6 months ago. He has had effusions noted from time to time on the right since the ear tube fell out. He has not been seen since the left ear tube fell out. His audiogram shows decreased hearing in the 1000, 2000 and 4000 ranges bilaterally. There is a slight tympanic bulge **on the right with a small effusion noted at the bottom of a moderately red TM. Left TM is quite full, red and bulging with a large amount of purulent fluid behind the membrane.** Nares are patent with mild clear drainage. Oropharynx is moist and pink with the posterior pharynx displaying a cobblestone appearance suggestive of chronic allergies. Patient is prescribed Zithromax x 5 days for the bilateral ear infection. He is also prescribed Nasonex nasal spray and Zyrtec to see if his ear symptoms improve by treating the suspected allergies. RTC in 3 weeks for follow up.

Diagnosis: **Chronic exudative otitis media.**

Diagnosis Code(s)

H65.493 Other chronic nonsuppurative otitis media, bilateral

Coding Note(s)

In ICD-10-CM, the Index entry for exudative otitis media directs the coder to see Otitis, media, nonsuppurative. Otitis, media, nonsuppurative, chronic identifies H65.49- Other chronic nonsuppurative otitis media. Chronic exudative otitis media is listed as an included condition under subcategory H65.49.

Peripheral Vertigo

Vertigo occurs due to a disturbance in the vestibular system—the body's balance system. Vertigo is the sensation that surroundings are spinning or moving, and the term vertigo is often inaccurately used interchangeably with "dizziness."

Vertigo is related to diseases of the nervous system or a disturbance in the normal systems of balance and position (e.g., positional vertigo). There are two main types of vertigo, central and peripheral. Central vertigo is due to central nervous system impairment or disease. Peripheral vertigo, also known as labyrinthitis, occurs when there is a problem with the part of the inner ear that controls balance (vestibular labyrinth or semicircular canals) or with the vestibular nerve, which connects the inner ear to the brainstem.

An acute attack of vertigo is usually due to inflammation of the semicircular canals of the inner ear. In fact, benign paroxysmal positional vertigo (also called benign positional vertigo) is estimated to be the most common cause of vertigo in the United States. Vertigo related to the vestibular labyrinth or semicircular canals may also be caused by drugs, injury (such as head injury), or Meniere's disease.

Caution is needed when coding vertigo. Disorders of vestibular function (H81) are classified with diseases of the inner ear (H80-H83). Vertigo that is not otherwise specified in the medical record documentation is coded to symptoms and signs in Chapter 18.

ICD-10-CM Coding and Documentation Requirements

Identify type of peripheral vertigo:

- Aural vertigo
- Other peripheral vertigo, which includes:
  - Lermoyez' syndrome
  - Otogenic vertigo

Identify laterality:

- Right external ear
- Left external ear
- Bilateral
- Unspecified

Aural Vertigo		Other peripheral vertigo	
H81.311	Right ear	H81.391	Right ear
H81.312	Left ear	H81.392	Left ear
H81.313	Bilateral	H81.393	Bilateral
H81.319	Unspecified	H81.399	Unspecified

Documentation and Coding Example

Forty-year old Caucasian female presents to Urgent Care with new onset dizziness and ringing in her ears. PMH is noncontributory. She takes no medications. She denies recent URI symptoms or any type of injury. She noticed the dizziness when she went to bed last night but was able to fall asleep. On awakening this morning, she experienced waves of dizziness just turning over in bed and it took her several minutes to be able to stand after sitting up on the edge of the bed. The ringing sound was soft when lying down, intensified when sitting up and then seemed to diminish, stopping completely within an hour of standing. She denies nausea or vomiting. T 98.0, P 68, R 12, BP 122/64. On examination, this is a well-developed, well-nourished woman who looks younger than her stated age. PERRL, negative for nystagmus. TMs clear. Neck supple without lymphadenopathy. Cranial nerves grossly intact. Gentle head positioning elicits short waves of dizziness with upward and downward movement but not from side to side. Heart rate is regular without murmur, bruit, gallop or rub. Breath sounds clear and equal bilaterally. Abdomen soft, non-distended with active bowel sounds. Peripheral pulses intact with normal reflexes in the extremities. No edema noted. Gait is normal. Impression: **Vertigo, aural in nature.** Plan: Meclizine 25 mg PO q 8 hours as needed. Patient is advised to follow up with PMD. As a courtesy this note has been electronically transmitted to her physician.

Diagnosis: **Aural vertigo.**

Diagnosis Code(s)

H81.319 Aural vertigo, unspecified

Coding Note(s)

Aural vertigo has a specific code in ICD-10-CM, but because the documentation does not specify whether one or both ears are affected, the unspecified code is assigned.

Summary

Best practices in documentation of diseases of the ear and mastoid process require more detailed information on the diagnosis and treatment of these conditions. In addition to standard documentation requirements such as the acuity of the disease, the etiology, the affected site, and any secondary or underlying disease process, there are specific diseases and disorders that require greater detail in medical record documentation to ensure optimal code assignment.

ICD-10-CM includes specificity regarding the type and cause of ear disorders which must be documented in the medical record. Many codes require more specific documentation of the site including right, left, or bilateral. ICD-10-CM also includes updated and specific terminology so understanding the terminology and more detailed documentation of the patient's condition will also be necessary.

Resources

Documentation checklists are available in Appendix A for the following conditions:

- Hearing loss
- Otitis media

Chapter 8 Quiz

1. What information is needed in order to report the most specific code for ear disorders?
   a. The external cause code to identify the cause of the condition
   b. The laterality (right, left, bilateral) of the affected site
   c. The specific cause and effect of the condition
   d. All of the above
2. Which of the following ear disorders are NOT classified with diseases of the ear in Chapter 8?
   a. Endocrine diseases with ear manifestations
   b. Infectious and parasitic ear diseases
   c. Neoplastic ear disorders
   d. All of the above
3. The physician documents the patient's diagnosis as otitis media in influenza. How is this coded?
   a. In Chapter 1 Certain infectious and parasitic diseases (A00-B99)
   b. In Chapter 8 Diseases of the ear and mastoid process (H60-H95)
   c. In Chapter 10 Diseases of the respiratory system (J00-J99)
   d. In Chapter 18 Symptoms, signs and abnormal clinical and laboratory findings, not elsewhere classified (R00-R99)
4. What diagnosis describes a type of noninfectious otitis externa?
   a. Acute actinic otitis externa
   d. Diffuse otitis externa
   c. Swimmer's ear
   d. Malignant otitis externa
5. Which of the following types of hearing loss is coded as unspecified sensorineural hearing loss?
   a. Central hearing loss
   b. Congenital deafness
   c. Perceptive hearing loss
   d. All of the above
6. How are postprocedural complications of the ear and mastoid process classified in ICD-10-CM?
   a. In Chapter 19 with Complications of surgical and medical care, not elsewhere classified
   b. In Chapter 20 with Complications of medical and surgical care or Misadventures to patients during surgical and medical care
   c. In Chapter 21 Factors Influencing Health Status and Contact with Health Services, in a separate code block the end of the chapter
   d. In Chapter 8 Diseases of the ear and mastoid process in a separate code block the end of the chapter
7. What instructions are included for nonsuppurative otitis media?
   a. Use additional code for any associated perforated tympanic membrane
   b. Use additional code to identify exposure to environmental tobacco smoke
   c. Use additional code to identify the infectious agent
   d. All of the above
8. If the physician documents the patient's diagnosis as vertigo, how is this coded?
   a. H81.8X- Other disorders of vestibular function
   b. H82.- Vertiginous syndromes in diseases classified elsewhere
   c. R42 Dizziness and giddiness
   d. All of the above
9. The code for an abscess of the external ear includes which of the following conditions?
   a. Boil of external ear
   b. Carbuncle of auricle or external auditory canal
   c. Furuncle of external ear
   d. All of the above
10. The physician documents the patient's bilateral hearing impairment as both conductive and sensorineural hearing loss. How is this classified?
    a. With one code for Central hearing loss, bilateral
    b. With one code for Mixed conductive and sensorineural hearing loss, bilateral
    c. With one code for Sensorineural hearing loss, asymmetrical
    d. With two codes, one for Conductive hearing loss, bilateral and one for Sensorineural hearing loss, bilateral

See next page for answers and rationales.

Chapter 8 Answers and Rationales

1. What information is needed in order to report the most specific code for ear disorders?

    b. The laterality (right, left, bilateral) of the affected site

    Rationale: *Coding diseases of the ear to the highest level of specificity available in ICD-10-CM requires specific documentation of the affected site including laterality (right, left, bilateral).*

2. Which of the following ear disorders are NOT classified with diseases of the ear in Chapter 8?

    d. All of the above

    Rationale: *According to the exclusion note at the beginning of Chapter 8, diseases of the ear and mastoid process (H60-H95) exclude: certain infectious and parasitic diseases (A00-B99); endocrine, nutritional and metabolic diseases (E00-E88); and neoplasms (C00-D49) in addition to other conditions.*

3. The physician documents the patient's diagnosis as otitis media in influenza. How is this coded?

    c. In Chapter 10 Diseases of the respiratory system (J00-J99)

    Rationale: *According to the Excludes1 note in the Tabular List at the code category for otitis media in diseases classified elsewhere, otitis media in influenza is coded to J09.X9, J10.83, or J11.83.*

4. What diagnosis describes a type of noninfectious otitis externa?

    a. Acute actinic otitis externa

    Rationale: *Acute actinic otitis externa is listed under the subcategory H60.5 Acute noninfective otitis externa. The other three conditions (diffuse otitis externa, swimmer's ear, malignant otitis externa) are all types of infectious otitis externa.*

5. Which of the following types of hearing loss is coded as unspecified sensorineural hearing loss?

    d. All of the above

    Rationale: *The Index entry for Loss of hearing without further specification directs the coder to H90.5, which lists central hearing loss, congenital deafness, and perceptive hearing loss not otherwise specified, as included conditions.*

6. How are postprocedural complications of the ear and mastoid process classified?

    d. In Chapter 8 Diseases of the ear and mastoid process in a separate code block the end of the chapter

    Rationale: *ICD-10-CM has a separate code block at the end of Chapter 8 (H95) which groups together in one category all intraoperative and postprocedural complications from treatment of ear and mastoid process disorders.*

7. What instructions are included for nonsuppurative otitis media?

    d. All of the above

    Rationale: *In ICD-10-CM, under category H65, there are instructional notes directing the coder to use additional codes for any associated perforated tympanic membrane and to identify any infectious agent, or exposure to environmental tobacco smoke (Z77.22), which may also be occupational (Z57.31), or in the perinatal period (P96.81).*

8. If the physician documents the patient's diagnosis as vertigo, how is this coded?

    c. R42 Dizziness and giddiness

    Rationale: *Vertigo that is not otherwise specified in the medical record documentation is coded with signs and symptoms in Chapter 18. Vertigo without further specification is indexed to the code for dizziness and giddiness (R42) and "Vertigo NOS" is listed as an included condition under that code.*

9. The code for an abscess of the external ear includes which of the following conditions?

    d. All of the above

    Rationale: *Code H60.0 Abscess of external ear lists boil of external ear, carbuncle of auricle or external auditory canal and furuncle of external ear as included conditions.*

10. The physician documents the patient's bilateral hearing impairment as both conductive and sensorineural hearing loss. How is this classified?

    b. With one code for Mixed conductive and sensorineural hearing loss, bilateral

    Rationale: *When both conductive and sensorineural types of hearing losses are present in the same ear, the term mixed hearing loss is used. ICD-10-CM contains specific codes to report mixed conductive and sensorineural hearing loss.*

Chapter 9
DISEASES OF THE CIRCULATORY SYSTEM

Introduction

Diseases of the circulatory system are found in Chapter 9. Some of the most frequently diagnosed circulatory system diseases and conditions have undergone significant changes from how they were historically reported including hypertension, coronary atherosclerosis, myocardial infarction, and cardiac arrhythmias. Essential hypertension is no longer designated as benign, malignant, or unspecified and is reported with code I10 Essential hypertension. However, secondary hypertension codes have been expanded and will require specific documentation. Coronary atherosclerosis codes are combination codes that report the presence or absence of angina as well as the atherosclerosis. The definition of the acute phase of treatment for myocardial infarction has been recently changed and is shortened to 4 weeks from 8 weeks There are no fifth digits identifying the myocardial infarction encounter as the initial episode of care or a subsequent episode of care. Instead, there are two code categories. A code from category I21 ST elevation (STEMI) and non-ST elevation (NSTEMI) myocardial infarction is assigned for the acute phase of care or for myocardial infarctions with a stated duration of 4 weeks (28 days) or less. A code from category I22 Subsequent ST elevation (STEMI) or non-ST elevation (NSTEMI) myocardial infarction is assigned for a subsequent acute (new) myocardial infarction at either the same or a different site in the heart occurring within the 4-week time frame of the initial acute myocardial infarction.

Cardiac arrhythmias are specific as to type. For example, a left bundle branch hemiblock, is designated as a left fascicular block must be documented as left anterior, left posterior, or other specified left fascicular block. Below is a table of sections in ICD-10-CM.

ICD-10-CM Chapter Blocks	
I00-I02	Acute Rheumatic Fever
I05-I09	Chronic Rheumatic Heart Diseases
I10-I15	Hypertensive Diseases
I20-I25	Ischemic Heart Diseases
I26-I28	Pulmonary Heart Disease and Diseases of Pulmonary Circulation
I30-I52	Other Forms of Heart Disease
I60-I69	Cerebrovascular Diseases
I70-I79	Diseases of Arteries, Arterioles and Capillaries
I80-I89	Diseases of Veins, Lymphatic Vessels and Lymph Nodes, Not Elsewhere Classified
I95-I99	Other and Unspecified Disorders of the Circulatory System

Coding Note(s)

Some chapters in ICD-10-CM contain chapter level instructions in the form of different types of coding notes, including Includes notes. However, for Chapter 9 Diseases of the Circulatory System, the only chapter level instructions are contained in an Excludes2 note, which is discussed below.

Exclusions

The specific conditions listed in the Excludes2 note appearing for this chapter are listed in the following table:

Excludes1	Excludes2
None	Certain conditions originating in the perinatal period (P04-P96) Certain infectious and parasitic diseases (A00-B99) Complications of pregnancy, childbirth and the puerperium (O00-O9A) Congenital malformations, deformations, and chromosomal abnormalities (Q00-Q99) Endocrine, nutritional, and metabolic diseases (E00-E88) Injury, poisoning and certain other consequences of external causes (S00-T88) Neoplasms (C00-D49) Symptoms, signs and abnormal clinical and laboratory findings, not elsewhere classified (R00-R94) Systemic connective tissue disorders (M30-M36) Transient cerebral ischemic attacks and related syndromes (G45.-)

Chapter Guidelines

Guidelines for coding diseases of the circulatory system cover five conditions which include:

- Hypertension
- Atherosclerotic coronary artery disease and angina
- Intraoperative and postprocedural cerebrovascular accident
- Sequelae of cerebrovascular disease
- Acute myocardial infarction

Hypertension

Hypertension is not classified as benign, malignant, or unspecified. Hypertension without associated heart or kidney disease is reported with the code I10 Essential hypertension.

Hypertension with Heart Disease

Causal relationship between hypertension and heart disease:

- Heart conditions classified to category I50 Heart failure and subcategories I51.4 Myocarditis, unspecified; I51.5 Myocardial degeneration; I51.7 Cardiomegaly; I51.89 Other ill-defined heart diseases, and I51.9 Heart disease, unspecified, are assigned to category I11 Hypertensive heart disease, when a causal relationship is stated, such as "left ventricular heart failure due to hypertension," or implied, such as "hypertensive left ventricular heart failure." When a causal relationship between hypertensive heart disease and these conditions is stated or implied, only the code for the hypertensive heart disease is reported. (See includes note under category I11)
- When a causal relationship between hypertensive heart disease and heart failure is stated or implied, the hypertensive heart disease with heart failure (I11.0) is sequenced first followed by a code from category I50 to identify the type of heart failure

No causal relationship between hypertension and heart disease:

- Heart conditions classified to category I50 Heart failure and subcategories I51.4 Myocarditis, unspecified; I51.5 Myocardial degeneration; I51.7 Cardiomegaly; I51.89 Other ill-defined heart diseases, and I51.9 Heart disease, unspecified, without a stated or implied causal relationship to the hypertension are coded separately. The same heart conditions with hypertension are also coded separately when the provider has documented they are unrelated to the hypertension. The hypertension is reported with code I10 Essential hypertension, and the heart disease is reported with a code from category I50 or subcategories I51.4-I51.7, I51.89, I51.9
- The codes are sequenced based on the documentation related to the circumstances of the admission/encounter

Hypertensive Chronic Kidney Disease

A causal relationship between the hypertension and the chronic kidney disease is always presumed and documentation of hypertension with chronic kidney disease is always reported as hypertensive chronic kidney disease.

A code from category I12 Hypertensive chronic kidney disease is assigned first when there is documented hypertension and a condition classifiable to category N18 Chronic kidney disease (CKD). CKD should not be coded as hypertensive if the provider indicates the CKD is not related to the hypertension.

A code from category N18 is reported secondarily to identify the stage of chronic kidney disease.

If the patient has hypertensive chronic kidney disease and acute renal failure, an additional code for the acute renal failure is also assigned. Codes are sequenced according to the circumstances of the admission or encounter.

Hypertensive Heart and Chronic Kidney Disease

Codes in category I13, Hypertensive heart and chronic kidney disease, are combination codes that include hypertension, heart disease and chronic kidney disease. The includes note at I13 states that the conditions reported in categories I11 and I12 are included in I13. If a patient has hypertension, heart disease, and chronic kidney disease, then a code from I13 should be used, not individual codes for each, or codes from I11 or I12.

If heart failure is also present, assign an additional code from category I50 to identify the type of heart failure.

A code from category N18 Chronic kidney disease should also be assigned to identify the stage of chronic kidney disease. If both acute renal failure and chronic kidney disease are present, the acute renal failure should also be coded and sequenced according to the circumstances of the admission or encounter.

Hypertensive Cerebrovascular Disease

Assign the appropriate code from categories I60-I69 first, followed by the appropriate hypertension code.

Hypertensive Retinopathy

A code from subcategory H35.0 Background retinopathy and retinal vascular changes is reported with a code from categories I10-I15 for the systemic hypertension. Sequencing depends on the reason for the encounter.

Secondary Hypertension

Two codes are required for secondary hypertension, one for the underlying etiology and one from category I15 to identify the hypertension. Sequencing depends on the reason for the encounter.

Transient Hypertension

A code for hypertension is NOT assigned unless the patient has a documented, established diagnosis of hypertension. Assign code R03.0 Elevated blood pressure reading without diagnosis of hypertension.

If the diagnosis is transient hypertension of pregnancy, assign a code from category O13 Gestational [pregnancy-induced] hypertension without significant proteinuria, or one from category O14 Pre-eclampsia, depending on the documentation.

Controlled Hypertension

This diagnosis typically refers to hypertension under control with medication. Assign the appropriate code from categories I10-I15.

Uncontrolled Hypertension

Generally, a diagnosis of uncontrolled hypertension refers to untreated hypertension or to hypertension that is not responding to medication therapy. Uncontrolled hypertension is assigned a code from categories I10-I15 as appropriate to identify the type of hypertension.

Pulmonary Hypertension

Pulmonary hypertension is classified as Other pulmonary heart diseases, category I27. For secondary cases, code also any associated conditions or adverse effects of drugs or toxin. Sequencing depends on the circumstances of the encounter.

Atherosclerotic Coronary Artery Disease and Angina

There are combination codes used reporting atherosclerotic coronary artery disease with angina pectoris. When the two conditions are documented, they are reported with codes from subcategories I25.11 Atherosclerotic heart disease of native coronary artery with angina pectoris, and I25.7 Atherosclerosis of coronary artery bypass graft(s) and coronary artery of transplanted heart with angina pectoris.

- It is not necessary to assign a separate code for angina pectoris when both conditions are documented because the combination code captures both conditions
- A causal relationship between the atherosclerosis and angina is assumed unless documentation specifically indicates that the angina is due to a condition other than atherosclerosis
- If a patient is admitted with an acute myocardial infarction (AMI) and coronary artery disease, the AMI is sequenced first

Intraoperative and Postprocedural Cerebrovascular Accident

A cause and effect relationship between a cerebrovascular accident (CVA) and a procedure cannot be assumed. The physician must document that a cause and effect relationship exists between the procedure and the CVA.

- Documentation must clearly identify the condition as an intraoperative or postoperative event
- The condition must also be clearly documented as an infarction or hemorrhage
- For a cerebrovascular infarction, see the following subcategories:
  - I97.81 Intraoperative cerebrovascular infarction
  - I97.82 Postprocedural cerebrovascular infarction

For a cerebrovascular hemorrhage, code assignment depends on the type of procedure performed. See the following subcategories:

- G97.3 Intraoperative hemorrhage and hematoma of a nervous system organ or structure complicating a procedure
- G97.5 Postprocedural hemorrhage and hematoma of a nervous system organ or structure complicating a procedure

Sequelae of Cerebrovascular Disease

Category I69 Sequelae of cerebrovascular disease is used to report conditions classifiable to categories I60-I67 as the cause of the late effect, particularly neurological deficits, which are themselves classified elsewhere. Guidelines are as follows:

- Sequelae/late effects are conditions that persist after the initial onset of the conditions classifiable to categories I60-I67
- The neurologic deficits may be present at the onset of the cerebrovascular disease or may arise at any time after the onset
- If the patient currently has cerebrovascular disease and deficits from an old cerebrovascular disease, codes from category I69 and categories I60-I67 may be reported together
- Transient ischemic attack (TIA) is reported instead of a code from category I69 to identify the history of the cerebrovascular disease.
- Some sequelae codes such as those for hemiplegia, hemiparesis and monoplegia which are found in category I69 require specification as to whether the affected side is dominant or nondominant. When the affected side is documented, but not specified as the patient's dominant or nondominant side, the left side is reported as nondominant and the right side is reported as dominant

Acute Myocardial Infarction

Acute myocardial infarction (AMI) is reported with codes that identify the AMI by type. Type 1 are those related to coronary artery disease and are defined based upon ECG changes as ST elevation myocardial infarction (STEMI) and non-ST elevation myocardial infarction (NSTEMI). STEMI is further classified based upon the site such as posterior or anterolateral wall. Type 2 AMI is due to ischemia not related to coronary artery disease. Types 3-5 are classified in a single category with instructions to code any related complications.

Initial acute myocardial infarction:

- Assign codes from category I21 for AMIs not documented as subsequent or not occurring within 28 days of a previous myocardial infarction
- Type 1 STEMI is reported with codes in subcategories I21.0-I21.2 and code I21.3
- Type 1 NSTEMI is reported with code I21.4, which is also used for "nontransmural" MIs
- If a Type 1 NSTEMI evolves to STEMI, the code for STEMI is reported
- If a Type 1 STEMI converts to NSTEMI due to thrombolytic therapy, it is still reported as a STEMI
- Encounters for care of the AMI during the first four weeks (equal to or less than 4 full weeks/28 days), are assigned a code from category I21. Examples of when reporting of a code from category I21 is appropriate include:
  - Transfers to another acute care setting for continued care of the AMI
  - Any encounter within the 4-week time frame for care related to the myocardial infarction
- Encounters related to the myocardial infarction after 4 full weeks of care are reported with the appropriate aftercare code
- Old or healed myocardial infarctions are assigned code I25.2 Old myocardial infarction
- Acute myocardial infarction, unspecified
  - I21.9 is the default code for a myocardial infarction documented only as acute MI, or unspecified type
  - If only Type 1 STEMI or transmural MI is documented without the site, query the provider. If the provider cannot be queried, assign code I21.3
- Nontransmural or subendocardial MI with site documented
  - Code as a nontransmural/subendocardial (NSTEMI) myocardial infarction I21.4
  - Codes for nontransmural/subendocardial myocardial infarction are not specific to site

- Subsequent acute myocardial infarction occurring within 28 days of a previous acute myocardial infarction:
  - Assign a code from category I22 for a new STEMI/NSTEMI documented as occurring within 4 weeks (28 days) of a previous type 1 or unspecified myocardial infarction, regardless of site
  - Codes in category I22 are never reported alone
    - » Assign a code from category I21 in conjunction with the code from I22
    - » Codes from categories I21 and I22 are sequenced based on the circumstances of the encounter
  - Assign a code from category I22 only for type 1 or unspecified subsequent myocardial infarctions
  - For subsequent type 2 MIs, assign only code I21.A1
  - For subsequent type 4 or 5 MIs, assign only code I21.A9
  - If a subsequent MI of one type occurs within 4 weeks of a MI of a different type, assign the appropriate codes from category I21 to identify each type. Do not report a code from category I22. Codes in category I22 are only assigned if both the initial and subsequent MIs are type 1 or unspecified
- Other types of myocardial infarction
  - ICD-10-CM provides codes for different types of myocardial infarction. Type 1 MIs are reported with I21.0-I21.4 and I21.9
  - Type 2 MIs, and MIs due to demand ischemia or secondary to ischemic imbalance, are reported with I21.A1 Myocardial infarction type 2 with the underlying cause coded first
    - » Do not assign code I24.8 Other forms of acute ischemic heart disease for the demand ischemia
    - » When a type 2 AMI code is described as NSTEMI or STEMI, assign only code I21.A1. Codes I21.01-I21.4 are only ever assigned for type 1 AMIs
  - Acute type 3, 4a, 4b, 4c and 5 MIs are reported with code I21.A9 Other myocardial infarction type.
  - Follow "Code also" and "Code first" notes related to complications, and for coding postprocedural MIs during or following cardiac surgery
- See coding guidelines for Chapter 21 Factors Influencing Health Status and Contact with Health Services (Z00-Z99) for information on reporting tPA (rtPA) in a different facility within the last 24 hours

General Documentation Requirements

In ICD-10-CM, codes for diseases of the circulatory system are becoming much more specific. The increasing specificity requires more complete documentation regarding the condition, site, and often the laterality as well. Assigning the most specific intraoperative and postoperative complication codes requires precise documentation by the physician. In addition, there are combination codes for some conditions that frequently occur together and assignment of these combination codes requires documentation of both conditions when they occur together, such as coronary atherosclerosis with angina pectoris.

Laterality

Laterality is required for many conditions including cerebrovascular diseases (I60-I69), diseases of the arteries, arterioles, and capillaries when pertaining to the extremities (I70-I79), and diseases of the veins of the extremities (I80-I87).

Intraoperative and Postprocedural Complications

Subcategory I97.1 captures other postprocedural cardiac functional disturbances. Functional disturbances are those that affect heart function and include conditions such as cardiac insufficiency, cardiac arrest, and heart failure. Documentation is required as to whether the functional disturbance occurred after a cardiac procedure or after a surgery performed on a site other than the heart and great vessels. Intraoperative cardiac functional disturbances are captured by codes in subcategory I97.7 with specific codes for intraoperative cardiac arrest occurring during cardiac surgery (I97.710) or during other surgery (I97.711). All other intraoperative functional disturbances are captured by codes in subcategory I97.79.

Hemorrhage and hematoma complicating a procedure are specific to whether the complication occurred during the procedure (intraoperative) or following the procedure (postoperative), and whether the hemorrhage or hematoma involving a circulatory system organ or structure was incurred as a result of a circulatory system procedure or a procedure on another organ or body system. For hemorrhage and hematoma resulting from a circulatory system procedure, the complication must be documented as complicating cardiac catheterization, cardiac bypass, or another circulatory system procedure. Accidental puncture or laceration of a circulatory system organ or structure during a procedure is specific to whether the procedure was being performed on a circulatory system organ or structure or on another organ or body system.

Combination Codes

Some conditions that frequently occur together are now reported with combination codes. Combination codes for diseases of the circulatory system include:

- Coronary atherosclerosis and angina (I25.1-). When coronary atherosclerosis and angina occur together, a cause and effect relationship is assumed unless documentation specifically states otherwise and a combination code is reported
  - For atherosclerotic heart disease of native coronary artery with angina pectoris, (see subcategory I25.11)
  - For atherosclerosis of coronary artery bypass graft(s) and coronary artery of transplanted heart with angina pectoris (see subcategory I25.7)
- Pulmonary embolism with acute cor pulmonale. (see subcategory I26.0)

There are additional combination codes that are reviewed in the code-specific examples.

Code-Specific Documentation Requirements

In this section, some of the more commonly reported diseases of the circulatory system are reviewed. The corresponding codes are listed with the documentation requirements identified. The focus is on frequently reported conditions with additional and more specific clinical documentation requirements. Though not all of the codes are discussed, this section will provide a representative sample of the type of additional documentation required for coding diseases of the circulatory system.

Angina Pectoris

Angina pectoris is chest pain caused by decreased blood flow to the heart muscle, usually from a spasm or partial occlusion in the coronary arteries. Angina pectoris can be further defined as stable, when pain is triggered by exertion or stress and resolves with rest or sublingual nitroglycerine, or unstable (crescendo), where pain occurs at rest or with minimal exertion and follows a pattern of increasing severity and duration.

In ICD-10-CM, category I20 contains codes for angina with four subcategories, I20.0 Unstable angina, I20.1 Angina pectoris with documented spasm, I20.8 Other forms of angina pectoris, and I20.9 Angina pectoris unspecified. In addition to these changes, there are now combination codes for atherosclerotic heart disease with angina pectoris.

Coding and Documentation Requirements

Identify angina related to atherosclerotic heart disease:

- Complicating atherosclerotic heart disease (see atherosclerotic heart disease)
- Not complicating atherosclerotic heart disease

If no diagnosis of atherosclerotic heart disease with angina, identify the type of angina pectoris:

- Unstable angina, which includes:
  - Accelerated angina
  - Crescendo angina
  - De novo effort angina
  - Intermediate coronary syndrome
  - Preinfarction syndrome
  - Worsening effort angina
- Angina with documented spasm, which includes:
  - Angiospastic angina
  - Prinzmetal angina
  - Spasm-induced angina
  - Variant angina
- Other forms of angina pectoris, which includes:
  - Angina equivalent
  - Angina of effort
  - Coronary slow flow syndrome
  - Stenocardia
- Unspecified angina pectoris, which includes:
  - Angina NOS
  - Anginal syndrome
  - Cardiac angina
  - Ischemic chest pain
  - Lipid rich plaque
  - Angina Pectoris

ICD-10-CM Code/Documentation	
I20.0	Unstable angina
I20.1	Angina pectoris with documented spasm
I20.8	Other forms of angina pectoris
I20.9	Angina pectoris, unspecified

Documentation and Coding Example

Fifty-six-year-old Caucasian female presents to her PMD with C/O new onset burning pain in her left shoulder and jaw lasting 5-10 minutes. She can go days without symptoms or have 3-6 episodes in a day. She often feels lightheaded or dizzy with the pain and sometimes feels like her heart is "skipping beats." She is divorced, her only child has just gone off to college and she also admits to job stress as the superintendent of an elementary school district faced with severe budget cuts. On examination, this is an extremely thin, immaculately groomed woman who looks her stated age. Her weight is down 12 lbs. since her last visit 7 months ago. She states she has not been interested in cooking with her son gone and often skips meals. Temperature 98.2, HR 70, RR 12, BP 124/82. PERRL, neck supple with no lymphadenopathy. ROM in jaw, shoulders, and arms WNL. HR regular without murmur. Breath sounds clear, equal bilaterally. Abdomen soft, non-tender with bowel sounds present in all quadrants. Peripheral pulses intact with no edema noted. Reflexes are normal in extremities. 12 lead EKG is WNL. Impression: Anxiety vs. Angina. Patient is given a sample of NTG 0.3 mg with instructions on use and a prescription for Xanax 0.5 mg. First available echocardiogram and stress EKG are tomorrow afternoon but patient has to prepare for a School Board meeting and declines this time. She is to schedule them the following day and will return for results immediately after.

Follow up visit PMD: Patient states she had symptoms before the Board meeting last night and took the NTG. She felt better immediately but did have a slight headache for a few hours. She has not filled the Xanax prescription. The echocardiogram and stress EKG were unremarkable per cardiologist. It is his opinion this is **stable angina**. He agrees with treating symptoms with NTG and Xanax. RTC in 3 months, sooner if symptoms progress or are not responsive to NTG, Xanax.

Diagnosis Code(s)

I20.9 Angina pectoris, unspecified

Coding Note(s)

Stable angina without any additional qualifiers is reported with an unspecified code in ICD-10-CM.

Atherosclerosis of Extremities

Atherosclerosis of the extremities is characterized by inflammation and accumulation of macrophage white blood cells and low-density lipoproteins along the arterial walls. This leads to narrowing of the vessels and decreased blood flow.

Lack of blood flow to the extremities can cause a number of complications including pain, ulceration, and gangrene.

Atherosclerosis of the extremities is reported with codes from 6 subcategories: I70.2, I70.3, I70.4, I70.5, I70.6, and I70.7. Atherosclerosis of the extremities is first classified by whether the blood vessel is a native artery or a bypass graft and the fourth character subcategory level identifies the type of graft. The type of bypass graft must be documented as: autologous vein bypass graft, nonautologous biological bypass graft, nonbiological bypass graft, other specified type of bypass graft, or unspecified type of bypass graft. The fifth character identifies any complications. For ulceration of the legs, this level also captures laterality. For other complications, laterality is captured by the sixth character. The sixth character for ulceration identifies the site more specifically as the thigh, calf, ankle, heel and midfoot, other part of foot, other part of leg, or unspecified site of leg.

Coding and Documentation Requirements

Identify atherosclerosis of the extremity as affecting:

- Native artery
- Bypass graft
  - Autologous vein
  - Nonautologous biological
  - Nonbiological
  - Other specified type
  - Unspecified graft
- Identify complications/manifestations:
  - Gangrene
  - Intermittent claudication
  - Rest pain
  - Ulceration
  - Other complication/manifestation
  - Unspecified or without complication/manifestation

Identify extremity:

- Arm
- Leg
  - Right
  - Left
  - Bilateral
- Unspecified extremity

For atherosclerosis of the arm with ulceration, use additional code (L98.49-) to identify severity:

- Limited to breakdown of skin
- Fat layer exposed
- Necrosis of muscle
- Necrosis of bone
- muscle involvement without evidence of necrosis
- bone involvement without evidence of necrosis
- other specified severity
- Unspecified severity

For atherosclerosis of the leg with ulceration:

- Identify site:
  - Thigh
  - Calf
  - Ankle
  - Midfoot
  - Heel
  - Other part of foot
  - Other part of leg
  - Unspecified site of leg
- Use additional code (L97.-) to identify severity of ulcer:
  - Limited to breakdown of skin
  - Fat layer exposed
  - Necrosis of muscle
  - Necrosis of bone
  - muscle involvement without evidence of necrosis
  - bone involvement without evidence of necrosis
  - other specified severity
  - Unspecified severity
- Use additional code to identify any:
  - Exposure to environmental tobacco smoke (Z77.22)
  - History of tobacco use (Z87.891)
  - Occupational exposure to environmental tobacco smoke (Z57.31)
  - Tobacco dependence (F17.-)
  - Tobacco use (Z72.0)

Atherosclerosis of Native Artery of Left Leg with Ulceration

ICD-10-CM Code/Documentation	
I70.241	Atherosclerosis of native arteries of left leg with ulceration of thigh
I70.242	Atherosclerosis of native arteries of left leg with ulceration of calf
I70.243	Atherosclerosis of native arteries of left leg with ulceration of ankle
I70.244	Atherosclerosis of native arteries of left leg with ulceration of heel and midfoot
I70.245	Atherosclerosis of native arteries of left leg with ulceration of other part of foot
I70.248	Atherosclerosis of native arteries of left leg with ulceration of other part of lower left leg
I70.249	Atherosclerosis of native arteries of left leg with ulceration of unspecified site

Documentation and Coding Example

Patient presents to Wound Care Clinic for continuing treatment of **left calf ulceration due to atherosclerosis of native vessels**. This sixty-one-year-old gentleman is well known to us. He has been disabled from a back injury since age forty-eight and was diagnosed with Peripheral Vascular Disease **(PVD) 10 years ago**. He is a **long-time smoker, has elevated cholesterol, and Type II diabetes**. Medications include Cilostazol for **leg pain and claudication**, Crestor for cholesterol, and Glucophage for

9. Diseases of the Circulatory System

diabetes. On examination, of both lower legs, he has muscle wasting, hair loss, thickened toenails, and bluish red discoloration from toes to knee. Pulses are weak but palpable on the right, present only by Doppler on the left. Unna Boot dressing carefully removed from **left lower leg to expose a crater like wound measuring 2 cm by 3 cm with a depth of 1.5 cm in the center. Skin is gone, fat pad exposed**. The bottom of the wound has a small slough of yellow tissue. Wound is gently debrided and cleaned with betadine and water. Unna Boot reapplied. Patient will return to clinic in 10 days for re-evaluation and continued treatment.

Diagnosis Code(s)

I70.242	Atherosclerosis of native arteries of left leg with ulceration of calf
L97.222	Non-pressure chronic ulcer of left calf with fat layer exposed
E11.622	Type II diabetes mellitus with other skin ulcer
Z72.0	Tobacco use

Coding Note(s)

The only condition treated at this visit is the leg ulcer; however, both the Type II diabetes and the smoking affect healing of chronic ulcers so these conditions should be reported secondarily. The elevated cholesterol is not coded because it is not evaluated or treated at this visit.

Subcategory I70.24 includes any condition classifiable to I70.212 and I70.222 so the leg pain and claudication are not reported additionally. Atherosclerosis requires documentation of the blood vessel as a native artery or bypass graft and also requires the type of bypass graft. Atherosclerosis codes with ulceration are specific to the right leg, left leg, or other extremities (arms). For ulceration of the legs, the site of the ulcer must also be documented to capture the most specific code. An additional code is required to identify the severity of the ulcer (category L97). The type II diabetes code also reflects a skin ulcer complication. Tobacco use and tobacco dependence are clearly differentiated in ICD-10-CM. The code for tobacco use is reported because the documentation does not specify tobacco dependence.

Bundle Branch Blocks: Left Hemiblock/ Right Branch Block

Left bundle branch hemiblock and right bundle branch block are types of conduction disorders of the heart. Conduction refers to electrical impulses that move through heart tissue and cause the heart to beat. Conduction disorders affect heart rhythm and rate. In some instances, rhythm and rate disturbances produce physiological symptoms, but sometimes they can only be identified when an electrocardiogram (ECG) is obtained. The following are some of the more common types of conduction disorders:

Left anterior fascicular block: Left anterior fascicular block (LAFB), also referred to as left anterior hemiblock, is the most common partial block of the left bundle branch and involves electrical conduction of impulses from the atrioventricular node. In a left anterior fascicular block, the anterior half of the left bundle branch is defective causing the impulse to pass first to the posterior area of the ventricle which delays activation of the anterior and upper ventricle. It can be observed on an ECG tracing as left axis deviation.

Left posterior fascicular block: Left posterior fascicular block, also referred to as left posterior hemiblock, is a less common partial block of the left bundle branch and involves electrical conduction of impulses from the atrioventricular node. In left posterior fascicular block, the posterior half of the left bundle branch is defective causing the impulse to pass first to the anterior and upper ventricle which delays activation of the posterior ventricle. It can be observed on an ECG tracing as right axis deviation.

Right fascicular block: This is a defect in the heart's electrical conduction system in which the right ventricle is not activated by an impulse from the right bundle branch but does depolarize when impulses from the left bundle branch travel through the myocardium. It can be observed on an ECG tracing as a wide QRS complex.

In ICD-10-CM, conduction disorders are found in two categories, I44 Atrioventricular and left bundle branch block, and I45 Other conduction disorders. Conditions in these two categories that have specific documentation requirements include left bundle branch hemiblock and right bundle branch block. Left bundle branch hemiblock must be specified as left anterior fascicular block, left posterior fascicular block, or other specified fascicular block to avoid assigning the code for an unspecified fascicular block. Right bundle branch block must be specified as right fascicular block or other specified right bundle branch block to avoid assigning the code for unspecified right bundle branch block.

Coding and Documentation Requirements

For left bundle branch hemiblock, identify fascicular block:

- Left anterior fascicular block
- Left posterior fascicular block
- Other fascicular block
- Unspecified fascicular block

For right bundle branch block, identify fascicular block:

- Right fascicular block
- Other right bundle branch block
- Unspecified right bundle branch block

Bundle Branch (Hemi) Block

ICD-10-CM Code/Documentation	
I44.4	Left anterior fascicular block
I44.5	Left posterior fascicular block
I44.69	Other fascicular block
I44.60	Unspecified fascicular block
I45.0	Right fascicular block
I45.19	Other right bundle branch block
I45.10	Unspecified right bundle-branch block

Documentation and Coding Example

Patient is a 45 year-old Caucasian male referred to cardiology after a routine preoperative EKG showed an abnormal rhythm. He is scheduled for an elective left shoulder arthroscopy in 5 days and anesthesia requests cardiology clearance prior to the procedure. Temperature 97.2, HR 62, RR 12, BP 128/70, Ht. 71 inches, Wt. 172 lbs. On examination, this is an athletic appearing, well-groomed gentleman who looks younger than his stated age. He states he is left handed, an avid tennis player and runner and began having left shoulder pain and stiffness a few months ago. MRI showed a small rotator cuff tear and he hopes surgery will help improve his ROM and allow him to resume tennis. He denies chest pain, SOB, dizziness, or palpitations. PERRL, neck supple. Carotid arteries without bruit. Extremities are without clubbing, pulses are full. HR regular without gallop, rub, bruit, or murmur. Breath sounds clear and equal. Abdomen soft, non-tender without bruit. EKG shows a left deviation in the QRS axis of -45 degrees and slight widening of the QRS complex. Also noted on EKG is a mild deviation of qR complex in the lateral limb leads of I, aVL. An abnormal rS pattern in inferior leads II, III, aVF and a 0.055 sec. delay of the intrinsicoid deflection in aVL. Results are consistent with a **benign left anterior hemiblock**. He is cleared for surgery. Cardiology note electronically transmitted to his orthopedist and to the anesthesia group.

Diagnosis Code(s)

I44.4 Left anterior fascicular block

Coding Note(s)

A hemiblock refers to an arrest of the electrical impulses in one of the two main divisions of the left branch of the atrioventricular bundle, either the anterior or posterior. The term hemiblock is synonymous with a fascicular or divisional block. In this case, the block is in the anterior portion, so code I44.4 is reported.

Cardiac Arrest

Cardiac arrest is the failure of the heart muscle to contract effectively which impedes the normal circulation of blood and prevents oxygen delivery to the body.

Cardiac arrest is not synonymous with a myocardial infarction. A myocardial infarction refers to a loss of blood supply to an area of the heart usually due to blockage of a coronary artery which causes the heart tissue to die (necrosis).

There are three codes for reporting a cardiac arrest. These codes identify the cardiac arrest as due to an underlying cardiac condition (I46.2); due to an underlying other (noncardiac) condition (I46.8); or due to an unspecified cause (I46.9). Codes in category I46 are not used to report a myocardial infarction, which is reported with codes from categories I21 and I22. There is also an Excludes2 note for cardiogenic shock which is reported with code R57.0.

Coding and Documentation Requirements

Identify cardiac arrest as due to:

- Underlying cardiac condition
- Other underlying condition
- Unspecified cause

Cardiac Arrest

ICD-10-CM Code/Documentation	
I46.2	Cardiac arrest due to underlying cardiac condition
I46.8	Cardiac arrest due to other underlying condition
I46.9	Cardiac arrest, cause unspecified

Documentation and Coding Example

Thirty-six-year-old Caucasian female brought in by EMS after suffering a **witnessed cardiac arrest**. Patient was **training for a recreational 5K run** with a group of friends when she suddenly collapsed on the **high school track** where they were training. Bystanders rushed to her side and an off-duty nurse assessed her to be pulseless and breathless and started CPR. EMS was called and an AED on the premises was activated. She was defibrillated x 2 and had a pulse by the time paramedics arrived on scene. She is conscious on arrival in ED, oriented only to self and has no recall of the incident. Sinus tach on monitor, 12 lead EKG shows prolonged QT interval. Blood drawn for CBC, electrolytes, and cardiac enzymes. Patient admitted to CCU for observation.

CCU Note: Patient had an uneventful night. She is alert and oriented x 3. She c/o chest discomfort during the night and was medicated twice with intravenous morphine sulfate with good relief. Patient was able to provide cardiologist with a history significant for syncopal episodes in adolescence which were attributed to low blood sugars, a family history of SIDS in a sibling, and a niece with congenital hearing loss. She is scheduled for echocardiogram to r/o cardiomyopathy or congenital heart defect. She was started on Propranolol 40 mg BID last evening. Transfer to telemetry floor following echo.

Telemetry Floor Note: Stable overnight with no evidence of tachycardia, improving QT interval although it is still prolonged. Echocardiogram was negative for cardiomyopathy or congenital defect. Genetic work up initiated given the family history of SIDS and congenital HL. Patient is discharged home on Propranolol. Appointment with cardiologist in 1 week. She is advised not to return to her job until cleared by cardiology and is forbidden to engage in any strenuous exercise.

Impression: **Sudden cardiac arrest brought on by exercise with underlying long QT syndrome.**

Diagnosis Code(s)

I45.81 Long QT syndrome

I46.2 Cardiac arrest due to underlying cardiac condition

Y93.02 Activity, running

Y92.39 Other specified sports and athletic area as the place of occurrence of the external cause

Y99.8 Other external cause status

Coding Note(s)

Long QT syndrome is a hereditary defect of the heart's electrical conduction system characterized by an abnormally long gap in the time it takes for the ventricles to contract.

The long QT syndrome is the principal/first-listed diagnosis followed by code I46.2 which identifies the cardiac arrest as due to an underlying cardiac condition. An external cause code should also be reported because the cardiac arrest has been documented as due to strenuous exercise (running) and the underlying cardiac condition. Code Y93.02 is reported to identify the activity as running; Y99.8 identifies the external cause status as a leisure activity; and Y92.39 identifies the place of occurrence.

Coronary Atherosclerosis

Coronary atherosclerosis is a condition affecting arterial blood vessels in the heart, characterized by inflammation and accumulation of macrophage white blood cells and low-density lipoproteins along the arterial walls. This leads to narrowing of the vessels and decreased blood flow to the heart muscle and may cause angina (chest pain).

In ICD-10-CM, there are combination codes for when coronary atherosclerosis and angina occur together. Codes for atherosclerotic heart disease are listed in category I25 Chronic ischemic heart disease, in subcategories I25.1, I25.7, and I25.8. Other conditions listed in this category include: old myocardial infarction (I25.2), aneurysm of heart (I25.3), coronary artery aneurysm and dissection (I25.4), ischemic cardiomyopathy (I25.5), and silent myocardial ischemia (I25.6).

Coding and Documentation Requirements

Identify site of coronary atherosclerosis:

- Native coronary artery
- Graft
  - Autologous
    - » Artery bypass graft
    - » Vein bypass graft
  - Nonautologous biological bypass graft
  - Other specified type of bypass graft
  - Unspecified type of bypass graft
- Transplanted heart
  - Native coronary artery of transplanted heart
  - Bypass graft (artery/vein) of transplanted heart

Identify presence or absence and type of angina pectoris:

- With angina pectoris
  - Unstable
  - With documented spasm
  - With other documented form of angina pectoris
  - Unspecified type of angina pectoris
- Without angina pectoris

Identify also any of the following conditions (assign additional code):

- Chronic total occlusion of coronary artery
- Coronary atherosclerosis due to
  - Calcified coronary lesion
  - Lipid rich plaque

Use additional code to identify any:

- Exposure to environmental tobacco smoke (Z77.22)
- History of tobacco use (Z87.891)
- Occupational exposure to environmental tobacco smoke (Z57.31)
- Tobacco dependence (F17.-)
- Tobacco use (Z72.0)

Atherosclerosis Native Coronary Artery

ICD-10-CM Code/Documentation	
I25.10	Atherosclerotic heart disease of native coronary artery without angina pectoris
I25.110	Atherosclerotic heart disease of native coronary artery with unstable angina pectoris
I25.118	Atherosclerotic heart disease of native coronary artery with other forms of angina pectoris
I25.111	Atherosclerotic heart disease of native coronary artery with angina pectoris with documented spasm
I25.118	Atherosclerotic heart disease of native coronary artery with other forms of angina pectoris
I25.119	Atherosclerotic heart disease of native coronary artery with unspecified angina pectoris

Documentation and Coding Example

Patient is a seventy-five-year-old Black male well known to us in Cardiac Clinic. He has a **history of AMI 3 years ago with 4 vessel aortocoronary bypass grafts using saphenous vein left leg**. He is a retired train engineer, recently widowed, and is accompanied today by his daughter. He complains of **increasing SOB and chest tightness with exertion**. EKG shows abnormal ST segments unchanged from previous tracings. Oxygen saturation is 97% on RA. There is a well healed midline chest scar. HR regular without bruit, murmur, or rubs. Breath sounds decreased in bases with fine wheezes scattered over bronchus. He has a history of asthma well controlled with Symbicort daily, Xopenex when symptoms flare. Current medications also include Crestor and Atenolol. Pulses full in all extremities. **Well healed scar from groin to ankle left leg**. Patient and daughter agree to noninvasive cardiac testing to evaluate cardiac function and possible angiogram or nuclear medicine thallium study to assess the coronary graft sites. He is scheduled for OP echocardiogram, stress test. Further tests to be determined by those results.

Cardiac Testing Lab Note: Patient tolerated echocardiogram well but **developed CP during bicycle stress test** and the test had to be aborted. He was admitted to Telemetry floor and scheduled for an angiogram in the AM. Labs drawn for CBC, cardiac enzymes, PT and PTT, blood type and hold.

Cardiac Catheterization Lab: Under monitored anesthesia care patient is prepped and draped and procedure is carried out through a cut down in right groin. The angiogram shows clean vascular grafts with good coronary blood flow in the anterior wall. There is a **new atherosclerotic lesion along the left circumflex coronary artery with almost total occlusion of this artery**. Patient tolerated procedure well and was transferred back to Telemetry floor for overnight observation.

Impression: **Chronic occlusion of native left circumflex artery with angina on exertion.**

Discharge Note: Test results were discussed with patient and daughter. They decline surgery for the blocked artery and prefer to treat symptoms if possible. He will return to cardiac clinic in 1 week for post angio checkup. We will review his medications at that time and make changes as appropriate. He is discharged home in the care of his daughter.

Diagnosis Code(s)

I25.118	Atherosclerotic heart disease of native coronary artery with other forms of angina pectoris
I25.2	Old myocardial infarction
Z95.1	Presence of aortocoronary bypass graft

Coding Note(s)

Angina on exertion or angina of effort is classified as an "other form of angina." Code I25.82 is not reported because this code requires a diagnosis of "chronic total occlusion" and the documentation states that there is "almost total occlusion" but not "total occlusion."

Hemorrhage, Nontraumatic: Intracerebral, Intracranial, Subarachnoid

Intracerebral

An intracerebral hemorrhage is defined as bleeding inside the brain. In ICD-1Ø-CM, nontraumatic intracranial hemorrhage (I61) is specific to the region where the hemorrhage occurred. To assign the most specific code, documentation must identify the site as subcortical or cortical hemisphere, brain stem, cerebellum, or intraventricular. Alternatively, the documentation may state that there are multiple localized intracerebral hemorrhages as this condition also has a specific code.

Coding and Documentation Requirements

Identify the region of the nontraumatic cerebral hemorrhage:

- Brain stem
- Cerebellum
- Hemispheric
  - Cortical
  - Subcortical
  - Unspecified
- Intraventricular
- Multiple localized sites
- Other specified site
- Unspecified site

Nontraumatic Intracerebral Hemorrhage

ICD-1Ø-CM Code/Documentation	
I61.Ø	Nontraumatic intracerebral hemorrhage in hemisphere, subcortical
I61.1	Nontraumatic intracerebral hemorrhage in hemisphere, cortical
I61.2	Nontraumatic intracerebral hemorrhage in hemisphere, unspecified
I61.3	Nontraumatic intracerebral hemorrhage in brain stem
I61.4	Nontraumatic intracerebral hemorrhage in cerebellum
I61.5	Nontraumatic intracerebral hemorrhage, intraventricular
I61.6	Nontraumatic intracerebral hemorrhage, multiple localized
I61.8	Other nontraumatic intracerebral hemorrhage
I61.9	Nontraumatic intracerebral hemorrhage, unspecified

Documentation and Coding Example

Seventy-four-year-old Caucasian male presents to neurologist with new onset confusion and speech difficulties. The patient is widowed and is accompanied today by his housekeeper/caregiver. Patient was diagnosed with **cerebral amyloid angiopathy** several years ago after suffering seizures. The seizures have been well controlled with Tegretol. His caregiver reports he was well until yesterday when he had a headache and vomiting. They thought he had the flu and symptoms seemed to resolve with fluids and rest. She went in to his bedroom this morning when he did not come down to breakfast and found him sitting in a chair, dressed but unable to figure out where he was and what he should be doing. He is oriented to person and recognizes his caregiver and this physician. VSS. There is **no history of a fall or injury to the head**. He is transferred to ED with orders for blood draw to include CBC, electrolyte panel, coagulation studies, Type and Cross, IV of NS and head CT to r/o intracranial bleed or tumor. Admit to floor after CT scan.

Radiology Note: Patient underwent a CT scan of the brain which showed a **small cerebellar hemorrhage**. He developed bradycardia and hypotension during the scan, which resolved after administration of IV atropine. He was transferred to neurosurgical floor for observation and is scheduled for MRI in the morning.

Floor Note: Patient is oriented x 3 after an uneventful night. He has a wry sense of humor and likes joking with the staff. He ate breakfast but complained that the hospital food is atrocious and he will surely wither away to nothing if his housekeeper cannot bring him in home cooked meals. Neurosurgical Team will evaluate him after the MRI.

Neurosurgical Note: Patient tolerated MRI well and scan reveals a **small hemorrhage in the lateral cerebellum** with no obstructive hydrocephalus present. Labs are WNL. Plan is to monitor one more day and discharge if symptoms continue to improve.

Discharge Note: Patient is discharged home in the care of his housekeeper. His only medication is Tegretol and he has an appointment with his neurologist in 1 week. Recommend he have a repeat MRI in 2-4 weeks.

Diagnosis Code(s)

I61.4	Nontraumatic intracerebral hemorrhage in cerebellum
E85.4	Organ-limited amyloidosis
I68.Ø	Cerebral amyloid angiopathy

Coding Note(s)

Cerebral amyloid angiopathy is a neurological condition that is characterized by the build-up of proteins, specifically amyloid, on the artery walls in the brain. Typically, the protein is deposited only in the cerebral arteries and not elsewhere in the body. The condition increases the risk of hemorrhagic stroke and dementia. The cause is unknown. The cerebral amyloid angiopathy is reported additionally because it is related to the intracerebral hemorrhage and affects the management of the patient.

The code for the nontraumatic intracerebral hemorrhage is specific to the cerebellum.

Intracranial

The brain is covered by three membranes. The dura mater is the outer membrane, the arachnoid is the middle membrane, and the pia mater is the inner membrane. Nontraumatic extradural hemorrhage, also called epidural hemorrhage, refers to spontaneous bleeding between the dura mater and the skull. Extradural bleeding is usually arterial. Nontraumatic subdural hemorrhage refers to spontaneous bleeding between the dura mater and the arachnoid. A subdural hemorrhage most often arises from bridging veins that cross the subdural space. Both extradural and subdural hemorrhage increase intracranial pressure and compress brain tissue.

In ICD-10-CM, other and unspecified nontraumatic intracranial hemorrhage, category I62, contains codes for subdural hemorrhage which must be documented as acute, subacute, or chronic; a code for extradural (epidural) nontraumatic hemorrhage; and one for unspecified intracranial hemorrhage.

Coding and Documentation Requirements

Identify site of other and unspecified intracranial hemorrhage:

- Extradural
- Subdural
  - Acute
  - Chronic
  - Subacute
  - Unspecified
- Unspecified intracranial hemorrhage

Nontraumatic Intracranial Hemorrhage

ICD-10-CM Code/Documentation	
I62.1	Nontraumatic extradural hemorrhage
I62.00	Nontraumatic subdural hemorrhage, unspecified
I62.01	Nontraumatic acute subdural hemorrhage
I62.02	Nontraumatic subacute subdural hemorrhage
I62.03	Nontraumatic chronic subdural hemorrhage
I62.9	Nontraumatic intracranial hemorrhage, unspecified

Documentation and Coding Example

Fifty-five-year-old Caucasian female presents to PMD with c/o difficulty with balance and lower extremity weakness x 1 week. She has a **history of bioprosthetic aortic valve replacement 2 years ago and is on Coumadin therapy**. INR has been within target range except for one elevated level about a month ago thought to be due to dietary changes when she was visiting her daughter. She is a self-employed interior designer and also works part time in an antiques store. She denies recent illness or exposure to chemicals/paints and can recall no injury that might account for her symptoms. She lives with her husband. Their daughter is married, with a new baby and lives quite a distance away.

Temperature 99, HR 80, RR 12, BP 136/80. On examination, this is a well-groomed, tired appearing woman who looks a little older than her stated age. PERRL, neck supple, cranial nerves grossly intact. No weakness appreciated in upper extremities. Apical pulse is regular with ejection click audible, PMI at apex. No rubs or gallop appreciated. Breath sounds clear, equal bilaterally. Abdomen soft, mildly obese. Liver at RCM, spleen not palpated. Negative for bruit over abdominal vessels. Lower extremity pulses are weak bilaterally. DTR of medial hamstring, patellar and Achilles are 1+ with a very slight positive Babinski. Muscle tone is decreased and balance is poor both on 2 feet and single footed, gait is slow and unsteady. There is no appreciated foot drop. Her symptoms are perplexing. She is sent to lab for blood draw, CBC, electrolytes, INR. Scheduled for noncontrast CT of head tomorrow to r/o tumor.

Admit Note: Patient is admitted to Neurosurgical service for evacuation of **subdural hematoma caused by her Coumadin therapy**. Her head CT revealed **a large crescent shaped bleed in the frontal lobe consistent with an evolving liquefaction of a chronic subdural hemorrhage**. She is clinically stable and can safely be an add on case today or tomorrow.

Post-Operative Note: Patient was taken to OR and under monitored anesthesia care, 2 Burr holes were placed through the frontal bone and the hematoma evacuated. Patient tolerated the procedure well and will be observed overnight in Neurosurgical ICU. INR 2.5 prior to procedure. She will be monitored closely for bleeding.

Post Op Day 1: Uneventful night. Patient is awake, oriented X3, tolerating liquid diet. Has required no pain medication. She will be transferred to rehabilitation unit for 3 days of intensive PT to ensure she regains strength in lower extremities. She will have a repeat head CT prior to discharge.

Rehab Discharge Note: Patient did well with inpatient rehab. She feels she is almost back to her baseline level of strength and functioning. Repeat cranial CT shows no re-accumulation of blood in the frontal lobe subdural space. She is discharged home and will continue PT in OP clinic. INR this morning is 3.1. PMD will assume care to monitor INR, Coumadin dose. Follow up appointment in Neurosurgical Clinic in 10 days.

Diagnosis Code(s)

I62.03	Nontraumatic chronic subdural hemorrhage
T45.515A	Adverse effect of anticoagulants, initial encounter
Z95.2	Presence of prosthetic heart valve
Z79.01	Long term use of anti-coagulants

Coding Note(s)

A mechanical heart valve is one made from synthetic materials. This type of heart valve requires continuous use of blood thinners, such as Coumadin. The subdural hemorrhage has been documented as an adverse effect of the Coumadin therapy. An adverse effect code is assigned as a secondary diagnosis for a drug that is correctly prescribed and properly administered. The adverse effect, in this case the chronic subdural hemorrhage, is the principal diagnosis. Additional codes are assigned for the presence of the prosthetic heart valve and the long-term use of anti-coagulants.

In ICD-1Ø-CM, there are specific codes for subdural hematoma which must be documented as acute, subacute, or chronic. The supplementary code identifying the presence of a heart valve is more specific and requires documentation of the type of heart valve as prosthetic (mechanical), xenogeneic (bovine, porcine), or other type of heart valve.

Subarachnoid

A subarachnoid hemorrhage is defined as bleeding between the middle (arachnoid) and inner (pia mater) membranes covering the brain. In ICD-1Ø-CM, nontraumatic subarachnoid hemorrhage, category I6Ø, is specific to site and must be documented as involving the carotid siphon or bifurcation, middle cerebral artery, anterior communicating artery, posterior communicating artery, basilar artery, vertebral artery, or other specified intracranial artery. For all sites except the basilar artery, laterality (right, left) is also required.

Coding and Documentation Requirements

Identify the site of the nontraumatic subarachnoid hemorrhage:

- Anterior communicating artery
- Basilar artery
- Carotid siphon and bifurcation
- Middle cerebral artery
- Posterior communicating artery
- Vertebral artery
- Other specified intracranial artery
- Unspecified intracranial artery
- Other specified site, which includes:
  - Meningeal hemorrhage
  - Rupture of arteriovenous malformation
- Unspecified subarachnoid hemorrhage

Identify laterality (except for basilar artery, other specified intracranial artery, and unspecified intracranial artery):

- Right
- Left
- Unspecified

Nontraumatic Subarachnoid Hemorrhage

ICD-1Ø-CM Code/Documentation	
Carotid Siphon & Bifurcation	
I6Ø.ØØ	Nontraumatic subarachnoid hemorrhage from unspecified carotid siphon and bifurcation
I6Ø.Ø1	Nontraumatic subarachnoid hemorrhage from right carotid siphon and bifurcation
I6Ø.Ø2	Nontraumatic subarachnoid hemorrhage from left carotid siphon and bifurcation
Posterior Communicating Artery	
I6Ø.3Ø	Nontraumatic subarachnoid hemorrhage from unspecified posterior communicating artery
I6Ø.31	Nontraumatic subarachnoid hemorrhage from right posterior communicating artery
I6Ø.32	Nontraumatic subarachnoid hemorrhage from left posterior communicating artery
Middle Cerebral Artery	
I6Ø.1Ø	Nontraumatic subarachnoid hemorrhage from unspecified middle cerebral artery
I6Ø.11	Nontraumatic subarachnoid hemorrhage from right middle cerebral artery
I6Ø.12	Nontraumatic subarachnoid hemorrhage from left middle cerebral artery
Vertebral Artery	
I6Ø.5Ø	Nontraumatic subarachnoid hemorrhage from unspecified vertebral artery
I6Ø.51	Nontraumatic subarachnoid hemorrhage from right vertebral artery
I6Ø.52	Nontraumatic subarachnoid hemorrhage from left vertebral artery
Basilar Artery	
I6Ø.4	Nontraumatic subarachnoid hemorrhage from basilar artery
Anterior Communicating Artery	
I6Ø.2	Nontraumatic subarachnoid hemorrhage from anterior communicating artery
Other/Unspecified Intracranial Arteries	
I6Ø.6	Nontraumatic subarachnoid hemorrhage from other intracranial arteries
I6Ø.7	Nontraumatic subarachnoid hemorrhage from unspecified intracranial artery
Other/Unspecified Subarachnoid Hemorrhage	
I6Ø.8	Other nontraumatic subarachnoid hemorrhage
I6Ø.9	Nontraumatic subarachnoid hemorrhage, unspecified

Documentation and Coding Example

Fifty-year-old Black female presents to ER with a two-hour history of worsening headache and weakness in her left leg. **PMH is significant for poorly controlled hypertension largely due to financial constraints to obtaining her medication.** She states she has taken her BP meds consistently for the past month. Temperature 97.8, HR 96, RR 14, BP 182/104. On examination, this is a thin, quiet woman who apologizes for bothering us today. She is accompanied by her son and his wife. She squints and attempts to shade her eyes with her hand stating the light bothers them. Fundoscopic exam is difficult because of light sensitivity but pupils appear to be equal and reactive to light. Neck supple without lymphadenopathy, no nuchal rigidity. Cranial nerves grossly intact. Upper extremities with normal CSM. Apical pulse regular with a soft S3 gallop. Breath sounds clear, equal bilaterally. Abdomen soft, flat with active BS. Lower extremity pulses intact with a marked decrease in reflexes and muscle strength in the left leg. IV started and blood drawn for CBC, coagulation studies, comprehensive metabolic panel. She is sent emergently to CT to r/o cerebral vascular accident.

Neurology Note: Called to examine patient in radiology. A noncontrast CT shows **bleeding in the subarachnoid space**. CT angiography was then performed and confirms a **non-traumatic subarachnoid bleed from the right middle cerebral artery into the interhemispheric fissure and extending to the surface of the right frontal lobe**. She is transferred to Neuro ICU in good condition for observation and conservative care.

Neuro ICU Note: Patient had an uneventful night with BP stable on Lotrel. No progression of weakness in her left lower extremity. Headache and light sensitivity have decreased in intensity but are still present. She was offered pain medication but has refused. Transfer to floor. PT evaluation requested to determine safety for ambulation and possible adaptive equipment.

Floor Note: PT evaluated patient and she is using a cane for assisted ambulation. Headache is described as very mild and light sensitivity has resolved. Plan discharge tomorrow after repeat CT scan.

Discharge Note: Subarachnoid hemorrhage from right middle cerebral artery. Hypertension. Resolving left leg weakness caused by subarachnoid hemorrhage. Repeat CT scan without contrast shows no extension of subarachnoid bleed. Patient is discharged home on Lotrel for BP regulation and a cane for ambulation. She will continue PT as an outpatient and follow up in Neurology Clinic in 1 week.

Diagnosis Code(s)

I60.11	Nontraumatic subarachnoid hemorrhage from right middle cerebral artery
I10	Essential hypertension

Coding Note(s)

In ICD-10-CM, there is a code also note indicating that hypertension is reported additionally when documented. The left leg weakness is a symptom of the current subarachnoid hemorrhage and is documented as resolving, so no additional codes are reported. In the PMH, it is noted that the patient's hypertension has been poorly controlled in the past due to economic hardship, but the patient has been taking her medication for the past month. The physician did not document that the subarachnoid hemorrhage was due to underdosing of hypertension medication, so a code for underdosing would not be reported.

Hypertensive Diseases

Hypertensive disease is classified into two broad types, essential hypertension and secondary hypertension. Essential hypertension, also called primary or idiopathic hypertension, refers to abnormally elevated blood pressure levels that have no underlying cause. Essential hypertension is often associated with an increase in age and there may be familial, genetic, and environmental factors to developing the disorder. The following conditions are associated with increased risk of developing essential hypertension: obesity, sodium sensitivity, elevated renin levels, insulin resistance, and vitamin D deficiency. Hypertension increases an individual's risk for cerebral, cardiac, and renal problems. Secondary hypertension refers to abnormally elevated blood pressure levels due to an underlying condition or cause. These can include: renal disease, adrenal gland tumors, congenital malformations of blood vessels, sleep apnea, medications (hormone contraceptives, decongestants, steroids), recreational drug use (cocaine), and thyroid and parathyroid gland disorders.

Hypertension is reported with codes from categories I10-I15. Categories I10-I14 classify essential hypertension as follows: I10 Essential hypertension; I11 Hypertensive heart disease; I12 Hypertensive chronic kidney disease; and I13 Hypertensive heart and chronic kidney disease. Secondary hypertension is reported with codes in category I15. ICD-10-CM no longer differentiates hypertension as benign, malignant, or unspecified. An additional instructional guideline has been added to ICD-10-CM to use an additional code to identify exposure to environmental and occupational tobacco smoke, any history of tobacco use, or current use of or dependence on tobacco.

Hypertension, Essential

Even though coding for essential hypertension has been made simpler with the elimination of historical subcategories for malignant, benign, and unspecified severity. Coding and documentation requirements related to hypertension are covered here because essential hypertension is one of the most common cardiovascular diseases.

Coding and Documentation Requirements

For essential hypertension, identify presence/absence of hypertensive heart and/or chronic kidney disease:

- Essential hypertension only
- Hypertensive heart disease
  - With heart failure
  - Without heart failure
- Hypertensive chronic kidney disease
  - With Stage 1-4 (I-IV) or unspecified chronic kidney disease
  - With Stage 5 (V) or end stage chronic kidney disease
- Hypertensive heart and chronic kidney disease
  - With heart failure
    - With Stage 1-4 (I-IV) or unspecified chronic kidney disease
    - With Stage 5 (V) or end stage chronic kidney disease
  - Without heart failure
    - With Stage 1-4 (I-IV) or unspecified chronic kidney disease
    - With Stage 5 (V) or end stage chronic kidney disease

For essential hypertensive heart disease with heart failure, use an additional code to specify the type of heart failure (I50.-).

For essential hypertensive chronic kidney disease, use an additional code to specify the stage of chronic kidney disease (N18.1-N18.9).

Use additional code to identify any:

- Exposure to environmental tobacco smoke (Z77.22)
- History of tobacco use (Z87.891)
- Occupational exposure to environmental tobacco smoke (Z57.31)
- Tobacco dependence (F17.-)
- Tobacco use (Z72.0)

ICD-10-CM Code/Documentation	
I10	Essential hypertension
I11.9	Hypertensive heart disease without heart failure
I11.0	Hypertensive heart disease with heart failure
I12.9	Hypertensive chronic kidney disease with stage 1 through stage 4 chronic kidney disease, or unspecified chronic kidney disease
I12.0	Hypertensive chronic kidney disease with stage 5 chronic kidney disease or end stage renal disease
I13.10	Hypertensive heart and chronic kidney disease without heart failure, with stage 1 through stage 4 chronic kidney disease, or unspecified chronic kidney disease
I13.0	Hypertensive heart and chronic kidney disease with heart failure and stage 1 through stage 4 chronic kidney disease, or unspecified chronic kidney disease
I13.11	Hypertensive heart and chronic kidney disease without heart failure, with stage 5 chronic kidney disease, or end stage renal disease
I13.2	Hypertensive heart and chronic kidney disease with heart failure and with stage 5 chronic kidney disease, or end stage renal disease

Documentation and Coding Example

Thirty-one-year-old Asian female is seen for **follow up of hypertension**. Patient initially presented for annual physical exam six months ago and was found to have a BP of 158/94. She was asked to monitor her BP daily at home for 1 month and readings were consistently above 140/90. She was resistant to go on medication and agreed to some dietary changes while continuing her usual exercise routine. Patient teaches jazz dance 2-4 hours a day, 4 days week. Of interest her Vitamin D, 25 OH level was low (8 ng/ml) and she was started on supplemental Vit D 5000 units/day. She also cut down on her sodium intake, which was quite high as she eats a lot of take-out food. BP readings improved for a few months with SBP ranging from 130-144 and DBP in the range of 82-92. However, in the last month her SBP is in the 140-150 range and DBP in the 90-100 range despite a much healthier diet. Her most recent Vit D level was 18 ng/ml. Patient is counseled on the long-term effects of **hypertension** and risks of not treating. She agrees to start medication and is given samples of Cozaar 25 mg. She will begin with 1 tablet in the evening and if she has no side effects she will increase the dose to 1 tablet in the evening and 1 in the AM. Patient will continue to monitor her BP daily. RTC in 1 month to report BP readings and any side effects of the medication.

Diagnosis Code(s)

I10 Essential hypertension

Coding Note(s)

There is a single code for reporting essential hypertension that is not complicated by hypertensive heart and/or chronic kidney disease. There is no documentation of exposure to tobacco smoke or any history of or current use or dependence on tobacco, so no additional codes are assigned.

Hypertension, Secondary

Secondary hypertension (I15) has five subcategories which include: renovascular hypertension, hypertension secondary to other renal disorders, hypertension secondary to endocrine disorders, other secondary hypertension, and unspecified secondary hypertension.

An additional code is required for secondary hypertension to identify the underlying condition, and an additional code should be reported for any documented exposure to tobacco smoke or any history of or current use or dependence on tobacco.

Coding and Documentation Requirements

Identify cause/type of secondary hypertension:

- Renovascular
- Due to other renal disorders
- Due to endocrine disorders
- Other secondary type
- Unspecified

Code also underlying condition

Use additional code to identify any:

- Exposure to environmental tobacco smoke (Z77.22)
- History of tobacco use (Z87.891)
- Occupational exposure to environmental tobacco smoke (Z57.31)
  - Tobacco dependence (F17.-)
  - Tobacco use (Z72.0)

Secondary Hypertension

ICD-10-CM Code/Documentation	
I15.0	Renovascular hypertension
I15.1	Hypertension secondary to other renal disorders
I15.2	Hypertension secondary to endocrine disorders
I15.8	Other secondary hypertension
I15.9	Secondary hypertension, unspecified

Documentation and Coding Example

Forty-eight-year-old Hispanic female presents to ED with c/o dizziness and "tightness" around her head for the past 2 hours. Patient is a kindergarten teacher with a strong **family history of early onset hypertension** in females. Her BP was moderately elevated at her last PE and she has been going to the school nurse twice a week for BP checks and reporting them to her doctor. She states that today was a fairly typical day but her symptoms began just before lunch. She waited until her students were dismissed to visit the school nurse who checked her BP and found it be 190/120. Triage nurse at PMD office directed her to ED where she was driven by a school staff member. Temperature 97.8, HR 88, RR 16, BP 202/122. On examination, this is an anxious appearing, slim, well-groomed woman who looks significantly younger than her stated age. PERRL, with no evidence of papilledema. Neck supple, without masses. Carotid arteries without bruit. HR regular without murmur, gallop, rub, or bruit.

Breath sounds clear and equal bilaterally. Abdomen soft and flat with active bowel sounds, soft bruit present in the midline. Reflexes are brisk and pulses bounding in all four extremities. EKG obtained and shows NSR without ectopy. IV started in left forearm, blood drawn for CBC, comprehensive metabolic panel, renin, and aldosterone levels. Labetalol 10 mg administered IVP with BP down to 150/100 and resolution of her headache and dizziness. Labetalol 100 mg given PO with orders to repeat PO dose q 12 hours and to repeat IV Labetalol for SPB>180 or DBP>110. Patient transferred to telemetry for observation. Doppler US of renal arteries scheduled for AM to **evaluate for renal artery stenosis**.

Telemetry Note Day 1: BP has been stable on PO Labetalol. **Doppler US shows renal artery stenosis with mild ischemic renal atrophy**.

Diagnosis: **Renovascular hypertension due to fibromuscular dysplasia**.

Plan: Continue Labetalol. Check renal function in 3 months, repeat renal US in 6 months. Discharge home today. Patient to check BP daily and f/u with PMD in 1 week.

Diagnosis Code(s)

I15.0	Renovascular hypertension
I77.3	Arterial fibromuscular dysplasia

Coding Note(s)

Fibromuscular dysplasia is a disease of the arteries that affects medium sized arteries, most often the renal arteries causing renal artery stenosis and renal atrophy from the reduced blood supply to the kidney. The renovascular disease may then cause secondary hypertension.

Because the secondary hypertension is due to the renovascular disease it is reported with code I15.0. The renal artery stenosis and resulting renal ischemia and atrophy are due to fibromuscular dysplasia, which is also referred to as fibromuscular hyperplasia. Fibromuscular hyperplasia of the renal artery is reported with code I77.3.

Myocardial Infarction

Myocardial infarction (MI) is an interruption of blood flow to an area of the heart muscle leading to cell damage or death. Type 1 myocardial infarctions are those related to coronary artery disease such as atherosclerotic plaque erosion or rupture and are defined based upon ECG changes as ST elevation myocardial infarction (STEMI) and non-ST elevation myocardial infarction (NSTEMI). STEMI stands for ST segment elevation myocardial infarction and is the more severe type.

STEMI occurs when a coronary artery is totally occluded and virtually all the heart muscle dependent on blood supplied by the affected artery begins to die. STEMI is further classified based upon the site such as posterior or anterolateral wall. NSTEMI is the milder form of myocardial infarction and stands for non-ST segment elevation myocardial infarction. In NSTEMI, the coronary artery is only partially occluded, and only the inner portion of the heart muscle supplied by the affected artery dies. NSTEMI is also referred to as a subendocardial infarction.

Historically the type of MI, (STEMI, NSTEMI), site, and the episode of care were required.

Codes for initial and subsequent type 1 acute ST elevation myocardial infarction (STEMI) are specific to site requiring identification of the affected coronary artery. Codes for the initial type 1 AMI should be used only for an AMI that is equal to or less than 4 weeks old (category I21). Codes for subsequent type 1 AMI are used only when the patient suffers a new AMI within 4 weeks (28 days) of a previous AMI. The codes for NSTEMI are used for initial or subsequent type 1 AMI documented as nontransmural or subendocardial. There is additional instruction to code also any documented exposure to tobacco smoke or any history of or current use or dependence on tobacco.

Coding and Documentation Requirements

Identify initial or subsequent AMI:

- Initial
- Subsequent (new AMI occurring within the 4-week time frame of the initial AMI)

Identify type of myocardial infarction:

- Type 1 ST elevation myocardial infarction (STEMI)
- Type 1 Non-ST elevation myocardial infarction (NSTEMI)
- Other type
  - Type 2
  - Other type (type 3, 4a, 4b, 4c, 5)
  - Unspecified acute MI

For type 1 STEMI identify site:

- Initial
  - Anterior wall
    - » Left main coronary artery
    - » Left anterior descending artery
    - » Other coronary artery of anterior wall
  - Inferior wall
    - » Right coronary artery
    - » Other coronary artery of inferior wall
  - Other specified sites
    - » Left circumflex coronary artery
    - » Other specified site
  - Unspecified site
- Subsequent
  - Anterior wall
  - Inferior wall
  - Other sites

For type 1 NSTEMI:

- No site-specific information required
- Identify as initial or subsequent

Identify any current complications of STEMI or NSTEMI (within initial 28-day period) and report additionally:

- Hemopericardium
- Atrial septal defect

- Ventricular septal defect
- Rupture of cardiac wall
- Rupture of chordae tendineae
- Rupture of papillary muscle
- Thrombosis of
  - Atrium
  - Auricular appendage
  - Ventricle
- Postinfarction angina
- Other specified type of current complication of AMI

Use additional code to identify any:

- Exposure to environmental tobacco smoke (Z77.22)
- History of tobacco use (Z87.891)
- Occupational exposure to environmental tobacco smoke (Z57.31)
- Tobacco dependence (F17.-)
- Tobacco use (Z72.0)
- Status post administration of tPA in a different facility within the last 24 hours prior to admission to current facility (Z92.82)

For Type 2, code first the underlying cause, if known and appropriate, such as:

- Anemia (D50.0-D64.9)
- Chronic obstructive pulmonary disease (J44.-)
- Paroxysmal tachycardia (I47.0-I47.9)
- Shock (R57.0-R57.9)

For other types of AMI:

- Code first, if applicable, causation:
  - Following cardiac surgery (I97.190)
  - During cardiac surgery (I97.790)
- Code also any known and applicable complication:
  - (Acute) stent occlusion (T82.897-)
  - (Acute) stent stenosis (T82.857-)
  - (Acute) stent thrombosis (T82.867-)
  - Cardiac arrest due to underlying cardiac condition (I46.2)
  - Complication of PCI (I97.89)
  - Occlusion of coronary artery bypass graft (T82.218-)

Acute Myocardial Infarction

ICD-10-CM Code/Documentation	
I21.01	ST elevation (STEMI) myocardial infarction involving left main coronary artery
I21.02	ST elevation (STEMI) myocardial infarction involving left anterior descending coronary artery
I21.09	ST elevation (STEMI) myocardial infarction involving other coronary artery of anterior wall
I21.11	ST elevation (STEMI) myocardial infarction involving right coronary artery
I21.19	ST elevation (STEMI) myocardial infarction involving other coronary artery of inferior wall
I21.21	ST elevation (STEMI) myocardial infarction involving left circumflex coronary artery
I21.29	ST elevation (STEMI) myocardial infarction involving other sites
I21.3	ST elevation (STEMI) myocardial infarction of unspecified site
I21.4	Non-ST elevation (NSTEMI) myocardial infarction
I21.9	Acute myocardial infarction, unspecified
I21.A1	Myocardial infarction type 2
I21.A9	Other myocardial infarction type
I22.0	Subsequent ST elevation (STEMI) myocardial infarction of anterior wall
I22.1	Subsequent ST elevation (STEMI) myocardial infarction of inferior wall
I22.2	Subsequent non-ST elevation (NSTEMI) myocardial infarction
I22.8	Subsequent ST elevation (STEMI) myocardial infarction of other sites
I22.9	Subsequent ST elevation (STEMI) myocardial infarction of unspecified site

Documentation and Coding Example 1

Sixty-eight-year-old Caucasian male presents to Urgent Care with a 24-hour history of nausea, vomiting, dizziness. Temperature 97.8, HR 52, RR 16, BP 132/90. On examination, this is a pale appearing, mildly diaphoretic gentleman who looks his stated age. On cardiac monitor he is in sinus bradycardia. 12-lead EKG obtained and shows ST elevation. O2 saturation is 96 % on RA. He denies chest pain but says he did have some pressure when he first started to feel ill. He describes waves of nausea but no vomiting. Oxygen started at 2 L NC, IV placed in right hand and blood drawn for cardiac enzymes, CBC, coagulation studies, comprehensive metabolic panel. Nitroglycerin 0.3 mg sublingual causes a drop in BP but patient feels no change in his symptoms. Impression: Acute myocardial infarction. Transport to ER with direct admit to CCU. Cardiologist is expecting him.

CCU Note 1: Patient admitted from Urgent Care. Initial cardiac enzymes show elevated Troponin I and T, myoglobin, CK and CK-MB. EKG with ST elevation. Bedside echocardiogram shows decreased blood flow to inferior wall. Bradycardia is resolving. HR 68. Denies chest, jaw, or arm pain. Skin color is pink, warm and dry to touch. Breaths sounds clear and equal bilaterally. Patient has an unremarkable medical history. He is a retired financial analyst, has regular medical checkups, has never had elevated BP, cholesterol, or triglycerides. He takes low dose ASA, Enzyme CoQ10, and Saw Palmetto for mild BPH. Patient is scheduled for Thallium study tomorrow to assess cardiac damage.

CCU Note 2: Uneventful night. Tolerating a liquid diet.

Pain has subsided. Serial cardiac enzymes show stable CK and CK-MB, Troponins still rising. Thallium nuclear scan of heart is positive for ischemic changes to the inferior wall and narrowing in multiple areas of the right coronary artery.

Diagnosis: **STEMI, inferior wall, right coronary artery**.

Diagnosis Code(s)

I21.11 ST elevation (STEMI) myocardial infarction involving right coronary artery

Coding Note(s)

Code I21.11 is the correct code because this AMI has not been preceded by a previous admission for an AMI. Subsequent AMI codes are assigned only when the patient has had a documented admission for an AMI during the previous 28 days.

Documentation and Coding Example 2

Fifty-five-year-old Caucasian male presents to ED with C/O midsternal chest discomfort and nausea. He states the pain occurred during sexual intercourse and was not relieved by NTG. He walked 2 blocks from his apartment to the hospital and appears pale and slightly diaphoretic. PMH is significant for **acute MI three weeks ago with angioplasty and stent placement**. Patient admits to being **non-compliant with cardiac rehabilitation, including making changes to his diet or starting an exercise program**. Medications include Lopressor for **HTN**, Lipitor for **hyperlipidemia** and NTG for **postinfarction angina**. His previous records are available. The EKG shows changes consistent with **old STEMI involving left anterior descending coronary artery and new changes possibly indicating an inferolateral transmural infarction**.

Plan: Cardiac enzymes, CBC w/diff, comprehensive electrolyte panel. IV has been started in his left forearm with #18 angio and D5W is infusing at TKO rate. MS 2 mg IVP has alleviated most of his chest pain. O2 started at 2 L/min per NC, O2 saturation is 97%. Patient has been seen by Cardiology fellow and is on call to cardiac cath lab.

Procedure Note: Successful coronary angiography with balloon angioplasty and stent placement of left circumflex artery. He was admitted to CCU following the procedure.

Discharge Summary: Patient had an uneventful hospital course and was discharged home. He has a follow up visit scheduled in 2 days with his cardiologist and will meet with the cardiac rehabilitation nurse at that time.

Diagnosis Code(s)

I22.1	Subsequent ST elevation (STEMI) myocardial infarction of inferior wall
I21.02	ST elevation (STEMI) myocardial infarction involving left anterior descending coronary artery
I23.7	Postinfarction angina
I10	Essential (primary) hypertension
E78.5	Hyperlipidemia, unspecified
Z91.11	Patient's noncompliance with dietary regimen
Z91.19	Patient's noncompliance with other medical treatment and regimen
Z95.5	Presence of coronary angioplasty implant and graft

Coding Note(s)

The patient was admitted for treatment of a second ST elevation acute MI at a different site from an ST elevation acute MI 3 weeks prior.

When a patient who suffered an acute myocardial infarction (AMI) has a new AMI within 4 weeks of the initial AMI, a code from category I22 Subsequent ST elevation (STEMI) and non-ST elevation (NSTEMI) myocardial infarction must be used in conjunction with a code from category I21 ST elevation (STEMI) and non-ST elevation (NSTEMI) myocardial infarction. The sequencing of the I22 and I21 codes depends on the circumstances of the encounter. In this case, the subsequent AMI is the reason for the admission so the code from category I22 is sequenced first. Codes in category I21 (initial AMI) and category I22 (second AMI) describe the specific site. There is a code block level instructional note for ischemic heart diseases (I20-I25) directing the coder to assign an additional code to identify presence of hypertension (I10-I15). Postinfarction angina is also reported additionally.

Occlusion of Cerebral Arteries

The cerebral arteries are those located within the cranium or brain. Occlusion of the cerebral arteries due to embolism or thrombosis and/or narrowing of the cerebral arteries affects blood flow to the region of the brain fed by the affected artery. Any interruption in blood flow can cause either transient ischemia or infarction.

Codes for occlusion and stenosis of the cerebral arteries are found in two categories. Category I63 identifies cerebral infarction of the precerebral and cerebral arteries. Subcategories I63.3, I63.4, and I63.5 are specific to the cerebral arteries. Documentation must identify the specific cerebral artery as anterior, middle, or posterior cerebral; cerebellar; other specified cerebral artery; or unspecified cerebral artery. The etiology of the cerebral infarction must be specified as due to thrombosis, embolism, or unspecified occlusion and stenosis. Laterality is also required. Category I66 reports occlusion and stenosis of the cerebral arteries not resulting in stroke. Documentation requirements for this category are the same as for category I63 except that etiology of the obstruction and stenosis is not required.

Coding and Documentation Requirements

Identify infarction status of occlusion and stenosis of cerebral arteries:

- With cerebral infarction
- Without cerebral infarction

With infarction

Identify etiology:

- Embolism
- Thrombosis
- Unspecified occlusion or stenosis

Identify site:

- Cerebral
  - Anterior
  - Middle
  - Posterior
- Cerebellar
- Other specified cerebral artery
- Unspecified cerebral artery

Identify laterality:

- Right
- Left
- Unspecified

Without infarction

Identify site:

- Cerebral artery
  - Anterior
  - Middle
  - Posterior
- Cerebellar artery
- Other specified cerebral artery
- Unspecified cerebral artery

Identify laterality:

- Right
- Left
- Bilateral
- Unspecified

Occlusion and Stenosis of Cerebral Arteries without Infarction

ICD-10-CM Code/Documentation	
Middle Cerebral Artery	
I66.01	Occlusion and stenosis of right middle cerebral artery
I66.02	Occlusion and stenosis of left middle cerebral artery
I66.03	Occlusion and stenosis of bilateral middle cerebral arteries
I66.09	Occlusion and stenosis of unspecified middle cerebral artery
Anterior Cerebral Artery	
I66.11	Occlusion and stenosis of right anterior cerebral artery
I66.12	Occlusion and stenosis of left anterior cerebral artery
I66.13	Occlusion and stenosis of bilateral anterior cerebral arteries
I66.19	Occlusion and stenosis of unspecified anterior cerebral artery
Posterior Cerebral Artery	
I66.21	Occlusion and stenosis of right posterior cerebral artery
I66.22	Occlusion and stenosis of left posterior cerebral artery
I66.23	Occlusion and stenosis of bilateral posterior cerebral arteries
I66.29	Occlusion and stenosis of unspecified posterior cerebral artery
Cerebellar Arteries	
I66.3	Occlusion and stenosis of cerebellar arteries
Other/Unspecified Arteries	
I66.8	Occlusion and stenosis of other cerebral arteries
I66.9	Occlusion and stenosis of unspecified cerebral artery

Documentation and Coding Example

Fifty-eight-year-old Caucasian female brought in by EMS after her speech became nonsensical while working. She is an Assistant DA and was in court arguing a case when she suddenly could not word find. She had no other symptoms but became extremely anxious and combative with people who tried to come to her aid. The judge had to have a bailiff subdue her and then ordered her to the hospital before she stopped resisting EMS. On arrival she is almost 15 minutes post onset of symptoms and she is regaining her speech although it is slow and measured. Temperature 98, HR 100, RR 14, BP 150/88. PERRL, neck supple. Cranial nerves grossly intact. Upper and lower extremities without weakness, reflexes normal. She denies headache, dizziness, visual changes. Blood drawn for CBC, coagulation study, electrolytes, toxicology screen. EKG normal. IV started in left forearm. Impression: Possible TIA, r/o vascular accident. On call for CT scan.

Radiology Note: CT was non-conclusive. Cranial angiography performed under MAC and reveals **a 40% occlusion of the right middle cerebral artery, no infarction or bleeding present**. Neurology consult ordered and she is admitted to floor overnight.

Neurology Note: This is thin, intensely energetic woman who is alert and oriented on examination. PMH is significant for **elevated cholesterol** identified 3 years ago for which she takes Lipitor 20 mg. She drinks 2-3 glasses of red wine daily. She works very long hours, eats irregular meals. She is started on clopidogrel 300 mg x 1 and ASA 325 mg. Consult with PMD to increase Lipitor dose.

Discharge Note: Uneventful night. She has no residual speech difficulties. Discharge home on clopidogrel 75 mg and ASA 325 mg daily, increase Lipitor to 40 mg/day. She is anxious to return to work and is advised to discuss that with her PMD at the appointment scheduled in 1 week. She has orders for a blood draw prior to that appointment to check CBC, platelets, coagulation, cholesterol, triglycerides, and LFT.

Diagnosis: **Single TIA due to 40% MCA occlusion**.

Plan: Conservative medical management.

Diagnosis Code(s)

I66.01	Occlusion and stenosis of right middle cerebral artery
G45.9	Transient cerebral ischemic attack, unspecified
E78.0	Pure hypercholesterolemia

Coding Note(s)

In ICD-10-CM, the same code is assigned regardless of whether the documentation indicates an occlusion or stenosis of the cerebral artery. Under Stenosis, artery, cerebral in the Alphabetic Index, the coder is directed to Occlusion, artery, cerebral. The code for cerebral atherosclerosis is not assigned without a specific diagnosis of atherosclerosis of the cerebral arteries. While the patient does have elevated cholesterol, the physician has documented only that the patient has occlusion/stenosis. In this case, the ischemia was temporary and did not lead to infarction so code I66.01 Occlusion and stenosis of right middle cerebral artery is reported.

Occlusion and Stenosis

Precerebral Arteries

The precerebral arteries, such as the common carotid, vertebral, and basilar arteries, are arteries that lead to the brain but are not contained within the cranium or skull. These arteries can become blocked by a thrombus or embolus or they can become narrowed, affecting blood flow to the brain.

In ICD-10-CM, codes for occlusion and stenosis of the precerebral arteries are found in two categories. Category I63 identifies cerebral infarction of the precerebral and cerebral arteries. Subcategories I63.0, I63.1, and I63.2 are specific to the precerebral arteries. Documentation must identify the specific precerebral artery as vertebral, basilar, carotid, or other specified artery, along with the etiology of the cerebral infarction as due to thrombosis, embolism, or unspecified occlusion and stenosis. Laterality is required for the vertebral and carotid arteries. Category I65 reports occlusion and stenosis of the precerebral arteries not resulting in stroke. Documentation requirements for this category are the same as for category I63 except that etiology of the obstruction and stenosis is not required.

Coding and Documentation Requirements

Identify infarction status of occlusion and stenosis of precerebral arteries:

- With cerebral infarction
- Without cerebral infarction

With cerebral infarction

Identify etiology:

- Embolism
- Thrombosis
- Unspecified occlusion or stenosis

Identify site:

- Basilar
- Carotid
- Vertebral
- Other specified precerebral artery
- Unspecified precerebral artery

Identify laterality for carotid and vertebral arteries:

- Right
- Left
- Bilateral
- Unspecified

Without cerebral infarction

Identify site:

- Basilar
- Carotid
- Vertebral
- Other specified precerebral artery
- Unspecified precerebral artery

Identify laterality for carotid and vertebral arteries:

- Right
- Left
- Bilateral
- Unspecified

Occlusion and Stenosis of Precerebral Arteries with Infarction

ICD-10-CM Code/Documentation	
Thrombosis	
I63.011	Cerebral infarction due to thrombosis of right vertebral artery
I63.012	Cerebral infarction due to thrombosis of left vertebral artery
I63.013	Cerebral infarction due to thrombosis of bilateral vertebral arteries
I63.019	Cerebral infarction due to thrombosis of unspecified vertebral artery
Embolism	
I63.111	Cerebral infarction due to embolism of right vertebral artery
I63.112	Cerebral infarction due to embolism of left vertebral artery
I63.113	Cerebral infarction due to embolism of bilateral vertebral arteries
I63.119	Cerebral infarction due to embolism of unspecified vertebral artery
Unspecified Occlusion/Stenosis	
I63.211	Cerebral infarction due to unspecified occlusion or stenosis of right vertebral artery
I63.212	Cerebral infarction due to unspecified occlusion or stenosis of left vertebral artery
I63.213	Cerebral infarction due to unspecified occlusion or stenosis of bilateral vertebral arteries
I63.219	Cerebral infarction due to unspecified occlusion or stenosis of unspecified vertebral artery

Documentation and Coding Example

Discharge summary: Patient is a thirty-six-year-old Caucasian female who was admitted for **left vertebral artery thrombotic event with cerebral infarction**. She presented initially to her PMD with a 3-day history of occipital headache and posterior nuchal stiffness and pain. Her symptoms were attributed to an unusually intense yoga workout and she was prescribed a muscle relaxant. When her symptoms escalated to include numbness in the left side of her face, loss of taste, vocal hoarseness, and distorted vision she presented to the ER where she was evaluated and sent for imaging studies. CT scan and duplex studies confirmed a **clot located in Segment I of the left vertebral artery**. She was admitted for anticoagulation therapy and observation. Initially treated with heparin and then switched to Coumadin. She is being discharged today after 5 days of observation and treatment with some improvement in her symptoms. Today her VS are normal, Temperature 97.4, HR 66, RR 12, BP 102/70 and INR stable at 3.0 on 7 mg Coumadin daily. She continues to have mild tingling/numbness on the left side of her face and oscillopsia. Vocal hoarseness and loss of taste has resolved. Plan: Repeat duplex study in 3 months. Monitor INR monthly with Coumadin adjustments as needed.

Impression: **Stable left vertebral artery thrombosis with cerebral infarction**.

Diagnosis Code(s)

I63.012	Cerebral infarction due to thrombosis of left vertebral artery

Coding Note(s)

In ICD-10-CM, codes in category I63 are specific to cerebral infarction. The infarction must be identified as due to thrombosis, embolism, or unspecified occlusion or stenosis. In this case, the documentation indicates that this was a thrombotic event so the code for thrombosis is assigned. The code is specific to the vertebral artery and laterality is documented as left, so code I63.012 is assigned.

Paroxysmal Tachycardia

Tachycardia refers to rapid beating of the heart, usually applied to rates over 90 beats per minute. Paroxysmal tachycardia refers to recurrent attacks of rapid heart rate, usually with abrupt onset and often with abrupt return to a normal heart rate. The condition originates from an abnormal electrical focus in the atrium, atrioventricular node, or ventricle.

There is a single code for supraventricular tachycardia (I47.1), but ventricular tachycardia must now be identified as re-entry ventricular arrhythmia (I47.0) or ventricular tachycardia (I47.2). There is also a code for unspecified paroxysmal tachycardia (I47.9).

Coding and Documentation Requirements

Identify type of paroxysmal tachycardia:

- Re-entry ventricular arrhythmia
- Supraventricular
- Ventricular
- Unspecified

Paroxysmal Tachycardia

ICD-10-CM Code/Documentation	
I47.1	Supraventricular tachycardia
I47.0	Re-entry ventricular arrhythmia
I47.2	Ventricular tachycardia
I47.9	Paroxysmal tachycardia, unspecified

Documentation and Coding Example

Patient is a 75-year-old Asian male **S/P anterior wall MI 1 year ago**. He is seen in Cardiology Clinic for routine follow up. He states he is feeling well, swimming daily in the local pool or the ocean when the weather is warm. He denies chest pain or SOB but does state in recent weeks he occasionally has short episodes of a "fast" heartbeat that makes him feel dizzy and he has to sit down. Episodes rarely last more than 5 minutes and then he feels fine. Current medications include ASA, Zocor, and Captopril. On examination, HR 86, RR 14, BP 138/80. Color pink, skin warm, dry with good turgor. Upper extremities without clubbing, pulses intact. Left carotid artery has a very soft bruit. Apical pulse regular without bruit, rub, gallop, or murmur. Breath sounds clear, equal bilaterally. Abdomen soft, non-distended, liver palpated at 2 cm below RCM, spleen is not palpated. No bruit appreciated over abdominal vessels. Femoral pulses full. Lower extremities without clubbing or edema, pulses intact. EKG shows occasional unifocal PVCs and broad Q waves in precordial leads and poor R wave progression from V1-3 to V4-6. QR waves consistent with his history of old anterior wall MI and previous EKGs. **Stress echocardiogram is initiated, patient goes into a run of V-tach and becomes dizzy**. Test aborted and he is observed and recovers in 6 minutes without intervention. Blood drawn for CBC, electrolytes, cardiac enzymes. RTC in 3 days for test results and possible medication adjustment. Patient is cautioned to call clinic or go to ED if episodes last longer than 10 minutes and to call 911 if he has syncope, nausea, chest pain, shortness of breath.

Impression: **New onset ventricular tachycardia**, possibly due to scar tissue formation at old MI site or electrolyte imbalance.

Diagnosis Code(s)

I47.2	Ventricular tachycardia
I25.2	Old myocardial infarction

The code for ventricular tachycardia is reported along with the code for the old myocardial infarction. Historically the term paroxysmal was used in the description for the ventricular tachycardia and is no longer the common terminology, therefor does not appear in the ICD-10-CM description. The physician is ruling out electrolyte imbalance, but since this is an outpatient visit the r/o condition is not reported.

Phlebitis and Thrombophlebitis of Lower Extremities

Phlebitis is the inflammation of a vein. Thrombophlebitis is vein inflammation with formation of a blood clot within the vessel. Causes of phlebitis and thrombophlebitis include: bacteria, chemicals, mechanical injury, prolonged immobilization, certain medications, genetic disorders, and alcohol and drug abuse. Phlebitis and thrombophlebitis of superficial veins are usually characterized by tenderness, redness, warmth and swelling over the inflamed vessel. Deep vein phlebitis and thrombophlebitis usually manifest with widespread pain and swelling in the affected limb. Thrombophlebitis poses a risk of the blood clot breaking free of the vessel wall and circulating to other areas of the body including the lungs and brain.

In ICD-10-CM, category I80 Phlebitis and thrombophlebitis lists codes for all sites, but only lower extremities codes are specific to superficial or deep vessels and only the lower extremities have some codes that are also specific to certain veins. There is a subcategory for superficial vessels, which includes the greater and lesser saphenous veins and the femoropopliteal vein. Codes for the iliac vein are listed in the subcategory for phlebitis and thrombophlebitis of the deep vessels of the extremities and there are also specific codes for the femoral, iliac, popliteal, and tibial veins. Laterality must be documented as right, left, or bilateral.

Coding and Documentation Requirements

Identify phlebitis or thrombophlebitis of lower extremity as affecting:

- Deep vessels
  - Calf muscle vein (gastrocnemius/soleal)

  - Iliac vein (common/external/internal)
  - Peroneal vein
  - Popliteal vein
  - Tibial vein (anterior/posterior)
  - Other specified deep vessel
  - Unspecified deep vessel
- Femoral vein (common/deep)
- Superficial vessels
- Unspecified lower extremity blood vessel

Specify laterality:

- Right
- Left
- Bilateral
- Unspecified

Phlebitis and Thrombophlebitis of Deep Vessels of Lower Extremities

ICD-1Ø-CM Code/Documentation	
Femoral Vein	
I8Ø.1Ø	Phlebitis and thrombophlebitis of unspecified femoral vein
I8Ø.11	Phlebitis and thrombophlebitis of right femoral vein
I8Ø.12	Phlebitis and thrombophlebitis of left femoral vein
I8Ø.13	Phlebitis and thrombophlebitis of femoral vein, bilateral
Unspecified Deep Vessels	
I8Ø.2Ø1	Phlebitis and thrombophlebitis of unspecified deep vessels of right lower extremity
I8Ø.2Ø2	Phlebitis and thrombophlebitis of unspecified deep vessels of left lower extremity
I8Ø.2Ø3	Phlebitis and thrombophlebitis of unspecified deep vessels of lower extremities, bilateral
I8Ø.2Ø9	Phlebitis and thrombophlebitis of unspecified deep vessels of unspecified lower extremity
Iliac Vein	
I8Ø.211	Phlebitis and thrombophlebitis of right iliac vein
I8Ø.212	Phlebitis and thrombophlebitis of left iliac vein
I8Ø.213	Phlebitis and thrombophlebitis of iliac vein, bilateral
I8Ø.219	Phlebitis and thrombophlebitis of unspecified iliac vein
Popliteal Vein	
I8Ø.221	Phlebitis and thrombophlebitis of right popliteal vein
I8Ø.222	Phlebitis and thrombophlebitis of left popliteal vein
I8Ø.223	Phlebitis and thrombophlebitis of popliteal vein, bilateral
I8Ø.229	Phlebitis and thrombophlebitis of unspecified popliteal vein
Tibial Vein	
I8Ø.231	Phlebitis and thrombophlebitis of right tibial vein
I8Ø.232	Phlebitis and thrombophlebitis of left tibial vein
I8Ø.233	Phlebitis and thrombophlebitis of tibial vein, bilateral
I8Ø.239	Phlebitis and thrombophlebitis of unspecified tibial vein
Peroneal Vein	
I8Ø.241	Phlebitis and thrombophlebitis of right peroneal vein
I8Ø.242	Phlebitis and thrombophlebitis of left peroneal vein
I8Ø.243	Phlebitis and thrombophlebitis of peroneal vein, bilateral
I8Ø.249	Phlebitis and thrombophlebitis of unspecified peroneal vein
Calf Muscular Vein	
I8Ø.251	Phlebitis and thrombophlebitis of right calf muscular vein
I8Ø.252	Phlebitis and thrombophlebitis of left calf muscular vein
I8Ø.253	Phlebitis and thrombophlebitis of calf muscular vein, bilateral
I8Ø.259	Phlebitis and thrombophlebitis of unspecified calf muscular vein
Other Deep Vessels of Lower Extremities	
I8Ø.291	Phlebitis and thrombophlebitis of other deep vessels of right lower extremity
I8Ø.292	Phlebitis and thrombophlebitis of other deep vessels of left lower extremity
I8Ø.293	Phlebitis and thrombophlebitis of other deep vessels of lower extremity, bilateral
I8Ø.299	Phlebitis and thrombophlebitis of other deep vessels of unspecified lower extremity

Documentation and Coding Example

Sixty-five-year-old female presents to PMD with **pain and swelling in her right leg**. The patient is recently retired and she and a friend just returned from a dream vacation to the South Pacific. The trip included almost 24 hours of airplane travel in each direction. She states she took ASA as a prophylactic, stayed hydrated, did seat exercises and walked around on the plane because she was aware of the dangers of blood clots. On examination, her right leg is edematous from toes to knee, posterior leg is exquisitely tender to palpation with positive Homans sign. Pulses are intact from groin to toes bilaterally, weaker on the right. Arrangements made for emergent Doppler US of bilateral lower extremities to be done outpatient at the hospital. She will be admitted if it is positive for blood clots.

Admit Note: Doppler US shows an **extensive thrombophlebitis of the right lower leg involving the popliteal vein, anterior and posterior tibial veins, and the soleus muscle sinus**. She is placed on BR. Blood drawn for CBC, PT, PTT, INR, D-dimer, comprehensive metabolic panel. IV Heparin therapy initiated. Fitted with compression stockings bilaterally.

Diagnosis Code(s)

I80.221	Phlebitis and thrombophlebitis of right popliteal vein
I80.231	Phlebitis and thrombophlebitis of right tibial vein
I80.251	Phlebitis and thrombophlebitis of right calf muscular vein

Coding Note(s)

There are no codes that capture phlebitis and thrombophlebitis for multiple vessels, so each site is coded separately. The codes are, however, specific to site and laterality. The thrombophlebitis of the tibial veins is reported with a single code because there are no separate codes for anterior and posterior, which are both included in category I80.23-. The soleus muscle sinus is captured by the code for right calf muscular vein, which includes both the soleus and gastrocnemius vein.

Premature Beats (Depolarization)

Premature heart beats, also referred to as ectopic beats, extrasystoles, or premature contractions, is a type of a heart rate irregularity caused by extra or skipped heart beats. This results in an irregular pulse. The condition often has no known cause and is usually harmless (benign).

The historical term premature beats has been replaced with premature depolarization and a code has been added to report ventricular premature depolarization (I49.3) which was previously reported using a nonspecific code for other premature beats/ depolarization. There is also a specific code for atrial premature depolarization (I49.1) and codes for other premature depolarization (I49.49) and unspecified premature depolarization (I49.40).

Coding and Documentation Requirements

Identify type of premature depolarization:

- Atrial (supraventricular)
- Ventricular
- Other specified premature beats
- Unspecified type

Premature Beats (Depolarization)

ICD-10-CM Code/Documentation	
I49.40	Unspecified premature depolarization
I49.1	Atrial premature depolarization
I49.3	Ventricular premature depolarization
I49.49	Other premature depolarization

Documentation and Coding Example

Twenty-four-year-old female presents to ER with c/o "heart beating crazy." Patient states this has been going on for a few days but in the past hour it has gotten much worse. HR 92, RR 14, BP 144/90. On examination, this is an anxious appearing young woman, clean, well groomed, and articulate. She states she is getting married in 2 days and has been overwhelmed with last minute details and entertaining out of town guests. She admits to only four hours sleep in the past 30 hours and has been consuming coffee and energy drinks non-stop. Hands are tremulous, cool to touch. PERRL, neck supple, mucus membranes moist and pink. Apical pulse is regularly irregular and cardiac monitor shows a steady run of bigeminy. 12 lead EKG obtained and **confirms multifocal ventricular premature beats**. Blood drawn for CBC, electrolytes, and cardiac enzymes. Patient is medicated with 1.0 mg Lorazepam PO and transferred to ER holding area for monitoring.

Holding Area Note: Patient slept for 3 hours in HA and awakes feeling less anxious. Only occasional multifocal PVCs are observed on monitor. She denies dizziness or chest pain. Blood tests all WNL. Patient is counseled regarding her caffeine intake and lack of sleep. She is given a prescription for Lorazepam to be used for anxiety and sleep. She admits to not having a PMD other than her gynecologist and is encouraged to establish with an internist when she returns from her honeymoon. She is discharged home accompanied by her fiancé.

Diagnosis: **Benign premature ventricular contractions.**

Diagnosis Code(s)

I49.3 Ventricular premature depolarization

Coding Note(s)

In ICD-10-CM, the term premature contraction is synonymous with depolarization and premature beats. The correct code can be found by referencing Contraction, premature, ventricular in the Alphabetic Index. It should be noted that the ICD-10-CM Alphabetic Index does not list ventricular under the main term Beats, premature, so if the diagnosis was stated as ventricular premature beats it would be necessary to reference synonymous terms such as contraction, depolarization, ectopic, or extrasystole to identify the correct code I49.3.

Pulmonary Embolism

Pulmonary embolism occurs when a blood clot or other intravascular material migrates and forms a blockage in the main artery to the lungs or arterial branches in the lungs. The most common cause of blockage is a blood clot from the legs due to deep vein thrombosis, but air, fat, amniotic fluid, and talc seen in intravenous drug users can also cause a pulmonary embolism. Symptoms include difficulty breathing, low oxygen saturation levels, chest pain (especially with inspiration), cough, and elevated heart and respiratory rates.

In ICD-10-CM, pulmonary embolism (I26.-) includes a diagnosis of pulmonary infarction, pulmonary thromboembolism, and pulmonary thrombosis. Documentation should include whether or not the condition is complicated by acute cor pulmonale. Pulmonary embolism should also be documented as septic embolism, saddle embolus, or other type of pulmonary embolism. For pulmonary embolism without acute cor pulmonale, subsegmental should also be identified and reported as either single or multiple emboli, with single subsegmental pulmonary embolism as the unspecified default. Pulmonary embolism due to complications of surgical and medical care (iatrogenic pulmonary embolism) is reported with codes from Chapter 19 Injury, Poisoning, and Certain Other Consequences of External Causes, categories T80-T88. Complications of surgical and medical care not classified elsewhere. Iatrogenic pulmonary embolism must be documented as pulmonary air embolism following infusion, transfusion, and therapeutic injection (T80.0-); pulmonary artery embolism following a procedure (T81.718); pulmonary embolism of vein following a procedure (T81.72-); pulmonary embolism as a complication of a cardiac prosthetic device, implant, or graft (T82.817-); pulmonary embolism as a complication of a vascular prosthetic device, implant, or graft (T82.818-).

Coding and Documentation Requirements

Identify type of pulmonary embolism and infarction

Identify if pulmonary embolism is care-related:

- Iatrogenic/post-operative/post-procedural
- Other pulmonary embolism (excludes pulmonary embolism complicating abortion, ectopic pregnancy, molar pregnancy, other pregnancy, childbirth, the puerperium, and trauma)

For iatrogenic/post-operative/post-procedural pulmonary embolism, specify as a complication due to:

- Infusion, transfusion, therapeutic injection
- Other medical or surgical procedure with pulmonary embolism of
  - Artery
  - Vein
- Prosthetic device, implant, or graft
  - Cardiac
  - Vascular

For other pulmonary embolism, specify type and presence/absence of acute cor pulmonale:

- Identify type
  - Septic pulmonary embolism
  - Single subsegmental pulmonary embolism
  - Multiple subsegmental pulmonary emboli
  - Saddle pulmonary embolism
  - Other pulmonary embolism

Identify presence/absence of acute cor pulmonale

- With acute cor pulmonale
- Without acute cor pulmonale

Pulmonary Embolisms

ICD-10-CM Code/Documentation	
T80.0-	Air embolism following infusion, transfusion and therapeutic injection
T81.718-	Complication of other artery following a procedure, not elsewhere classified
T81.72-	Complication of vein following a procedure, not elsewhere classified
T82.817-	Embolism of cardiac prosthetic devices, implants and grafts
T82.818-	Embolism of vascular prosthetic devices, implants and grafts
I26.01	Septic pulmonary embolism with acute cor pulmonale
I26.90	Septic pulmonary embolism without acute cor pulmonale
I26.02	Saddle embolus of pulmonary artery with acute cor pulmonale
I26.92	Saddle embolus of pulmonary artery without acute cor pulmonale
I26.09	Other pulmonary embolism with acute cor pulmonale
I26.99	Other pulmonary embolism without acute cor pulmonale
I26.93	Single subsegmental pulmonary embolism without acute cor pulmonale
I26.94	Multiple subsegmental pulmonary emboli without acute cor pulmonale

Documentation and Coding Example

A 36-year-old male presented with 1 week of fever, cough, chest pain, and difficulty walking. Computed tomography (CT) of the chest demonstrated bilateral pulmonary nodules and cavitation, consistent with **septic pulmonary emboli. Blood cultures grew MRSA on admission**. CT of the abdomen/pelvis, as well as magnetic resonance imaging (MRI) of the spine did not reveal thrombophlebitis or abscess. Pt started on IV vancomycin. Patient remained febrile with complaint of pain in left leg so on day 6 of the admission, a gallium scan was obtained which demonstrated increased uptake in the left thigh. CT of the lower extremities revealed an enhancing **fluid collection extending the full length of the left quadriceps muscle, consistent with pyomyositis,** without evidence of deep-vein thrombosis. Surgical drainage revealed gram-positive cocci in clusters on Gram stain; the culture (obtained during vancomycin therapy) was negative. The patient defervesced after drainage and recovered with 4 weeks of vancomycin therapy.

Diagnosis: **Sepsis due to MRSA complicated by septic pulmonary embolism. Pyomyositis, left quadriceps muscle, due to MRSA.**

Diagnosis Code(s)

A41.02	Sepsis due to Methicillin resistant Staphylococcus aureus
I26.90	Septic pulmonary embolism without acute cor pulmonale
M60.052	Infective myositis, left thigh
B95.62	Methicillin resistant Staphylococcus aureus infection as the cause of diseases classified elsewhere

Coding Note(s)

The reason for the admission is the sepsis which is complicated by septic pulmonary embolism.

The underlying infection, which is the sepsis, is coded first per the coding instructions under septic pulmonary embolism. Pulmonary embolism has a combination code to identify concurrent acute cor pulmonale. In this case, there is no documentation indicating the patient has acute cor pulmonale, so code I26.90 Septic pulmonary embolism without acute cor pulmonale is reported. The patient also has pyomyositis which is likely the cause of the sepsis, but the sepsis complicated by the septic pulmonary embolism is the reason for the admission, so the infective myositis is reported secondarily. An additional code, B95.62 is reported to identify the infectious organism causing the pyomyositis which is also documented as due to MRSA. Even though the cultures from the drainage did not show MRSA, this is due to the patient being on Vancomycin prior to obtaining the culture and the physician has documented the pyomyositis as due to MRSA so it is appropriate to code it as such.

Sequelae (late effect) of Cerebrovascular Disease

A late effect is the residual effect or condition that is present after the acute phase of an illness or injury has terminated. There is no time limit as to when a late effect code can be assigned. In some cases, the residual condition may be apparent early or it may occur months or years later. The term late effect has been replaced with the term sequela in ICD-1Ø-CM.

Category I69 Sequelae of cerebrovascular disease, captures both the condition that caused the sequela and the specific sequela being treated. Codes are first classified by the cause of the sequela. These conditions include: nontraumatic subarachnoid hemorrhage, nontraumatic intracerebral hemorrhage, other nontraumatic intracranial hemorrhage, cerebral infarction, other cerebrovascular diseases, and unspecified cerebrovascular diseases. Sequelae of nontraumatic cerebrovascular disease are then classified as cognitive deficits, speech and language deficits, hemiplegia/hemiparesis, monoplegia of upper and lower limbs, other paralytic syndromes, other late effects, and unspecified late effects.

The types of sequelae that require more specific documentation are monoplegia and hemiplegia/hemiparesis. These conditions require documentation related to the side affected by the sequela (right, left) and whether that side is dominant or non-dominant, (right side dominant, left side dominant, right side non-dominant, left side non-dominant). Note that alterations of sensation and visual disturbances do not have specific codes. Sequelae of traumatic intracranial injuries are not reported with codes from category I69.

Coding and Documentation Requirements

Identify the cause of the sequela(e) as nontraumatic:

- Cerebral infarction
- Intracerebral hemorrhage
- Intracranial hemorrhage
- Subarachnoid hemorrhage
- Other cerebrovascular disease
- Unspecified cerebrovascular disease

Identify the late effect of the cerebrovascular disease:

- Apraxia
- Ataxia
- Cognitive deficits
  - Attention and concentration deficit
  - Cognitive social or emotional deficit
  - Frontal lobe and executive function deficit
  - Memory deficit
  - Psychomotor deficit
  - Visuospatial deficit and spatial neglect
  - Other cognitive signs and symptoms
  - Unspecified cognitive symptoms and signs
- Dysphagia
- Facial weakness
- Hemiplegia/hemiparesis affecting
  - Right side dominant
  - Right side non-dominant
  - Left side dominant
  - Left side non-dominant
  - Unspecified side
- Monoplegia
  - Upper limb affecting
    - » Right side dominant
    - » Right side non-dominant
    - » Left side dominant
    - » Left side non-dominant
    - » Unspecified side
  - Lower limb affecting
    - » Right side dominant
    - » Right side non-dominant
    - » Left side dominant
    - » Left side non-dominant
    - » Unspecified side
- Other paralytic syndrome affecting
  - Bilateral (both sides)
  - Right side dominant
  - Right side non-dominant
  - Left side dominant
  - Left side non-dominant
  - Unspecified side
- Speech and language deficits
  - Aphasia
  - Dysphasia
  - Dysarthria
  - Fluency disorder
  - Other specified speech and language deficit
- Other sequelae
- Unspecified sequelae

Hemiplegia/Hemiparesis Dominant Side as Late Effect (Sequela) of Cerebrovascular Disease

ICD-1Ø-CM Code/Documentation	
I69.Ø51	Hemiplegia and hemiparesis following nontraumatic subarachnoid hemorrhage affecting right dominant side
I69.151	Hemiplegia and hemiparesis following nontraumatic intracerebral hemorrhage affecting right dominant side
I69.251	Hemiplegia and hemiparesis following other nontraumatic intracranial hemorrhage affecting right dominant side
I69.351	Hemiplegia and hemiparesis following cerebral infarction affecting right dominant side
I69.851	Hemiplegia and hemiparesis following other cerebrovascular disease affecting right dominant side
I69.951	Hemiplegia and hemiparesis following unspecified cerebrovascular disease affecting right dominant side
I69.Ø52	Hemiplegia and hemiparesis following nontraumatic subarachnoid hemorrhage affecting left dominant side
I69.152	Hemiplegia and hemiparesis following nontraumatic intracerebral hemorrhage affecting left dominant side
I69.252	Hemiplegia and hemiparesis following other nontraumatic intracranial hemorrhage affecting left dominant side
I69.352	Hemiplegia and hemiparesis following cerebral infarction affecting left dominant side

ICD-10-CM Code/Documentation	
I69.852	Hemiplegia and hemiparesis following other cerebrovascular disease affecting left dominant side
I69.952	Hemiplegia and hemiparesis following unspecified cerebrovascular disease affecting left dominant side

Documentation and Coding Example

Intake Note: Patient is a seventy-year-old gentleman who is admitted to Rehabilitation Center following stabilization and treatment of a **cerebral infarction due to small spontaneous intracerebral vertebro-basilar bleed**. On examination, this is a **right hand dominant**, thin Asian male who looks younger than his stated age. He has **right hemiparesis involving arm, leg, and trunk**. He also displays significant Pusher Syndrome with loss of postural balance and ataxia. There is some difficulty with processing verbal directions such as moving the correct side of his body when asked to lift his right and then left hand. There are no vestibular symptoms or visual field deficits. He has **no aphasia or cognitive impairments**. Patient will be evaluated by OT, PT, and ST and a plan of care will be instituted. Estimated length of stay is three weeks, possibly longer with Pusher Syndrome. He does not appear to be at risk for aspiration and may have a soft diet and thin liquids unless ST finds this to be contraindicated.

Diagnosis Code(s)

I69.151 Hemiplegia and hemiparesis following nontraumatic intracerebral hemorrhage affecting right dominant side

Coding Note(s)

Pusher syndrome is a symptom of stroke that is seen in approximately 10% of patients. Patients with Pusher syndrome push forcefully away from the stronger side while sitting or standing. The pushing is caused by an altered perception of the body's midline in relation to gravity. The patient believes his/her body is oriented upright when his/her body is actually leaning toward the hemiparetic side. When the patient is upright this causes the patient to push away from the stronger, nonhemiparetic side. There is not a code for Pusher syndrome in ICD-10-CM, so only the hemiparesis is reported.

The code identifies the hemiplegia as affecting the right side and identifies this as the dominant side. It also identifies the cause of the sequela as a nontraumatic intracerebral hemorrhage. The code for hemiparesis/hemiplegia as a sequela of cerebral infarction not otherwise specified (I69.351) is not used because code I69.151 identifying the intracerebral hemorrhage is a more specific code.

Transient Cerebral Ischemia/Other and Ill-Defined Cerebrovascular Disease

Transient cerebral ischemia is defined as a temporary loss of blood to an area in the brain. In ICD-10-CM, Diseases of the Circulatory System are found in Chapter 9 within subcategory I67.8 Other specified cerebrovascular diseases. Conditions in this subcategory include acute cerebrovascular insufficiency, cerebral ischemia, posterior reversible encephalopathy syndrome, cerebral vasospasm and constriction, and other cerebrovascular disease. However, additional codes for transient cerebral ischemic attacks and related syndromes are listed in Chapter 6 Diseases of the Nervous System. Category G45 lists codes for vertebro-basilar artery syndrome, carotid artery syndrome, multiple and bilateral precerebral artery syndromes, amaurosis fugax, transient global amnesia, and other and unspecified transient cerebral ischemic attacks.

Coding and Documentation Requirements

Identify the transient cerebral ischemia or related syndrome:

- Amaurosis fugax
- Carotid artery syndrome
- Multiple or bilateral precerebral artery syndrome
- Transient global amnesia
- Vertebro-basilar artery syndrome, which includes:
  - Basilar artery syndrome
  - Vertebral artery syndrome
- Other specified transient cerebral ischemic attacks and related syndromes, which includes:
  - Subclavian steal syndrome
- Unspecified transient cerebral ischemia, which includes:
  - Cerebral artery spasm
  - Intermittent cerebral ischemia
  - Transient ischemic attack (TIA)

Transient Cerebral Ischemia

ICD-10-CM Code/Documentation	
G45.3	Amaurosis fugax
G45.0	Vertebro-basilar artery syndrome
G45.8	Other transient cerebral ischemic attacks and related syndromes
G45.1	Carotid artery syndrome (hemispheric)
G45.2	Multiple and bilateral precerebral artery syndromes
G45.8	Other transient cerebral ischemic attacks and related syndromes
G45.9	Transient cerebral ischemic attack, unspecified
G45.4	Transient global amnesia

Documentation and Coding Example

Fifty-year-old Caucasian female presents to ED accompanied by her family who states that she woke this morning and appeared to have memory loss. On examination, this is a tall, slim, athletic appearing woman who is cooperative but anxious. She is oriented to person and place and recognizes her husband and daughter. Her last clear memory is being in her hot tub last evening. Her husband fills in that she worked yesterday as usual, went to a martial arts class (she is a black belt) in the late afternoon, returned home to cook dinner, clean kitchen. She swam laps in the pool for 30 minutes and then used the hot tub before going to bed. Her husband left for work before she awoke and it was her daughter who noticed she kept repeating questions and actions. She called her father who came home and they brought her to the ED. PERRL, neck supple, cranial nerves grossly intact. There is no weakness in her extremities, no involuntary movement noted. Semantic and syntax language is preserved. Attention is normal, visual/spatial skills intact. She is able to identify common objects and follow simple directions. Her husband doubts she could have received a head injury at her martial arts class yesterday. She has a PMH of migraine headaches and takes Lipitor for elevated cholesterol. Heplock placed and blood drawn for CBC, comprehensive metabolic panel, PT, PTT, INR. Brain MRI with diffusion weighted imaging is negative for bleeding, infarctions, or tumor. Phone consult obtained with neurologist on call who is able to view the MRI and discuss with radiologist. Their impression is **Transient Global Amnesia**. Neurologist can see patient in his office at 3 pm today. Patient and family are given information regarding TGA. They agree to follow up with neurologist this afternoon. She is discharged in good condition.

Diagnosis Code(s)

G45.4 Transient global amnesia

Coding Note(s)

In ICD-10-CM, transient global amnesia is classified as a transient cerebral ischemic attack and related syndrome in the nervous system chapter.

Valve Disorders – Nonrheumatic

Disorders of the heart valves relate to the inability of the valves to open and close properly, either not allowing blood to flow properly to other heart chambers or not allowing blood to flow properly to the pulmonary and aortic arteries. Valve disorders are classified as rheumatic, nonrheumatic, or congenital. Only nonrheumatic types are classified in categories I34-I37. Rheumatic heart disease, including valve disorders, is classified in categories I00-I09. Congenital anomalies of the heart valves are classified in categories Q22-Q23. Below is a discussion of the most common disorders of each heart valve and the most common causes of each disorder.

Aortic valve: The aortic valve is located between the left ventricle of the heart and the aorta and is formed by 3 leaflets. The most common disorder of the aortic valve is stenosis, which is a narrowing and stiffening of the valve that restricts the outflow of blood from the left ventricle into the aorta and systemic circulation. Stenosis can be due to degenerative calcification of the valve, damage from disease, or a congenital defect. Another disorder is valve insufficiency and regurgitation characterized by leakage of blood backward into the ventricle during diastole, the resting phase of the heartbeat.

Mitral valve: The mitral valve is located between the left atrium and the left ventricle of the heart and is formed by 2 leaflets. The most common disorder of the mitral valve is insufficiency and regurgitation of blood backward toward the atrium after systole, the atrial contraction phase of the heartbeat. Mitral valve insufficiency may be due to degenerative diseases that weaken the valve and supporting structures, infection, and congenital anomalies. Another disorder is mitral stenosis which restricts the forward flow of blood through the left atrium to the left ventricle. Mitral valve stenosis is most often caused by rheumatic fever which is an inflammatory disease following Group A Streptococcus infection that can affect the heart as well as other body organs.

Pulmonary valve: The pulmonary valve is located between the right ventricle of the heart and the pulmonary artery and is formed by 3 leaflets. Pulmonary valve disorders include atresia, a congenital anomaly in which the valve fails to develop, stenosis which restricts the forward flow of blood from the ventricle to the lungs, and insufficiency and regurgitation which is characterized by leakage of blood backward into the ventricle during diastole. Pulmonary valve disorders are rare and are almost always congenital.

Tricuspid valve: The tricuspid valve is located between the right atrium and the right ventricle of the heart and is formed by 3 leaflets. Tricuspid valve disorders include stenosis which restricts the forward flow of blood through the atrium to the ventricle, and insufficiency and regurgitation which is characterized by leakage of blood backward into the ventricle during diastole. Tricuspid valve disorders may be congenital or caused by infection, or rheumatic fever.

In ICD-10-CM, codes are classified first by site, which includes I34 Nonrheumatic mitral valve disorders; I35 Nonrheumatic aortic valve disorders; I36 Nonrheumatic tricuspid valve disorders; and I37 Nonrheumatic pulmonary valve disorders. Nonrheumatic valve disorders are then further classified by the specific type of disorder, which must be documented as insufficiency alone, stenosis alone, stenosis with insufficiency, or a specific other type of nonrheumatic valve disorder.

Coding and Documentation Requirements

Identify site of nonrheumatic valve disorder:

- Aortic
- Mitral
- Pulmonary
- Tricuspid

For mitral valve, specify condition:

- Insufficiency
- Prolapse
- Stenosis
- Other specified disorder
- Unspecified

For aortic, pulmonary, and tricuspid valve, specify condition:

- Insufficiency (without stenosis), which includes:
  - Incompetence
  - Regurgitation
- Stenosis
  - With insufficiency
  - Without insufficiency
- Other specified disorder
- Unspecified

Nonrheumatic Heart Valve Disorders

ICD-10-CM Code/Documentation	
I34.0	Nonrheumatic mitral (valve) insufficiency
I34.1	Nonrheumatic mitral (valve) prolapse
I34.2	Nonrheumatic mitral (valve) stenosis
I34.8	Other nonrheumatic mitral (valve) disorders
I34.9	Nonrheumatic mitral (valve) disorder, unspecified
I35.0	Nonrheumatic aortic (valve) stenosis
I35.1	Nonrheumatic aortic (valve) insufficiency
I35.2	Nonrheumatic aortic (valve) stenosis with insufficiency
I35.8	Other nonrheumatic aortic (valve) disorders
I35.9	Nonrheumatic aortic (valve) disorder, unspecified
I36.0	Nonrheumatic tricuspid (valve) stenosis
I36.1	Nonrheumatic tricuspid (valve) insufficiency
I36.2	Nonrheumatic tricuspid (valve) stenosis with insufficiency
I36.8	Other nonrheumatic tricuspid (valve) disorders
I36.9	Nonrheumatic tricuspid (valve)
I37.0	Nonrheumatic pulmonary (valve) stenosis
I37.1	Nonrheumatic pulmonary (valve) insufficiency
I37.2	Nonrheumatic pulmonary (valve) stenosis with insufficiency
I37.8	Other nonrheumatic pulmonary (valve) disorders
I37.9	Nonrheumatic pulmonary (valve) disorder, unspecified

Documentation and Coding Example

Eighteen-year-old Black female presents to Cardiology Clinic having been referred by Student Health. Patient is a freshman at the University on a full athletic scholarship, she plays basketball and sprints short distance for Track and Field. Temperature 97.4, HR 60, RR 12, BP 90/58, Pulse oximeter 99%. Ht. 70 inches, Wt. 123 lbs. According to patient she presented to SH a number of times with c/o heart palpitations and chest pain. She was told she had "anxiety" and prescribed Xanax. Those symptoms have continued and in the past month she has also experienced trouble catching her breath especially after exercise, mild fatigue, and a chronic cough. For the past two nights she wakes up suddenly feeling like she cannot breathe, sitting up seems to make the feeling go away. Her coach accompanied her to Student Health this morning and insisted she be referred to a specialist. On examination, this is a tall, thin, athletic appearing young woman who looks her stated age. PERRL, neck supple without lymphadenopathy, mucous membranes moist and pink. Carotid arteries without bruit. Extremities are without edema, clubbing, pulses are full. HR is regular with a mid-systolic click murmur that fades when upright, intensifies when supine. Breath sounds clear, equal bilaterally. She has a very mild scoliosis that she states has not progressed since it was diagnosed at age 11. She sees an orthopedist yearly for monitoring. Abdomen soft, non-distended with active bowel sounds. No bruit or rub appreciated over abdominal vessels. EKG is unremarkable at this time. Patient is fitted with a 24-hour Holter monitor and given directions for use. RTC tomorrow for echocardiogram and Holter monitor results.

Cardiology Follow Up: Holter monitor was significant for occasional runs of atrial fibrillation but overall shows a sinus bradycardia which would be expected in a young athlete. Echocardiogram at rest and during exercise was performed with results significant for mildly enlarged left ventricle and moderate decrease in ejection fraction.

Impression: **Mitral valve prolapse with significant regurgitation, no stenosis.** Results were discussed and shared with her father via phone call at the patient's request. She is prescribed Propranolol 20 mg BID. RTC in 1 week for recheck and medication dosage adjustment.

Diagnosis Code(s)

I34.1 Nonrheumatic mitral (valve) prolapse

Coding Note(s)

The condition is specified as mitral valve prolapse. The regurgitation is a symptom of the prolapse and is not reported additionally.

Varicose Veins of Lower Extremities

Varicose veins occur most often in the lower extremities but can occur anywhere in the body. Varicose veins result from valve incompetence. Leaflet valves in the vein which normally open and close to move blood forward do not function properly allowing retrograde (backward) flow and pooling of blood in the vessels. The vein then becomes enlarged, tortuous (twisted), and painful. The condition is more common in women, with pregnancy often a precipitating factor. Varicose veins may form following injury, as a sequela to deep vein thrombosis, or be present at birth.

In ICD-10-CM, varicose veins of lower extremities, category I83, are also classified based on whether the condition is asymptomatic or associated with complications such as ulcer, inflammation, both ulcer and inflammation, pain, or other complications. In addition, documentation of laterality is required for varicose veins complicated by ulcers either with or without inflammation. Documentation of the site of the ulcer is also required. Severity of the ulcer is captured by an additional code from category L97.

Coding and Documentation Requirements

Identify status of varicose veins of lower extremity:

- Asymptomatic
- Complicated by:
  - Inflammation
  - Pain
  - Ulcer
  - Ulcer and inflammation
  - Other complication (edema, swelling)
- Identify laterality:
  - Right
  - Left
  - Unspecified

With ulcer or ulcer and inflammation

- Identify site of ulcer:
  - Ankle

  - Calf
  - Foot
    - » Heel
    - » Midfoot
    - » Other part of foot
  - Thigh
  - Other part of leg
  - Unspecified site of leg
- Use additional code (L97.-) to identify severity of ulcer:
  - Limited to breakdown of skin
  - Fat layer exposed
  - Necrosis of muscle
  - Necrosis of bone
  - Unspecified severity

Varicose Veins of Lower Extremities with Other Complications

ICD-10-CM Code/Documentation	
Varicose Veins with Pain	
I83.811	Varicose veins of right lower extremity with pain
I83.812	Varicose veins of left lower extremity with pain
I83.813	Varicose veins of bilateral lower extremity with pain
I83.819	Varicose veins of unspecified lower extremity with pain
Varicose Veins with Other Complications	
I83.891	Varicose veins of right lower extremity with other complications
I83.892	Varicose veins of left lower extremity with other complications
I83.893	Varicose veins of bilateral lower extremity with other complications
I83.899	Varicose veins of unspecified lower extremity with other complications

Documentation and Coding Example

Patient is a twenty-seven-year-old Caucasian female who presents with complaint of **painful and swollen superficial veins in both legs**. She is one year post delivery of twins and states she developed the enlarged veins during her pregnancy. She is interested in having laser treatments. On examination, this is a healthy, athletic appearing woman, tan and well dressed. Patient states she swims and plays tennis and is very self-conscious of how her legs look. There are numerous dark red to purple superficial spider like varicosities on anterior and posterior thighs bilaterally, posterior knee, and anterior calf. They are also prominent over the dorsum of her left foot and just inside the left ankle. Additionally, there are areas of **bulging red varicosities along the left long and short saphenous veins, dorsal venous arch, calf perforator veins, and posterior arch vein. The right leg is less affected with only a few bulging red areas along the calf perforator veins**. The swelling abates in all areas when patient is supine, increases when standing. Patient is advised that a surface laser could be used effectively on the superficial spider type veins but she would need sclerotherapy injections to treat the larger veins. She is further advised that her insurance company may consider this a cosmetic procedure and refuse to cover the costs. She is interested in pursuing treatment. An appointment will be arranged for venous Doppler study of bilateral lower extremities to rule out any deep vein involvement and map the affected area. Patient will return once that has been completed and a detailed treatment plan will be discussed.

Diagnosis Code(s)

I83.813	Varicose veins of bilateral lower extremities with pain
I83.893	Varicose veins of bilateral lower extremities with other complications

Coding Note(s)

In ICD-10-CM, there is a specific code for varicose veins with pain, but swelling is captured by the code for varicose veins with other complications. The documentation must specify laterality, and there is a code for bilateral varicose veins.

Summary

Physicians and coders for all specialties will be affected by the new documentation requirements in the circulatory system chapter because these conditions are commonly evaluated and treated by primary care providers, cardiologists, neurologists, surgeons, emergency department physicians, and geriatricians as well as other specialties. Some of the areas to focus on include the guidelines that identify new definitions for the acute phase of a myocardial infarction and subsequent myocardial infarctions. Most code categories related to the blood vessels are more specific to site, often the specific blood vessel must be identified. Laterality is an important component of many codes including conditions affecting the cerebrovascular system such as cerebrovascular hemorrhage, infarction, and occlusion and stenosis. Laterality must also be documented for conditions affecting the arteries and veins of the legs such as atherosclerosis, phlebitis and thrombophlebitis, and varicosities.

Resources

Documentation checklists are available in Appendix A for the following condition(s):

- Angina
- Coronary atherosclerosis
- Myocardial infarction
- Varicose veins of lower extremities

Chapter 9 Quiz

1. The physician documentation indicates that the patient is status post recent acute myocardial infarction (AMI) and is now being seen for a new STEMI of left anterior descending artery. What information is needed to assign the correct code for the new AMI?
   a. Documentation of the amount of time that has elapsed since the first acute myocardial infarction
   b. Documentation of whether or not the first AMI has healed
   c. Documentation of whether the new AMI is transmural or nontransmural
   d. Documentation of whether this patient is being transferred from another facility
2. How is atherosclerosis of a native coronary artery with angina pectoris reported?
   a. Two codes are needed, one for the coronary artery disease and one for the angina pectoris
   b. Since angina pectoris is a symptom of atherosclerosis only the code for atherosclerosis is reported
   c. A combination code is used that captures both the coronary artery disease and the angina pectoris
   d. None of the above
3. What information is NOT needed to assign the most specific code for hypertension?
   a. Documentation of the hypertension as primary or secondary
   b. Documentation of any related heart disease
   c. Documentation of any chronic kidney disease
   d. Documentation of the hypertension as benign or malignant
4. There is not a specific code for varicose veins of the lower extremities with which of the following complications?
   a. Pain
   b. Swelling
   c. Inflammation and ulcer
   d. Ulcer alone
5. Atherosclerosis of the native arteries of the lower extremities documented as complicated by ulcer, claudication, and rest pain is assigned codes as follows:
   a. A separate code is assigned for each complication
   b. A combined code is assigned for the claudication and rest pain and an additional code is assigned for the ulcer
   c. A code is assigned for the atherosclerosis with the ulcer and an additional code is assigned to identify the severity of the ulcer
   d. Three separate codes are assigned for atherosclerosis with claudication, atherosclerosis with rest pain, and atherosclerosis with ulcer, and a fourth code is assigned to identify the severity of the ulcer.
6. A patient who has undergone a cardiovascular surgical procedure has a postoperative cerebrovascular accident (CVA). Identify the correct guideline related to coding of the postoperative CVA.
   a. A cause and effect relationship between a CVA and a procedure cannot be assumed. The physician must specify that a cause and effect relationship exists between the procedure and the CVA
   b. A cause and effect relationship between a CVA and a cardiovascular procedure is always assumed and code G97.52 Postprocedural hemorrhage and hematoma of a nervous system organ or structure following other procedure is assigned
   c. A cause and effect relationship between a CVA and a cardiovascular procedure is always assumed and code I97.820 Postprocedural cerebrovascular infarction during cardiac surgery is assigned
   d. There are no guidelines related to CVAs occurring after a procedure. Use the correct code from category I63 to identify the cerebral infarction.
7. The physician has documented that the patient has a left posterior bundle branch block. How is this reported?
   a. I44.5 Left posterior fascicular block
   b. I44.60 Unspecified fascicular block
   c. I44.69 Other fascicular block
   d. I44.7 Left bundle branch block, unspecified
8. The physician has documented the reason for the encounter as prinzmetal angina. How is this reported?
   a. I20.0 Unstable angina
   b. I20.1 Angina pectoris with documented spasm
   c. Since there is not a specific code for prinzmetal angina, code I20.8 Other forms of angina pectoris is reported
   d. The physician must be queried for a more specific diagnosis
9. Subcategory I97.1 captures postprocedural cardiac functional disturbances. Which of the following is not classified as a postprocedural cardiac functional disturbance?
   a. Cardiac insufficiency
   b. Cardiac arrest
   c. Hemorrhage of a circulatory system organ
   d. Heart failure
10. Which condition would not be reported with a code from category I69 sequelae of cerebrovascular disease?
    a. Hemiparesis due to nontraumatic subarachnoid hemorrhage
    b. Monoplegia following traumatic brain injury
    c. Cognitive deficit due to nontraumatic intracerebral hemorrhage
    d. Aphasia due to cerebral infarction

See next page for answers and rationales.

Chapter 9 Answers and Rationales

1. The physician documentation indicates that the patient is status post recent acute myocardial infarction (AMI) and is now being seen for a new STEMI of left anterior descending artery. What additional information is needed to assign the correct code for the new AMI?

   a. **Documentation of the amount of time that has elapsed since the first acute myocardial infarction**

   Rationale: *Information on the amount of time that has elapsed since the first AMI is needed. If less than 4 weeks (28 days) has elapsed, a code from category I22 Subsequent STEMI and NSTEMI myocardial infarction is assigned. If more than 4 weeks (28 days) has elapsed, a code from category I21 STEMI and NSTEMI myocardial infarction is assigned. Whether the first AMI is documented as healed or not has no bearing on code assignment for the current MI. The AMI has been documented as a STEMI, which is the same thing as a transmural MI. Transfer of the patient from another facility does not affect code assignment for the new MI.*

2. How is atherosclerosis of a native coronary artery with angina pectoris reported?

   c. **A combination code is used that captures both the coronary artery disease and the angina pectoris**

   Rationale: *In ICD-10-CM a combination code is reported that captures both the atherosclerosis of the native coronary artery and the angina pectoris.*

3. What information is NOT needed to assign the most specific code for hypertension?

   d. Documentation of the hypertension as benign or malignant

   Rationale: *Hypertension codes are no longer classified as benign or malignant in ICD-10-CM, so these qualifiers are no longer required. There are specific codes for secondary hypertension, hypertension with related heart disease, and hypertension with chronic kidney disease, so these conditions must be documented to allow for assignment of the most specific code.*

4. There is not a specific code for varicose veins of the lower extremities with which of the following complications?

   b. **Swelling**

   Rationale: *There are specific codes for varicose veins with inflammation and ulcer, ulcer alone, and pain. There is also a specific code for varicose veins with inflammation alone. However, varicose veins documented as complicated by swelling are reported with a code from subcategory I83.89 Varicose veins of lower extremities with other complications, which includes edema and swelling but is not specific to either of these conditions.*

5. Atherosclerosis of the native arteries of the lower extremities documented as complicated by ulcer, claudication, and rest pain is assigned codes as follows:

   c. **A code is assigned for the atherosclerosis with the ulcer and an additional code is assigned to identify the severity of the ulcer**

   Rationale: *There is an Includes note to indicate that the atherosclerosis of the native arteries with ulceration includes any condition in subcategory I70.21 (intermittent claudication) and I70.22 (rest pain), so only the code for the atherosclerosis with ulceration is reported. There is a note indicating that an additional code is needed to identify the severity of the ulcer.*

6. A patient who has undergone a cardiovascular surgical procedure has a postoperative cerebrovascular accident (CVA). Identify the correct guideline related to coding of the postoperative CVA.

   a. **A cause and effect relationship between a CVA and a procedure cannot be assumed. The physician must specify that a cause and effect relationship exists between the procedure and the CVA**

   Rationale: *The guidelines for Chapter 9 Circulatory System Diseases specifically address CVA following a procedure and state that a cause and effect relationship cannot be assumed. The physician must document that a cause and effect relationship exists.*

7. The physician has documented that the patient has a left posterior bundle branch block. How is this reported in ?

   a. **I44.5 Left posterior fascicular block**

   Rationale: *Code I44.5 Left posterior fascicular block is used. The terms left posterior bundle branch block and left posterior fascicular block are synonymous.*

8. The physician has documented the reason for the encounter as prinzmetal angina. How is this reported?

   b. I20.1 Angina pectoris with documented spasm

   Rationale: *Angina with documented spasm includes angina documented as angiospastic angina, prinzmetal angina, spasm-induced angina, and variant angina.*

9. Subcategory I97.1 captures postprocedural cardiac functional disturbances. Which of the following is not classified as a postprocedural cardiac functional disturbance?

   c. Hemorrhage of a circulatory system organ

   Rationale: *Functional disturbances are those that affect heart function and include conditions such as cardiac insufficiency, cardiac arrest, and heart failure. Documentation is required as to whether the functional disturbance occurred after a cardiac procedure or after a surgery performed on a site other than the heart and great vessels.*

10. Which condition would not be reported with a code from category I69 sequelae of cerebrovascular disease?

    b. Monoplegia following traumatic brain injury

    Rationale: *Category I69 Sequelae of cerebrovascular disease, reports sequelae of nontraumatic conditions, such as nontraumatic subarachnoid hemorrhage, nontraumatic intracerebral hemorrhage, other nontraumatic intracranial hemorrhage, cerebral infarction, other cerebrovascular diseases, and unspecified cerebrovascular diseases. Sequelae of traumatic intracranial injuries are not reported with codes from category I69. In these cases, the specific type of sequela is reported first, such as monoplegia, followed by the code for the traumatic injury with 7th character 'S' to identify the condition as a sequela of the injury.*

Chapter 1Ø
DISEASES OF THE RESPIRATORY SYSTEM

Introduction

Diseases of the respiratory system are found in Chapter 1Ø. This chapter includes conditions affecting the nose and sinuses, throat, tonsils, larynx and trachea, bronchi, and lungs. The chapter is organized by the general type of disease or condition and by site with diseases affecting primarily the upper respiratory system or the lower respiratory system housed in separate sections or blocks. The table below shows how this chapter is organized for each coding system.

ICD-1Ø-CM Blocks	
JØØ-JØ6	Acute Upper Respiratory Infections
JØ9-J18	Influenza and Pneumonia
J2Ø-J22	Other Acute Lower Respiratory Infections
J3Ø-J39	Other Diseases of Upper Respiratory Tract
J4Ø-J47	Chronic Lower Respiratory Diseases
J6Ø-J7Ø	Lung Diseases Due to External Agents
J8Ø-J84	Other Respiratory Diseases Principally Affecting the Interstitium
J85-J86	Suppurative and necrotic conditions of the lower respiratory tract
J9Ø-J94	Other Diseases of the Pleura
J95	Intraoperative and Postprocedural Complications and Disorders of the Respiratory System, Not Elsewhere Classified
J96-J99	Other Diseases of the Respiratory System

Coding Note(s)

Chapter level instructions include a note related to reporting respiratory conditions occurring in more than one site and is not specifically indexed. In this instance, the code for the lower anatomic site is reported. The example given is a diagnosis of tracheobronchitis. Since there is no code for tracheobronchitis, the code for bronchitis (category J4Ø) is reported. There is also a chapter level note related to using an additional code when there is documented exposure to tobacco smoke, history of tobacco use, or current tobacco use and dependence.

Exclusions

There is only an Excludes2 note for Chapter 1Ø.

Excludes1	Excludes2
None	Certain conditions originating in the perinatal period (PØ4-P96) Certain infectious and parasitic diseases (AØØ-B99) Complications of pregnancy, childbirth and the puerperium (OØØ-O9A) Congenital malformations, deformations and chromosomal abnormalities (QØØ-Q99) Endocrine, nutritional and metabolic diseases (EØØ-E88) Injury, poisoning and certain other consequences of external causes (SØØ-T88) Neoplasms (CØØ-D49) Smoke inhalation (T59.81-) Symptoms, signs and abnormal clinical and laboratory findings, not elsewhere classified (RØØ-R94)

Chapter Guidelines

There are several guidelines for Chapter 1Ø. The guidelines cover COPD and asthma, acute respiratory failure and influenza. Guidelines for influenza are specific to influenza due to avian influenza virus. Finally, there are guidelines for ventilator associated pneumonia.

COPD and Asthma

Category J44 Other chronic obstructive pulmonary disease includes asthma with COPD. However, when reporting COPD with asthma, a second code from category J45 Asthma is required to identify the type of asthma. Codes in category J44 differentiate between uncomplicated cases and those with an acute exacerbation, which is a worsening or decompensation of a chronic condition. An acute exacerbation is not the same as an infection superimposed on a chronic condition, although an exacerbation may be triggered by an infection. This can be better understood by looking at the Includes, Excludes, Code also, and Use additional code notes in category J44. Under J44.1 Chronic obstructive pulmonary disease with (acute) exacerbation, there is an Excludes2 note indicating that COPD with acute bronchitis is reported with J44.Ø Chronic obstructive pulmonary disease with (acute) lower respiratory infection. However, because this is an Excludes2, if the patient has an exacerbation triggered by the infection, then both codes (J44.Ø and J44.1) are reported along with an additional code to identify the infection.

Acute Respiratory Failure

Guidelines for reporting acute respiratory failure (J96.0) and acute and chronic respiratory failure (J96.2) relate to sequencing of these codes. Sequencing guidelines are as follows:

- Acute or acute and chronic respiratory failure as principal diagnosis. Assign J96.0 or J96.2 as the principal diagnosis when:
  - It is established after study to be chiefly responsible for occasioning the admission to the hospital
  - Assignment of J96.0 or J96.2 is supported based on the Alphabetic Index and Tabular List
  - Chapter specific guidelines such as those for obstetrics, poisoning, HIV, and newborns support the assignment of J96.0 or J96.2 as the principal diagnosis. If chapter specific guidelines provide different sequencing direction, the chapter specific guidelines take precedence
- Acute or acute and chronic respiratory failure as secondary diagnosis. Assign as a secondary diagnosis if:
  - The condition occurs after admission
  - The condition is present on admission but does not meet the definition of principal diagnosis
- Acute or acute and chronic respiratory failure and another acute condition:
  - Sequencing will not be the same for every situation. This applies whether the other acute condition is a respiratory or non-respiratory condition
  - Sequencing will be dependent on the circumstances of the admission
  - If both conditions meet the definition of the principal diagnosis, either of the two conditions may be sequenced first
  - If documentation is not clear as to which condition was responsible for the admission, query the provider

Influenza Due to Avian Influenza Virus (Avian Influenza)

There are three code categories for reporting influenza which are as follows:

- J09 Influenza due to certain identified influenza viruses:
  - All codes in this category report influenza due to identified novel influenza A virus with various complications or manifestations such as pneumonia, other respiratory conditions, gastrointestinal manifestations, or other manifestations. Identified novel influenza A viruses include: avian (bird) influenza, swine influenza (2009 H1N1), influenza A/H5N1, and influenza of other animal origin (not bird or swine)
- J10 Influenza due to other identified influenza virus:
  - This category includes Influenza A/H1N1 or H3N2 viruses that are not identified as variant or novel
- J11 Influenza due to unidentified influenza virus

Guidelines for reporting avian influenza are as follows:

- Code only confirmed cases of avian influenza and other certain identified or specific types of influenza reported with codes from category J09 and J10. This is an exception to the inpatient guideline related to uncertain diagnoses
- Confirmation does not require a positive laboratory finding. Documentation by the provider that the patient has avian influenza, or influenza due to other identified novel influenza A virus, is sufficient to report J09 Influenza due to certain identified influenza viruses
- Documentation of "suspected", "possible", or "probable" avian influenza or other novel influenza A virus is reported with a code from category J11 Influenza due to unidentified influenza virus

Ventilator Associated Pneumonia

Ventilator associated pneumonia (VAP) is listed in category J95 Intraoperative and postprocedural complications and disorders of respiratory system, not elsewhere classified. As with all procedural and postprocedural complications, the provider must document the relationship between the condition and the procedure. Guidelines for reporting VAP are as follows:

- Code J95.851 Ventilator associated pneumonia should be assigned only when the provider has documented the condition as VAP
- An additional code should be assigned to identify the organism (from categories B95-B97)
- Codes from categories J12-J18 are not assigned additionally to identify the type of pneumonia for VAP
- If the provider has not documented that a patient with pneumonia who is on a mechanical ventilator has VAP, do not assign code J95.851
- If the documentation is unclear as to whether or not the patient has VAP, query the provider
- VAP developing after admission is reported as a secondary diagnosis
- If the patient is admitted for one type of pneumonia and subsequently develops VAP, the appropriate code from J12-J18 is reported as the principal diagnosis and code J95.851 is reported as an additional diagnosis

General Documentation Requirements

When documenting diseases of the respiratory system there are a number of general documentation requirements of which providers should be aware. In this section we will discuss codes for acute recurrent conditions, combination codes, and intraoperative and postprocedural complications and disorders of the respiratory system.

Acute Recurrent Conditions

Acute sinusitis (J01.-) and acute streptococcal tonsillitis (J03.0-) differentiate between an acute unspecified condition and an acute recurrent condition. If the patient has an acute recurrent condition, documentation should specifically identify the condition as such. If the condition is not documented as acute recurrent, the default code for acute unspecified is reported.

Combination Codes

There are many combination codes for acute conditions and the infectious organism. Codes for acute bronchitis and acute bronchiolitis include the infectious organism.

There are also combination codes for influenza with specific manifestations. In categories J10 Influenza due to other identified influenza virus, and J11 Influenza due to unidentified influenza virus, associated complications and manifestations captured by the combination code include:

- Encephalopathy
- Gastrointestinal manifestations
- Myocarditis
- Otitis media
- Pneumonia
  - With same other identified influenza virus pneumonia
  - Other specified type of pneumonia
  - Unspecified type of pneumonia
- Other respiratory manifestations
- Other specified manifestations

Intraoperative and Postprocedural Complications and Disorders of the Respiratory System

Most complications or disorders of the respiratory system occurring during or following a procedure are reported with codes listed in the respiratory system chapter. These codes are found in category J95. Complications and conditions reported with codes from this chapter include:

- Chemical pneumonitis due to anesthesia
- Complication of respirator or ventilator
  - Mechanical
  - Ventilator associated pneumonia
  - Other complication
- Intraoperative
  - Accidental puncture or laceration of a respiratory system organ or structure
    - » During a respiratory system procedure
    - » During a procedure not being performed on the respiratory system
  - Hemorrhage or hematoma of a respiratory system organ or structure
    - » During a respiratory system procedure
    - » During a procedure not being performed on the respiratory system
  - Other respiratory system complications, not elsewhere classified

Postprocedural
  - Air leak
  - Hemorrhage or hematoma of a respiratory system organ or structure
    - » Following a respiratory system procedure
    - » Following a procedure not being performed on the respiratory system
  - Pulmonary insufficiency (acute or chronic)
    - » Following thoracic surgery
    - » Following nonthoracic surgery
  - Pneumothorax
  - Respiratory failure
  - Subglottic stenosis
    - » Other respiratory system complications, not elsewhere classified
- Tracheostomy complications
  - Hemorrhage from stoma
  - Infection of stoma
  - Malfunction of stoma
  - Tracheoesophageal fistula
  - Other tracheostomy complication
  - Unspecified complication
- Transfusion related acute lung injury (TRALI)

Intraoperative and post-procedural hemorrhage/hematoma and laceration/puncture are specific to the procedure being performed. If the complication occurs during a procedure being performed on the respiratory system, code J95.61 is reported for hemorrhage/hematoma or code J95.71 for laceration/puncture. If the respiratory complication occurs during a procedure that is not being performed on the respiratory system, code J95.62 is reported for hemorrhage/hematoma or code J95.72 for laceration/puncture.

Postprocedural hemorrhage and hematoma follow a similar coding concept. Unlike intraoperative bleeding complications however, the postoperative complication separates hemorrhage and hematoma. Postprocedural hemorrhage of a respiratory system organ or structure following a respiratory system procedure is coded as J95.830 while a postoperative hematoma of a respiratory system organ or structure is coded as J95.860. Postprocedural hemorrhage of a respiratory system organ following a non- respiratory system procedure is coded as J95.831 and postprocedural hematoma as J95.861.

Code-Specific Documentation Requirements

While the documentation requirements for coding diseases of the respiratory system are not as extensive as those for diseases affecting other body systems, documentation requirements for some of the more commonly reported conditions do require additional information. In this section, the following conditions will be reviewed: acute sinusitis, acute bronchitis and bronchiolitis, viral and bacterial pneumonia, influenza, emphysema, asthma, bronchiectasis, acute respiratory distress syndrome, and acute and chronic respiratory failure.

Acute Bronchitis and Bronchiolitis

Bronchitis is an inflammation of the mucous membranes lining the bronchi. Bronchi are the large to medium-size airways that branch from the trachea carrying air to the lungs. Bronchitis may be acute or chronic. Acute bronchitis usually occurs with a viral or bacterial infection with symptoms that include cough with production of mucus.

Bronchiolitis is the inflammation and swelling of the mucous membranes lining the bronchioles, the smallest airways in the lungs. Bronchiolitis is most often caused by a viral infection and primarily affects infants and children under the age of 2 years. Symptoms can include productive cough, wheezing, tachypnea (fast breathing), nasal flaring, and intercostal retractions.

Codes for acute bronchitis (category J20) are combination codes specific to the infectious organism when the infectious organism is known. There is also a code for acute bronchitis, unspecified. Codes for acute bronchiolitis (category J21) include specific codes for acute bronchiolitis due to RSV, human metapneumovirus, and other specified organisms as well as a code for acute bronchiolitis, unspecified. Bronchospasm with either acute bronchitis or acute bronchiolitis is included in the code category.

Coding and Documentation Requirements

Identify condition:

- Acute bronchitis
- Acute bronchiolitis

Identify the organism:

- Acute bronchitis due to
  - *Mycoplasma pneumoniae*
  - *Haemophilus influenzae*
  - Streptococcus
  - Coxsackievirus
  - Parainfluenza virus
  - Respiratory syncytial virus (RSV)
  - Rhinovirus
  - Echovirus
  - Other specified organisms
- Acute bronchiolitis due to
  - Respiratory syncytial virus (RSV)
  - Human metapneumovirus
  - Other specified organisms
- Acute bronchitis, unspecified
- Acute bronchiolitis, unspecified

ICD-10-CM Code/Documentation	
J20.0	Acute bronchitis due to Mycoplasma pneumoniae
J20.1	Acute bronchitis due to Haemophilus influenzae
J20.2	Acute bronchitis due to streptococcus
J20.3	Acute bronchitis due to coxsackievirus
J20.4	Acute bronchitis due to parainfluenza virus
J20.5	Acute bronchitis due to respiratory syncytial virus (RSV)
J20.6	Acute bronchitis due to rhinovirus
J20.7	Acute bronchitis due to echovirus
J20.8	Acute bronchitis due to other specified organisms
J20.9	Acute bronchitis, unspecified
J21.0	Acute bronchiolitis due to respiratory syncytial virus
J21.1	Acute bronchiolitis due to human metapneumovirus
J21.8	Acute bronchiolitis due to other specified organisms
J21.9	Acute bronchiolitis, unspecified

Documentation and Coding Example

Five-month-old female infant is brought to pediatrician's office for worsening cold symptoms. According to mother, infant was well until 3 days ago when she developed clear nasal drainage and a cough. Both parents work and infant goes to a fairly large daycare center where many of the children have been sick this winter. Temperature 100.4, HR 122, RR 24, BP 70/54 O2 sat 96%. On examination, infant is alert and active, PERRL, TMs mildly red, not bulging. Copious clear nasal drainage, sample obtained and sent to lab for culture including rapid RSV antigen test. Oral mucosa moist and pink, pharynx red without exudates. Breath sounds have wheezes throughout, no distinct areas of consolidation. Mild intercostal retractions noted. Abdomen soft with active bowel sounds. Mother states baby has been breastfeeding and taking expressed breast milk from a bottle but has not been interested in solid food.

Chest x-ray obtained and shows few areas of hyperinflation and patchy infiltrates, some peribronchial cuffing. Nebulizer treatment with Xopenex and ipratropium bromide given with some improvement in respiratory symptoms, including decreased wheezing and retractions. **Rapid RSV is positive.**

Impression: **RSV infection with bronchiolitis.**

Plan: Discharge home with nebulizer loaner. Xopenex and ipratropium bromide q 4 hours. Continue breast feeding on demand. Tylenol for fever > 100 degrees. Parent advised to notify daycare of confirmed RSV so they can alert other parents if necessary.

Recheck scheduled for tomorrow afternoon. Parent given detailed explanation of signs and symptoms that would indicate respiratory compromise with instructions to call office or go to ED.

Diagnosis Code(s)

J21.0 Acute bronchiolitis due to respiratory syncytial virus

Coding Note(s)

For coding respiratory syncytial virus infection, assignment of the most specific code requires identification of the site/ manifestation as bronchitis (J20.5), bronchiolitis (J21.0), or pneumonia (J12.1).

Asthma

Asthma is a chronic inflammatory condition that causes narrowing of the bronchi, which are the large upper airways connecting the trachea to the lungs. The disease is characterized by swelling, increased mucus production, and muscle tightness. Triggers can include allergens, smoke, exercise, stress, and respiratory infections. Genetic and environmental factors may contribute to asthma. Symptoms include cough, wheeze, chest tightness, and difficulty breathing.

Asthma is coded and reported as mild, moderate, or severe and then further differentiated as to whether it is uncomplicated, with acute exacerbation, or with status asthmaticus. Mild cases are further differentiated by whether they are documented as intermittent or persistent. Chronic obstructive asthma is not listed in the category for asthma but is under category J44 Other chronic obstructive pulmonary disease. Other forms of asthma include both exercise induced bronchospasm and cough variant with an additional code available for other specified types of asthma.

Coding and Documentation Requirements

Identify type of asthma:

- Mild
  - Intermittent
  - Persistent
- Moderate persistent
- Severe persistent
- Other specified type
  - Exercise induced bronchospasm
  - Cough variant
  - Other
- Unspecified type

Identify complications (except for other specified types):

- Uncomplicated
- With acute exacerbation
- With status asthmaticus

Identify also tobacco exposure, use, dependence, or history of dependence

Asthma with Exacerbation

ICD-10-CM Code/Documentation	
J45.21	Mild intermittent asthma with (acute) exacerbation
J45.31	Mild persistent asthma with (acute) exacerbation
J45.41	Moderate persistent asthma with (acute) exacerbation
J45.51	Severe persistent asthma with (acute) exacerbation

Documentation and Coding Example

Fifty-two-year-old Black female presents to ED with acute asthma episode. She is SOB, anxious, using accessory muscles in neck and chest to try and move air. Expiratory wheezes can be heard without using a stethoscope. Medications include Qvar, Singulair daily, and Xopenex last used 1 hour ago. HR 120, RR 22, BP 150/90. O2 saturation 92% on RA when she arrived and is now 95% on O2 4 L/m via mask that is also delivering Xopenex and Ipratropium bromide via nebulizer. IV started in left hand, 100 mg Solu-Cortef administered IVP. Patient is less anxious and able to speak in complete sentences following breathing treatment and oxygen therapy. She is placed on O2 via NC and maintains O2 saturation at 95%. Patient is able to give a medical history, which includes **asthma/allergies since the age of 2. Triggers include animal dander, pollen, mold, cold weather, and URI.** She has used **oral and inhaled steroids** extensively with documented osteoporosis on bone density study 2 years ago. Chest x-ray obtained and pneumonia is R/O.

Impression: **Moderate persistent asthma with acute exacerbation** most likely due to weather change/temperature drop.

Plan: Admit overnight for breathing treatments and IV steroids.

Diagnosis code(s)

J45.41	Moderate persistent asthma with (acute) exacerbation
Z79.51	Long term (current) use of inhaled steroids
Z79.52	Long term (current) use of systemic steroids

Coding Note(s)

Both extrinsic and intrinsic asthma are reported with codes from category J45. The code is selected based on the severity of the asthma, which in this case is documented as moderate. Long term use of steroids is differentiated as systemic use or inhaled use. Since the patient has used both types, codes for both are assigned.

Bacterial Pneumonia

Like many codes in Chapter 10, many of the pneumonias caused by bacteria have a combination code. The most common cause of bacterial pneumonia is *Streptococcus pneumoniae*, also called pneumococcal pneumonia. Lobar pneumonia of unspecified organism is not reported with the code for pneumonia due to *S. pneumoniae* (J13); it is reported with code J18.1 Lobar pneumonia, unspecified organism. Most of the more common types of bacterial pneumonia have specific codes. There are also a few bacterial causes of pneumonia that are classified in Chapter 1 Infectious and Parasitic Diseases, so it is important to use the Alphabetic Index to locate the correct code.

Mycoplasma pneumoniae is classified as bacterial pneumonia. Legionnaires' disease is classified in Chapter 1 Infectious and Parasitic Diseases

Documentation and Coding Requirements

Identify the causative organism:

- *Escherichia coli*
- *Haemophilus influenzae*
- Klebsiella
- Legionnaires' disease
- Mycoplasma
- Other (aerobic) gram negative
- Pneumococcal [streptococcus]
- Pseudomonas
- Staphylococcus
  - Methicillin resistant
  - Methicillin susceptible
  - Other specified staphylococcus
  - Unspecified staphylococcus
- Streptococcus
  - Group B
  - Pneumoniae [pneumococcal]
  - Other specified/unspecified streptococci
- Other specified bacteria
- Unspecified bacteria

Identify any associated influenza, if applicable

Identify any associated abscess, if present

Bacterial Pneumonia

ICD-10-CM Code/Documentation	
A48.1	Legionnaires' disease
J13	Pneumonia due to Streptococcus pneumonia
J14	Pneumonia due to Haemophilus influenzae
J15.0	Pneumonia due to Klebsiella pneumoniae
J15.1	Pneumonia due to Pseudomonas
J15.20	Pneumonia due to staphylococcus, unspecified
J15.211	Pneumonia due to Methicillin susceptible Staphylococcus aureus
J15.212	Pneumonia due to Methicillin resistant Staphylococcus aureus
J15.29	Pneumonia due to other staphylococcus
J15.3	Pneumonia due to streptococcus, group B
J15.4	Pneumonia due to other streptococci
J15.5	Pneumonia due to Escherichia coli
J15.6	Pneumonia due to other Gram-negative bacteria
J15.7	Pneumonia due to Mycoplasma pneumoniae
J15.8	Pneumonia due to other specified bacteria
J15.9	Unspecified bacterial pneumonia
J18.1	Lobar pneumonia, unspecified organism

Documentation and Coding Example

Eighteen-month-old Caucasian male is brought into ED by EMS after suffering a febrile seizure at home. Grandparents provide a sketchy medical history as they are caring for the child while his parents are away. Attempts to contact the parents are being made. Grandparents state the child had a cough and congestion when they assumed care 2 days ago. He was a little tired and his appetite was decreased but he was taking fluids. Grandparents do not know if he has received childhood vaccinations. He seemed feverish this afternoon but there was no Tylenol or ibuprofen in the house so the grandmother gave him a sponge bath with cool water. A short time later he had a generalized motor seizure and since they are unfamiliar with the community they called 911 and an ambulance was dispatched. EMS crew states their ETA was 4 minutes and the child was unresponsive and still having a motor seizure when they arrived. He was administered Diastat in the field, intravenous line was placed, oxygen was started and he was transported to the ED. On arrival the child was sedated without seizure activity. T 104, P 116, R 18, BP 78/50, O2 saturation on O2 at 2 L/min via mask is 99%. Color pale, mucous membranes dry and pink. PERRLA. Throat red, without exudate. TMs pink but not bulging, fluid is visible in the left middle ear. Breath sounds are decreased in the left base, with scattered rales and wheezes throughout. He was administered acetaminophen 80 mg PR and cooling blanket applied. Blood drawn for CBC w/diff, metabolic panel and blood culture, LAT for Hib was also drawn given his unknown immunization status. Chest x-ray obtained and shows left lower lobe infiltrates.

Impression: **Acute pneumonia.**

Plan: Admit to PICU. Start IV Ampicillin, Gentamycin, and Ceftriaxone.

PICU Day 1: Afebrile with acetaminophen. Cooling blanket dc'd. No recurrence of seizure and EEG was WNL. **LAT blood testing for Hib is positive,** waiting for sensitivities on blood culture. O2 saturation 98% on RA, supplemental O2 discontinued. Continue antibiotic therapy. Advance diet as tolerated. Transfer to Pediatric Floor when bed is available. Repeat chest x-ray in AM.

Admit Day 2: Continues to do well. Repeat chest x-ray shows clearing infiltrates in lungs. **Hib is sensitive to Ceftriaxone,** Ampicillin and Gentamycin dc'd. Parents are at bedside.

Final Diagnosis: **Pneumonia due to H. influenza, febrile seizure, underimmunization status.**

Diagnosis Code(s)

J14	Pneumonia due to Haemophilus influenzae
R56.00	Simple febrile convulsions
Z28.3	Underimmunization status

Coding Note(s)

There is a combination code for the pneumonia due to H. influenzae. The febrile convulsion is reported additionally. Febrile convulsions are classified as simple or complex. If the febrile confusion is not specified as simple or complex, the default is simple. In this case, there is documentation describing the seizure as generalized motor seizure, the seizure lasted under 15 minutes, and did not recur within 24 hours. To be classified as complex, the seizure must last for more than 15 minutes, recur within 24 hours, or involve only one side of the body. So, the diagnosis would be simple febrile convulsions. The underimmunization status is also coded.

Bronchiectasis

Bronchiectasis refers to destruction and widening of the large airways. It most often occurs following recurrent, severe lower respiratory tract infection or inflammation. It may also occur following inhalation of a foreign object. Category J47 Bronchiectasis, differentiates between uncomplicated bronchiectasis and bronchiectasis with acute lower respiratory infection or exacerbation.

Coding and Documentation Requirements

Specify bronchiectasis and complications:

- With acute lower respiratory infection
- With exacerbation
- Uncomplicated

Identify tobacco exposure, use, dependence, or history of dependence

Bronchiectasis

ICD-10-CM Code/Documentation	
J47.0	Bronchiectasis with acute lower respiratory infection
J47.1	Bronchiectasis with (acute) exacerbation
J47.9	Bronchiectasis, uncomplicated

Documentation and Coding Example

Twenty-six-year-old Caucasian male arrives in ED accompanied by Street Medicine Team. He is well known to the street doctors, works as a day laborer, lives out of his car, and is usually in good health. He has a **history of tobacco use since late teens, smokes a few cigarettes a day** when he can afford to buy them. He also drinks 1-2 beers almost daily. Temperature 100.8, HR 78, RR 18, BP 106/66, O2 saturation 95% on RA. On examination, this is a thin, ill-appearing young man with good hygiene, wearing clean clothes and well spoken. He states he was well until about 4 days ago when his normally dry, chronic cough became productive of yellow sputum. Today he is breathless and feels like he is drowning in secretions. PERRL, TMs clear. Neck supple. Breath is malodorous, teeth are clean and in good repair. Mucous membranes moist, pink. Nares patent with thin clear secretions. Oropharynx mildly red, moist with a cobblestone appearance. Heart rate regular without gallop or rub. No clubbing or cyanosis present. Breath sounds have fine scattered rales and wheezes on the right with decreased sounds in right middle and lower lobes. Left breath sounds are relatively clear and equal. Abdomen soft, non-distended. Bowel sounds present in all quadrants. Spleen is not palpated, liver is at the RCM. IV started in left arm and blood drawn for CBC, comprehensive metabolic panel, quantitative immunoglobulin levels. Sputum sent for analysis including gram stain, culture. Chest x-ray obtained and shows **right lower lobe consolidation consistent with pneumonia**. Patient will be admitted to medical floor for antibiotics and respiratory therapy. Pulmonology fellow requests high resolution CT scan of chest to further evaluate lung disease due to his history of tobacco use and chronic cough.

Pulmonology Note: CT scan shows bulbous appearing dilated bronchus on the right with areas of constriction and obstructive scarring. There is a **postobstructive pneumonitis in the right middle and lower lobes of the lung**. These findings are consistent with **bronchiectasis exacerbated by acute lower respiratory infection**. Preliminary sputum gram stain and **culture positive for Klebsiella species, sensitive to current antibiotics**.

Diagnosis code(s)

J15.0	Pneumonia due to Klebsiella pneumoniae
J47.0	Bronchiectasis with acute lower respiratory infection
Z72.0	Tobacco use

Coding Note(s)

In the documentation above, the ED physician has described the condition as pneumonia while the pulmonologist has described it as pneumonitis. In the Alphabetic Index under pneumonitis there is a note to "see also Pneumonia." Since codes for acute bacterial lower respiratory tract infections are not listed under pneumonitis, the main term pneumonia is referenced for the correct code. The code for the pneumonia is the first listed or principal diagnosis because that is the condition that occasioned the ED visit. The bronchiectasis is a concurrent chronic condition that is reported additionally.

There is a code for reporting bronchiectasis with acute lower respiratory infection which is a complicating factor in bronchiectasis. There is a code also note for reporting tobacco use. Code Z72.0 is assigned rather than a code for tobacco dependence because there is no documentation indicating that the patient is dependent on tobacco.

Bronchitis/Chronic Bronchitis

Chronic bronchitis is an inflammation of the linings of the bronchi, also called the bronchial tubes, that has been present for more than a year with symptoms occurring most days of the month for at least three months. There are four categories of bronchitis that define non-acute bronchitis, J40 Bronchitis not specified as acute or chronic, J41 Simple and mucopurulent chronic bronchitis, J42 Unspecified chronic bronchitis, and J44 Other chronic obstructive pulmonary disease. Obstructive chronic bronchitis, is referred to as chronic obstructive pulmonary disease and is reported with codes in category J44. Conditions listed as included under category J44 are:

- Asthma with chronic obstructive pulmonary disease
- Chronic asthmatic (obstructive) bronchitis
- Chronic bronchitis with airways obstruction
- Chronic bronchitis with emphysema
- Chronic emphysematous bronchitis
- Chronic obstructive asthma
- Chronic obstructive bronchitis
- Chronic obstructive tracheobronchitis

Documentation and Coding Requirements

Identify type of non-acute bronchitis:

- Chronic
  - Mixed simple and mucopurulent chronic bronchitis
  - Mucopurulent
  - Simple
  - Unspecified chronic bronchitis
- Chronic obstructive pulmonary disease
  - With acute lower respiratory infection
    - » Type of organism
  - With (acute) exacerbation
  - Unspecified
- Not specified as acute or chronic

Identify tobacco exposure, use, dependence, or history of dependence

Chronic Bronchitis

ICD-10-CM Code/Documentation	
J40	Bronchitis, not specified as acute or chronic
J41.0	Simple chronic bronchitis
J41.1	Mucopurulent chronic bronchitis
J41.8	Mixed simple and mucopurulent chronic bronchitis
J42	Unspecified chronic bronchitis
J44.0	Chronic obstructive pulmonary disease with (acute) lower respiratory infection
J44.1	Chronic obstructive pulmonary disease with (acute) exacerbation
J44.9	Chronic obstructive pulmonary disease, unspecified

Documentation and Coding Example

Seventeen-year-old Black male presents to Urgent Care with 4 day history of fever and chills, shortness of breath, and a productive cough. The patient is well known to the clinic as he does community service and is mentored by a physician on staff. He plans to study medicine when he goes to college in the fall. Patient has a history of chronic asthmatic bronchitis from second hand smoke exposure. Current medications include Qvar Inhaler BID. T 101.8, P 100 R 22, BP 110/72, O2 Saturation on RA 95%. On examination, this is a thin, but muscular, well groomed, articulate but somewhat anxious young male. Eyes are clear, PERRLA. Nares patent with thin secretions, oral mucosa moist and pink. Posterior pharynx red, without exudate. Tonsils and adenoids are not enlarged. TM's clear. Neck supple without lymphadenopathy. Apical pulse regular, peripheral pulses full but not bounding, no clubbing or cyanosis in extremities. Breath sounds have wheezes and scattered rales that do not clear with coughing, decreased sounds in the right middle and lower lobes. Abdomen soft with hypoactive bowel sounds. Liver palpated at 2 cm below the RCM, spleen at 1 cm below that LCM. He admits to decreased appetite x 2 days and mild nausea today. Cough is productive of thick, greenish mucous and a specimen is collected and sent to the lab. He was given an updraft treatment of albuterol and NS with supplemental O2 at 40%. O2 saturation improved during treatment and he was placed on O2 at 2 L/min via NC when it was completed. Chest x-ray obtained and shows changes consistent with chronic bronchitis and infiltrates in the right lung suggestive of pneumonia. IV started in right hand with LR infusing. Blood drawn for CBC, comprehensive metabolic panel, blood cultures. Gram stain of sputum shows gram negative rods. Suspect Pseudomonas infection. He will be admitted for updraft treatments and antibiotics.

In Patient Day 1: He remains febrile with temperature spike to 102.2. He is comfortable with ibuprofen and appetite is improving. Blood culture is negative at 24 hours. Sputum has heavy growth of P. aeruginosa, waiting for sensitivities. He continues to require oxygen at 2 L/min to maintain an oxygen saturation of >97%. Updraft nebulizer treatments of albuterol continue q 4 hours. Repeat chest x-ray confirms pneumonia in right middle and lower lobes. IV antibiotics of Tobramycin and Ampicillin will continue until sensitivities are back, consider monotherapy as soon as possible.

Final Diagnosis: Acute and chronic obstructive bronchitis with superimposed pneumonia due to P. aeruginosa.

Diagnosis Code(s)

J44.0	Chronic obstructive pulmonary disease with (acute) lower respiratory infection
J15.1	Pneumonia due to Pseudomonas
Z77.22	Contact with and (suspected) exposure to environmental tobacco smoke (acute) (chronic)

Coding Note(s)

Classifications for chronic bronchitis include a code specific for COPD with acute lower respiratory infection. The superimposed infection is due to P. aeruginosa which is a Pseudomonas infection so the code for pneumonia due to Pseudomonas is assigned. There is a use additional code note for exposure to environmental tobacco smoke so code Z77.22 is reported additionally to indicate a specified circumstance presenting hazards to health.

Emphysema

Emphysema is a type of chronic obstructive pulmonary disease (COPD) characterized by the slow destruction of elastic tissue forming the alveoli (air sacs) in the lungs. This leads to an increase in alveoli size and subsequent wall collapse with expiration which traps carbon dioxide in the lung and limits oxygen availability. Causes include smoking, pollution, and exposure to coal or silica dust. A genetic condition that causes a deficiency of the protein, alpha 1-antitrypsin, can also lead to emphysema. Symptoms include shortness of breath and cough.

There are five codes that differentiate between different morphological types of emphysema including: unilateral emphysema, also called MacLeod's syndrome; panlobular emphysema, also called panacinar emphysema; and centrilobular emphysema, also called centriacinar emphysema. There are also codes for other specified type of emphysema, which would include paraseptal emphysema, and unspecified emphysema. Centrilobular emphysema begins in the bronchioles, spreads peripherally, involves primarily the upper half of the lungs, and is associated with long-term cigarette smoking. Panlobular emphysema destroys the entire alveolus, occurs primarily in the lower half of the lungs, and is seen primarily in individuals with a genetic condition that causes alpha1-antitrypsin (AAT) deficiency.

Coding and Documentation Requirements

Identify type of emphysema:

- Unilateral [MacLeod's syndrome]
- Panlobular
- Centrilobular
- Other emphysema
- Unspecified emphysema

Identify tobacco exposure, use, dependence, or history of dependence

Emphysema

ICD-10-CM Code/Documentation	
J43.0	Unilateral pulmonary emphysema [MacLeod's syndrome]
J43.1	Panlobular emphysema
J43.2	Centrilobular emphysema
J43.8	Other emphysema
J43.9	Emphysema, unspecified

Documentation and Coding Example

Twenty-five-year-old Caucasian male presents to pulmonary specialist with a six-month history of left upper chest discomfort when flying and shortness of breath with physical exercise. Patient is an avid recreational pilot and had a recent physical to renew his pilot's license, mentioned his symptoms to the examining physician who found them puzzling and suggested he see a lung specialist. Temperature 97.4, HR 60, RR 16, BP 110/60, O2 saturation 97% on RA. On examination, this is a well-developed, well-nourished pleasant young man. PMH is non-contributory. Usual childhood illnesses including colds, flu, strep throat, and infectious mononucleosis in high school. He does recall having a few URIs in the past year, the last about a month before he noticed the chest discomfort and SOB. Fingernails pink, good capillary refill, no clubbing. PERRL, neck supple without lymphadenopathy. Nares patent, mucous membranes moist and pink. Oral pharynx clear. TMs clear. HR regular without gallop or rub. Breath sounds are diminished on the left upper lobe with fine scattered rales throughout left lung fields. Patient denies pain at this time and describes the discomfort he has when flying as an achy tightness in left upper chest and back. PFT indicate mild obstructive pulmonary disease that improves with a bronchodilator. Chest x-ray shows unilateral hyperlucency of left lung, upper lobe. CT confirms hyperlucent left lung and shows a mediastinal shift to the right on inspiration and expiration.

Diagnosis: **MacLeod's Emphysema.**

Plan: Sample of Spiriva inhaler and Singulair tablets given to patient with instruction for use. He will return in 2 weeks for repeat PFT and chest x-ray.

Diagnosis Code(s)

J43.0 Unilateral pulmonary emphysema [MacLeod's syndrome]

Coding Note(s)

The documentation specifies the specific type of emphysema as MacLeod's for which there is a specific code.

Influenza

Influenza is a common viral illness characterized by fever, chills, sore throat, headache, body aches, cough, and fatigue. Gastrointestinal symptoms such as nausea and vomiting may be present with some strains of the influenza virus. The virus is very contagious and is spread by respiratory droplets in the air, on contaminated surfaces, and via direct (person to person) contact with an infected individual. Complications of influenza can include pneumonia, bronchitis, and sinus and ear infections. Encephalopathy and myocarditis are rare complications.

There are three categories—J09 Influenza due to certain identified influenza viruses; J10 Influenza due to other identified influenza virus; and J11 Influenza due to unidentified influenza virus. There is no category or subcategory specific to the Type A/H1N1 virus, which is included within category J10. However, swine Influenza virus (viruses that normally cause infections in pigs) should be reported with a code from J09.X-. Codes are specific as to manifestations with codes for influenza with pneumonia, other respiratory manifestations, gastrointestinal manifestations, encephalopathy, myocarditis, otitis media, and other manifestations.

Coding and Documentation Requirements

Identify type of influenza and manifestations/complications:

- Novel influenza A virus
  - With gastrointestinal manifestations
  - With pneumonia
  - With other respiratory manifestations
  - With other specified manifestations, which includes:
    - Encephalopathy
    - Myocarditis
    - Otitis media
- Other identified influenza virus
  - With encephalopathy
  - With gastrointestinal manifestations
  - With myocarditis
  - With otitis media
  - With pneumonia
    - With same other identified virus pneumonia
    - With other specified type of pneumonia
    - With unspecified type of pneumonia
  - With other respiratory manifestations
  - With other specified manifestations
- Unidentified type of influenza virus
  - With encephalopathy
  - With gastrointestinal manifestations
  - With myocarditis
  - With otitis media
  - With pneumonia
    - Specified type
    - Unspecified type
  - With other respiratory manifestations
  - With other specified manifestations

Influenza

ICD-10-CM Code/Documentation	
J09.X1	Influenza due to identified novel influenza A virus with pneumonia
J09.X2	Influenza due to identified novel influenza A virus with other respiratory manifestations
J09.X3	Influenza due to identified novel influenza A virus with gastrointestinal manifestations
J09.X9	Influenza due to identified novel influenza A virus with other manifestations
J10.00	Influenza due to other identified influenza virus with unspecified type of pneumonia
J10.01	Influenza due to other identified influenza virus with the same other identified influenza pneumonia
J10.08	Influenza due to other identified influenza virus with other specified pneumonia
J10.1	Influenza due to other identified influenza virus with other respiratory manifestations

ICD-10-CM Code/Documentation	
J10.2	Influenza due to other identified influenza virus with gastrointestinal manifestations
J10.81	Influenza due to other identified influenza virus with encephalopathy
J10.82	Influenza due to other identified influenza virus with myocarditis
J10.83	Influenza due to other identified influenza virus with otitis media
J10.89	Influenza due to other identified influenza virus with other manifestations
J11.00	Influenza due to unidentified influenza virus with unspecified type of pneumonia
J11.08	Influenza due to unidentified influenza virus with specified pneumonia
J11.1	Influenza due to unidentified influenza virus with other respiratory manifestations
J11.2	Influenza due to unidentified influenza virus with gastrointestinal manifestations
J11.81	Influenza due to unidentified influenza virus with encephalopathy
J11.82	Influenza due to unidentified influenza virus with myocarditis
J11.83	Influenza due to unidentified influenza virus with otitis media
J11.89	Influenza due to unidentified influenza virus with other manifestations

Documentation and Coding Example

Patient is a 20-year-old female who presents to Urgent Care Clinic with worsening flu symptoms. Patient was seen one week ago for sudden onset of fever, chills, headache and was diagnosed with influenza. She was prescribed ibuprofen, fluids and rest, offered reassurance and sent home. Patient states her symptoms progressed with body aches, malaise, sore throat, and dry cough. Fever was gone by day 3 at which time she developed nasal congestion with copious clear drainage. Today she has fever of 102 and chills. Her cough is productive of thick white mucus. She has pain in her left lower rib area, worse with inspiration. Temperature 101.6, HR 94, RR 18, BP 98/52. Neck supple with palpable cervical and supraclavicular lymph nodes. Oral mucosa red with patchy white exudates, enlarged tonsils. HR regular without murmur, rub, gallop. Breath sounds decreased in left base, fine rales and wheezes throughout. Abdomen soft, non-distended. O2 sat 98% on RA. Chest x-ray shows scattered infiltrates in both lungs and an area of consolidation in left base.

Impression: **Pneumonia secondary to influenza.** Blood drawn for CBC. Sputum sent for culture. She is prescribed Azithromycin, advised to continue ibuprofen for pain and fever. RTC in 3 days for recheck and test results.

Diagnosis Code(s)

J11.00 Influenza due to unidentified influenza virus with unspecified type of pneumonia

Coding Note(s)

The influenza virus has not been identified nor has the type of pneumonia been identified so the correct code is for influenza due to an unidentified influenza virus with an unspecified type of pneumonia.

Respiratory Failure and Acute Respiratory Distress Syndrome

Respiratory failure and acute respiratory distress syndrome (ARDS) are two devastating conditions that affect the respiratory system. These conditions are found in separate categories and code blocks in Chapter 10 but will be discussed together here. Category code J80 Acute respiratory distress syndrome (ARDS) is listed in the code block J80-J84 Other Respiratory Diseases Principally Affecting the Interstitium. Category J96 Respiratory failure, not elsewhere classified is listed in code block J96-J99 Other Diseases of the Respiratory System and includes codes for respiratory failure documented as acute, chronic, acute and chronic, or unspecified except for those conditions in the newborn or when the respiratory failure is documented as postprocedural. Codes for respiratory failure are further differentiated by whether the condition is documented as with hypoxia, with hypercapnia, or whether there is no mention of hypoxia or hypercapnia.

Respiratory failure may occur when the respiratory system fails in one or both of its gas exchange functions: oxygenation and carbon dioxide elimination. It may be classified as either acute or chronic and as either hypoxemic or hypercapnic.

Hypoxemic respiratory failure, also referred to as Type I respiratory failure, is characterized by an arterial oxygen tension (PaO2) lower than 60 mm Hg with a normal or low arterial carbon dioxide tension (PaCO2) and is the most common form of respiratory failure. It is most often associated with acute diseases of the lung that involve fluid filling or collapse of alveolar units. Conditions that may result in hypoxemic respiratory failure include pneumonia, pulmonary edema, and pulmonary hemorrhage.

Hypercapnic respiratory failure, also referred to as Type II respiratory failure, is characterized by a PaCO2 higher than 50 mm Hg. Hypoxemia may be seen with hypercapnia in patients who are breathing room air. The duration of the hypercapnic respiratory failure affects the level of bicarbonate which in turn affects the pH. Common causes of hypercapnic respiratory failure include drug overdose, neuromuscular disease, chest wall abnormalities, and severe airway disorders, such as asthma and chronic obstructive pulmonary disease (COPD).

In order to understand these conditions better, definitions are listed below.

Acute Respiratory Distress Syndrome (ARDS): A life threatening condition caused by injury, inflammation, or infection of the lungs. It is characterized by low levels of oxygen in the blood and can occur alone or with systemic organ failure (heart, liver, kidney).

Acute Respiratory Failure: An acute condition characterized by low levels of oxygen and/or high levels of carbon dioxide in circulating blood caused by impaired exchange of gas (oxygen, carbon dioxide) at the alveolar level. The condition typically develops over minutes or hours.

Chronic Respiratory Failure: A chronic condition characterized by low levels of oxygen and/or high levels of carbon dioxide in circulating blood caused by impaired exchange of gas (oxygen, carbon dioxide) at the alveolar level. The condition typically develops over days, weeks, or months.

Acute and Chronic Respiratory Failure: These conditions may occur together when an individual with an underlying chronic condition causing low levels of oxygen and/or high levels of carbon dioxide in circulating blood develops an acute problem worsening the symptoms. For example: Respiratory failure in a patient with emphysema (chronic condition) with bacterial pneumonia (acute condition).

Hypoxia: Decreased levels of oxygen in circulating blood (PaO2 <60 to 80 mm Hg).

Hypercapnia: Increased levels of carbon dioxide in circulating blood (PaCo2 >50 to 55 mm Hg).

Coding and Documentation Requirements

Identify respiratory condition:

- Respiratory failure
- Respiratory distress or insufficiency

For respiratory failure, identify:

- Temporal factors
  - Acute
  - Chronic
  - Acute and chronic
- Type
  - With hypercapnia
  - With hypoxia
  - Unspecified whether with hypercapnia or hypoxia

Respiratory failure

ICD-10-CM Code/Documentation	
J80	Acute respiratory distress syndrome
J96.00	Acute respiratory failure, unspecified whether with hypoxia or hypercapnia
J96.01	Acute respiratory failure with hypoxia
J96.02	Acute respiratory failure with hypercapnia
J96.10	Chronic respiratory failure, unspecified whether with hypoxia or hypercapnia
J96.11	Chronic respiratory failure with hypoxia
J96.12	Chronic respiratory failure with hypercapnia
J96.20	Acute and chronic respiratory failure, unspecified whether with hypoxia or hypercapnia
J96.21	Acute and chronic respiratory failure with hypoxia
J96.22	Acute and chronic respiratory failure with hypercapnia
J96.90	Respiratory failure, unspecified, unspecified whether with hypoxia or hypercapnia
J96.91	Respiratory failure, unspecified with hypoxia
J96.92	Respiratory failure, unspecified with hypercapnia

Documentation and Coding Example

Twenty-year-old Asian male referred to pulmonary clinic by his neurologist for nocturnal dyspnea and increasing daytime sleepiness. Patient was diagnosed with **limb girdle muscular dystrophy 3 years ago with weakness impacting primarily the upper extremities.** On examination, this is a small stature, thin young man, well-groomed and articulate. Temperature 98.6, HR 92, RR 20, BP 108/58, O2 Sat on RA 92 %. Color pale, skin warm, dry to touch. Mucous membranes moist and pale pink. TMs clear. Voice has a somewhat nasal quality. Nares patent, moist membranes without drainage. Mouth and throat are benign with no enlargement of lymph tissue. Neck supple. HR regular without murmur, an S3 gallop is appreciated. Patient had a routine EKG and echocardiogram 3 months ago which showed mild right axis deviation and right atrial enlargement. He is followed by cardiology q 6 months. Breath sounds decreased in bases but clear throughout. PFT shows a TV 0.24, VC 1.2, NIF -50. ABG on RA shows a pH 7.4, **PaCO2 51, PaO2 65,** HCO3 33, O2 Sat. 91%. Chest x-ray reveals basilar atelectasis. Patient is scheduled for a sleep study.

Sleep Study Note: Patient returns to clinic for sleep study. Procedure explained including possible use of non-invasive positive pressure nasal mask. A 6-hour monitored polysomnogram revealed 32 episodes of apnea and >200 periods of hypopnea with an average duration of 27 seconds. These occurred primarily during REM sleep with O2 saturation decreasing from an average of 82% to 35%. Nasal Bi-PAP was initiated during test with a marked improvement in O2 saturation and an 80% decrease in apnea and hypopnea episodes.

Impression: **Chronic hypercapnic respiratory failure due to underlying neuromuscular disease complicated by sleep related hypoventilation.**

Plan: Nasal Bi-PAP nightly. RTC in 1 month for recheck

Diagnosis code(s)

G71.09	Other specified muscular dystrophies
J96.12	Chronic respiratory failure with hypercapnia
G47.36	Sleep related hypoventilation in conditions classified elsewhere

Coding Note(s)

The cardiac conditions are not coded even though they are noted here, because the only problems being addressed are the pulmonary conditions.

While the patient does have decreased PaO2 levels, the code for respiratory failure with hypoxemia is not reported. According to the definition of hypercapnic respiratory failure, hypoxemia may be seen in a patient breathing room air. Also, the clinical indicator for hypoxemia is PaO2 less than 60-80. Since this is a range, and a diagnosis of hypoxemia is dependent on all the blood gas variables, some individuals might be considered hypoxemic at levels lower than 80 but other individuals may not be considered hypoxemic until PaO2 levels are below 60. Since the patient's PaO2 is 65 which is still above the lower threshold for hypoxemia, and the physician has not diagnosed the patient as having respiratory failure with hypoxemia, the diagnosis is chronic respiratory failure with hypercapnia (J96.12).

Sinusitis

Sinusitis is an inflammation or infection of the nasal/accessory sinuses of the respiratory tract. The condition may be acute or chronic. Acute sinusitis is classified in category J01 and chronic sinusitis is classified in category J32. Both acute and chronic sinusitis are differentiated by site as maxillary, frontal, ethmoidal, or sphenoidal. There is a specific code for pansinusitis and a code for other sinusitis which is used to report sinusitis involving more than one sinus but not documented as involving all sinuses. In addition, acute sinusitis documented as recurrent has a specific code for each sinus. For acute sinusitis not specified as recurrent, the default is the unspecified code.

Documentation and Coding Requirements

Identify temporal factors:

- Acute
- Chronic

Identify affected sinus(es):

- Ethmoidal
- Frontal
- Maxillary
- Sphenoidal
- Pansinusitis
- Other acute/chronic sinusitis (includes more than one sinus but not pansinusitis)
- Unspecified acute/chronic sinusitis

Identify acute as recurrent or unspecified:

- Recurrent
- Unspecified (not recurrent)

Use additional code to identify infectious organism when documented.

For chronic sinusitis, use additional code to identify:

- Exposure to environmental tobacco smoke
- Exposure to tobacco smoke in the perinatal period
- History of tobacco use
- Occupational exposure to environmental tobacco smoke
- Tobacco dependence
- Tobacco use

Sinusitis

ICD-10-CM Code/Documentation	
Acute Sinusitis	
J01.00	Acute maxillary sinusitis, unspecified
J01.01	Acute recurrent maxillary sinusitis
J01.10	Acute frontal sinusitis, unspecified
J01.11	Acute recurrent frontal sinusitis
J01.20	Acute ethmoidal sinusitis, unspecified
J01.21	Acute recurrent ethmoidal sinusitis
J01.30	Acute sphenoidal sinusitis, unspecified
J01.31	Acute recurrent sphenoidal sinusitis
J01.40	Acute pansinusitis, unspecified
J01.41	Acute recurrent pansinusitis
J01.80	Other acute sinusitis
J01.81	Other acute recurrent sinusitis
J01.90	Acute sinusitis, unspecified
J01.91	Acute recurrent sinusitis, unspecified
Chronic Sinusitis	
J32.0	Chronic maxillary sinusitis
J32.1	Chronic frontal sinusitis
J32.2	Chronic ethmoidal sinusitis
J32.3	Chronic sphenoidal sinusitis
J32.4	Chronic pansinusitis
J32.8	Other chronic sinusitis
J32.9	Chronic sinusitis, unspecified

Documentation and Coding Example

Twenty-two-year-old Hispanic female returns to clinic for **follow up of sinusitis**. Patient has a history of **allergic rhinitis** for which she uses Rhinocort AQ when her symptoms flare. She has had occasional episodes of sinusitis usually following URI that cleared with Zithromax, but this year she has had **4 episodes, the last one did not respond to the usual treatment**. A CT scan one week ago showed consolidation with minimal air in the maxillary and ethmoid sinuses and blockage of the ostia consistent with acute sinusitis. A sterile tap of the maxillary sinus was performed with culture positive for **H. influenzae and M. catarrhalis**, both sensitive to Augmentin. Patient states she has been on the antibiotic for 3 days. On examination: T 98.8, P 68, R 14, BP 100/66. Conjunctiva mildly red and eyes have a clear, watery drainage. She continues to have tenderness in the eye orbits, upper jaw, and teeth. Nares swollen with scant amount of thick mucus, no polyps or septal deviation. Oral mucosa is moist and pink, posterior pharynx has a cobblestone appearance consistent with **chronic allergies** and thick purulent mucus coats the tissue. Neck supple with lymph node enlargement appreciated in the parotid, mandibular, and cervical areas. She denies problems swallowing but states she has completely lost her sense of smell. Breath sounds are clear and equal bilaterally.

Impression: **Recurrent acute infection of the maxillary and anterior ethmoid sinuses due to H. influenzae and M. catarrhalis**, on appropriate antibiotic therapy. **Allergic rhinitis.**

Plan: Continue Augmentin x 14 days. Patient has run out of her Rhinocort AQ and it is not covered by her new insurance. She is given samples of Flonase with instructions for use. She is also given an Rx for guaifenesin to take as needed for cough and congestion. RTC in 2 weeks, sooner if symptoms worsen or do not improve.

Diagnosis Code(s)

J01.81	Other acute recurrent sinusitis
B96.3	Haemophilus influenzae [H.influenzae] as the cause of diseases classified elsewhere
B96.89	Other specified bacterial agents as the cause of diseases classified elsewhere
J30.9	Allergic rhinitis, unspecified

Coding Note(s)

The acute sinusitis is documented as recurrent and is present in more than one sinus but not all four so the code for other acute recurrent sinusitis is assigned. There are two infectious organisms, both bacteria, that have caused the sinusitis. There is a specific code for the *H. influenzae*, but the *M. catarrhalis* must be reported with the other specified code because there is not a specific code for this organism. The physician has also diagnosed allergic rhinitis but has not specified the cause so the unspecified code is assigned.

Streptococcal Sore Throat

Streptococcal sore throat like many codes in Chapter 10 is classified as a combination code indicating the organism as well as the anatomic location. It is further classified based upon anatomic involvement of pharyngitis vs. tonsillitis. And finally, the codes are classified as to whether they are acute or recurrent.

Coding and Documentation Requirements

Identify condition:

- Pharyngitis
- Tonsillitis

For tonsillitis identify:

- Not recurrent/unspecified
- Recurrent

ICD-10-CM Code/Documentation	
J02.0	Streptococcal pharyngitis
J03.00	Acute streptococcal tonsillitis, unspecified
J03.01	Acute recurrent streptococcal tonsillitis

Documentation and Coding Example

Patient presents with sudden onset of sore throat, headache, fever, and complaints of difficulty swallowing. Tonsils are red and enlarged. Rapid strep test positive. **This is the third visit in the past three months for acute streptococcal tonsillitis.** Prescription for ten-day course of antibiotics.

Diagnosis: **Acute recurrent streptococcal tonsillitis**

ICD-10-CM Diagnosis Code(s)

J03.01 Acute recurrent streptococcal tonsillitis

Viral Pneumonia

Pneumonia is an infection or inflammation of the lungs that can be caused by a variety of microorganisms including viruses, bacteria, fungi, and other microorganisms. Viral pneumonia may be caused by the influenza virus, viruses that cause the common cold (adenovirus, parainfluenza virus, and coronaviruses), and respiratory syncytial virus (RSV). Other less common causes of viral pneumonia include varicella and herpes viruses.

Specific codes exist for adenoviral pneumonia (J12.0), RSV pneumonia (J12.1), parainfluenza virus pneumonia (J12.2), and SARS-associated corona-virus pneumonia (J12.81). The latter is not the same as the newly discovered 2019 novel coronavirus that emerged in December of 2019 officially named "SARS-CoV-2", causing "coronavirus disease 2019", abbreviated COVID-19. This newer virus is genetically related to the virus causing the outbreak of SARS-associated coronavirus pneumonia in 2003, but causes a different illness and is currently reported with temporary code U07.1. Additionally, there is a specific code for human metapneumovirus (hMPV) pneumonia (J12.3).

Human metapneumovirus (hMPV) is a family of viruses that was first identified in 2001, but it most likely has been causing respiratory illnesses for decades worldwide. Human metapneumoviruses cause upper respiratory infections, such as colds, and lower respiratory tract infections, such as pneumonia or bronchitis in people of all ages. Most people with hMPV infection have mild upper respiratory symptoms including cough, runny nose, nasal congestion, sore throat, and fever. A small percentage of people will develop more serious lower respiratory illnesses. Most often those experiencing more serious illnesses are the very young, the very old, and immune compromised individuals.

Instructions for influenza complicated by pneumonia require reporting the appropriate influenza code first with an additional code for the pneumonia when the pneumonia is not caused by the influenza virus and the specific causative agent of the pneumonia is identified.

Documentation and Coding Requirements

Identify cause of viral pneumonia:

- Adenovirus
- Human metapneumovirus (hMPV)
- Parainfluenza virus
- Respiratory syncytial virus (RSV)
- SARS-associated coronavirus
- Other specified virus (excludes some viral infections complicated by pneumonia and influenza complicated by pneumonia caused by the same influenza virus)
- Unspecified

Note: Pneumonia caused by the 2019 novel coronavirus (COVID-19), is reported with codes U07.1 COVID-19 and J12.89 Other viral pneumonia.

Viral Pneumonia

ICD-10-CM Code/Documentation	
J12.0	Adenoviral pneumonia
J12.1	Respiratory syncytial virus pneumonia
J12.2	Parainfluenza virus pneumonia
J12.3	Human metapneumovirus pneumonia
J12.81	Pneumonia due to SARS-associated coronavirus
J12.89	Other viral pneumonia
J12.9	Viral pneumonia, unspecified

Documentation and Coding Example

Forty-six-year-old Caucasian male presents to ED with a 3-day history of cough, congestion, and low grade fever. **PMH is significant for renal failure on dialysis x 10 years with kidney transplant 18 months ago. He takes daily Imuran and Methylprednisolone to prevent rejection and Nexium for GI symptoms related to steroid use**. Patient states he was seen yesterday by his PMD who diagnosed a viral URI and prescribed rest, fluids, and ibuprofen. He developed a sore throat, wheeze and shortness of breath in the past few hours and his PMD advised him to go immediately to the ED. On examination: T 99.8, P 90, R 20, BP 140/92, O2 saturation 92% on RA, increased to 98% on supplemental O2 at 4 L/min via NC. Alert, oriented, somewhat anxious adult male with mild respiratory distress. Breath sounds are decreased in bases bilaterally with scattered rales throughout the lungs that do not clear with coughing. Wheezing is appreciated over the bronchi. He is given a nebulizer treatment of Xopenex and budesonide with some improvement in air flow. IV started in left arm and blood drawn for CBC/diff, PT, PTT, metabolic panel, respiratory secretions for culture. D5W infusing at 100 cc/hr. Chest x-ray obtained and shows scattered infiltrates throughout right and left lungs consistent with a viral pneumonia.

Impression: **Viral pneumonia in an immune compromised patient**.

Plan: Admit to medical floor under care of Renal Transplant Service and Infectious Disease.

Inpatient Day 1: Stable. Continues to receive respiratory treatments of Xopenex and budesonide q 4 hours. Taking oral fluids but has nausea and no appetite. Remains on IV D5.45 NS with 10 mEq KCL. **Suspect viral infection is caused by hMPV**. Waiting for lab confirmation.

Inpatient Day 2: **Lab confirms human Metapneumovirus infection**. Repeat chest x-ray shows improvement with infiltrates in left and right bases and right middle lobe. Respiratory status much improved with breathing treatments q 6 hours and O2 saturation 98% on RA. Plan discharge tomorrow if he continues to improve.

Diagnosis Code(s)

J12.3	Human metapneumovirus pneumonia
Z94.0	Kidney transplant status
Z79.52	Long term (current) use of systemic steroids
Z79.899	Other long term (current) drug therapy

Coding Note(s)

There is a specific code for metapneumovirus pneumonia. The patient's kidney transplant status is reported additionally as are the long-term use of systemic steroids and the long term use of the anti-rejection drug Imuran. There is not a specific code for long term use of Imuran so the other specified code is assigned.

Summary

Diseases of the respiratory system have fewer documentation requirements than other chapters, but the documentation requirements affect some of the more common conditions seen in the outpatient setting, including influenza, strep throat, and strep tonsillitis. Respiratory failure is another condition with significant documentation requirements. Capturing this complication requires an understanding of the definitions of acute and chronic respiratory failure and the difference between respiratory failure described as hypoxic or hypercapnic. If the patient has documentation of clinical laboratory values indicative of hypoxemia or hypercapnia, without specific documentation of respiratory failure, it will be necessary for coders to identify those values and query the physician to determine if a diagnosis of respiratory failure is warranted.

Resources

Documentation checklists are available in Appendix A for the following condition(s):

- Asthma
- Bronchitis/Bronchiolitis, Acute Infection
- Influenza
- Pharyngitis/Tonsillitis, Acute
- Pneumonia

Clinical indicator checklists are available in Appendix B for the following condition(s):

- Chronic Obstructive Pulmonary Disease
- Pneumonia

Chapter 10 Quiz

1. What factor influencing health status should be additionally coded when documented for diseases of the respiratory system?
   a. The infectious organism
   b. Other related health conditions
   c. Any exposure to tobacco smoke or use of tobacco
   d. All of the above
2. To assign the most specific code for asthma, which of the following documentation elements must be provided?
   a. The condition must be described as acute or chronic
   b. The asthma must be specified as mild, moderate, or severe
   c. The condition must be specified as childhood asthma or adult asthma
   d. The condition must be described as extrinsic or intrinsic
3. What acute conditions differentiate between an acute and an acute recurrent condition?
   a. Paranasal sinusitis and streptococcal tonsillitis
   b. Sinusitis, pharyngitis, and tonsillitis
   c. Sinusitis and streptococcal pharyngitis
   d. Sinusitis and unspecified upper respiratory infection
4. How is acute respiratory distress syndrome reported?
   a. With a nonspecific code from category J96.9- Respiratory failure unspecified
   b. With the code for acute respiratory failure unspecified whether with hypoxia or hypercapnia (J96.00)
   c. With a code from block J80-J84 Other respiratory diseases principally affecting the interstitium
   d. With code J99 Respiratory disorders in diseases classified elsewhere
5. Acute type I respiratory failure documented as present on admission is reported as follows:
   a. As the first-listed or principal diagnosis using code J96.01
   b. As a secondary diagnosis using code J96.01
   c. As the first-listed or principal diagnosis using code J96.02
   d. As the principal or a secondary diagnosis depending on the circumstances of the admission as documented by the physician using code J96.01
6. When chronic obstructive pulmonary disease (category J44) is complicated by viral pneumonia, the following coding guidelines and instructions are applicable:
   a. The code for COPD with acute exacerbation is assigned (J44.1)
   b. The code for COPD with acute lower respiratory infection is assigned along with a code identifying the organism (J44.0, B97.89)
   c. The code for COPD with acute lower respiratory infection is assigned along with a code for the viral pneumonia (J44.0, J12.9)
   d. The code for COPD with acute lower respiratory infection is assigned (J44.0)
7. A condition documented as severe persistent asthma with COPD is reported as follows:
   a. J44.9 Chronic obstructive pulmonary disease, unspecified
   b. J45.50 Severe persistent asthma, uncomplicated
   c. J45.998 Other asthma
   d. J44.9 Chronic obstructive pulmonary disease, unspecified and J45.50 Severe persistent asthma, uncomplicated
8. What additional information is required to assign the most specific code for lower respiratory syncytial virus infection?
   a. The site/manifestation of the infection must be documented as bronchitis, bronchiolitis, or pneumonia
   b. The infection must be documented as acute or subacute
   c. RSV bronchitis or bronchiolitis must be documented as with or without bronchospasm
   d. All of the above
9. Some manifestations of influenza are reported with a combination code. What manifestation does not need to be reported with an additional code for J09.X Influenza due to identified novel influenza A virus?
   a. Gastrointestinal manifestations
   b. Encephalopathy
   c. Otitis media
   d. Myocarditis
10. Streptococcal tonsillitis requires documentation as:
    a. Acute or subacute
    b. Acute or acute recurrent
    c. Type A or Type B
    d. Acute or other specified type

See next page for answers and rationales.

Chapter 10 Answers and Rationales

1. What factor influencing health status should be additionally coded when documented for diseases of the respiratory system?

    c. **Any exposure to tobacco smoke or use of tobacco**

    Rationale: *Exposure to tobacco smoke and use of tobacco are classified as factors influencing health status and there is a note to use an additional code where applicable to identify these factors. While it may be appropriate to code the infectious organism and/or related health conditions, these are not considered factors influencing health status for coding purposes, so the only correct answer is c.*

2. To assign the most specific code for asthma, which of the following documentation elements must be provided?

    b. **The asthma must be specified as mild, moderate, or severe**

    Rationale: *The condition must be described as mild, moderate, or severe. It is also necessary to document any exacerbation and whether the condition is complicated by status asthmaticus. For mild asthma, it is also necessary to document the condition as either intermittent or persistent.*

3. What acute conditions differentiate between an acute and an acute recurrent condition?

    a. **Paranasal sinusitis and streptococcal tonsillitis**

    Rationale: *Paranasal sinusitis (maxillary, frontal, ethmoidal, sphenoidal, pansinusitis, other sinusitis, and unspecified paranasal sinusitis) and streptococcal tonsillitis require documentation of the acute condition as acute or acute recurrent. Acute pharyngitis, including streptococcal pharyngitis, does not have a separate code for acute recurrent conditions nor does an unspecified acute upper respiratory infection.*

4. How is acute respiratory distress syndrome reported?

    c. **With a code from block J80-J84 Other respiratory diseases principally affecting the interstitium**

    Rationale: *There is a specific code for acute respiratory distress syndrome (J80) that is listed in the code block J80-J84.*

5. Acute type I respiratory failure documented as present on admission is reported as follows:

    d. **As the principal or a secondary diagnosis depending on the circumstances of the admission as documented by the physician using code J96.01**

    Rationale: *Type 1 respiratory failure is another name for hypoxemic respiratory failure. When described as acute respiratory failure, it is reported with code J96.01. There should also be clinical documentation and blood gas values to support this diagnosis. Whether or not the condition is reported as the principal or a secondary diagnosis is dependent on the circumstances of the admission.*

6. When chronic obstructive pulmonary disease (category J44) is complicated by viral pneumonia, the following coding guidelines and instructions are applicable:

    c. **The code for COPD with acute lower respiratory infection is assigned along with a code for the viral pneumonia (J44.0, J12.9)**

    Rationale: *According to the coding guidelines, codes in category J44 differentiate between uncomplicated cases and those with an acute exacerbation, which is a worsening or decompensation of a chronic condition. An acute exacerbation is not the same as an infection superimposed on a chronic condition, though an exacerbation may be triggered by an infection. This is why there is a third option, code J44.0 COPD with (acute) lower respiratory infection. There is a note under J44.0 indicating that an additional code should be reported to identify the infection. In this case, the infection is specified as viral pneumonia so the J12.9 Viral pneumonia unspecified is reported. Nothing more is documented related to the viral pneumonia so it is not possible to identify the organism more specifically.*

7. A condition documented as severe persistent asthma with COPD is reported as follows:

    d. **J44.9 Chronic obstructive pulmonary disease, unspecified and J45.50 Severe persistent asthma, uncomplicated**

    Rationale: *The alphabetic index identifies J44.9 as the correct code. Under J44, there is a note to code also the type of asthma, if applicable. The asthma has been documented as severe, persistent asthma so code J45.50 is also reported.*

8. What additional information is required to assign the most specific code for lower respiratory syncytial virus infection?

    a. **The site/manifestation of the infection must be documented as bronchitis, bronchiolitis, or pneumonia**

    Rationale: *Assignment of the most specific code requires identification of the site/manifestation as bronchitis (J20.5), bronchiolitis (J21.0), or pneumonia (J12.1). The same code is used whether the condition is described as acute or subacute and whether it is described as with or without bronchospasm.*

9. Some manifestations of influenza are reported with a combination code. What manifestation does not need to be reported with an additional code for J09.X Influenza due to identified novel influenza A virus?

    a. **Gastrointestinal manifestations**

    Rationale: *Gastroenteritis is the only manifestation listed above that has a specific combination code (J09.X3) for influenza due to identified novel influenza A virus. The other three conditions are reported with code J09.X9 Influenza due to identified novel influenza A virus with other manifestations and require an additional code to identify the specific manifestation.*

10. Streptococcal tonsillitis requires documentation as:

    b. **Acute or acute recurrent**

    Rationale: *Codes are available for acute and acute recurrent streptococcal tonsillitis.*

Chapter 11
DISEASES OF THE DIGESTIVE SYSTEM

Introduction

Diseases of the digestive system are found in Chapter 11 of ICD-10-CM. Some of the most frequently diagnosed digestive system diseases and conditions, such as cholecystitis, cholelithiasis, hernias, and colitis require specific documentation for more than one axis of information in order to assign the proper code(s). For example, when reporting cholecystitis, documentation must specify the cholecystitis as acute, chronic, or acute and chronic, whether the cholecystitis occurs alone or with cholelithiasis, and whether or not obstruction is present. The combination codes for cholelithiasis with cholecystitis further identify the site of the calculus as being in the gallbladder, the bile duct, or both. There are also combination codes for calculus of the bile duct documented as with cholangitis. Many conditions require documentation of site in addition to type. Ulcerative (chronic) colitis is reported by location of the inflammation in the colon, occurring as pancolitis, proctitis, rectosigmoiditis, left sided hemicolitis, or other location, in addition to any specific complications or without complications. Another coding consideration is that conditions complicating a disease are often captured with combination codes instead of being reported separately.

Within the digestive system chapter, diseases of the liver, gallbladder, biliary tract, and pancreas are subdivided with specific code blocks for Diseases of the Liver (K70-K77) and Disorders of the Gallbladder, Biliary Tract, and Pancreas (K80-K87). Below is a table of the digestive system blocks in ICD-10-CM:

ICD-10-CM Blocks	
K00-K14	Diseases of Oral Cavity and Salivary Glands
K20-K31	Diseases of Esophagus, Stomach, and Duodenum
K35-K38	Diseases of Appendix
K40-K46	Hernia
K50-K52	Noninfective Enteritis and Colitis
K55-K64	Other Diseases of Intestines
K65-K68	Diseases of Peritoneum and Retroperitoneum
K70-K77	Diseases of Liver
K80-K87	Disorders of Gallbladder, Biliary Tract, and Pancreas
K90-K95	Other Diseases of the Digestive System

Coding Note(s)

Some chapters contain chapter level coding instructions in the form of notes. However, there are no chapter level instructions for diseases of the digestive system.

Exclusions

In addition to general chapter level notes that provide coding instructions, many chapters have chapter level exclusions. In the digestive system chapter, there are only Excludes2 notes, which are listed in the table below.

Excludes1	Excludes2
None	Certain conditions originating in the perinatal period (P04-P96) Certain infectious and parasitic diseases (A00-B99) Complications of pregnancy, childbirth, and the puerperium (O00-O9A) Congenital malformations, deformations, and chromosomal abnormalities (Q00-Q99) Endocrine, nutritional, and metabolic diseases (E00-E88) Injury, poisoning, and certain other consequences of external causes (S00-T88) Neoplasms (C00-D49) Symptoms, signs, and abnormal clinical and laboratory findings, not elsewhere classified (R00-R94)

Chapter Guidelines

There are currently no chapter guidelines for diseases of the digestive system. This means that the general guidelines and the notes and instructions contained in the Alphabetic Index and Tabular List should be followed when assigning codes for diseases of the digestive system.

General Documentation Requirements

Some important considerations related to documentation for diseases of the digestive system include:

- Designation of concomitant conditions as acute and/or chronic
- Designation of some acute conditions as recurrent, or not specified as recurrent
- Specificity related to intraoperative vs. postprocedural complications
- Combination codes requiring specific documentation of related complications. Examples include:
  - Regional enteritis/Crohn's disease (K50) and ulcerative colitis (K51) – Combination codes capture the following complications:
    - » Abscess
    - » Fistula
    - » Intestinal obstruction
    - » Rectal bleeding
  - Diverticular disease (K57) must be documented as:

    » With or without perforation and abscess
    » With or without bleeding
  - Calculus of bile duct – Combination codes capture the condition with cholangitis or cholecystitis

Code-Specific Documentation Requirements

In this section, documentation requirements for some of the more frequently reported digestive system diseases are discussed. The ICD-10-CM codes are listed and the documentation requirements are identified. Although not all conditions are covered, this section provides a representative sample of the types of documentation needed to assign codes at the highest level of specificity.

Abscess of Anal and Rectal Regions

An anal or rectal (anorectal) abscess is an inflammation and infection near the anal opening or inside the anus or rectum. The condition usually occurs in the presence of an anal fissure or as a result of a blocked anal gland. Symptoms can include pain, swelling, and drainage from the anal area. Fistula development is common following anorectal abscess.

Anorectal abscesses are classified by their anatomic location. Abscesses with superficial pockets of infection beneath the anal skin are the most common. Ischiorectal abscesses occur when the purulent material crosses the external anal sphincter into the ischiorectal space. If it moves to the contralateral side, a horseshoe abscess is formed. Intrasphincteric abscesses are suppurative infection contained between the internal and external anal sphincters and may remain within the anal canal. When it extends further above the levator ani, a supralevator abscess forms, which is the least common type.

An includes note indicates that the codes for anal and/or rectal abscesses include cellulitis of these sites.

Documentation must clearly identify the site as anal (excludes intrasphincteric) (K61.0), rectal (excludes ischiorectal) (K61.1), anorectal (K61.2), ischiorectal (K61.3-), intrasphincteric (KI61.4) or supralevator (K61.5).

Coding and Documentation Requirements

Identify site of abscess:

- Anal
- Anorectal
- Intrasphincteric
- Ischiorectal
  - Horseshoe
  - Other ischiorectal
- Rectal
- Supralevator

ICD-10-CM Code/Documentation	
K61.0	Anal abscess
K61.1	Rectal abscess
K61.2	Anorectal abscess
K61.31	Horseshoe abscess
K61.39	Other ischiorectal abscess
K61.4	Intrasphincteric abscess
K61.5	Supralevator abscess

Documentation and Coding Example

Three-year-old Hispanic male brought into ED by parents with severe constipation and inconsolable crying. There is a history of anal fissure during infancy that resolved without treatment. Father states the child's last BM was 4 days ago and normal size and consistency. He usually defecates daily. Appetite decreased x 2 days. Unable to examine child in present condition. Anesthesia and Pediatric Surgery called to consult. Patient medicated with IM Versed by anesthesiologist and placed on cardiac monitor. Temperature 99.4, HR 126, RR 16, BP 60/46. IV started in right antecubital fossa and secured on armboard. Examine under MAC is significant for a **large fecal impaction**, which is manually removed to reveal a small lump in the posterior wall of the anal canal.

Impression: **Anal abscess.**

Pediatric Surgery Note: Patient was taken to OR for anoscopic exam which confirms an **intrasphincteric abscess in the posterior anus**. A transverse incision was made between the internal and external sphincter to the dentate line. The abscess was drained and culture sent to lab. A de Pezzer catheter was sutured into place. Iodophor gauze was used to pack the area and patient was taken to recovery in good condition. EBL 10 cc.

Diagnosis Code(s)

K61.4 Intrasphincteric abscess

K56.41 Fecal impaction

Coding Note(s)

The initial impression was an anal abscess, but on anoscopic exam the abscess was more specifically identified as being an intrasphincteric abscess, so the more specific code is assigned. Fecal impaction is reported additionally for the ED visit.

Anal Fissure

An anal fissure is a linear break or tear in the skin surrounding the anal opening. A fissure may be superficial or extend into the sphincter muscle. The condition usually heals on its own but may become chronic if blood supply to the anal mucosa is impaired.

Anal fissures must be documented as acute (K60.0) or chronic (K60.1). There is also a code for an unspecified anal fissure (K60.2). Anal fissures complicated by anal abscess or cellulitis are reported with codes from category K61. Anal fissures must also be clearly differentiated from anal sphincter tears, which are reported with code K62.81.

Coding and Documentation Requirements

Identify status of anal fissure:

- Acute
- Chronic
- Unspecified

ICD-10-CM Code/Documentation	
K60.0	Acute anal fissure
K60.1	Chronic anal fissure
K60.2	Anal fissure, unspecified

Documentation and Coding Example

Patient is a 22-year-old Caucasian male who presents for recheck of a **chronic anal fissure**. He was initially seen three months ago with rectal pain and bleeding following anal intercourse with a new partner. He was screened for STDs including HIV, all negative. He was prescribed sitz baths, Miralax, high fiber diet, increased fluids, and advised to refrain from recipient intercourse. He was compliant with treatment but continued to have pain and occasional bleeding with bowel movements. An anoscopic exam one month ago revealed a **nonhealing fissure** with the appearance of a chronic linear ulcer in the posterior midline of the anal opening. Fibers of the internal anal sphincter could be visualized at the base of the fissure. He was prescribed 0.2% Nitroglycerin cream to be applied topically BID. Patient states his symptoms have resolved and he has been pain free for two weeks. On examination the fissure shows significant healing with granulation tissue at the base of the ulcer covering the previously exposed internal sphincter. Patient denies experiencing nitroglycerin side effects such as headaches or dizziness. He does state he stopped using Miralax one week ago because he is getting adequate fiber in his diet and his stools have remained soft and regular since making that change. He is advised to continue using nitroglycerine cream and to schedule a follow-up appointment in one month. Anticipate complete healing will have been achieved and Nitroglycerin cream can be discontinued at that time.

Diagnosis Code(s)

K60.1 Chronic anal fissure

Anal and Rectal Fistula

An anal or rectal fistula is an abnormal, inflammatory connection between the anal canal or rectum and the skin surrounding the anal opening. Fistulas usually originate in the anal glands located between the layers of the anal sphincter muscles and are frequently a complication of an anal or rectal (anorectal) abscess. Symptoms include pain, itching, and drainage.

Anal/rectal fistulas must be documented as anal (K60.3), rectal (K60.4), or anorectal (K60.5). These codes are reported only for fistulas documented as extending from the anus or rectum to the skin. If documentation describes a fistula from the rectum to the bladder or to the vagina, a code from the genitourinary system would be reported. Anal, rectal, and anorectal fistulas complicated by abscess or cellulitis are reported with codes from category K61.

Coding and Documentation Requirements

Identify site of fistula:

- Anal
- Anorectal
- Rectal

ICD-10-CM Code/Documentation	
K60.3	Anal fistula
K60.4	Rectal fistula
K60.5	Anorectal fistula

Documentation and Coding Example

Sixty-year-old Black male is seen in clinic for c/o rectal pain and itching. He has a history of hemorrhoids and occasional constipation but his usual remedies of increased fiber and fluids have not helped relieve his present symptoms. PMH is noncontributory. Patient is a school bus driver currently on his summer break.

Perianal area is examined carefully with patient in a dorsal lithotomy position. **External hemorrhoidal skin tags are noted.** There is **moderate swelling around the anterior anal opening with a fistula** opening in the skin at the 1 o'clock position. A small blunt lachrymal probe inserted through the external opening is easily manipulated in a straight tract to the internal opening. DRE shows good sphincter tone, prostate is normal size and smooth. There is no evidence of abscess either in the perianal area or rectum. Anoscopy is performed with good visualization of the rectum. There is a **large internal hemorrhoid** present but no polyps or inflammation noted. The **internal fistula opening is observed just past the internal sphincter in the rectum.**

Diagnosis: **Anorectal fistula. Internal hemorrhoid. External hemorrhoidal skin tags.**

Plan: Findings are discussed with patient and his wife. Plan is for elective fistulotomy under general anesthesia. He is sent to surgery scheduler to make the necessary arrangements.

Diagnosis Code(s)

K60.5 Anorectal fistula

K64.8 Other hemorrhoids

K64.4 Residual hemorrhoidal skin tags

Coding Note(s)

Codes for anal, anorectal, and rectal fistulas are specific to site. Internal hemorrhoid codes require documentation of the degree. Since the degree is not documented in this scenario, the code for other hemorrhoids is used since this code includes internal hemorrhoids without mention of degree.

Anal and Rectal Polyp

An anal or rectal polyp is a common type of tissue growth arising from the wall of the anus or rectum. Polyps can be benign or malignant. There may be a hereditary predisposition to the development of polyps, a condition referred to as familial polyposis, and polyps also occur more frequently in the presence of inflammatory bowel disease. The condition is largely asymptomatic but bleeding, cramping, abdominal pain, diarrhea, and intestinal obstruction may occur, particularly when the polyps are large.

Documentation must be carefully reviewed when coding polyps of the rectum and anus as some types of polyps are classified as benign neoplasms and are reported with codes from the neoplasm chapter. For example, adenomatous polyps and familial polyposis are not classified in the digestive system chapter; instead these conditions are reported with codes for benign neoplasms. Polyp codes are specific to site and should be documented as anal polyp (K62.0) or rectal polyp (K62.1).

Coding and Documentation Requirements

Identify site of polyp:

- Anal
- Rectal

ICD-10-CM Code/Documentation	
K62.0	Anal polyp
K62.1	Rectal polyp

Documentation and Coding Example

Fifty-five-year-old Caucasian female presents for screening colonoscopy. Her PMH is significant for mild asthma and hypothyroidism. Medications include Synthroid 50 mcg daily and Albuterol inhaler PRN asthma symptoms. There is no family history of colon cancer. Informed consent is obtained and IV started in left hand, LR infusing. Patient is medicated with Versed 2 mg and Fentanyl 25 mcg IVP, DRE shows good sphincter tone and scope is passed easily into rectum. Excellent bowel prep allows good visualization of the intestine and a **single polyp is noted in the rectum** just below the rectosigmoid junction. Exam continues to be unremarkable through the sigmoid colon, descending colon, transverse colon, and cecum. Patient became uncomfortable and was given another 25 mcg of Fentanyl to complete the exam. The **single polyp in the rectum** was re-examined and appears to be 0.5 cm in size and hyperplastic in appearance. It is removed without incident and sent to pathology. Patient tolerated the procedure well and was taken to recovery in good condition. She was discharged home and told to expect a call within one week with biopsy results.

Diagnosis Code(s)

K62.1 Rectal polyp

Coding Note(s)

The polyp is described as being hyperplastic in appearance. Hyperplastic polyps are the most common type of rectal polyps and this type of benign polyp is reported with code K62.1. A type of benign rectal polyp not reported with code K62.1 is an adenomatous polyp, which is reported with the code for a benign neoplasm (D12.8).

Acute Pancreatitis

Acute pancreatitis is a sudden inflammation of the pancreas. The pancreas produces enzymes and the hormones insulin and glucagon. Pancreatitis occurs when the enzymes it produces become active while still in the pancreas and begin to digest the pancreatic tissue, which causes inflammation, bleeding, and damage to the pancreas and pancreatic blood vessels. The condition is most often due to alcoholism or alcohol abuse (alcohol-induced), but may also be caused by blockage of the pancreatic or common bile ducts (biliary), certain drugs (drug-induced), or other conditions such as autoimmune disorders. In some cases, the cause of the pancreatitis is not known (idiopathic).

Category K85 Acute pancreatitis differentiates between acute pancreatitis of unknown cause (idiopathic), due to gallstones (biliary acute pancreatitis), alcohol-induced, drug-induced, and other specified types. There is also a code for unspecified acute pancreatitis. The second axis of coding identifies the acute pancreatitis as occurring either with infected necrosis, with uninfected necrosis, or without necrosis or infection.

Coding and Documentation Requirements

Identify type of acute pancreatitis:

- Alcohol-induced
- Biliary (gallstone)
- Drug-induced
- Idiopathic
- Other specified type
- Unspecified

Identify presence or absence of necrosis/infection:

- Without necrosis or infection
- With uninfected necrosis
- With infected necrosis

ICD-10-CM Code/Documentation	
K85.00	Idiopathic acute pancreatitis without necrosis or infection
K85.01	Idiopathic acute pancreatitis with uninfected necrosis
K85.02	Idiopathic acute pancreatitis with infected necrosis
K85.10	Biliary acute pancreatitis without necrosis or infection
K85.11	Biliary acute pancreatitis with uninfected necrosis
K85.12	Biliary acute pancreatitis with infected necrosis
K85.20	Alcohol induced acute pancreatitis without necrosis or infection
K85.21	Alcohol induced acute pancreatitis with uninfected necrosis
K85.22	Alcohol induced acute pancreatitis with infected necrosis
K85.30	Drug induced acute pancreatitis without necrosis or infection
K85.31	Drug induced acute pancreatitis with uninfected necrosis
K85.32	Drug induced acute pancreatitis with infected necrosis
K85.80	Other acute pancreatitis without necrosis or infection
K85.81	Other acute pancreatitis with uninfected necrosis
K85.82	Other acute pancreatitis with infected necrosis
K85.90	Acute pancreatitis without necrosis or infection, unspecified
K85.91	Acute pancreatitis with uninfected necrosis, unspecified
K85.92	Acute pancreatitis with infected necrosis, unspecified

Documentation and Coding Example

Nineteen-year-old Asian female presents to ED with 2-day history of fever, anorexia, and abdominal pain. Patient states her symptoms came on suddenly while driving back to her college campus after Spring Break. She admits to binge drinking, little sleep, and a lot of junk food during the vacation. PMH is noncontributory, her only medications are oral contraceptive pills and occasional Claritin for seasonal allergies. Temperature 99, HR 96, RR 14, BP 92/62. On examination, this is a petite young woman who is resting rather comfortably on a gurney. She states her symptoms are relieved somewhat by lying flat and describes her abdominal pain as starting suddenly as a sharp pain that radiated into her back, gradually changing into a dull, throbbing pain localized right below her sternum. The pain is fairly constant and she has no appetite, mild waves of nausea, but no vomiting. PERRL, neck supple without lymphadenopathy. HR regular, pulses full. Breath sounds have few scattered rales in the bases bilaterally. Bowel sounds are decreased in all quadrants. There is guarding and tenderness in the RUQ and LUQ but especially over the epigastric area. Patient is menstruating and pelvic exam is deferred at this time. Ultrasound of abdomen is completely benign. Blood drawn for CBC, CRP, comprehensive metabolic panel, liver enzymes including amylase and lipase. IV started in right hand, D5LR infusing. Medicated with MS for pain which allows her to sleep.

Internal Medicine Admit Note: Labs are significant for 14,000 WBC with predominate PMNs, mildly elevated CRP, AST, ALT, calcium, and glucose. Amylase and lipase are significantly elevated. Patient is admitted for **alcohol induced acute pancreatitis**. Orders for NPO, IV hydration, and analgesics. Advance diet to low fat when anorexia/nausea resolves. Monitor electrolytes, lipase, and amylase daily. Finger stick blood glucose monitoring QID. Notify on call resident for BGL >160.

Diagnosis Code(s)

K85.20 Alcohol induced acute pancreatitis without necrosis or infection

Coding Note(s)

A single code captures both the acute pancreatitis and the cause as alcohol induced as well as the presentation without infection or necrosis.

Appendicitis

Appendicitis is an inflammation of the appendix. Also called the vermiform or cecal appendix, this structure is a finger-shaped, blind pouch that extends from the intestine in the area of the cecum near the junction of the large and small intestine. The condition may be acute or chronic. Symptoms can include abdominal pain often starting in the midline and localizing to the right lower quadrant, anorexia, nausea, vomiting, and fever.

Acute appendicitis is subclassified as with generalized peritonitis (K35.2-) or with localized peritonitis (K35.3-). Acute appendicitis with generalized peritonitis may occur with (K35.21) or without (K35.20) abscess. Acute appendicitis with localized peritonitis must be coded more specifically by presentation either with perforation with or without abscess, or without perforation but with or without gangrene. Other codes for appendicitis include unspecified acute appendicitis (without peritonitis) (K35.80), other acute appendicitis without perforation or gangrene (K35.890) or without perforation, with gangrene, other appendicitis (K36) which includes appendicitis documented as chronic or recurrent, and unspecified appendicitis (K37).

Coding and Documentation Requirements

Identify type and presentation of appendicitis:

- Acute appendicitis
  - With generalized peritonitis
    - With abscess
    - Without abscess
  - With localized peritonitis
    - With perforation, with abscess
    - With perforation, without abscess
    - Without perforation or gangrene
    - Without perforation, with gangrene
  - Other acute appendicitis
    - Without perforation or gangrene
    - Without perforation, with gangrene
  - Unspecified acute appendicitis (includes acute appendicitis without peritonitis)
- Other appendicitis, which includes:
  - Chronic
  - Healed (obliterative)
  - Interval
  - Neurogenic
  - Obstructive
  - Recurrent
  - Relapsing
  - Subacute (adhesive)
  - Subsiding
- Unspecified appendicitis

ICD-10-CM Code/Documentation	
K35.20	Acute appendicitis with generalized peritonitis, without abscess
K35.21	Acute appendicitis with generalized peritonitis, with abscess
K35.30	Acute appendicitis with localized peritonitis, without perforation or gangrene
K35.31	Acute appendicitis with localized peritonitis and gangrene, without perforation
K35.32	Acute appendicitis with perforation and localized peritonitis, without abscess
K35.33	Acute appendicitis with perforation and localized peritonitis, with abscess
K35.80	Unspecified acute appendicitis
K35.890	Other acute appendicitis, without perforation or gangrene
K35.891	Other acute appendicitis without perforation, with gangrene
K36	Other appendicitis
K37	Unspecified appendicitis

Documentation and Coding Example

Thirty-six-year-old Caucasian female presents to ED with twelve-hour history of worsening abdominal pain. She states she awoke this morning with mild epigastric pain and no appetite. Her children have had a stomach bug and when she passed some loose stools she thought she probably had the same virus. However, the pain has worsened throughout the day, localized more to the right side and she has nausea but no vomiting. Temperature 99, HR 92, RR 14, BP 126/60. LMP was 3 weeks ago, she is sexually active with her husband and currently uses an IUD for contraception. She has three children ages 1, 4, and 6, all pregnancies uncomplicated and delivered vaginally. On examination, this is a tired appearing woman who looks her stated age. PERRL, neck supple. Mucous membranes dry, pink. HR regular, breath sounds clear. Abdomen is mildly obese and covered with shiny pink striae. Bowel sounds are hypoactive in all quadrants. She has some guarding with palpation but no rebound tenderness. Dunphy, obturator, and psoas signs negative. Pelvic and rectal exams are noncontributory. Blood drawn for CBC, CRP, and electrolytes. Urine sample obtained for UA, beta HCG, 5-HIAA. IV started in left forearm with LR infusing for hydration. Consider ultrasound pending labs.

ED Interim Note: CBC shows elevated WBCs with 75% neutrophils. CRP elevated, electrolytes show mild dehydration. Urine HCG negative, 5-HIAA positive. MANTRELS score is 6. Symptoms are unchanged with hydration. Ultrasound will be obtained. Consider CT if negative.

Four-hour reassessment: Ultrasound unremarkable. Patient has now developed positive Dunphy sign, rebound tenderness. Abdominopelvic **CT reveals periappendicular abscess with localized peritonitis**. Surgical service called to evaluate.

Surgical Service Note: Patient was seen in ED almost 24 hours post onset of abdominal symptoms. She was started on IV Timentin for acute abdomen and taken to the OR mid-morning for an uneventful laparoscopic appendectomy under general anesthesia. Appetite has returned and she tolerates a regular diet, she has also had a normal bowel movement. Discharged home on oral antibiotics and Vicodin for pain. Follow up in Surgery Clinic in 1 week.

Discharge Diagnosis: **Acute appendicitis with periappendicular abscess and localized peritonitis**.

Diagnosis Code(s)

K35.30 Acute appendicitis with localized peritonitis, without perforation or gangrene

Coding Note(s)

Code K35.30 is reported for acute appendicitis with localized peritonitis and includes the condition documented as with a peritoneal abscess as long as the peritonitis is documented as localized. A periappendicular abscess is an abscess around the appendix and it also codes to K35.30 which can be verified using the Alphabetic Index and referencing Abscess, periappendicular. Peritonitis that is not specified as either generalized or localized, stated as occurring with appendicitis, is reported with code K35.2 Acute appendicitis with generalized peritonitis.

Barrett's Esophagus

Barrett's esophagus refers to changes in the lining of the esophagus caused by gastroesophageal reflux. The stomach acid that is refluxed into the esophagus causes the esophageal mucosa to become more like the lining of the stomach. Patients with Barrett's esophagus may develop dysplasia which increases the risk of developing esophageal cancer.

Barrett's esophagus is subclassified as without dysplasia (K22.70) or with dysplasia (K22.71-). For Barrett's esophagus with dysplasia, the dysplasia must be documented as low grade (K22.710) or high grade (K22.711). Documented malignant neoplasm of the esophagus is excluded from the subcategory for Barrett's esophagus and should be reported instead with a code from category C15. Also excluded from this subcategory is Barrett's ulcer (subcategory K22.1).

Coding and Documentation Requirements

Identify presentation of Barrett's esophagus:

- With dysplasia
  - Low grade
  - High grade
  - Unspecified
- Without dysplasia

ICD-10-CM Code/Documentation	
K22.70	Barrett's esophagus without dysplasia
K22.710	Barrett's esophagus with low grade dysplasia
K22.711	Barrett's esophagus with high grade dysplasia
K22.719	Barrett's esophagus with dysplasia, unspecified

Documentation and Coding Example

Forty-five-year-old Hispanic male presents to Gastroenterology Clinic one week following his annual endoscopic evaluation. This pleasant gentleman was diagnosed with Barrett's esophagus four years ago which had been stable with no evidence of dysplasia. He states he feels well and experienced only a few hours of mild throat irritation following the procedure. He confirms that he is taking Prilosec daily and calcium carbonate antacids when he experiences heartburn or upset stomach. He admits that those symptoms have been more frequent in the past few months. Biopsy report is reviewed and findings shared with patient. He has **low grade dysplasia on three of eight tissue samples**. The abnormal samples are all in the area of the distal esophagus within 2 cm of the LES. Advise repeat endoscopy in 6 months with biopsies. We will switch his PPI from Prilosec to Protonix and add a 500 mg calcium carbonate tablet QID, following meals and at bedtime. Patient agrees to this plan, he is given samples of Protonix and a written prescription. He will receive a reminder in the mail in 5 months to schedule his next appointment. He agrees to call sooner should his symptoms change or if he has questions or concerns.

Diagnosis Code(s)

K22.710 Barrett's esophagus with low grade dysplasia

Coding Note(s)

The tissue samples from the esophagus have identified low grade dysplasia in this patient with previously diagnosed Barrett's esophagus. The presence or absence of dysplasia and the severity of the dysplasia is captured by a single code for Barrett's esophagus.

Cholelithiasis

Cholelithiasis refers to the presence of stones or calculi in the gallbladder. Cholelithiasis may occur alone or with cholecystitis, which is an inflammation of the gallbladder most often caused by the presence of calculi or sludge that blocks the flow of bile. Calculi in the bile ducts (choledocholithiasis) may also cause inflammation of the bile ducts, referred to as cholangitis. Cholecystitis may be acute or chronic and chronic cases may be complicated by an acute inflammation.

Codes for cholelithiasis are found in category K80. The site of the calculus is identified along with the presence or absence of any cholecystitis. When cholecystitis is present, specific codes identify it as acute, chronic, acute and chronic, or other.

There are also combination codes for calculus of the bile duct with cholangitis, with cholecystitis, and without cholangitis or cholecystitis. These combination codes also identify the cholangitis or cholecystitis, when present, as acute, chronic, acute and chronic, or unspecified. Other subcategories provide codes for calculus of both the gallbladder and the bile duct with cholecystitis (acute, chronic, acute and chronic, unspecified) and without cholecystitis. The condition of with or without obstruction is also a component of all the cholelithiasis combination codes.

Coding and Documentation Requirements

Identify site of calculus (cholelithiasis):

- Bile duct only
- Gallbladder only
- Gallbladder and bile duct
- Other

For calculus of gallbladder only, identify:

- With cholecystitis
  - Acute
  - Acute and chronic
  - Chronic
  - Other
- Without cholecystitis

For calculus of bile duct only, identify:

- With cholangitis
  - Acute
  - Acute and chronic
  - Chronic
  - Unspecified
- With cholecystitis
  - Acute
  - Acute and chronic
  - Chronic
  - Unspecified
- Without cholangitis or cholecystitis

For calculus of gallbladder and bile duct, identify:

- With cholecystitis
  - Acute
  - Acute and chronic
  - Chronic
  - Unspecified
- Without cholecystitis

Identify as with or without obstruction:

- With obstruction
- Without obstruction

ICD-10-CM Code/Documentation	
K80.30	Calculus of bile duct with cholangitis, unspecified, without obstruction
K80.31	Calculus of bile duct with cholangitis, unspecified, with obstruction
K80.32	Calculus of bile duct with acute cholangitis without obstruction
K80.33	Calculus of bile duct with acute cholangitis with obstruction
K80.34	Calculus of bile duct with chronic cholangitis without obstruction
K80.35	Calculus of bile duct with chronic cholangitis with obstruction
K80.36	Calculus of bile duct with acute and chronic cholangitis without obstruction
K80.37	Calculus of bile duct with acute and chronic cholangitis with obstruction

Documentation and Coding Example

Fifty-two-year-old Caucasian female presents to ED with a two-day history of fever, chills, and right upper quadrant pain that now radiates to her right shoulder and upper back. She states she has a history of gallstones and is scheduled for surgical removal of her gallbladder next month. Temperature 101, HR 102, RR 16, BP 100/50. On examination, this is an acutely ill, mildly obese woman. PERRL, there is no evidence of jaundice in eyes or skin. Neck supple without lymphadenopathy. Mucous membranes moist and pink. Good ROM in upper extremities, reflexes intact, pulses are weak. Apical pulse has a gallop murmur present. Breath sounds have scattered rales throughout. Abdomen is soft, flat with marked tenderness, and guarding in the URQ. Liver is difficult to palpate due to guarding but is below the RCM. Spleen is at the LCM. IV started in left forearm, infusing LR. Blood drawn for CBC, ESR, CRP, comprehensive metabolic panel, liver enzymes. Her surgeon is notified and orders an abdominal ultrasound.

Surgical service note: Patient is seen in ED following abdominal US which shows **dilation of the bile duct with stones present**. Labs are significant for elevated bilirubin, alanine transaminase, and aspartate transaminase. WBC 18,000 with left shift. CRP, ESR elevated.

Impression: **Acute cholangitis with gallstones**. Patient is admitted for IV hydration and antibiotics. Consider ERCP if patient is not improved in 24 hours on ciprofloxacin and metronidazole.

Diagnosis Code(s)

K80.32 Calculus of bile duct with acute cholangitis without obstruction

Coding Note(s)

Code K80.32 captures both the calculus in the bile duct and the cholangitis and more specifically identifies the cholangitis as acute.

Chronic Hepatitis

Hepatitis is an inflammation of the liver that may be an acute or chronic condition. Chronic hepatitis is generally defined as any type of hepatitis lasting longer than 6 months. It is characterized by hepatocellular necrosis with infiltration of inflammatory cells. The condition may be asymptomatic but common symptoms include jaundice (yellow discoloration of eyes and skin), anorexia (loss of appetite), and fatigue.

The difference between chronic persistent hepatitis and chronic active hepatitis is the histological presence of cell necrosis in the active type versus no cell necrosis present in the persistent type. Chronic active hepatitis is also known as chronic aggressive type in which the inflammatory changes in the liver are associated with ongoing necrosis of cells. In chronic persistent hepatitis, the inflammation is confined to the portal tracts and no necrosis is seen. Chronic lobular hepatitis presents a histological pattern in which the portal tracts are inflamed with patches of inflammatory lymphocytic infiltration appearing in the adjacent parenchyma.

Category K73 Chronic hepatitis, not elsewhere classified reports chronic hepatitis as persistent, lobular, active, other specific type, and unspecified. Specified causative types of chronic hepatitis documented as due to viral diseases, alcohol, drugs, toxins, or granulomatous disease have more specific codes and are not reported in category K73. Autoimmune hepatitis is not classified under chronic hepatitis, but is instead listed in category K75 under other inflammatory liver diseases.

Coding and Documentation Requirements

Identify type of chronic hepatitis, not specified as to cause:

- Active
- Lobular
- Persistent
- Other specified type
- Unspecified

ICD-10-CM Code/Documentation	
K73.0	Chronic persistent hepatitis, not elsewhere classified
K73.1	Chronic lobular hepatitis, not elsewhere classified
K73.2	Chronic active hepatitis, not elsewhere classified
K73.8	Other chronic hepatitis, not elsewhere classified
K73.9	Chronic hepatitis, unspecified
K75.4	Autoimmune hepatitis

Documentation and Coding Example

Eleven-month-old Black female presents to Pediatric Gastroenterology Clinic for routine monitoring of her liver function. This delightful infant had a **congenital coarctation of the aorta**, identified on prenatal ultrasound and repaired one month after birth. While her initial postoperative recovery appeared entirely benign, she was found to have abnormal liver function tests one month post surgery. After ruling out viral, autoimmune, or granulomatous diseases, and drugs and toxic exposure, it is believed her **chronic hepatitis has an etiology of ischemic insult related to her cardiac condition**. On examination, her eyes are clear without evidence of jaundice. Her skin pigmentation is relatively light with no underlying jaundice noted. She has a well healed surgical scar in the midline of her chest. Breath sounds are clear and equal bilaterally. Abdomen is soft and round with liver palpated at 2 cm below the RCM. Spleen is palpated at the LCM. There is no ascites appreciated. She was bagged for urine upon arrival and there is a clear light yellow sample, dipstick UA WNL. Blood was drawn upon arrival in clinic today and results are discussed with parents. CBC normal, albumin is low, ALT and AST remain elevated. Bilirubin and PT are in the high normal range as is GGT and APT. Overall her liver function is stable and slightly improved from last month. Plan liver ultrasound prior to next appointment and repeat labs.

Diagnosis: **Chronic hepatitis due to ischemic insult. Status post repair of congenital coarctation of aorta**.

Diagnosis Code(s)

K73.8	Other chronic hepatitis, not elsewhere classified
Z87.74	Personal history of (corrected) congenital malformation of the heart and circulatory system

Coding Note(s)

Category K73 contains codes for chronic hepatitis not elsewhere classified. Codes from this category are reported only when the type of chronic hepatitis does not have a more specific code. There are no specific codes for chronic hepatitis due to ischemic insult, so a code from category K73 is appropriate. There are no additional descriptors other than the etiology of ischemic insult, so the code for other chronic hepatitis not elsewhere classified is assigned. An additional code is assigned to identify the personal history of repair of congenital coarctation of the aorta.

Fibrosis/Sclerosis/Cirrhosis of Liver

Liver fibrosis is a histological change in liver cells caused by liver inflammation. This change is characterized by an increase in collagen fiber deposits in the extra-cellular spaces of the liver causing a decrease in blood perfusion and leading to hardening of the liver cells, or hepatic sclerosis. Liver cirrhosis arises as a late stage of chronic liver fibrosis and sclerosis. It is characterized by progressive changes to the liver's fundamental structure as normal cells are lost and replaced with irreversible scar tissue in the terminal stages of chronic liver disease which may be of alcoholic, nonalcoholic, toxic (drug-induced), or biliary causes. Biliary cirrhosis is a more rare form of cirrhosis caused by inflammation, disease, or defects in the biliary ducts within the liver.

There are specific codes for hepatic fibrosis (K74.00-K74.02), hepatic sclerosis (K74.1), and hepatic fibrosis with sclerosis (K74.2). Codes for cirrhosis include unspecified cirrhosis (K74.60), other cirrhosis (K74.69), alcoholic cirrhosis (K70.3), and codes for reporting biliary cirrhosis. Biliary cirrhosis must be documented as primary (K74.3) or secondary (K74.4) and if primary or secondary is not specified, the code for unspecified biliary cirrhosis must be used (K74.5).

Coding and Documentation Requirements

Identify the condition:

- Cirrhosis
  - Alcoholic
    - » With ascites
    - » Without ascites
  - Biliary
    - » Primary
    - » Secondary
    - » Unspecified
  - Other specified type, nonalcoholic, which includes:
    - » Cryptogenic
    - » Macronodular
    - » Micronodular
    - » Mixed type
    - » Portal
    - » Postnecrotic
  - Unspecified
- Fibrosis and Sclerosis
  - Alcoholic
  - Nonalcoholic
    - » Fibrosis alone
    - » Sclerosis alone

ICD-10-CM Code/Documentation	
K70.2	Alcoholic fibrosis and sclerosis of liver
K70.30	Alcoholic cirrhosis of liver without ascites
K70.31	Alcoholic cirrhosis of liver with ascites
K74.00	Hepatic fibrosis, unspecified
K74.01	Hepatic fibrosis, early fibrosis
K74.02	Hepatic fibrosis, advanced fibrosis
K74.1	Hepatic sclerosis
K74.2	Hepatic fibrosis with hepatic sclerosis
K74.3	Primary biliary cirrhosis
K74.4	Secondary biliary cirrhosis
K74.5	Biliary cirrhosis, unspecified
K74.60	Unspecified cirrhosis of liver
K74.69	Other cirrhosis of liver

Documentation and Coding Example

Thirty-seven-year-old female presents to clinic with complaints of ongoing fatigue, dry itchy skin and eyes, swollen feet and ankles. She has also experienced some digestive problems in the past week, particularly bloating, gas, and loose stools. Patient is a poor historian, losing her train of thought and struggling to understand simple questions. Her twenty-year-old daughter has accompanied her to the appointment and tries to provide more details. Daughter states the fatigue started one year ago right after her mother finished college and was promoted to a new position. She lost interest in cooking and baking, something she was passionate about all of her life. She began to complain about dry skin and itching, trying dozens of lotions to relieve the symptoms. She mentioned her dry itchy eyes to her eye doctor at a routine exam a few months ago and was prescribed Pataday and Zyrtec which have not been helpful. The poor concentration and memory problems are very recent changes and are the primary reason her family insisted she seek medical care. Temperature 97.4, HR 70, RR 12, BP 138/82. Wt. 128 lbs. Ht. 66 inches. On examination, this is a well-developed, well-nourished female. PERRL, xanthoma lesions are present on eyelids. Neck supple without lymphadenopathy. There is no evidence of jaundice, skin warm, dry to touch. Mucous membranes are somewhat dry, good oral hygiene. Cranial nerves are grossly intact. Peripheral pulses full, reflexes normal. There is mild edema in her feet bilaterally with xanthoma lesions also present on the soles of her feet. HR is regular without bruit, rub, or murmur. Breath sounds clear, equal bilaterally. Abdomen is soft, flat with no evidence of ascites. Normal bowel sounds. Liver palpated at 2 cm below the RCM, spleen at LCM. Lab order for fasting CBC, comprehensive metabolic panel, lipid panel, AMA, PT, TSH, and Vitamin D3 level given to patient. RTC in 1 week for test results.

Clinic Follow-Up Note: Labs were significant for elevated AST, APT with positive anti-mitochondrial antibodies (AMA). D3 level 15, mildly decreased platelets, TSH normal. Patient returned for abdominal ultrasound with US guided liver biopsy which showed inflammation and scarring consistent with **primary biliary cirrhosis**. A baseline bone density is planned for next week. Patient was prescribed Actigall for her symptoms and will RTC in 2 weeks for recheck.

Diagnosis Code(s)

K74.3 Primary biliary cirrhosis

Coding Note(s)

The code for primary biliary cirrhosis is assigned as that was documented from the ultrasound findings. Secondary biliary cirrhosis would need to be documented as such if the cause of the bile duct obstruction, narrowing, or closure were caused by another identified condition, such as a tumor.

Gastrointestinal Ulcer

Ulcers of the gastrointestinal tract are a result of damage to the mucus producing cells in the gut. The mucous membrane cells protect the gut from pathogens and the corrosive acid the stomach produces to digest food. There is normally a balance between the acid and the protective mucus in the gut. However, when the balance is disrupted, the mucosal lining can become damaged. Inflammation of the gut lining occurs which may eventually result in ulceration of the underlying tissue. Gastrointestinal ulcers may also be caused by *Helicobacter pylori* infection and some medications. Excessive alcohol use may also predispose an individual to ulcers of the gastrointestinal tract.

Gastrointestinal ulcers are classified by site with different categories provided for gastric ulcers, duodenal ulcers, and gastrojejunal ulcers. Peptic ulcers are reported with codes from a separate category when the site of the gastrointestinal ulcer is not documented. Because some medications increase the risk for gastrointestinal ulcers, an additional code should be reported if there is documentation indicating that the ulcer was drug-induced, even though there is no "use additional code" instruction for drug induced gastrointestinal ulcers.

Codes for ulcers are combination codes that include complications of hemorrhage and/or perforation. However, since obstruction is not a common complication of gastrointestinal ulcers, it is not a component of gastrointestinal ulcer codes. There is a "use additional code" instruction to identify alcohol abuse and dependence.

Documentation and Coding Requirements

Identify site:

- Duodenal
- Gastric
- Gastrojejunal
- Peptic (site unspecified)

Identify as acute/chronic:

- Acute
- Chronic
- Unspecified

Identify complications:

- Both hemorrhage and perforation
- Hemorrhage only
- Perforation only
- Without hemorrhage or perforation

Use additional code to identify alcohol abuse or dependence.

ICD-10-CM Code/Documentation	
K26.0	Acute duodenal ulcer with hemorrhage
K26.1	Acute duodenal ulcer with perforation
K26.2	Acute duodenal ulcer with both hemorrhage and perforation
K26.3	Acute duodenal ulcer without hemorrhage or perforation
K26.4	Chronic or unspecified duodenal ulcer with hemorrhage
K26.5	Chronic or unspecified duodenal ulcer with perforation
K26.6	Chronic or unspecified duodenal ulcer with both hemorrhage and perforation
K26.7	Chronic duodenal ulcer without hemorrhage or perforation
K26.9	Duodenal ulcer, unspecified as acute or chronic, without hemorrhage or perforation

Documentation and Coding Example

Thirty-nine-year-old Caucasian female presents to GI Clinic for upper endoscopy after a one-month history of vague upper abdominal pain, nausea, anorexia, and a 10 lb. weight loss. She had vacationed in Bali prior to the onset of symptoms and saw her PMD who prescribed OTC ranitidine which was not helpful. CBC and electrolytes have all been WNL. She was referred to GI for consult. A blood test for ***H. pylori* was found to be positive.** She agreed to EGD before starting antibiotics and PPI to treat the *H. pylori* infection. She denies vomiting blood, passing dark or tarry stools. PMH: Seasonal allergies treated with Zyrtec when necessary. She does not smoke, but does drink alcohol, 1-2 glasses of wine 2-3 x week. Denies use of NSAIDs. Patient is single and works in public relations. The procedure was explained, questions answered, and informed consent was obtained. Patient was placed on cardiac monitor and pulse oximeter. An IV was started in her right hand with LR infusing, throat was sprayed with Cetacaine and she was sedated with Versed and Fentanyl. With the patient resting on her right side on the treatment table, the scope was easily passed down the esophagus which was entirely normal in appearance. The stomach was examined next and was also WNL. Transition though the pylorus was somewhat difficult due to very tight musculature and upon entering the **duodenum profuse inflammation was encountered in the duodenal bulb with a 1.5 cm ulceration noted** on the posterior surface just beyond the pylorus. The ulcer bed showed **no evidence of bleeding and involved only the superficial muscularis mucosae.** The inflammation diminished markedly at the descending duodenum and was completely gone by the turn of the ascending duodenum. Biopsies and brushings of the ulcer were obtained and the scope was withdrawn. Patient tolerated the procedure well and was discharged home 2 hours later.

Impression: **Acute duodenal ulcer due to *Helicobacter pylori* infection.**

Plan: Amoxicillin, Metronidazole and Pantoprazole x 2 weeks. Repeat EGD only if symptoms do not improve. Patient will call in 1 week for biopsy results.

Note electronically sent to PMD.

Diagnosis Code(s)

K26.3	Acute duodenal ulcer without hemorrhage or perforation
B96.81	Helicobacter pylori [H. pylori] as the cause of diseases classified elsewhere

Coding Note(s)

The physician has documented that the acute duodenal ulcer is due to *H. pylori* infection. The code for the acute duodenal ulcer is the first listed code and an additional code is assigned to identify the cause as *H. pylori.*

Inguinal Hernia

An inguinal hernia occurs when there is a weakness in the muscles in the groin area between the abdomen and thigh that allows the omentum or intestine to protrude through the weakened area. Inguinal hernias typically enlarge over time if they are not surgically repaired. This can cause pressure on surrounding tissues with resulting discomfort or pain. In men, a large inguinal hernia can extend into the scrotum causing pain and swelling in the scrotum. More serious complications of inguinal hernia include incarceration or strangulation of the intestine. Incarceration occurs when a loop of omentum or intestine becomes trapped in the weakened area of the muscle, which can lead to bowel obstruction. Strangulation occurs when the blood supply is cut off to the herniated portion of the intestine. This can lead to death of the strangulated bowel tissue and gangrene. For coding purposes, an incarcerated and/or strangulated hernia without gangrene is classified as a hernia with obstruction. Irreducible hernia is another term also used to describe an incarcerated hernia. For a hernia with documented gangrene with or without mention of obstruction, the code for hernia with gangrene is assigned.

Inguinal hernias are first classified as bilateral or unilateral and then as with obstruction without gangrene, with gangrene, or without obstruction or gangrene. At the fifth character level inguinal hernias are classified as recurrent or not specified as recurrent.

Documentation and Coding Requirements

Identify inguinal hernia as unilateral/bilateral:

- Bilateral
- Unilateral/Unspecified

Identify presence/absence of complications:

- Gangrene (and obstruction)
- Obstruction, without gangrene
- Without obstruction or gangrene

Identify as recurrent/not recurrent:

- Not specified as recurrent
- Recurrent

ICD-10-CM Code/Documentation	
K40.40	Unilateral inguinal hernia, with gangrene, not specified as recurrent
K40.41	Unilateral inguinal hernia, with gangrene, recurrent
K40.30	Unilateral inguinal hernia, with obstruction, without gangrene, not specified as recurrent
K40.31	Unilateral inguinal hernia, with obstruction, without gangrene, recurrent
K40.90	Unilateral inguinal hernia, without obstruction or gangrene, not specified as recurrent
K40.91	Unilateral inguinal hernia, without obstruction or gangrene, recurrent
K40.10	Bilateral inguinal hernia, with gangrene, not specified as recurrent
K40.11	Bilateral inguinal hernia, with gangrene, recurrent
K40.00	Bilateral inguinal hernia, with obstruction, without gangrene, not specified as recurrent
K40.01	Bilateral inguinal hernia, with obstruction, without gangrene, recurrent
K40.20	Bilateral inguinal hernia, without obstruction or gangrene, not specified as recurrent
K40.21	Bilateral inguinal hernia, without obstruction or gangrene, recurrent

Documentation and Coding Example

Twenty-four-year-old Black male presents to PMD with a lump in his left groin. Patient is an active duty police officer who first noticed the lump in the evening after a vigorous day on the job but it was gone in the morning. He noticed it again yesterday after a typical gym workout with weights and cardio and the lump was still present when he awoke this morning. He denies pain, changes in bowel habits, or any urinary symptoms. **PMH is significant for bilateral inguinal hernias, repaired in infancy and acute lymphocytic leukemia at age 7**. On examination, this is a healthy appearing Black male who looks his stated age. Eyes clear, PERRLA. Mucous membranes moist and pink. Cranial nerves grossly intact. Breath sounds clear, equal bilaterally. Heart rate regular without murmur, rub, or bruit. He has a 4 cm linear keloid scar in his left anterior chest which he states is from an old Port-A-Cath location. Abdomen soft, flat, and muscular. Liver palpated at RCM, spleen is not palpated. He has active bowel sounds in all quadrants. There are well healed keloid scars along both inguinal areas from his previous hernia repairs. Testicles are down, normal circumcised penis. With the patient standing, the right inguinal ring is examined and found to be intact with no evidence of hernia. The left inguinal ring is found to be compromised allowing the examiners fingertip to advance up into the inguinal canal with a protrusion striking the finger pad. The bulge enlarges with coughing but is **easily reduced**.

Impression: **Left inguinal hernia, recurrent**. Plan: Refer to general surgery for non-emergent repair. Patient is advised of symptoms that would require immediate treatment and he verbalizes understanding.

Diagnosis Code(s)

K40.91 Unilateral inguinal hernia, without obstruction or gangrene, recurrent

Z85.6 Personal history of leukemia

Coding Note(s)

The patient has an uncomplicated recurrent unilateral hernia which is the reason for the visit. The patient also has a history of lymphocytic leukemia, which is reported additionally. In ICD-10-CM, the personal history code identifies the condition only as a personal history of leukemia without identifying the type.

Irritable Bowel Syndrome

Irritable bowel syndrome (IBS) is a common, noninflammatory bowel disease characterized by abdominal pain and cramping, changes in bowel movements, and other symptoms. Onset is usually before age 35, with women affected more than men, and often there is a positive family history of the condition. Irritable bowel syndrome (K58.-) must be documented as with or without diarrhea, with constipation, or mixed alternating with diarrhea and constipation, and other irritable bowel syndrome.

Coding and Documentation Requirements

Identify as irritable bowel syndrome:

- With diarrhea
- Without diarrhea
- With constipation
- Mixed
- Other

ICD-10-CM Code/Documentation	
K58.0	Irritable bowel syndrome with diarrhea
K58.1	Irritable bowel syndrome with constipation
K58.2	Mixed irritable bowel syndrome
K58.8	Other irritable bowel syndrome
K58.9	Irritable bowel syndrome without diarrhea

Documentation and Coding Example

Twenty-four-year-old female presents today for annual medical exam. She admits to having a stressful year with her marriage 6 months ago and starting a new business 2 months ago. She states her symptoms began with abdominal pain, vomiting, and diarrhea on her honeymoon cruise. There was a CDC confirmed norovirus outbreak on the ship. Her acute symptoms resolved with fluids and rest but she has continued to experience **abdominal cramps, gas, bloating, and bouts of diarrhea**. She has tried a dairy free diet, limiting caffeine and alcohol, and increasing dietary fiber. Her appetite is decreased. Temperature 98.2, HR 70, RR 12, BP 102/68, Wt. 110. On examination, this is a well-groomed, tired appearing young woman. PERRL, neck supple, cranial nerves grossly intact. HR regular without bruit, rubs, or murmur. Breath sounds clear, equal bilaterally. Abdomen is soft and flat. Bowel sounds high pitched and hyperactive. Liver palpated at 1 cm below RCM, spleen is not palpated. Pelvic exam is deferred as she saw her GYN just 3 months ago and the exam was normal. She is using a diaphragm for contraception.

Impression: **Irritable bowel syndrome**.

Plan: Blood drawn for CBC, comprehensive metabolic panel, TSH. Stool sample for O & P and cultures. Patient is prescribed hyoscyamine ½ hour before meals for abdominal cramps and **loperamide BID if needed for diarrhea.** F/U appointment in two weeks to see if symptoms have improved. Consider adding a low dose tricyclic antidepressant at that time if she is still exhibiting symptoms and lab work is normal.

Diagnosis Code(s)

K58.0	Irritable bowel syndrome with diarrhea

Coding Note(s)

There are separate codes for irritable bowel syndrome with diarrhea and without diarrhea, which is one of the common symptoms of the condition. The impression states only that the patient has irritable bowel syndrome; however, the physician has also documented diarrhea in the history and prescribed medication for the diarrhea so code K58.0 Irritable bowel syndrome with diarrhea is assigned.

Regional Enteritis (Crohn's Disease)

Regional enteritis, also called Crohn's disease, is a type of inflammatory bowel disease. It typically affects the intestines, but can occur anywhere from the mouth to the anus. The condition is characterized by abdominal pain, diarrhea, vomiting, and weight loss. The onset of Crohn's disease is believed to be influenced by an interaction between the environment, the immune system, and intestinal bacteria in genetically susceptible individuals. While often described as an autoimmune disorder, the condition is now thought to be an immune deficiency state. Crohn's disease is characterized by chronic inflammation and thickening of the gastrointestinal tract. Complications include bleeding, fistula formation, abscess, and obstruction.

Category K50 Crohn's disease is specific to site but contains information on complications of the disease. Medical record documentation must identify any complications, which include rectal bleeding, intestinal obstruction, fistula, abscess, and other specified complications. There is also a code for Crohn's disease identified as without complications and one for Crohn's disease identified as with complications but with no documentation as to the specific type of complication.

Coding and Documentation Requirements

Identify site of regional enteritis/Crohn's disease:

- Small intestine
- Large intestine
- Both small and large intestine
- Unspecified site

Identify as with or without complications:

- With complication
  - Abscess
  - Fistula
  - Intestinal obstruction
  - Rectal bleeding
  - Other specific complication
  - Unspecified complication
- Without complication

ICD-10-CM Code/Documentation	
K50.10	Crohn's disease of large intestine without complications
K50.111	Crohn's disease of large intestine with rectal bleeding
K50.112	Crohn's disease of large intestine with intestinal obstruction
K50.113	Crohn's disease of large intestine with fistula
K50.114	Crohn's disease of large intestine with abscess
K50.118	Crohn's disease of large intestine with other complication
K50.119	Crohn's disease of large intestine with unspecified complications

Documentation and Coding Example

Fifteen-year-old Caucasian male is referred to Pediatric Gastroenterology Clinic by his PMD with a 3-month history of crampy abdominal pain and intermittent **diarrhea which has become bloody in the past few days**. Patient is seen with his mother who does most of the talking. She states his symptoms came on gradually and they have been to the pediatrician numerous times. He was initially treated for gastroenteritis with a BRAT diet. When symptoms persisted, he was put on a dairy free diet and stool samples were checked for parasites. Upon request mother allows the patient to be examined in private. Temperature 98.8, HR 66, RR 14, BP 98/59, Ht. 68", Wt. 131 lbs. Patient is more relaxed and answers questions readily with his mother out of the room. He admits to extreme fatigue and disappointment that he has been unable to play baseball this semester due to his illness. He feels his social life has suffered and he admits he may be a little depressed. On examination, this is a thin young man with good hygiene, clear skin, minimal face and body hair but a thick, curly head of hair. PERRL, neck supple without lymphadenopathy. Cranial nerves grossly intact. TMs clear, mucous membranes moist and pink. Nares patent and pharynx clear. HR regular without murmur, bruit, or rubs. Breath sounds clear, equal bilaterally. Peripheral pulses full with normal reflexes. Abdomen concave, with good muscle definition, prominent hip and rib bones. Bowel sounds are hyperactive. Liver is palpated at the RCM and spleen at the LCM. There is minimal guarding to deep palpation on the left side, none on right. Testicles are descended bilaterally, no evidence of inguinal hernia. Penis is circumcised and there is no drainage from the urethra. DRE shows good sphincter tone.

Impression: Probable inflammatory bowel disease.

Plan: Upper endoscopy followed by colonoscopy. Blood drawn for CBC, comprehensive metabolic panel, serum albumin, CRP, ESR, ASCA, and p-ANCA antigen. Repeat stool sample for culture, O & P.

GI Clinic Follow up Note: Upper endoscopy unremarkable. Findings on colonoscopy were significant for **patchy areas of inflammation from anus to cecum with an area just below the ileocecal junction that is actively bleeding**. CBC showed mildly elevated WBC, no anemia. Elevated CRP, ESR. ASCA positive, p-ANCA antigen negative. Findings are consistent with **Crohn's Disease**. Patient is started on Mesalamine for the inflammation. He will return to clinic in 2 weeks for recheck and will have a repeat colonoscopy in 3 months, sooner if symptoms are not improved on this treatment regimen.

Diagnosis Code(s)

K50.111 Crohn's disease of large intestine with rectal bleeding

Coding Note(s)

The patient has areas of inflammation from the anus to the cecum so the Crohn's disease is confined to the large intestine. The condition is complicated by rectal bleeding and that is captured by code K50.111.

Sialadenitis

Sialadenitis is an infection of one or more of the salivary glands. Infections are relatively common and may be either viral or bacterial. Infections may also be recurrent. The parotid glands are the largest pair of salivary glands, and infection of the parotid gland may be documented as parotitis. The other two pairs of salivary glands that may become infected are the submandibular and sublingual glands.

Instead of one single code for infection of the salivary glands, sialadenitis (K11.2-) is subclassified as acute, acute recurrent, and chronic. Infections of the parotid glands due to mumps virus (B26.) and uveoparotid fever (D86.89) are excluded from conditions reported with codes in subcategory K11.2-.

Coding and Documentation Requirements

Identify status of sialadenitis:

- Acute
- Acute recurrent
- Chronic
- Unspecified

ICD-10-CM Code/Documentation	
K11.20	Sialadenitis, unspecified
K11.21	Acute sialadenitis
K11.22	Acute recurrent sialadenitis
K11.23	Chronic sialadenitis

Documentation and Coding Example

Twelve-year-old female presents to pediatrician with painful swelling along her cheek and right jaw. Child was on a school sponsored camping trip and states she became ill 1 day ago with fever and pain in front of her ear and along her right jaw. She was given Tylenol by her teacher. Her mother noticed swelling on the right side of her face and neck as soon as she got off the bus last night. Temperature 101, HR 92, RR 14, BP 98/50. On examination, this is a slim, ill-appearing adolescent female. PERRL. Neck supple. The left side of the face is normal without swelling or tenderness. There is obvious swelling over the right cheek and jaw and the right parotid gland is enlarged and firm to touch. She complains of acute tenderness over and around the right parotid gland. The preauricular and supraclavicular lymph nodes on the right side are also enlarged. The buccal mucosa on the left is normal. The buccal mucosa of the right cheek is red and inflamed. Breath is quite foul smelling despite good oral hygiene. Purulent drainage is noted from Stensen's duct on the right. Breath sounds clear, equal bilaterally. HR regular. Swab of drainage from right Stensen's duct sent to lab for culture and sensitivity.

Diagnosis: **Acute sialadenitis right parotid gland.**

Plan: Will treat with one dose of IV Clindamycin followed by oral antibiotics for 10 days.

Addendum: Lab results indicate ***S. aureus* infection** sensitive to prescribed antibiotics.

Diagnosis Code(s)

K11.21 Acute sialadenitis

B95.61 Methicillin susceptible Staphylococcus aureus infection (MSSA) as the cause of diseases classified elsewhere

Coding Note(s)

The default code for *S. aureus* infection not specified as methicillin resistant or methicillin susceptible is the code for methicillin susceptible. Methicillin is a beta lactam antibiotic and *S. aureus* that is susceptible to any beta lactam is classified as MSSA. Clindamycin is a commonly prescribed antibiotic for anaerobic bacterial infections of the mouth, including dental infections. Clindamycin is not a beta lactam antibiotic; however, because there is no documentation indicating resistance to beta lactam antibiotics, the infection is classified as methicillin susceptible.

Code K11.21 is specific for acute sialadenitis that is not documented as recurrent.

Toxic Liver Disease

The liver plays a key role in concentrating and metabolizing ingested nutrients and chemicals. Many substances can cause damage to the liver in both therapeutic doses and overdose amounts. When the liver is damaged by a drug or toxic substance, it is referred to as toxic liver disease. Damage may be widespread but is more commonly confined to a zone or liver lobule. The condition may be asymptomatic although common symptoms include jaundice (yellow discoloration of eyes and skin), anorexia (loss of appetite), and fatigue.

Category K71 includes codes for toxic liver disease with cholestasis, necrosis, active, chronic and other forms of hepatitis, fibrosis and cirrhosis, and other liver disorders. Chronic hepatitis in toxic liver disease is brought on by constant exposure to toxic substances such as drugs and chemicals that the liver must break down and remove from the bloodstream. Such toxic substances include over-the-counter pain relievers, prescription medications, industrial chemicals such as cleaning solvents and herbicides, and even overuse of certain herbal supplements.

Toxic liver disease (K71) is its own category. Codes in this category are combination codes that identify both the condition as toxic liver disease and the manifestation, such as cholestasis, hepatic necrosis, hepatitis, fibrosis and cirrhosis, or other specified disorders of the liver, as well as additional complications such as coma and ascites.

Coding and Documentation Requirements

Identify the toxic liver disease with its manifestations/complications:

- Cholestasis
- Fibrosis/cirrhosis
- Hepatic necrosis
  - » With coma
  - » Without coma
- Hepatitis
  - Acute
  - Chronic
    - » Active
    - » With ascites
    - » Without ascites
    - » Lobular
    - » Persistent
  - Not elsewhere classified
- Other specified disorders of liver, which include:
  - Focal nodular hyperplasia
  - Hepatic granulomas
  - Peliosis hepatis
  - Veno-occlusive disease
- Unspecified disorder

Assign a code from T36-T65 with fifth or sixth character 1-4 or 6 as the first-listed code when applicable for poisoning:

- Identify drug or toxin
- Identify intent
  - Accidental (unintentional)
  - Assault
  - Intentional self harm
  - Underdosing
  - Undetermined

If condition was due to an adverse effect of a drug used therapeutically (right drug, right dose, right route of administration), use an additional code from T36-T65 with fifth or sixth character 5.

ICD-10-CM Code/Documentation	
K71.0	Toxic liver disease with cholestasis
K71.10	Toxic liver disease with hepatic necrosis, without coma
K71.11	Toxic liver disease with hepatic necrosis, with coma
K71.2	Toxic liver disease with acute hepatitis
K71.3	Toxic liver disease with chronic persistent hepatitis
K71.4	Toxic liver disease with chronic lobular hepatitis
K71.50	Toxic liver disease with chronic active hepatitis without ascites
K71.51	Toxic liver disease with chronic active hepatitis with ascites
K71.6	Toxic liver disease with hepatitis, not elsewhere classified
K71.7	Toxic liver disease with fibrosis and cirrhosis of liver
K71.8	Toxic liver disease with other disorders of liver
K71.9	Toxic liver disease, unspecified

Documentation and Coding Example

Twenty-year-old Caucasian male presents to PMD with a few months history of weight loss, fatigue, and a scaly yellow rash. In the past few days he has developed yellow discoloration in his eyes and dark brown urine. He recently returned from a 6-month study abroad program in Fiji. He denies acute illness or recent injury. He states he was living on a fairly remote island and ate mostly fresh fish and native plants. He developed a taste for Kava root and being unable to find a plant to grow and harvest from, he bought some **Kava root** powder off the internet and has been brewing it as a tea. On examination, this is an ill appearing young man, thin, with noticeable muscle wasting. Temperature 99, HR 100, RR 14, BP 114/70, Wt. 142, Ht. 70 inches. Sclera is dull and yellow, PERRL. Neck supple with a few enlarged supraclavicular lymph nodes. Mucous membranes pale pink and dry. Nares patent. He has noticeable plaque buildup on his teeth and there are scattered herpes-like mouth sores on gums, buccal mucosa, and soft palate. Skin is very dry with raised areas of yellow discoloration and flaking/scaling of the epidermis. Heart rate regular, soft S2 murmur present, no bruit or rub. Breath sounds clear, equal bilaterally. Abdomen is mildly distended and tender with a faint fluid shift on palpation. Liver is 4 cm below the RCM. Femoral pulses intact, no hernia appreciated. Testicles down and penis uncircumcised with easily retracted foreskin and no drainage noted from urethra. DRE shows good sphincter tone and stool negative for occult blood. Patient is sent to ER for blood tests and IV hydration. Admit pending lab results.

Impression: **Acute hepatitis, possibly due to Kava poisoning.**

Floor Note Day 1: Patient was observed in ED for 4 hours while receiving IV hydration with LR and then admitted to medical floor. His initial lab results were significant for macrocytosis of RBCs, low platelets, elevated LFTs. Hepatitis Panel is negative for viral infection. Herpes virus also negative. Family member brought in a sample of Kava which is still being analyzed. Abdominal ultrasound showed thickening in the area of the center lobe of the liver, negative for ascites. US guided liver biopsy was performed with pathology still pending. VS are stable.

Floor Note Day 2: Liver biopsy revealed inflammatory cells but no evidence of fibrosis or cirrhosis. Preliminary chemical analysis of Kava sample did not show any gross contaminants but does appear to be a very potent extract of the plant. Nutrition consult ordered. Plan discharge in AM if patient remains stable.

Diagnosis: **Acute hepatitis due to P. methysticum ingestion**.

Diagnosis Code(s)

T62.2X1A Toxic effect of other ingested (parts of) plant(s), accidental (unintentional), initial encounter

K71.2 Toxic liver disease with acute hepatitis

Coding Note(s)

There is no specific code for toxic effects of Kava or for the chemical methysticum, which is responsible for the sedative effects of the plant. A nonspecific code for toxic effect of a plant is assigned. The external cause is accidental because the patient did not intend to harm himself with the Kava tea.

There is a note for codes in category K71 indicating that the drug or toxin is coded first. Code T62.2x1- requires a 7th character to identify the episode of care, which in this case is the initial encounter because the patient is receiving care for the acute phase of the illness. The 7th character 'A' is appended to the code to designate the initial encounter. The code for toxic liver disease, K71.2, is specific to acute hepatitis and is sequenced after the toxic effect code.

Ulcerative Colitis

Ulcerative colitis is a chronic inflammatory bowel disease that affects the large intestine including the rectum. The condition is usually intermittent with exacerbation of symptoms consisting of diarrhea with or without blood and/or mucus, and then extended periods without symptoms. The disease is treated as an autoimmune disorder with a presumed genetic susceptibility for development and certain environmental factors that trigger the immune response. Foods and diet do not usually influence the disease but stress is often a factor with exacerbations.

Ulcerative colitis (K51) requires documentation of both the site and any complications. Documentation should identify the condition as the following:

- Inflammatory polyps (K51.4-) – Small localized areas of inflammation
- Left sided colitis (K51.5-) – Also called left hemicolitis, involving the rectum, sigmoid colon, and descending colon
- Pancolitis (K51.0-) – Includes ulcerative (chronic) colitis involving the small intestine and colon (enterocolitis); ileum and colon (ileocolitis), also called backwash ileitis; and universal colitis
- Proctitis (K51.2-) – Ulcerative colitis involving only the rectum
- Rectosigmoiditis (K51.3-) – Ulcerative colitis involving only the rectum and sigmoid colon
- Other ulcerative colitis (K51.8-) – Other specified site or sites
- Unspecified colitis (K51.9-) – Site is not specified in the documentation

Coding and Documentation Requirements

Identify the site of ulcerative colitis or condition:

- Inflammatory polyps
- Left sided colitis
- Pancolitis (enterocolitis, ileocolitis, universal colitis)
- Proctitis
- Rectosigmoiditis (proctosigmoiditis)
- Other specified site
- Unspecified site

Identify as with or without complications:

- With complication
  - Abscess
  - Fistula
  - Intestinal obstruction
  - Rectal bleeding
  - Other specified complication
  - Unspecified complication
- Without complication

ICD-10-CM Code/Documentation	
K51.40	Inflammatory polyps of colon without complications
K51.411	Inflammatory polyps of colon with rectal bleeding
K51.412	Inflammatory polyps of colon with intestinal obstruction
K51.413	Inflammatory polyps of colon with fistula
K51.414	Inflammatory polyps of colon with abscess
K51.418	Inflammatory polyps of colon with other complication
K51.419	Inflammatory polyps of colon with unspecified complications

Documentation and Coding Example

Fifty-year-old Caucasian female presents to her gastroenterologist with a 4-day history of abdominal pain and bloating. She is having 4-6 loose stools per day that contain blood and mucus. PMH is significant for ulcerative colitis diagnosed in college and treated with sulfazine for a few years. On review of her records, her last flare was almost 10 years ago and resolved with cortisone enemas. She was advised to schedule a colonoscopy at that time but did not return until today. She admits to being under considerable stress right now. Her son will have his Bar Mitzvah in two weeks and it is a huge affair for her family both religiously and socially. Temperature 100.2, HR 88, RR 12, BP 128/70, Wt. 103. On examination, this is a thin, almost emaciated appearing woman, impeccably groomed who looks somewhat younger than her stated age. Oral mucosa is moist, pink with a few scattered aphthous ulcers noted on the posterior pharynx. Abdomen appears slightly distended; bowel sounds are high pitched and hyperactive. There is tenderness and guarding with deep palpation over the left upper and lower quadrants. DRE causes marked tenesmus. Informed consent obtained and patient is sedated for colonoscopy without bowel prep. **Visual exam is significant for inflammation with multiple areas of ulceration involving the rectum and descending colon. At the junction of the transverse and descending colon is a large pseudopolyp causing significant obstruction of the bowel lumen.** This is removed without difficulty and sent for pathology. Patient tolerated the procedure well and after adequate recovery she is discharged home with a prescription for Azathioprine orally and cortisone enemas. RTC in 1 week for recheck.

Diagnosis: **Chronic ulcerative colitis with large pseudopolyp causing obstruction at junction of transverse and descending colon.**

Diagnosis Code(s)

K51.412 Inflammatory polyps of colon with intestinal obstruction

Coding Note(s)

In the Alphabetic Index under Colitis, ulcerative, pseudopolyp, there is a note to see polyps, colon, inflammatory. When this reference is checked, the code provided is K51.40 which is reported for uncomplicated inflammatory polyps. However, the inflammatory polyps are complicated by intestinal obstruction so code K51.412 is reported.

Summary

The most important documentation issues to be aware of in the digestive system chapter include:

- Identification of conditions as acute, chronic, or acute and chronic. Example: Anal fissure requires documentation of the condition as acute or chronic.
- Identification of any acute conditions that are recurrent as acute recurrent. Example: Sialadenitis requires documentation of the condition as acute, acute recurrent, or chronic.
- Clearly identifying any complications that are often associated with specific conditions. Example: Combination codes for Crohn's disease and regional enteritis require clear documentation of any complications.
- Specifically identifying the site. Example: Anal and rectal abscesses now require documentation of site as anal, rectal, anorectal, ischiorectal, or intrasphincteric.
- Precisely documenting the etiology of some diseases. Example: Acute pancreatitis should be documented as alcohol-induced, biliary (gallstone), drug-induced, idiopathic, or other specific type.
- Documenting diseases and disorders with specific concomitant conditions. Example: Toxic liver disease should now be documented as with cholestasis, with hepatic necrosis with or without coma, with acute hepatitis, with chronic persistent hepatitis, with chronic lobular hepatitis, with chronic active hepatitis with or without ascites, with other specified hepatitis, with fibrosis and cirrhosis, or with other specific liver disorders.

Resources

Documentation checklists are available in Appendix A for the following condition(s):

- Cholecystitis, Cholelithiasis, Choledocholithiasis, and Cholangitis

Chapter 11 Quiz

1. The physician has documented the diagnosis as cholelithiasis with cholecystitis. What additional information is required to capture the most specific code for cholelithiasis with cholecystitis?
   a. Documentation of the cholecystitis as acute and/or chronic
   b. Documentation of cholelithiasis as with or without obstruction
   c. Documentation of the site of the calculus as gallbladder and/or bile duct
   d. All of the above
2. The term pseudopolyposis of the colon is synonymous with what term?
   a. Polyposis of colon
   b. Adenomatous polyp of colon
   c. Inflammatory polyps of colon
   d. Polyps of colon
3. What disorder due to toxic liver disease would not be reported with code K71.8?
   a. Peliosis hepatis
   b. Chronic lobular hepatitis
   c. Hepatic granulomas
   d. Focal nodular hyperplasia
4. What additional information must be documented related to acute pancreatitis to capture the most specific code?
   a. Etiology
   b. Complications
   c. Manifestations
   d. Both a. and b.
5. When a patient has toxic liver disease caused by ingestion of a toxic plant, what is the principle or first listed diagnosis code?
   a. The code for the toxic liver disease
   b. The code for the adverse effect of the toxic plant
   c. The toxic effect code that identifies the plant
   d. It depends on the circumstances surrounding the admission
6. The physician has documented left sided ulcerative colitis. What additional information is required to assign the most specific code?
   a. The specific sites in the left side must be identified as the rectum, sigmoid colon, and descending colon
   b. Any complications must be documented, or the documentation must be specific enough for the coder to know that there are no associated complications
   c. Rectal bleeding can be assumed but other complications must be specifically documented
   d. The condition must be specified as acute or chronic
7. The physician has documented that the patient has sialoadenitis. What additional information is needed to capture the most specific code?
   a. Identification of the specific salivary gland as parotid, submandibular, or sublingual
   b. Documentation of laterality (right, left, bilateral)
   c. Documentation of acute, acute recurrent, or chronic
   d. Documentation of with or without complications
8. What type of chronic hepatitis is classified in the category for other inflammatory liver diseases?
   a. Autoimmune hepatitis
   b. Chronic persistent hepatitis
   c. Chronic lobular hepatitis
   d. Chronic active hepatitis
9. What condition is not reported with a code from Chapter 11 Diseases of the Digestive System?
   a. Parotitis due to mumps
   b. Dental caries
   c. Indigestion
   d. Retroperitoneal abscess
10. What is NOT a documentation consideration for reporting codes within the digestive system chapter?
    a. Designation of additional conditions as acute and/or chronic
    b. Designation of some recurrent conditions as acute recurrent
    c. Combination codes requiring more specific documentation of complications related to certain conditions
    d. Infectious or parasitic etiologies

See next page for answers and rationales.

Chapter 11 Answers and Rationales

1. The physician has documented the diagnosis as cholelithiasis with cholecystitis. What additional information is required to capture the most specific code for cholelithiasis with cholecystitis?

   d. All of the above

   Rationale: *To assign the most specific code, the cholecystitis must be documented as acute, chronic, or acute and chronic; the site of the calculus must be documented as gallbladder, bile duct, or gallbladder and bile duct; and the physician must indicate whether the calculus is obstructing the flow of bile.*

2. The term pseudopolyposis of the colon is synonymous with what term?

   c. Inflammatory polyps of colon

   Rationale: *Pseudopolyposis of the colon is synonymous with inflammatory polyps of the colon which is reported with a code from subcategory K62.1. The other conditions are excluded from subcategory K62.1. Polyposis and adenomatous polyps are reported with code D12.6 and polyps not otherwise specified are reported with K63.5.*

3. What disorder due to toxic liver disease would not be reported with code K71.8?

   b. Chronic lobular hepatitis

   Rationale: *Code K71.8 reports toxic liver disease with other disorders of the liver which includes peliosis hepatis, hepatic granulomas, focal nodular hyperplasia, and veno-occlusive disease of the liver. Toxic liver disease with chronic lobular hepatitis is reported with code K71.4.*

4. What additional information must be documented related to acute pancreatitis to capture the most specific code?

   d. Both a. and b.

   Rationale: *Etiology refers to the cause of the acute pancreatitis and must be documented as idiopathic (unknown cause), biliary (gallstone), alcohol-induced, drug-induced, or of other specified cause. If the etiology is not documented, the code for unspecified acute pancreatitis (K85.9) must be assigned. The second axis of coding is the absence or presence of complications such as infected necrosis, uninfected necrosis, and without necrosis or infection.*

5. When a patient has toxic liver disease caused by ingestion of a toxic plant, what is the principle or first listed diagnosis code?

   c. The toxic effect code that identifies the plant

   Rationale: *There is a note for codes in category K71 indicating that the drug or toxin is coded first. All codes in categories T51-T65 are related to toxic effects and capture the intent as accidental, intentional self-harm, assault, or undetermined. There are no codes for adverse effects because adverse effects refer to drugs and medicinal substances only, not to nonmedicinal substances.*

6. The physician has documented left sided ulcerative colitis. What additional information is required to assign the most specific code?

   b. Any complications must be documented, or the documentation must be specific enough for the coder to know that there are no associated complications

   Rationale: *There are now combination codes for ulcerative colitis and specific complications, so any complications must be documented or the code for ulcerative colitis without complications is assigned. No additional information is required related to site because left sided or left hemicolon ulcerative colitis is defined as involving the rectum, sigmoid colon, and descending colon. While rectal bleeding is a common symptom of ulcerative colitis, the physician must document the presence of rectal bleeding – it cannot be assumed. Ulcerative colitis is not differentiated as acute or chronic.*

7. The physician has documented that the patient has sialoadenitis. What additional information is needed to capture the most specific code?

   c. Documentation of acute, acute recurrent, or chronic

   Rationale: *The only additional information required to capture the most specific code is documentation of the condition as acute, acute recurrent or chronic*

8. What type of chronic hepatitis is classified in the category for other inflammatory liver diseases?

   a. Autoimmune hepatitis

   Rationale: *Autoimmune hepatitis has been classified in K75 Other inflammatory liver diseases.*

9. What condition is not reported with a code from Chapter 11 Diseases of the Digestive System?

   a. Parotitis due to mumps

   Rationale: *There is a chapter level Excludes2 note indicating that certain infectious and parasitic diseases are not reported with codes from the digestive system chapter. Under sialoadenitis, the code for mumps (B26.-) is specifically excluded with an Excludes1 note.*

10. What is NOT a documentation consideration for reporting codes within the digestive system chapter?

    d. Infectious or parasitic etiologies

    Rationale: *Documentation specifically related to acute and chronic conditions, designation for some acute conditions as acute recurrent, and combination codes requiring documentation of the concomitant condition as well are all considerations when assigning codes from the digestive system chapter. Digestive conditions known to be caused by particular infectious agents or pathogens are normally reported with codes from Chapter 1.*

Chapter 12

DISEASES OF THE SKIN AND SUBCUTANEOUS TISSUE

Introduction

Diseases of the skin and subcutaneous tissue include diseases affecting the epidermis, dermis, and hypodermis, subcutaneous tissue, nails, sebaceous glands, sweat glands, and hair and hair follicles. Common conditions of the skin and subcutaneous tissue include boils, cellulitis, abscess, pressure ulcers, lymphadenitis, and pilonidal cysts.

Codes for diseases of the skin and subcutaneous tissue are located in Chapter 12. Integumentary system diseases span nine code blocks in ICD-10-CM with most code categories expanded to the fourth- or fifth-character level. Chapter 12 in ICD-10-CM classifies conditions into related disease groups.

Integumentary system codes include additional detail and specificity about various conditions of skin and subcutaneous tissue such as laterality and site designation, or type and cause. Codes for pressure ulcers, for example, are combination codes that include site, laterality, and severity in the code description. These codes classify the four stages of pressure ulcers as well as unstageable pressure ulcers. The laterality of the affected site is also specified in the codes for carbuncle, furuncle, abscess, cellulitis, and non-pressure ulcers.

ICD-10-CM captures a level of specificity for disease coding that requires precise clinical information documented in the medical record. Contact dermatitis for example, is specified as allergic or irritant and the substance causing the condition must also be specifically identified.

In addition to more specificity, updated and standardized terminology is used in ICD-10-CM. For example, dermatitis and eczema are common conditions coded to this chapter. ICD-10-CM includes a note indicating that the terms dermatitis and eczema are used synonymously and interchangeably.

Other clinical terms are commonly used interchangeably in medical record documentation. Various terms are used to describe pressure ulcers, and instructional notes are provided to clarify that codes for pressure ulcers include diagnoses documented as:

- Bed sore
- Decubitus ulcer
- Plaster ulcer
- Pressure area
- Pressure sore

Understanding the coding and documentation requirements for diseases of the skin and subcutaneous tissue begins with a review of the code blocks in ICD-10-CM, which are displayed in the table below.

ICD-10-CM Blocks	
L00-L08	Infections of the Skin and Subcutaneous Tissue
L10-L14	Bullous Disorders
L20-L30	Dermatitis and Eczema
L40-L45	Papulosquamous Disorders
L49-L54	Urticaria and Erythema
L55-L59	Radiation-Related Disorders of the Skin and Subcutaneous Tissue
L60-L75	Disorders of Skin Appendages
L76	Intraoperative and Postprocedural Complications of Skin and Subcutaneous Tissue
L80-L99	Other Disorders of the Skin and Subcutaneous Tissue

Diseases of the skin and subcutaneous tissue include:

- Infections of the skin and subcutaneous tissues
- Noninfectious inflammatory conditions of the skin classified in five code blocks:
  - L10-L14 Bullous Disorders
  - L20-L30 Dermatitis and Eczema
  - L40-L45 Papulosquamous Disorders
  - L49-L54 Urticaria and Erythema
  - L55-L59 Radiation-Related Disorders of the Skin and Subcutaneous Tissue
- Other diseases of the skin in two code blocks, one for other disorders of the skin and subcutaneous tissues and one for disorders of the skin appendages such as hair, nails and glands.
- Intraoperative and postprocedural complications of the skin and subcutaneous tissues in code block L76.

Exclusions

To assign the most specific code possible, close attention must be paid to the coding and sequencing instructions in the Tabular List and Alphabetic Index, particularly the exclusion notes. There are no Excludes 1 notes for Chapter 12; however, there are multiple Excludes 2 notes which are listed in the table below.

Excludes1	Excludes2
None	Certain conditions originating in the perinatal period (P04-P96) Certain infectious and parasitic diseases (A00-B99) Complications of pregnancy, childbirth and the puerperium (O00-O9A) Congenital malformations, deformations, and chromosomal abnormalities (Q00-Q99) Endocrine, nutritional and metabolic diseases (E00-E88) Lipomelanotic reticulosis (I89.8) Neoplasms (C00-D49) Symptoms, signs and abnormal clinical and laboratory findings, not elsewhere classified (R00-R94) Systemic connective tissue disorders (M30-M36) Viral warts (B07.-)

Chapter Guidelines

The coding guidelines include the coding conventions, the general coding guidelines, and the chapter-specific coding guidelines. Coding and sequencing guidelines for integumentary diseases and complications due to the treatment of integumentary conditions are incorporated into the Alphabetic Index and the Tabular List.

The *ICD-10-CM Official Guidelines for Coding and Reporting* specifically address the need for consistent, complete documentation in the medical record, calling complete and accurate documentation "essential" for code assignment and reporting of diagnoses and procedures.

Chapter specific guidelines for Diseases of the Skin and Subcutaneous Tissue all relate to detailed instruction for pressure ulcers and non-pressure chronic ulcers.

ICD-10-CM Official Guidelines for Coding and Reporting

Pressure ulcer stage codes

- Pressure ulcer stages:
  - Codes from category L89 Pressure ulcer are combination codes that identify the site of the pressure ulcer as well as the stage of the ulcer. The ICD-10-CM classifies pressure ulcer stages based on severity, which is designated by stages 1-4, unspecified stage, and unstageable. Assign as many codes from category L89 as needed to identify all the pressure ulcers the patient has, if applicable.
- Unstageable pressure ulcers:
  - Assignment of the code for unstageable pressure ulcer (L89.--0) should be based on the clinical documentation. These codes are used for pressure ulcers whose stage cannot be clinically determined (e.g., the ulcer is covered by slough or eschar or has been treated with a skin or muscle graft).
  - These codes should not be confused with the codes for unspecified stage (L89.--9). When there is no documentation regarding the stage of the pressure ulcer, assign the appropriate code for unspecified stage (L89.--9).
- Documented pressure ulcer stage:
  - Assignment of the pressure ulcer stage code should be guided by clinical documentation of the stage or documentation of the terms found in the Alphabetic Index.
  - For clinical terms describing the stage that are not found in the Alphabetic Index, and when there is no documentation of the stage, the provider should be queried.
- Patients admitted with pressure ulcers documented as healed:
  - No code is assigned if the documentation states that the pressure ulcer is completely healed.
- Patients admitted with pressure ulcers documented as healing:
  - Pressure ulcers described as healing should be assigned the appropriate pressure ulcer stage code based on the documentation in the medical record. If the documentation does not provide information about the stage of the healing pressure ulcer, assign the appropriate code for unspecified stage.
  - If the documentation is unclear as to whether the patient has a current (new) pressure ulcer or if the patient is being treated for a healing pressure ulcer, query the provider.
- Patient admitted with pressure ulcer evolving into another stage during the admission:
  - If a patient is admitted to an inpatient hospital with a pressure ulcer at one stage and it progresses to a higher stage, assign the code for the highest stage reported for that site.

Non-pressure chronic ulcers

- No code is assigned when documentation states the non-pressure chronic ulcer is healed
- Patient admitted with non-pressure ulcers documented as healing:
  - Non-pressure ulcers described as healing should be assigned the appropriate non-pressure ulcer code based on the documentation in the medical record. If the documentation does not provide information about the severity of the healing non-pressure ulcer, assign the appropriate code for unspecified severity
  - If the documentation is unclear as to whether the patient has a current (new) non-pressure ulcer or if the patient is being treated for a healing non-pressure ulcer, query the provider.
  - For ulcers present on admission but healed at the time of discharge, assign the code for the site and severity of the non-pressure ulcer at the time of admission
- Patient admitted with non-pressure ulcer progressing into another severity level during the admission:
  - If a patient is admitted to an inpatient hospital with a non-pressure ulcer at one severity level and it progresses to a higher severity level, two codes should be assigned: one for the site and severity of the ulcer on admission and a second one for the same ulcer site and the highest severity level reported during the stay.

General Documentation Requirements

Documentation requirements depend on the particular disease or disorder affecting the integumentary system. Some of the new general documentation requirements are discussed here, but greater detail for some of the more common integumentary system diseases will be provided in the next section.

In general, basic medical record documentation requirements include the severity or status of the disease (e.g., acute or chronic), as well as the site, etiology, and any secondary disease process. Physician documentation of the significance of any findings or confirmation of any diagnosis found in laboratory or other diagnostic test reports is necessary for code assignment. Provider documentation should also clearly specify any cause-and-effect relationship between medical treatment and an integumentary disorder.

Many of the codes in Chapter 12 require site specificity for accurate and detailed code assignment. For example, the location of an abscess of the trunk must be identified as the chest wall, abdominal wall, umbilicus, back, groin, or perineum in order to code to the highest level of specificity available. Laterality must be documented for abscess as well as for cellulitis, carbuncle, furuncle, and pressure and non-pressure ulcers.

In addition to these general documentation requirements, there are specific diseases and disorders that require greater detail in documentation to ensure optimal code assignment.

Code-Specific Documentation Requirements

In this section, ICD-10-CM code categories, subcategories, and subclassifications for some of the more frequently reported integumentary diseases are reviewed. Although not all codes with significant documentation requirements are discussed, this section will provide a representative sample of the type of documentation needed for integumentary diseases. The section is organized alphabetically by the code category, subcategory, or subclassification.

Acne

Acne is an inflammatory eruption of the skin appearing most commonly on the face, neck, chest, back, and shoulders. Acne may also occur on the trunk, arms, legs, and buttocks. Acne occurs when hair follicles become clogged with oil and dead skin cells. Acne varioliformis is an infection involving the follicles and the production of pus occurring primarily on the forehead and temples. It is also referred to as acne necrotica miliaris.

Cystic acne (or acne vulgaris) is characterized by scaly red skin, blackheads and whiteheads (comedones), papules, and pustules. The "cysts," that accompany cystic acne, can appear on the buttocks, groin, and armpit area where sweat collects in hair follicles. Codes for acne are categorized in Chapter 12 under Disorders of skin appendages.

Coding and Documentation Requirements

Identify type:

- Acne conglobata
- Acné excoriée des jeunes filles, which includes:
  - Picker's acne
- Acne tropica
- Acne varioliformis, which includes:
  - Acne necrotica miliaris
- Acne vulgaris
- Infantile acne
- Other specified acne
- Unspecified acne

Acne

ICD-10-CM Code/Documentation	
L70.0	Acne vulgaris
L70.1	Acne conglobata
L70.2	Acne varioliformis
L70.3	Acne tropica
L70.4	Infantile acne
L70.5	Acné excoriée des jeunes filles
L70.8	Other acne
L70.9	Acne, unspecified

Documentation and Coding Example

A 19-year-old female presents with complaints of acne on her chin and left temple locally, due to frequent cell phone use where the receiver rubs on her face. She indicates the problem is worsening.

Medications: Patient is currently taking oral contraceptives, started last year, prescribed by her gynecologist. Allergic to penicillin, results in difficulty breathing.

History: Menses onset 13 y.o., light flow, regular, no complications. Positive for birth control pill use. Vaccination status is current. History of childhood chickenpox. No previous surgeries. Family history is non-contributory. Patient reports good dietary habits, regular exercise. Patient consumes 3-5 servings of caffeine per day. Non-smoker, admits to social alcohol use. Denies STD history.

Review of Systems: Reddening of face, acne problems, no allergic or immunologic symptoms. Denies fever, headache, nausea, dizziness.

Physical Exam: Patient is a pleasant 19-year-old female, in no apparent distress, well-developed, well-nourished and with good attention to hygiene and body habitus. Skin: Examination of scalp shows no abnormalities. Hair growth and distribution is normal. Inspection of skin outside of affected area reveals no abnormalities. Palpation of skin shows no abnormalities. Inspection of eccrine and apocrine glands shows no evidence of hyperhidrosis, chromhidrosis or bromhidrosis. Face shows keratotic papule.

Impression/Plan: **Acne vulgaris.**

Recommended treatment is antibiotic therapy. Tetracycline 250 mg capsule, BID. Discussed with the patient the prescription for Tetracycline and gave her information regarding the side effects and the proper method of ingestion. Patient received extensive counseling about acne and literature regarding acne vulgaris. She understands the course of acne treatment is long-term. Patient to return for follow-up in 4 weeks.

Diagnosis: **Acne vulgaris.**

Diagnosis code(s)

L70.0 Acne vulgaris

Coding Note(s)

ICD-10-CM provides a specific code for acne vulgaris.

Alopecia

Alopecia is a skin disease characterized by loss of hair. The condition may be localized or there may be loss of hair on all hair bearing skin. One of the more common types of alopecia is alopecia areata. This is an acquired skin disease believed to be caused by an autoimmune disorder which causes the immune system to attack the hair follicles disrupting normal hair formation. Alopecia areata may occur on any part of the body, but most often hair loss is limited to patchy areas on the scalp. When the hair loss occurs in a band-like or wave-like pattern, usually on the temporal (side) and/or occipital (back) region of the scalp, and hair remains on the top of the scalp, it is referred to as ophiasis or ophiasis patterned alopecia areata. When hair loss occurs on the entire scalp, the condition is referred to as alopecia totalis. When there is total loss of body hair, the condition is referred to as alopecia universalis. Hair loss may resolve and hair may regrow without medical treatment or hair loss may be permanent. There are a variety of medical treatments but not all treatments work for all individuals.

Another form of hair loss is referred to as effluvium, which means outflowing, and these types are caused by changes in the hair growth cycle. Hair follicles in the scalp go through two phases, a growth phase and a resting phase. In a normal hair growth cycle, 80-90% of hair follicles are in the growth phase called anagen and 10-20% are in the rest phase called telogen. In telogen effluvium, there is a significant increase in the number of hair follicles that are in the dormant or resting phase during which no hair growth occurs. This results in general shedding and thinning of hair which is typically more pronounced on the top of the scalp. Shedding and thinning may occur only on the scalp or may also be present on other parts of the body. In anagen effluvium, the pattern of hair loss is typically the same occurring diffusely over the entire scalp, but the hair loss occurs much more quickly. Instead of hair being shed and increased numbers of hair follicles being in the telogen stage, in anagen effluvium hair is shed rapidly while still in the growth phase. Anagen effluvium typically occurs as a side effect of cytotoxic drugs used to treat cancer. Once the cytotoxic drugs are discontinued hair growth resumes.

A third classification of hair loss is androgenic alopecia, also called androgenetic alopecia. Even though the condition is sometimes referred to as male-pattern baldness, it affects both men and women. Androgenic alopecia is a genetically determined disorder of the hair follicles. It is believed that damage to the hair follicle occurs when testosterone is converted into dihydrotestosterone (DHT) by an enzyme in the oil gland of the hair follicle. DHT causes damage to the hair follicle resulting in the inability of the follicle to grow normal hair. Normal adult hair is replaced with vellus hair which is the thin, fine, short hair present on the hair bearing surfaces of the body before puberty.

In ICD-10-CM, alopecia codes capture specific types of hair loss. Codes for nonscarring hair loss are organized into three categories including L63 Alopecia areata, L64 Androgenic alopecia, and L65 Other nonscarring hair loss. There is a fourth category in the code set for cicatricial alopecia (L66), which contains codes for scarring types of hair loss and includes several specified conditions. Hair is considered a skin appendage. Codes for alopecia are categorized in Chapter 12 under the section Disorders of skin appendages.

Coding and Documentation Requirements

Identify type of hair loss:

- Alopecia areata
  - Ophiasis
  - Totalis (capitis)
  - Universalis
  - Other specified type
  - Unspecified
- Androgenic alopecia
  - Drug-induced androgenic alopecia
  - Other specified type of androgenic alopecia
  - Unspecified
- Cicatricial alopecia (scarring type)
  - Folliculitis decalvans
  - Folliculitis ulerythematosa reticulata
  - Lichen planopilaris (follicular lichen planus)
  - Perifolliculitis capitis abscedens
  - Pseudopelade
  - Other cicatricial alopecia
  - Unspecified
  - Other nonscarring type:
  - Alopecia mucinosa
  - Anagen effluvium
  - Telogen effluvium
  - Other specified type of nonscarring hair loss
  - Unspecified nonscarring type
- Alopecia

ICD-10-CM Code Category	ICD-10-CM Code/Documentation	
Nonscarring hair loss	L63.0	Alopecia (capitis) totalis
	L63.1	Alopecia universalis
	L63.2	Ophiasis
	L63.8	Other alopecia areata
	L63.9	Alopecia areata, unspecified
	L64.0	Drug-induced androgenic alopecia
	L64.8	Other androgenic alopecia
	L64.9	Androgenic alopecia, unspecified
	L65.0	Telogen effluvium
	L65.1	Anagen effluvium
	L65.2	Alopecia mucinosa
	L65.8	Other specified nonscarring hair loss
	L65.9	Nonscarring hair loss, unspecified
Scarring hair loss	L66.0	Pseudopelade
	L66.1	Lichen planopilaris
	L66.2	Folliculitis decalvans
	L66.3	Perifollicular capitis abscedens
	L66.4	Folliculitis ulerythematosa reticulata
	L66.8	Other cicatricial alopecia
	L66.9	Cicatricial alopecia unspecified

Documentation and Coding Example

Follow-up visit for **ophiasis**. This 48-year-old female noted hair loss in the right temporal region approximately 6 months ago. Hair loss progressed and eventually extended around the occipital region and into the left temporal area in the typical wave pattern of ophiasis. She has undergone a regimen of cortisone shots into the bald regions. There is now fine, thin hair regrowth beginning in the regions of hair loss. New hair is completely white.

Impression: **Resolving ophiasis.**

Plan: Patient will monitor hair growth and examine scalp for any signs of new hair loss. If she notes that hair growth in the bald regions is not becoming thicker or not continuing or if she notes any new bald patches, she will return for re-evaluation.

Diagnosis Code(s)

L63.2 Ophiasis

Coding Note(s)

There is a specific code for ophiasis which is a form of alopecia areata.

Carbuncle/Furuncle

A furuncle, or boil, is an infection of a hair follicle. Individual furuncles may cluster together forming a carbuncle.

ICD-10-CM includes specific codes for furuncle, carbuncle, abscess, and cellulitis. Cutaneous abscess, furuncle, and carbuncle are found in category L02 while codes for cellulitis and acute lymphangitis are located in category L03. These codes further specify the affected site by identifying laterality, so it is essential that the medical record documentation fully describe the site. Coding and documentation requirements for carbuncle and furuncle are included here with the coding and documentation requirements and coding example for abscess and cellulitis to follow.

Coding and Documentation Requirements

Identify condition:

- Carbuncle
- Furuncle

Identify site:

- Buttock
- Face
- Foot
- Hand
- Limb (except hand/foot)
  - Lower limb
  - Upper limb
  - Axilla
  - Unspecified limb
- Neck
- Trunk
  - Abdominal wall
  - Back [any part, except buttocks]
  - Chest wall
  - Groin
  - Perineum
  - Umbilicus
  - Unspecified site of trunk
- Other site
  - Head (any part except face)
  - Other specified site
- Unspecified site

For upper and lower limbs/hand/foot identify laterality:

- Right
- Left
- Unspecified

Use additional code to identify any infectious organism (B95-B96).

Carbuncle/Furuncle

ICD-10-CM Code/Documentation			
Furuncle		**Carbuncle**	
L02.02	Furuncle of face	L02.03	Carbuncle of face
L02.12	Furuncle of neck	L02.13	Carbuncle of neck
L02.221	Furuncle of abdominal wall	L02.231	Carbuncle of abdominal wall
L02.222	Furuncle of back [any part, except buttock]	L02.232	Carbuncle of back [any part, except buttock]

12. Diseases of the Skin and Subcutaneous Tissue

ICD-10-CM Code/Documentation			
Furuncle		Carbuncle	
L02.223	Furuncle of chest wall	L02.233	Carbuncle of chest wall
L02.224	Furuncle of groin	L02.234	Carbuncle of groin
L02.225	Furuncle of perineum	L02.235	Carbuncle of perineum
L02.226	Furuncle of umbilicus	L02.236	Carbuncle of umbilicus
L02.229	Furuncle of trunk, unspecified	L02.239	Carbuncle of trunk, unspecified
L02.421	Furuncle of right axilla	L02.431	Carbuncle of right axilla
L02.422	Furuncle of left axilla	L02.432	Carbuncle of left axilla
L02.423	Furuncle of right upper limb	L02.433	Carbuncle of right upper limb
L02.424	Furuncle of left upper limb	L02.434	Carbuncle of left upper limb
L02.521	Furuncle right hand	L02.531	Carbuncle of right hand
L02.522	Furuncle left hand	L02.532	Carbuncle of left hand
L02.529	Furuncle unspecified hand	L02.539	Carbuncle of unspecified hand
L02.32	Furuncle of buttock	L02.33	Carbuncle of buttock
L02.425	Furuncle of right lower limb	L02.435	Carbuncle of right lower limb
L02.426	Furuncle of left lower limb	L02.436	Carbuncle of left lower limb
L02.621	Furuncle of right foot	L02.631	Carbuncle of right foot
L02.622	Furuncle of left foot	L02.632	Carbuncle of left foot
L02.629	Furuncle of unspecified foot	L02.639	Carbuncle of unspecified foot
L02.821	Furuncle of head [any part, except face]	L02.831	Carbuncle of head [any part, except face]
L02.828	Furuncle of other sites	L02.838	Carbuncle of other sites
L02.92	Furuncle, unspecified	L02.93	Carbuncle, unspecified

Documentation and Coding Example

HPI: This is a 58-year-old obese white male who presents to the clinic with an area of **tenderness, redness, and swelling in the neck area that has become pustular**. It began ten days ago as a small red lump on the skin, then the surrounding skin became swollen and inflamed and painful with visible pus filling the center of the lump. Self-treatment with warm compresses brought some temporary relief.

ROS: Patient denies vertigo, syncope, convulsions or headaches. No muscle or joint pain. Denies fever, shortness of breath, dyspnea on exertion, chest pain, cough or hemoptysis. Denies nausea, melena, rectal bleeding, he has occasional indigestion. Genitourinary is normal. No other complaints. All other systems negative on review.

Medications: None. No known drug allergies. Patient is single, lives alone. Denies use of alcohol. Former smoker, one pack of cigarettes per day, quit over 5 years. Past medical history is significant for right knee ACL repair six years ago. Mother is alive and well. Father died of cancer.

Physical Examination: Well-developed, obese white male in no acute distress. Pleasant, alert and oriented x3. Pulse 72 regular rate and rhythm, respirations 18, blood pressure 122/88. Normocephalic and atraumatic. PERRLA. Extraocular movements are intact. Neck is supple, no thyromegaly or cervical adenopathy. Pharynx is clear. Tympanic membranes are normal. Chest is symmetrical with equal expansion. Lungs clear to percussion and auscultation. No cardiomegaly. No thrills or murmurs. Normal sinus rate and rhythm. No guarding or rebound tenderness in the abdomen; bowel sounds are normal. No peripheral edema, cyanosis or varicosities. Inguinal area is normal. Skin is normal color, turgor and temperature with no ulcerations or rashes noted except in the neck area on the left side under the chin line. On examination, there is a **single hair follicle with pus, no multiple hair follicle involvement**. Exudate sent to lab for culture to rule out inclusion cysts or deep fungal infection.

Impression/Plan: **Solitary boil on neck**. No oral antibiotics or incision and drainage necessary at this time. Patient instructed to keep the skin clean using an antiseptic soap for washing the infected areas, to wash his hands carefully before and after touching the boil, and avoid greasy creams. Patient counseled not to share washcloths or towels with others. Apply warm compresses for 15 minutes several times a day to help the boil come to a head and drain followed by application of topical clindamycin cream. If resolved, no follow-up necessary; however, patient instructed to return to the clinic if it worsens or fever develops.

Diagnosis: **Single boil on neck.**

Diagnosis Code(s)

L02.12 Furuncle of neck

Coding Note(s)

The Alphabetic Index entry for Boil directs the user to see Furuncle, by site. Boil and folliculitis of neck are listed as included conditions under code L02.12.

Cellulitis/Abscess/Acute Lymphangitis

Cellulitis is a diffuse inflammation of the connective tissue causing severe inflammation of deeper dermal and subcutaneous layers of the skin. Cellulitis is a common bacterial infection usually caused by streptococcus or staphylococcus. A cutaneous abscess is an accumulation of pus surrounded by inflamed tissue resulting from an infection of the skin and subcutaneous tissue. Acute lymphangitis is caused by an infection involving the lymphatic vessels. The lymphatic vessels become inflamed and painful and there are visible red streaks below the skin surface. Acute lymphangitis is a serious condition that can evolve into a systemic infection and sepsis if not treated promptly.

ICD-10-CM provides specific codes for cutaneous abscess and for cellulitis. Cellulitis may be complicated by acute lymphangitis—an inflammation of the lymphatic vessels. There are distinct codes for cellulitis, cutaneous abscess, and for acute lymphangitis, so provider documentation of the presence of lymphangitis in cellulitis cases is needed in order to assign the most accurate codes. The provider documentation in the medical record should clearly distinguish lymphangitis from lymphadenitis, which is an inflammation of a lymph node.

The site affected by cellulitis, abscess, or acute lymphangitis is further specified by identifying laterality, so the site must be fully described in the medical record documentation in order to assign the most accurate codes.

Coding and Documentation Requirements

Identify condition:

- Acute lymphangitis
- Cellulitis, which includes:
  - Chronic
  - Diffuse
  - Phlegmonous
  - Septic
  - Suppurative
- Cutaneous abscess

Identify site:

- Abdominal wall
- Axilla
- Back (any part, except buttock)
- Buttock
- Chest wall
- Face
- Finger
- Foot (except toe)
- Groin
- Hand (except finger)
- Head (any part, except face)
- Lower limb
- Neck
- Perineum
- Toe
- Trunk, unspecified site
- Umbilicus
- Upper limb
- Other specified site
- Unspecified site

For abscess, cellulitis, or acute lymphangitis affecting the extremities, identify laterality:

- Right
- Left
- Unspecified

Cellulitis, Abscess, Acute Lymphangitis

ICD-1Ø-CM Code/Documentation	
Cutaneous Abscess	
LØ2.Ø1	Cutaneous abscess of face
LØ2.11	Cutaneous abscess of neck
LØ2.811	Cutaneous abscess of head [any part, except face]
LØ2.211	Cutaneous abscess of abdominal wall
LØ2.212	Cutaneous abscess of back [any part, except buttock]
LØ2.213	Cutaneous abscess of chest wall
LØ2.214	Cutaneous abscess of groin
LØ2.215	Cutaneous abscess of perineum
LØ2.216	Cutaneous abscess of umbilicus
LØ2.219	Cutaneous abscess of trunk, unspecified
LØ2.31	Cutaneous abscess of buttock
LØ2.411	Cutaneous abscess of right axilla
LØ2.412	Cutaneous abscess of left axilla
LØ2.413	Cutaneous abscess of right upper limb
LØ2.414	Cutaneous abscess of left upper limb
LØ2.511	Cutaneous abscess of right hand
LØ2.512	Cutaneous abscess of left hand
LØ2.519	Cutaneous abscess of unspecified hand
LØ2.415	Cutaneous abscess of right lower limb
LØ2.416	Cutaneous abscess of left lower limb
LØ2.419	Cutaneous abscess of limb, unspecified
LØ2.611	Cutaneous abscess of right foot
LØ2.612	Cutaneous abscess of left foot
LØ2.619	Cutaneous abscess of unspecified foot
LØ2.818	Cutaneous abscess of other sites
LØ2.91	Cutaneous abscess, unspecified
Cellulitis	
LØ3.211	Cellulitis of face
LØ3.221	Cellulitis of neck
LØ3.811	Cellulitis of head [any part, except face]
LØ3.311	Cellulitis of abdominal wall
LØ3.312	Cellulitis of back [any part except buttock]
LØ3.313	Cellulitis of chest wall
LØ3.314	Cellulitis of groin
LØ3.315	Cellulitis of perineum
LØ3.316	Cellulitis of umbilicus
LØ3.319	Cellulitis of trunk, unspecified
LØ3.317	Cellulitis of buttock
LØ3.111	Cellulitis of right axilla
LØ3.112	Cellulitis of left axilla
LØ3.113	Cellulitis of right upper limb
LØ3.114	Cellulitis of left upper limb
LØ3.Ø11	Cellulitis of right finger
LØ3.Ø12	Cellulitis of left finger
LØ3.Ø19	Cellulitis of unspecified finger
LØ3.119	Cellulitis of unspecified part of limb
LØ3.115	Cellulitis of right lower limb
LØ3.116	Cellulitis of left lower limb
LØ3.Ø31	Cellulitis of right toe
LØ3.Ø32	Cellulitis of left toe
LØ3.Ø39	Cellulitis of unspecified toe
LØ3.119	Cellulitis of unspecified part of limb
LØ3.818	Cellulitis of other sites
LØ3.9Ø	Cellulitis, unspecified
Lymphangitis	
LØ3.212	Acute lymphangitis of face
LØ3.222	Acute lymphangitis of neck

ICD-1Ø-CM Code/Documentation	
LØ3.891	Acute lymphangitis of head [any part, except face]
LØ3.321	Acute lymphangitis of abdominal wall
LØ3.322	Acute lymphangitis of back [any part except buttock]
LØ3.323	Acute lymphangitis of chest wall
LØ3.324	Acute lymphangitis of groin
LØ3.325	Acute lymphangitis of perineum
LØ3.326	Acute lymphangitis of umbilicus
LØ3.329	Acute lymphangitis of trunk, unspecified
LØ3.327	Acute lymphangitis of buttock
LØ3.121	Acute lymphangitis of right axilla
LØ3.122	Acute lymphangitis of left axilla
LØ3.123	Acute lymphangitis of right upper limb
LØ3.124	Acute lymphangitis of left upper limb
LØ3.Ø21	Acute lymphangitis of right finger
LØ3.Ø22	Acute lymphangitis of left finger
LØ3.Ø29	Acute lymphangitis of unspecified finger
LØ3.125	Acute lymphangitis of right lower limb
LØ3.126	Acute lymphangitis of left lower limb
LØ3.129	Acute lymphangitis of unspecified part of limb
LØ3.Ø41	Acute lymphangitis of right toe
LØ3.Ø42	Acute lymphangitis of left toe
LØ3.Ø49	Acute lymphangitis of unspecified toe
LØ3.898	Acute lymphangitis of other sites
LØ3.91	Acute lymphangitis, unspecified

Documentation and Coding Example

This 62-year-old male presents to the ED with complaints of pain and tenderness over the instep of his **left foot**. The patient is afebrile. On examination, the painful area is red and inflamed and there is fluctuance on palpation of the inflamed region.

Impression: **Subcutaneous abscess**

Treatment: The area was prepped and draped and a local anesthetic administered. A cruciate incision was made over the abscess site and the abscess drained. A sample of the fluid was sent to the lab for culture and sensitivity. The abscess cavity was flushed with sterile saline. The wound was left open to heal by secondary intention and a soft dressing was applied.

Plan: The patient was given instructions on care of the abscess site. Pros and cons of antibiotics were discussed and the patient elects not to take antibiotics at this time. Patient instructed to return for any increased pain, swelling, redness around or extending from the drainage site or for any fever, body aches or other symptoms that may suggest systemic infection.

Diagnosis Code(s)

LØ2.612 Cutaneous abscess of left foot

Coding Note(s)

Abscess of the foot is classified to category LØ2 Cutaneous abscess, furuncle, and carbuncle. The code is specific to site and laterality.

Contact Dermatitis

Contact dermatitis results when skin comes in direct contact with a substance that causes inflammation of the skin. Skin inflammation may be due to an allergy to the substance or due to irritants in the substance.

Contact dermatitis is classified by type. Allergic contact dermatitis is coded differently from irritant contact dermatitis so the medical record documentation must clearly identify the type of contact dermatitis as well as the cause. If the documentation does not specify whether the contact dermatitis is allergic or irritant, an unspecified code must be assigned. When contact dermatitis is an adverse effect of a drug, the documentation must identify the specific drug for accurate code assignment.

Coding and Documentation Requirements

Identify type:

- Allergic contact dermatitis
- Irritant contact dermatitis
- Unspecified contact dermatitis

Identify contact dermatitis as due to:

- Animal (cat) (dog) dander
- Adhesives
- Cosmetics
- Drugs in contact with skin
- Dyes
- Food in contact with skin
- Metals
- Plants [except food]
- Other chemical products, which include:
  - Cement
  - Insecticide
  - Plastic
  - Rubber
- Other specified agents
- Unspecified cause

Identify irritant contact dermatitis as due to:

- Cosmetics
- Detergents
- Drugs in contact with skin
- Food in contact with skin
- Metals
- Plants [except food]
- Oils and greases
- Solvents
- Other chemical products, which include:
  - Cement
  - Insecticide
  - Plastic
  - Rubber

- Other specified agents
- Unspecified cause

Identify unspecified contact dermatitis as due to:

- Cosmetics
- Drugs and medicines in contact with skin
- Dyes
- Food in contact with skin
- Other chemical products, which include:
  - Cement
  - Insecticide
  - Plastic
  - Rubber
- Plants [except food]
- Other specified agents
- Unspecified cause

Contact Dermatitis

ICD-10-CM Code/Documentation	
L23.1	Allergic contact dermatitis due to adhesives
L23.81	Allergic contact dermatitis due to animal (cat) (dog) dander
L23.5	Allergic contact dermatitis due to other chemical products
L24.5	Irritant contact dermatitis due to other chemical products
L25.3	Unspecified contact dermatitis due to other chemical products
L23.2	Allergic contact dermatitis due to cosmetics
L24.3	Irritant contact dermatitis due to cosmetics
L25.0	Unspecified contact dermatitis due to cosmetics
L24.0	Irritant contact dermatitis due to detergents
L23.3	Allergic contact dermatitis due to drugs in contact with skin
L24.4	Irritant contact dermatitis due to drugs in contact with skin
L25.1	Unspecified contact dermatitis due to drugs in contact with skin
L23.4	Allergic contact dermatitis due to dyes
L25.2	Unspecified contact dermatitis due to dyes
L23.6	Allergic contact dermatitis due to food in contact with the skin
L24.6	Irritant contact dermatitis due to food in contact with skin
L25.4	Unspecified contact dermatitis due to food in contact with skin
L24.1	Irritant contact dermatitis due to oils and greases
L23.89	Allergic contact dermatitis due to other agents
L24.89	Irritant contact dermatitis due to other agents
L25.8	Unspecified contact dermatitis due to other agents
L23.7	Allergic contact dermatitis due to plants, except food
L24.7	Irritant contact dermatitis due to plants, except food
L25.5	Unspecified contact dermatitis due to plants, except food
L23.0	Allergic contact dermatitis due to metals
L24.81	Irritant contact dermatitis due to metals
L24.2	Irritant contact dermatitis due to solvents
L23.9	Allergic contact dermatitis, unspecified cause
L24.9	Irritant contact dermatitis, unspecified cause
L25.9	Unspecified contact dermatitis, unspecified cause

Documentation and Coding Example

A 27-year-old white female referred for dermatology consultation of **eczema of her right hand**. Patient was treated with Cetaphil cream and Cetaphil cleansing lotion with increased moisturizing cream. She was referred for evaluation because she is flaring. Her hands are very dry and cracked. She started using hot, soapy water to wash her hands because she states the Cetaphil cleansing lotion is causing burning and pain because of the fissures in her skin.

No history of dermatological problems. No bad sunburns or blood pressure problems in the past. No known drug allergies. Current medications include daily Multivitamin and Tums PRN. She is a nonsmoker.

Vital Signs: Temperature 98.4, pulse 72, respirations 20, and blood pressure is 118/76. Head is normocephalic. Pupils are equal and reactive. The nares are patent. Oropharynx is clear without lesions. Neck is supple without lymphadenopathy. Heart, regular rate and rhythm. Lungs, positive breath sounds at the bases. No crackles or wheezes are heard. Abdomen is soft, nontender, nondistended, with positive bowel sounds heard. Neurologic intact. Extremities: Without cyanosis, clubbing or edema. Skin is warm and dry without any rash except for area of complaint. Examination reveals very dry, cracked hands bilaterally. Irritant contact dermatitis caused by over washing of the hands with harsh soap.

Impression: **Irritant contact dermatitis of both hands from harsh soap**.

Treatment: Discontinue hot soapy water and wash her hands with Cetaphil cleansing lotion. Aristocort ointment 0.1% and Polysporin ointment TID and PRN itch. Keflex 500 mg BID for two weeks with one refill. Return in one month if not better; otherwise, on a PRN basis. Consult letter sent to PCP.

Diagnosis: **Bilateral irritant contact dermatitis of hands**.

Diagnosis code(s)

L24.0 Irritant contact dermatitis due to detergents

Coding Note(s)

Contact dermatitis is classified by type and cause, so the provider documentation must identify both. In this case, the documentation specifies the type of contact dermatitis as irritant and the associated cause as detergent. There is no subclassification for location or laterality.

Psoriasis

Psoriasis is a common skin disorder that manifests with thick silvery scales and dry, red, itchy patches that are often painful. Patients typically experience periodic flare ups and periods of remission. Outbreaks may be triggered by infection, injury, stress, cold, or medications. Psoriasis is a chronic condition that can also affect other tissues such as the joints causing psoriatic arthritis or arthropathy.

Complete, accurate coding requires documentation identifying the presence of arthritis, arthropathy, or spondylitis.

Coding and Documentation Requirements

Identify type of psoriasis:

- Acrodermatitis continua
- Arthropathic psoriasis
  - Distal interphalangeal psoriatic arthropathy
  - Psoriatic arthritis mutilans
  - Psoriatic juvenile arthropathy
  - Psoriatic spondylitis
  - Other psoriatic arthropathy
  - Unspecified arthropathic psoriasis
- Generalized pustular psoriasis, which includes:
  - Impetigo herpetiformis
  - Von Zumbusch's disease
- Guttate psoriasis
- Psoriasis vulgaris
- Pustulosis palmaris et plantaris
- Other specified psoriasis, which includes:
  - Flexural psoriasis
- Unspecified psoriasis

Psoriasis and Psoriatic arthropathy

ICD-10-CM Code Category	ICD-10-CM Code/Documentation	
Psoriatic arthropathy	L40.50	Arthropathic psoriasis, unspecified
	L40.51	Distal interphalangeal psoriatic arthropathy
	L40.52	Psoriatic arthritis mutilans
	L40.53	Psoriatic spondylitis
	L40.54	Psoriatic juvenile arthropathy
	L40.59	Other psoriatic arthropathy
Psoriasis	L40.0	Psoriasis vulgaris
	L40.1	Generalized pustular psoriasis
	L40.2	Acrodermatitis continua
	L40.3	Pustulosis palmaris et plantaris
	L40.4	Guttate psoriasis
	L40.8	Other psoriasis
	L40.9	Psoriasis, unspecified

Documentation and Coding Example 1

Patient is a 12-year-old male suffering from **Psoriasis on elbows, knees, and hands.** His eruptions worsened in the past two weeks. He has erythematous eruptions with scaling and severe itching and burning. Itching is aggravated at night. There are many cracks with watery discharge and much bleeding. Patient also reports **asymmetrical joint stiffness of the knees** in the morning or after long periods of inactivity. At the onset of this severe aggravation, he was put on steroids and methotrexate by his dermatologist. There is a strong family history of psoriasis; his father, his paternal uncle both suffer from psoriasis and his paternal grandfather also suffers from psoriatic arthritis. The patient's psoriasis is aggravated in summer; he can't tolerate heat and desires a fan in all seasons. He complains of gastric upset for the past week to ten days. No recent upper respiratory infections or other viral infections or stressful events. History is also negative for physical trauma, vaccination, or sunburn.

Vitals: 110/75, 72, 98.6. Well-nourished white male, NAD, alert and oriented to person, place, and time. AT/NC; oropharynx clear with moist mucous membranes; and normal dentition and gums. Anicteric sclerae, moist conjunctiva; PERRLA, fundi clear with sharp disc margins and normal posterior segments. Trachea midline; FROM, neck supple, no lymphadenopathy, thyromegaly or carotid bruits; no JVD. Lungs CTA in front with no rales or crackles; normal respiratory effort; no dullness to percussion. CV: RRR. Abdomen: Soft, non-tender; no masses or HSM, normal abdominal aorta without bruits. Appetite is normal with cravings for spicy foods with previously noted complaints of gastric upset for 7-10 days. He drinks approximately 1-2 liters/day; urine and stool are normal.

Skin: Normal temperature, turgor, and texture. He has erythematous eruptions with scaling and several cracks with watery discharge. Psoriasis papules are sharply demarcated, erythematous, scaly, and pruritic. No extremity lymphadenopathy; brisk and symmetric pedal pulses; no digital cyanosis however, there is evidence of dactylitis in the toes and the toenails appear pitted. There is stiffness, swelling, and tenderness of the knee joints and surrounding ligaments and tendons. He has **psoriatic arthritis developing in both the knees.** Concomitant joint and nail involvement reinforces the diagnosis. The patient was started on Carcinosin 200 and saw improvement with reduced scaling within two weeks. The pain in his knees was also improving. New eruptions were under control and his gastric upset also reduced significantly.

Diagnosis: **Juvenile Psoriatic Arthritis.**

Diagnosis code(s)

L40.54 Psoriatic juvenile arthropathy

Coding Note(s)

Arthritic or arthropathic psoriasis is classified by type such as distal interphalangeal psoriatic arthropathy, psoriatic arthritis mutilans, psoriatic spondylitis and psoriatic juvenile arthropathy.

Documentation and Coding Example 2

This 26-year-old male presents today with complaints of psoriasis on his scalp. He has experienced periodic outbreaks since he was a child so he is familiar with the condition which typically flares when he is under stress. This flare started when he was finishing work on his master's degree and preparing for public presentations of his master's thesis. He has been using an over-the-counter medicated shampoo without relief of symptoms.

Examination: This is a well-developed, well-nourished, thin, athletic young man. Ht 5'10", Wt 139, T 98.2, B/P 108/70, P 66 and regular, R 18. Skin of face, trunk, and arms is clear. There are several small crusty and inflamed patches noted around the knees bilaterally. These are consistent with psoriasis. Examination of the neck is normal. Thyroid normal. There are no enlarged lymph nodes noted in the neck region. The top and sides of the scalp are clear but there is a large contiguous area of crusting and inflamed skin from the level of the ear to the base of the hairline on the back of the scalp.

Impression: **Plaque psoriasis flare**.

Plan: Patient will continue to use medicated shampoo. He was given prescriptions for corticosteroid ointment for the psoriasis outbreak on his legs and for corticosteroid scalp solution to treat the outbreak on his scalp as these have worked well in the past. He is to return in 4 weeks for re-evaluation or sooner if there is any exacerbation of symptoms.

Diagnosis Code(s)

L40.0 Psoriasis vulgaris

Coding Note(s)

Plaque psoriasis is synonymous with psoriasis vulgaris and is listed as an inclusion term under code L40.0. It can be found in the Alphabetic Index under psoriasis, plaque.

Skin Ulcer Chronic

A skin ulcer is a breakdown in the skin that may involve only the skin, extend into the subcutaneous tissue and fat layer, or even deeper into the muscle and bone. Classification of skin ulcers depends on whether the skin ulcer is documented as a pressure or non-pressure ulcer. In ICD-10-CM, skin ulcers that are caused by pressure are classified in category L89. Non-pressure ulcers are classified in category L97 and in subcategory L98.4. Precise documentation of the location, causation (pressure vs. chronic non-pressure) and severity of the chronic skin ulcer is imperative for proper code selection. Chronic ulcers documented as healing should be coded to the current stage of the ulcer. Both pressure and non-pressure ulcers will be reviewed with separate tables, documentation guidelines and documentation examples for each.

Pressure Ulcers

A pressure ulcer is an ulceration caused by prolonged pressure occurring most often over bony prominences of the body. The ulcer is caused by ischemia of the underlying structures of the skin, fat, and muscles as a result of the sustained and constant pressure. Documentation related to pressure ulcers is integral to coding, assessment, and measurement of quality of care. A pressure ulcer is sometimes documented as decubitus ulcer, bed sore, plaster ulcer, pressure area, or pressure sore.

In ICD-10-CM, a combination code that describes both the pressure ulcer site and the ulcer stage is defined for coding. Codes for decubitus ulcers also include laterality, and severity. These codes classify the four stages of pressure ulcers as well as unstageable and unspecified stage pressure ulcers. Pressure ulcer stages are classified based on severity and designated by stages I-IV (1-4) and unstageable.

A pressure ulcer coded as "unstageable" should not be confused with a pressure ulcer whose stage is unspecified. Assigning a code for an unstageable pressure ulcer must be based on the clinical documentation indicating that the pressure ulcer stage cannot be clinically determined. Unstageable pressure ulcers are advanced stage pressure ulcers that cannot have the extent of tissue damage confirmed due to being obscured by slough or eschar. After the slough or eschar is removed, either a stage 3 or stage 4 pressure ulcer is revealed. The code for unspecified pressure ulcer is assigned when there is no documentation regarding the stage of the pressure ulcer.

Deep tissue pressure injury (DTPI) is currently defined as "intact or non-intact skin with localized area of persistent non-blanchable deep red, maroon, purple discoloration or epidermal separation revealing a dark wound bed or blood filled blister". DTPIs often have both ischemic and pressure-induced etiologies, and arise from intense or prolonged pressure and shear forces at a bone and muscle interface. Unlike advanced pressure ulcers, deep tissue injury may resolve without tissue loss, or the wound may evolve to show the actual extent of tissue injury. These type of wounds are also reported in category L89 Pressure ulcer as pressure-induced deep tissue damage by site and laterality.

Coding and Documentation Requirements

Identify pressure ulcer or deep tissue pressure injury site:

- Ankle
- Back
  - Upper
  - Lower
  - Unspecified part
- Buttock
- Contiguous site of back, buttock, hip
- Elbow
- Head (includes face)
- Heel
- Hip
- Sacral region, which includes:
  - Coccyx
  - Tailbone
- Other specified site
- Unspecified site

Identify laterality:

- Right
- Left
- Unspecified

Identify pressure ulcer stage: (based upon clinical documentation)

- Pressure ulcer stage 1
  - Pre-ulcer skin changes with persistent focal edema
- Pressure ulcer stage 2
  - Abrasion
  - Blister
  - Partial thickness skin loss involving epidermis and/or dermis
- Pressure ulcer stage 3
  - Full thickness skin loss with damage or necrosis of subcutaneous tissue

- Pressure ulcer stage 4
  - Necrosis through to underlying muscle, tendon or bone
- Unstageable
- Unspecified stage

Pressure Ulcer of Heel

ICD-10-CM Code/Documentation	
Unspecified Heel	
L89.600	Pressure ulcer of unspecified heel, unstageable
L89.601	Pressure ulcer of unspecified heel, stage 1
L89.602	Pressure ulcer of unspecified heel, stage 2
L89.603	Pressure ulcer of unspecified heel, stage 3
L89.604	Pressure ulcer of unspecified heel, stage 4
L89.609	Pressure ulcer of unspecified heel, unspecified stage
Right Heel	
L89.610	Pressure ulcer of right heel, unstageable
L89.611	Pressure ulcer of right heel, stage 1
L89.612	Pressure ulcer of right heel, stage 2
L89.613	Pressure ulcer of right heel, stage 3
L89.614	Pressure ulcer of right heel, stage 4
L89.619	Pressure ulcer of right heel, unspecified stage
Left Heel	
L89.620	Pressure ulcer of left heel, unstageable
L89.621	Pressure ulcer of left heel, stage 1
L89.622	Pressure ulcer of left heel, stage 2
L89.623	Pressure ulcer of left heel, stage 3
L89.624	Pressure ulcer of left heel, stage 4
L89.629	Pressure ulcer of left heel, unspecified stage

Documentation and Coding Example

An 83-year-old female presented with a chief concern of an **ulcer on the posterior aspect of her left heel** which has recently gotten worse. The patient denies any trauma to the foot. **The ulceration developed following an extended period of bed rest**. She has no known allergies. There is no history of fever, rash, respiratory infection, or gastrointestinal symptomatology. There is no history of diabetes, psoriasis, skin cancers, or dysplastic nevi. Her medical history is otherwise unremarkable.

Vital Signs: BP = 120/80. Pulse = 80 Resp =12. Patient is afebrile. The neck is supple. There is no jugular venous distension. The thyroid is nontender. The lungs are clear to auscultation and percussion. There is a regular rhythm. S1 and S2 are normal. No abnormal heart sounds detected. Normal bowel sounds are present. The abdomen is soft, nontender, without organomegaly. There is no CVA tenderness. No hernias noted. There is no clubbing, cyanosis, or edema in the extremities. Skin is warm and dry. The left heel is covered by a bandage and, on examination, there is a **shallow, open ulcer located on the lateral aspect of the left heel, with blistering and partial thickness loss of epidermal tissue**. The ulcer is approximately 6 cm in size, with a red pink wound bed without slough.

Laboratory Studies: White blood cell count was unremarkable. Hematocrit 31.9. Sedimentation rate was 57. BUN 24 and Creatinine 1.6. Cultures showed no growth thus far.

Assessment: **Decubitus ulcer, left heel.**

Plan: Cover with vancomycin, pending the results of the cultures. Incision and drainage will depend on possibility of infected bone.

Diagnosis: **Decubitus ulcer, left heel with partial thickness epidermal skin loss.**

Diagnosis code(s)

L89.622 Pressure ulcer of left heel, stage 2

Coding Note(s)

When coding pressure ulcers, documentation of the ulcer size, location, eschar and granulation tissue, exudate, odor, sinus tracts, undermining, or infection and appropriate staging (I through IV) are essential. Codes for decubitus ulcers in ICD-10-CM include site, laterality, and severity—including the four stages of pressure ulcers so only one code is necessary to describe the patient's condition. Code L89.622 includes pressure ulcer with partial thickness skin loss involving the epidermis and/or dermis, left heel.

Non-Pressure Chronic Ulcer of Lower Limb/Other Sites/Unspecified Site

Non-pressure ulcers may also be referred to as atrophic, chronic, neurogenic, non-healing, non-infected sinus, perforating, trophic, or tropical ulcers. Non-pressure skin ulcers are typically caused by another condition which is usually vascular in nature. Common causal conditions include: atherosclerosis of the extremities, chronic venous hypertension, diabetes mellitus with circulatory complications, and postphlebitic syndrome.

In ICD-10-CM, non-pressure chronic skin ulcers of the lower extremities are classified in category L97 and non-pressure chronic skin ulcers of other sites are classified in subcategory L98.4. Codes in category L97 and subcategory L98.4 may be reported alone if the etiology is not known or they may be reported as secondary codes when the underlying condition is documented. For example, ulcers caused by circulatory system disease such as varicose veins, post-thrombotic syndrome, or chronic venous hypertension are first assigned a code from the circulatory system chapter of the Tabular List, and then a second code is assigned from category L97 or subcategory L98.4 to describe the specific anatomical location. Other causes of non-pressure chronic ulcers include diabetes mellitus and atherosclerosis. In addition to assigning the etiology as the first listed diagnosis, any gangrene is also listed before the code for the ulcer.

Non-pressure chronic ulcers are classified by anatomical location and codes further specify the severity of tissue damage, which ranges from breakdown of the skin only to necrosis of bone. Documentation of the specific anatomical site and a detailed description of the severity are necessary for optimal code assignment.

Coding and Documentation Requirements

Identify site of non-pressure chronic ulcer:

- Back
- Buttock
- Lower leg
  - Ankle
  - Calf
  - Heel and midfoot
  - Other part of foot (includes toe)
  - Other part of lower leg
  - Unspecified part of lower leg
- Thigh
- Other specified site / unspecified site

Identify ulcer severity as:

- Limited to breakdown of skin
- With fat layer exposed
- With necrosis of muscle
- With necrosis of bone
- With muscles involvement without evidence of necrosis
- With bone involvement without evidence of necrosis
- With other specified severity
- Unspecified severity

Identify laterality:

- Right
- Left
- Unspecified

Identify and code first any associated underlying condition:

- Atherosclerosis of the lower extremities
- Chronic venous hypertension
- Diabetic ulcers
- Gangrene
- Postphlebitic syndrome
- Post-thrombotic syndrome
- Varicose ulcer

Non-Pressure Chronic Ulcer – Calf

ICD-10-CM Code/Documentation	
Unspecified Calf	
L97.201	Non-pressure chronic ulcer of unspecified calf limited to breakdown of skin
L97.202	Non-pressure chronic ulcer of unspecified calf with fat layer exposed
L97.203	Non-pressure chronic ulcer of unspecified calf with necrosis of muscle
L97.204	Non-pressure chronic ulcer of unspecified calf with necrosis of bone
L97.205	Non-pressure chronic ulcer of unspecified calf with muscle involvement without evidence of necrosis
L97.206	Non-pressure chronic ulcer of unspecified calf with bone involvement without evidence of necrosis
L97.208	Non-pressure chronic ulcer of unspecified calf with other specified severity
L97.209	Non-pressure chronic ulcer of unspecified calf with unspecified severity
Right Calf	
L97.211	Non-pressure chronic ulcer of right calf limited to breakdown of skin
L97.212	Non-pressure chronic ulcer of right calf with fat layer exposed
L97.213	Non-pressure chronic ulcer of right calf with necrosis of muscle
L97.214	Non-pressure chronic ulcer of right calf with necrosis of bone
L97.215	Non-pressure chronic ulcer of right calf with muscle involvement without evidence of necrosis
L97.216	Non-pressure chronic ulcer of right calf with bone involvement without evidence of necrosis
L97.218	Non-pressure chronic ulcer of right calf with other specified severity
L97.219	Non-pressure chronic ulcer of right calf with unspecified severity
Left Calf	
L97.221	Non-pressure chronic ulcer of left calf limited to breakdown of skin
L97.222	Non-pressure chronic ulcer of left calf with fat layer exposed
L97.223	Non-pressure chronic ulcer of left calf with necrosis of muscle
L97.224	Non-pressure chronic ulcer of left calf with necrosis of bone
L97.225	Non-pressure chronic ulcer of left calf with muscle involvement without evidence of necrosis
L97.226	Non-pressure chronic ulcer of left calf with bone involvement without evidence of necrosis
L97.228	Non-pressure chronic ulcer of left calf with other specified severity
L97.229	Non-pressure chronic ulcer of left calf with unspecified severity

Documentation and Coding Example

Patient is a 42-year-old male with a **poor healing ulceration of the right lower extremity**. He states that the ulcer and surrounding redness has been present for approximately 6 months without significant improvement, but without significant worsening either. The patient denies any fevers or chills and denies any worsening redness or pain to the right lower extremity. He denies any cough or sputum. Has not had any chest pain, palpitations, or lightheadedness. He denies any orthopnea or PND. No chest pain on exertion or dyspnea on exertion. He has no trauma, headache, visual disturbances, focal weakness, numbness, or any gait disturbances. He denies any joint pain, rash, back pain, abdominal pain, vomiting, diarrhea, constipation, hematochezia, melena or any change in appetite. He has had no dysuria, hematuria, increased urinary frequency or urgency. Denies any upper respiratory infection symptoms, sore throat, or odynophagia. All other systems are reviewed and otherwise negative.

Past medical history is significant for this chronic non-healing right lower extremity ulcer. No previous surgeries. Denies tobacco, alcohol, or illicit drug use. Family history is noncontributory. Medications: NKDA; Daily multivitamin.

Vital Signs: Blood pressure 148/90, pulse 92, respirations 21, temperature 98.5 degrees Fahrenheit oral, O2 95% on room air.

This is a well-developed, well-nourished male, ambulating. Alert and oriented x3. In no acute respiratory distress. The patient is otherwise afebrile with stable vital signs and does not appear toxic otherwise. HEENT: Pupils equal, round, and reactive to light. Extraocular muscles are intact. Mucous membranes are moist. Oropharynx is clear. Neck: No JVD. Supple. Lungs: Clear to auscultation bilaterally. No wheezes or rales. Heart: Regular rate and rhythm. Normal S1, S2. Abdomen: Soft, nontender to deep palpation in all quadrants. No rebound or guarding. Normoactive bowel sounds. Neurological: Sensation is intact to light touch. Skin: Warm and dry.

Extremities: There is a chronic shallow nonhealing ulcer on the lateral aspect of the right calf with some surrounding erythema, however, without significant warmth. The wound is shallow, limited to breakdown of skin, and does appear to have clean granulation tissue at the base. There is no fluctuance or induration. No active drainage. No proximal lymphangitic streaking. No inguinal lymphadenopathy is present. Full range of motion in all joints.

Labs were unremarkable. Lab work does not show significant leukocytosis and the patient does not appear to have significant underlying diabetes to suggest an immunocompromised state. The blood culture so far is negative.

Clinical Impression: Chronic lower extremity nonhealing ulcer which has been ongoing for 6 months. The patient was treated with one dose of IV ciprofloxacin. Wound care protocol, dressings applied. A prescription was sent to pharmacy and the patient will be provided with a 3-day supply of antibiotics. He will follow up in 2 days for repeat wound check.

Disposition: Discharged to home, stable. Follow up with primary physician in 2 days for repeat wound check. He has been given antibiotics to take as directed and will return to the emergency department for any worsening symptoms including worsening redness, fevers, chills, vomiting, or any other concerning symptoms.

Diagnosis: **Chronic nonhealing ulcer, right lower leg**.

Diagnosis code(s)

L97.211 Non-pressure chronic ulcer of right calf limited to breakdown of skin

Coding Note(s)

ICD-10-CM codes for non-pressure ulcers specify the site as well as the severity of tissue damage from limited to breakdown of skin to necrosis of bone.

Summary

The ICD-10-CM codes include detail and specificity about various conditions of skin and subcutaneous tissue such as laterality and site designation. Provider documentation of the severity of the disease, the etiology and any secondary disease process, as well as the specific site is necessary for code assignment. Provider documentation of any cause-and-effect relationship between a medical treatment and an integumentary disorder is also required for accurate, complete code assignment.

Many combination codes exist that identify both the disorder and common manifestation. For example, decubitus ulcer codes are combination codes that include the site, laterality, and stages of pressure ulcers.

In addition to specificity, updated and standardized terminology is used in ICD-10-CM. Because the clinical information has been updated to include advances in medical diagnosis and treatment for conditions, an understanding of specific coding terms is needed along with more detailed documentation of the patient's condition.

Resources

Documentation checklists are available in Appendix A for the following condition(s):

- Dermatitis
- Skin ulcer, chronic, non-pressure
- Skin ulcer, pressure

Chapter 12 Quiz

1. Codes for diseases of the skin and subcutaneous tissue are classified in Chapter 12. In ICD-10-CM these conditions are organized into:
   a. Three subsections
   b. Nine code blocks
   c. Fourth-character subclassifications
   d. Fifth-character level subclassifications
2. Where are nail disorders classified in ICD-10-CM?
   a. With diseases of the connective tissue
   b. With diseases of the musculoskeletal system
   c. With diseases of the skin and subcutaneous tissue
   d. With infectious and parasitic diseases
3. Which codes are used for pressure ulcers when the clinical documentation indicates the stage cannot be clinically determined because the ulcer is covered by eschar?
   a. Assign the appropriate code for unspecified stage
   b. Assign the appropriate code for unstageable pressure ulcer
   c. Assign the code for the highest stage for that site
   d. The provider must be queried for additional information regarding the stage of the pressure ulcer
4. The physician documents the patient's diagnosis as boil of the neck. How is this coded?
   a. Boil of neck
   b. Furuncle of neck
   c. Folliculitis of neck
   d. All of the above
5. Which of the following statements is true regarding coding of chronic skin ulcers?
   a. Requires dual coding to identify the ulcer type and the ulcer stage
   b. A combination code is used to identify the ulcer type and the ulcer stage/severity.
   c. Anatomic location is not part of the code description.
   d. All codes require site and laterality.
6. The physician documents the patient's diagnosis as eczema. How is this coded?
   a. Acute dermatitis due to unspecified cause
   b. Dermatitis, unspecified
   c. Other specified dermatitis
   d. Psoriasis, unspecified
7. Cellulitis may be complicated by acute lymphangitis. Which of the following is true regarding coding of cellulitis with lymphangitis?
   a. There is no differentiation between cellulitis with lymphangitis and cellulitis without lymphangitis
   b. There are combination codes for cellulitis and acute lymphangitis
   c. There are distinct codes for cellulitis and acute lymphangitis
   d. None of the above
8. Which of the following is NOT coded as a pressure ulcer?
   a. Bed sore
   b. Chronic ulcer of skin of lower limb
   c. Decubitus ulcer
   d. Plaster ulcer
9. What information is specified in both the pressure ulcer and non-pressure ulcer codes?
   a. Laterality only
   b. Site only
   c. Site and laterality
   d. Etiology
10. A patient is admitted with sacral pressure ulcers documented as healed. How is this coded?
   a. Assign the appropriate code for unstageable ulcer
   b. Assign the appropriate code for unspecified stage only if the patient is being treated for the pressure ulcer
   c. Assign the appropriate personal history health status code (Z77-Z99)
   d. No code is assigned if the documentation states that the pressure ulcer is completely healed

See next page for answers and rationales.

Chapter 12 Answers and Rationales

1. Codes for diseases of the skin and subcutaneous tissue are classified in Chapter 12. In ICD-10-CM these conditions are organized into:

   b. Nine code blocks

   Rationale: *The beginning of the chapter notes code blocks contained in the chapter, followed by a list of the nine code blocks included in the chapter.*

2. Where are nail disorders classified in ICD-10-CM?

   c. With diseases of the skin and subcutaneous tissue

   Rationale: *Nail disorders are classified with disorders of skin appendages in the L60-L75 code block.*

3. Which codes are used for pressure ulcers when the clinical documentation indicates the stage cannot be clinically determined because the ulcer is covered by eschar?

   b. Assign the appropriate code for unstageable pressure ulcer

   Rationale: *According to the ICD-10-CM Official Guidelines for Coding and Reporting Section I.C.12.a.2: Assignment of the code for unstageable pressure ulcer (L89.--0) should be based on the clinical documentation. These codes are used for pressure ulcers whose stage cannot be clinically determined (e.g., the ulcer is covered by eschar or has been treated with a skin or muscle graft).*

4. The physician documents the patient's diagnosis as boil of the neck. How is this coded?

   d. All of the above

   Rationale: *The Index entry for Boil directs the user to see Furuncle, by site. Boil and Folliculitis of neck are listed as included conditions under code L02.12.*

5. Which of the following statements is true regarding coding of chronic skin ulcers?

   b. A combination code is used to identify the ulcer type and the ulcer stage/severity

   Rationale: *According to the ICD-10-CM Official Guidelines for Coding and Reporting Section I.C.12.a. Codes from category L89, L97 and L98.4 are combination codes that identify the type (pressure vs. non-pressure), site of the ulcer as well as the stage/severity of the ulcer and laterality, as appropriate.*

6. The physician documents the patient's diagnosis as eczema. How is this coded in ICD-10-CM?

   b. Dermatitis, unspecified

   Rationale: *Code L30.9 Dermatitis, unspecified lists Eczema, NOS as an included condition. The Index entry for Eczema directs the coder to code L30.9 and there is a note to see also Dermatitis.*

7. Cellulitis may be complicated by acute lymphangitis. Which of the following is true regarding coding of cellulitis with lymphangitis?

   c. There are distinct codes for cellulitis and acute lymphangitis

   Rationale: *Codes in category L03, Cellulitis and acute lymphangitis, include subcategories for cellulitis by site and acute lymphangitis by site.*

8. Which of the following is NOT coded as a pressure ulcer?

   b. Chronic ulcer of skin of lower limb

   Rationale: *According to the inclusion note, codes in category L89, Pressure ulcer, include bed sore, decubitus ulcer, plaster ulcer, pressure area, and pressure sore. Category L97 Non-pressure chronic ulcer of lower limb NEC, includes chronic ulcer of skin of lower limb.*

9. What information is specified in both the pressure ulcer and non-pressure ulcer codes?

   c. Site and laterality

   Rationale: *Codes in category L89 specify the site of the ulcer including laterality, and the ulcer stage as in Pressure ulcer of left heel, stage 1 (L89.621). Non-pressure ulcer codes do not identify the stage, but site and laterality. For example, code L97.421 Non-pressure chronic ulcer of left heel and midfoot limited to breakdown of skin.*

10. A patient is admitted with sacral pressure ulcers documented as healed. How is this coded?

    d. No code is assigned if the documentation states that the pressure ulcer is completely healed

    Rationale: *According to the coding guidelines, no code is assigned for patients admitted with pressure ulcers when the documentation states that the pressure ulcer is completely healed.*

Chapter 13

COMPLICATIONS OF PREGNANCY, CHILDBIRTH, AND THE PUERPERIUM

Introduction

Codes for complications of pregnancy, childbirth, and the puerperium are found in Chapter 13. There are no fifth digit subclassifications that identify the episode of care. Instead of episode of care designations, the majority of codes for complications that occur during pregnancy are organized to identify the trimester, which is captured by the fourth, fifth, or sixth character. In order to assign the most specific code, documentation will now need to provide the trimester or the weeks of gestation. The fourth, fifth, or sixth character may also capture the stage of pregnancy for complications that can occur at any point or at certain times in the pregnancy—during second or third trimester, childbirth, or postpartum, such as eclampsia in category O15. Some complications, specifically those that typically occur or are treated only in a single trimester, such as ectopic pregnancy (O00), do not identify the trimester. In addition, complications that occur only during childbirth or the puerperium contain that information in the code description, such as obstructed labor due to generally contracted pelvis (O65.1) or puerperal sepsis (O85).

Another key point in assigning pregnancy codes is the need for a 7th character identifying the fetus for which the complication code applies. For single gestation, or when the documentation is insufficient to identify the fetus, the 7th character '0' for not applicable/unspecified is assigned. For multiple gestations, each fetus should be identified with a number as fetus 1, fetus 2, fetus 3, etc. The fetus or fetuses affected by the condition should then be clearly identified using the number assigned to the fetus. For example, a triplet gestation in the third trimester with fetus 1 having no complications, fetus 2 in a separate amniotic sac having polyhydramnios, and fetus 3 having hydrocephalus with maternal pelvic disproportion would require reporting of the complications as follows: Fetus 1 – No codes; Fetus 2 – O40.3XX2 Polyhydramnios, third trimester, fetus 2; Fetus 3 – O33.6XX3 Maternal care for disproportion due to hydrocephalic fetus, fetus 3. An additional code identifying the triplet pregnancy would also be reported.

Coding Instructions

There are important coding notes and instructions at the chapter level. The first note indicates that codes from Chapter 15 are to be used only on maternal records, never on newborn records. Codes that capture conditions in the newborn that were caused by a maternal condition are found in Chapter 16 Certain Conditions Originating in the Perinatal Period, in code categories P00-P04, and these codes are reported only on the newborn record.

Codes in Chapter 15 are to be used for conditions related to or aggravated by the pregnancy, childbirth, or the puerperium, which may be either maternal causes or obstetric causes. While not specifically addressed in the chapter level instructions, it should also be noted that codes in Chapter 15 are sequenced first over codes from other chapters. Codes from other chapters are reported additionally following any instructions at the code level. For example, codes for diabetes mellitus in pregnancy, childbirth, and the puerperium (O24) are sequenced first followed by a code from categories E08-E13 to identify the specific type of diabetes and any complications or manifestations.

Because most complications related to pregnancy require identification of the trimester, there is also an explanation on how each trimester is calculated. Trimester is calculated using the first day of the last menstrual period. Calculations for trimesters are as follows:

- First trimester – less than 14 weeks 0 days
- Second trimester – 14 weeks 0 days to less than 28 weeks 0 days
- Third trimester – 28 weeks 0 days to delivery

There is also a note to use an additional code to identify weeks of gestation. Weeks of gestation codes are supplementary codes found in category Z3A.

Chapter Organization

The chapter is organized with categories for ectopic pregnancy, molar pregnancy, and pregnancy with abortive outcome listed first. Categories for complications primarily related to pregnancy are listed next, followed by codes related to labor and delivery, which includes both complications of labor and delivery and normal delivery. Complications related to the puerperium are the final listed codes. There are some exceptions. Conditions that have the potential to complicate pregnancy, childbirth, and/or the puerperium, such as edema, proteinuria, and hypertensive disorders (O10-O16) are listed together with fourth, fifth, or sixth characters that identify the stage of care. Codes for supervision of high risk pregnancy (O09) and abnormal findings on antenatal screening of the mother (O28) are also found within this chapter.

Multiple gestation placenta status is captured with a combination code for multiple gestation that includes information on the number of placentas and amniotic sacs (O30). Inconclusive fetal viability (O36.80) is also listed in Chapter 15 as are other codes for maternal care for other fetal problems. Refer to the table below for a complete list of the blocks of codes in ICD-10-CM.

ICD-10-CM Blocks	
O00-O08	Pregnancy with Abortive Outcome
O09	Supervision of High Risk Pregnancy
O10-O16	Edema, Proteinuria and Hypertensive Disorders in Pregnancy, Childbirth and the Puerperium
O20-O29	Other Maternal Disorders Predominantly Related to Pregnancy
O30-O48	Maternal Care Related to the Fetus and Amniotic Cavity and Possible Delivery Problems
O60-O77	Complications of Labor and Delivery
O80-O82	Encounter for Delivery
O85-O92	Complications Predominantly Related to the Puerperium
O94-O9A	Other Obstetric Conditions, Not Elsewhere Classified

Exclusions

In ICD-10-CM Chapter 15, the excludes notes are as follows:

Excludes1	Excludes2
Supervision of normal pregnancy (Z34.-)	Mental and behavioral disorders associated with the puerperium (F53) Obstetrical tetanus (A34) Postpartum necrosis of pituitary gland (E23.0) Puerperal osteomalacia (M83.0)

Supervision of normal pregnancy is a type 1 excludes note which means that codes in category Z34 cannot be reported in conjunction with codes from Chapter 15. Codes for supervision of normal pregnancy are used only for patients who have no conditions complicating maternal or obstetric care. Codes in category Z34 are sub-classified as normal first pregnancy (Z34.0), other normal pregnancy (Z34.8), and normal pregnancy unspecified (Z34.9). A fifth character is required to identify the trimester.

The Excludes2 note for mental and behavioral disorders associated with the puerperium refers to postpartum depression reported with code F53.0, and puerperal psychosis reported with F53.1. Because puerperal psychosis and postpartum depression are listed as a type 2 excludes note, codes F53.0 and F53.1 can be reported with other complications of the puerperium when the postpartum depression or psychosis occur together with other complications.

Chapter Guidelines

Chapter 15 guidelines include information covering general rules and sequencing of codes as well as coding rules for specific conditions. The guideline categories are as follows:

General rules for coding obstetric cases

- Selection of OB principle diagnosis
- Pre-existing conditions versus conditions due to the pregnancy
- Pre-existing hypertension in pregnancy
- Fetal conditions affecting the management of the mother
- HIV infection in pregnancy, childbirth, and the puerperium
- Diabetes mellitus in pregnancy
- Long term use of insulin
- Gestational (pregnancy-induced) diabetes
- Sepsis and septic shock complicating abortion, pregnancy, childbirth, and the puerperium
- Puerperal sepsis
- Alcohol, tobacco, and drug use during pregnancy, childbirth, and the puerperium
- Poisoning, toxic effects, adverse effects, and underdosing in a pregnant patient
- Normal delivery (O80)
- The peripartum and postpartum periods
- Sequelae of complications of pregnancy, childbirth, and the puerperium (O94)
- Termination of pregnancy and spontaneous abortions
- Abuse in a pregnant patient

General Rules for Coding Obstetric Cases

General rules cover sequencing priority, assigning a character for the trimester and special coding rules related to the trimester, and assigning a 7th character to identify the fetus.

Sequencing Priority

- Codes in Chapter 15 Complications of Pregnancy, Childbirth, and Puerperium (O00-O9A) have sequencing priority over codes from other chapters
- Additional codes from other chapters may be reported with Chapter 15 codes to specify the condition further
- Documentation that the pregnancy is incidental to the encounter is reported with code Z33.1 Pregnant state, incidental. It is the provider's responsibility to document that the condition being treated is not affecting the pregnancy

Use Chapter 15 Codes Only on the Maternal Record

- Use only on maternal records, never on newborn records
- Codes that capture conditions in the newborn that were caused by a maternal condition are found in Chapter 16 Certain Conditions Originating in the Perinatal Period, in code categories P00-P04, and these codes are reported only on the newborn record

Final Character for Identification of Trimester

- Most codes in Chapter 15 have a final character indicating the trimester
- Assignment of the final character for trimester is based on the provider's documentation which may identify the trimester or the number of weeks gestation for the current encounter
- Trimesters are calculated using the first day of the last menstrual period as follows:
  - First trimester – less than 14 weeks 0 days
  - Second trimester – 14 weeks 0 days to less than 28 weeks 0 days
  - Third trimester – 28 weeks 0 days to delivery

- The final character identifying the trimester may be the 4th, 5th, or 6th character
- Codes that do not identify the trimester include:
  - Conditions that only occur during a single specific trimester
  - Conditions for which the concept of trimester does not apply
- Conditions may have characters only for certain trimesters because the condition does not occur in all trimesters but does occur in more than one trimester. For example, category O14 Pre-eclampsia, has specific codes only for the second and third trimesters because pre-eclampsia does not occur in the first trimester (except in patients with pre-existing hypertension, and this condition is reported with codes from category O11)
- If a delivery occurs during the admission, and there is an "in childbirth" option for the complication, the code for "in childbirth" is assigned

Trimester Selection for Inpatient Admissions Encompassing More Than One Trimester

- When an inpatient admission encompasses more than one trimester, the code is assigned based on when the condition developed- not when the discharge occurred (e.g. if the condition developed during the second trimester and the patient was discharged during the third trimester, the code for the second trimester is assigned)
- If the condition being treated developed prior to the current admission/encounter, or was a pre-existing condition, the trimester character at the time of the admission/encounter is used

Unspecified Trimester

- Unspecified trimester character should be used only when the documentation is insufficient to determine the trimester and it is not possible to obtain clarification from the provider

7th Character for Fetus Identification

Some complications of pregnancy and childbirth occur more frequently in multiple gestation pregnancies. These complications may affect one or more fetuses and require a 7th character to identify the fetus or fetuses affected by the complication.

- The following categories/subcategories require identification of the fetus:
  - O31 Complications specific to multiple gestation
  - O32 Maternal care for malpresentation of fetus
  - O33.3 Maternal care for disproportion due to outlet contraction of pelvis
  - O33.4 Maternal care for disproportion of mixed maternal and fetal origin
  - O33.5 Maternal care for disproportion due to unusually large fetus
  - O33.6 Maternal care for disproportion due to hydrocephalic fetus
  - O35 Maternal care for known or suspected fetal abnormality and damage
  - O36 Maternal care for other fetal problems
  - O40 Polyhydramnios
  - O41 Other disorders of amniotic fluid and membranes
  - O60.1 Preterm labor with preterm delivery
  - O60.2 Term delivery with preterm labor
  - O64 Obstructed labor due to malposition and malpresentation of fetus
  - O69 Labor and delivery complicated by umbilical cord complications
- The 7th character identifies the fetus for which the complication code applies
- For multiple gestations, each fetus should be identified with a number as Fetus 1, Fetus 2, Fetus 3, etc. The fetus or fetuses affected by the condition should be documented using the number assigned to the fetus. The complication code is then assigned for each fetus affected by the complication
- The 7th character '0' for not applicable/unspecified is assigned in cases of single gestations, when the documentation is insufficient to identify the fetus affected and it is not possible to obtain clarification, or when it is not possible to determine clinically which fetus is affected

Selection of OB Principle or First-Listed Diagnosis

These guidelines relate to assignment and sequencing of codes for routine outpatient prenatal visits, prenatal visits for high-risk patients, and selection of principle or first-listed diagnosis for episodes of care when no delivery occurs, when delivery occurs, and for the outcome of delivery.

Routine Outpatient Prenatal Visits

- A code from category Z34 Encounter for supervision of normal pregnancy, should be used as the first listed diagnosis when there are no documented complications present
- A code from category Z34 should not be used with another code from Chapter 15
- Supervision of high risk pregnancy codes in category O09 are for use only during the prenatal period. For complications that occur during the labor and delivery episode as a result of a high risk pregnancy, assign the applicable complication code(s) from Chapter 15
- Assign code O80 Encounter for full-term uncomplicated delivery if there are no complications during labor and delivery

Supervision of High Risk Pregnancy

- A code from category O09 Supervision of high-risk pregnancy, should be assigned as the first-listed diagnosis for routine prenatal outpatient visits for patients with high-risk pregnancies
- Secondary codes from Chapter 15 may be used in conjunction with codes from category O09

Episodes When No Delivery Occurs

- The principle diagnosis should correspond to the principle complication of the pregnancy which necessitated the encounter as documented by the provider
- When more than one documented complication exists, and all are treated or monitored, any of the complications may be sequenced first

Episodes When a Delivery Occurs

- When an obstetric patient delivers during an admission, the condition prompting the admission is sequenced as the principal diagnosis
- If multiple conditions prompted the admission, the condition most related to the delivery is listed as the principal diagnosis. A code for any complication of the delivery should be assigned as an additional diagnosis
- If the patient was admitted with a condition that resulted in the performance of a cesarean procedure, that condition should be reported as the principal diagnosis
- If the reason for the admission/encounter was unrelated to the condition resulting in the cesarean delivery, the condition related to the reason for the admission/encounter should be selected as the principal diagnosis

Outcome of Delivery

- A code from category Z37 Outcome of delivery should be included on every maternal record when a delivery has occurred
- Codes from category Z37 are not used on subsequent maternal records
- Codes from category Z37 are not used on the newborn record

Pre-Existing Conditions Vs. Conditions Due to the Pregnancy

Certain categories in Chapter 15 distinguish between conditions of the mother that existed prior to pregnancy (pre-existing) and those that are a direct result of the pregnancy. Two examples are hypertension (O10, O11, O13) and diabetes mellitus (O24). The physician must provide clear documentation as to whether the condition existed prior to pregnancy or whether it developed during the pregnancy or as a result of the pregnancy.

Categories that do not distinguish between pre-existing conditions and pregnancy-related conditions may be used for either.

If a puerperal complication develops postpartum during the delivery encounter, and a specific code for the puerperal complication exists, it is acceptable to report the code for the puerperal complication with codes related to complications of pregnancy and childbirth.

Pre-Existing Hypertension in Pregnancy

Category O10 Pre-existing hypertension complicating pregnancy, childbirth and the puerperium includes codes for hypertensive heart and hypertensive chronic kidney disease. When one of these codes is assigned, it is necessary to add a secondary code from the appropriate hypertension category (I11-I13) to identify the type of hypertensive heart and/or chronic kidney disease.

Fetal Conditions Affecting the Management of the Mother

Two categories are available for reporting fetal conditions affecting the mother—O35 Maternal care for known or suspected fetal abnormality and damage; and O36 Maternal care for other fetal problems. Guidelines for assigning these codes are as follows:

- Assign a code from categories O35 or O36 only when the fetal condition is actually responsible for modifying the management of the mother. This may include:
  - Diagnostic studies
  - Additional observation
  - Special care
  - Termination of the pregnancy

In Utero Surgery

- When surgery is performed on the fetus, a diagnosis code from category O35 should be assigned to identify the fetal condition
- Codes from Chapter 16 Certain Conditions Originating in the Perinatal Period are not used on the maternal record to identify fetal conditions for in utero surgery. Surgery performed in utero on a fetus is still coded as an obstetric encounter

HIV Infection in Pregnancy

During pregnancy, childbirth, and the puerperium, HIV infection is reported as follows:

- A patient admitted because of an HIV-related illness should receive a principal diagnosis from subcategory O98.7- HIV disease complicating pregnancy, childbirth, and the puerperium followed by the code(s) for the HIV related illness(es) [B20 for symptomatic HIV disease/AIDs reported additionally along with specific codes identifying the HIV-related illness]
- Patients admitted with asymptomatic HIV infection status during pregnancy, childbirth, and the puerperium should receive codes from subcategories O98.7- and Z21 Asymptomatic HIV infection status

Diabetes Mellitus in Pregnancy

Diabetes mellitus is a significant complicating factor in pregnancy. All pregnant women with diabetes mellitus are considered to have a complication that affects maternal and obstetric care, so a code from category O24 Diabetes mellitus in pregnancy, childbirth, and the puerperium should be assigned for outpatient and inpatient encounters with one or more codes from categories E08-E13 to provide additional information about the type of diabetes and any specific complications and/or manifestations. Coding and sequencing are as follows:

- A code from category O24 is reported first
- A code or codes from the appropriate category (E08-E13) in Chapter 4 is assigned to identify specific complications/ manifestations

Long Term Use of Insulin

- If the diabetes is being treated with insulin or oral medications, assign code Z79.4 Long-term (current) use of insulin or code Z79.84 Long-term (current) use of oral hypoglycemic drugs.
- If the patient is treated with both oral medications and insulin, only the code for insulin-controlled should be assigned

Gestational (Pregnancy-Induced) Diabetes

Gestational diabetes can occur during the second and third trimesters in women who were not diabetic prior to pregnancy. Gestational diabetes can cause complications similar to those in patients with pre-existing diabetes. It also puts the woman at risk for developing diabetes after the pregnancy. Coding guidelines for reporting gestational diabetes are as follows:

- Assign a code from subcategory O24.4 Gestational diabetes mellitus
- Do not assign any other codes from category O24 Diabetes mellitus in pregnancy, childbirth and the puerperium in conjunction with a code from O24.4-.
- The provider must document whether the gestational diabetes is being controlled by diet, oral hypoglycemics, or insulin
- If documentation indicates the gestational diabetes is being controlled with both diet and insulin, report only the code for insulin-controlled
- If documentation indicates the gestational diabetes is being treated with both diet and oral hypoglycemic medications, report only the code for "controlled by oral hypoglycemic drugs".
- Do not assign code Z79.4 Long-term (current) use of insulin or code Z79.84 Long-term (current) use of oral hypoglycemic drugs with codes from subcategory O24.4
- An abnormal glucose tolerance test in pregnancy without specific documentation by the provider that the patient has gestational diabetes is assigned a code from subcategory O99.81 Abnormal glucose complicating pregnancy, childbirth, and the puerperium

Sepsis and Septic Shock Complicating Abortion, Pregnancy, Childbirth, and the Puerperium

There are specific codes for sepsis and septic shock complicating abortion, pregnancy, childbirth, and the puerperium in Chapter 15. When one of these codes is assigned, a code for the specific type of infection should be assigned as an additional diagnosis. When severe sepsis is present, a code from subcategory R65.2- Severe sepsis should be used along with codes for any documented organ dysfunction associated with the sepsis as additional diagnoses.

Puerperal Sepsis

Code O85 Puerperal sepsis should be assigned with a secondary code to identify the causal organism:

- For a bacterial infection, assign a code from categories B95-B96
- Do not assign a code from category A40 Streptococcal sepsis, or A41 Other sepsis
- If applicable, use an additional code (R65.2-) to identify severe sepsis
- Assign additional codes for any documented acute organ dysfunction associated with the sepsis
- Do not assign code O85 for sepsis following an obstetrical procedure

Alcohol, Tobacco, and Drug Use During Pregnancy, Childbirth, and the Puerperium

Alcohol use during pregnancy, childbirth, and the puerperium

- For documented alcohol use during the pregnancy or postpartum, assign a code from subcategory O99.31 Alcohol use complicating pregnancy, childbirth, and the puerperium
- Assign a secondary code from category F10 Alcohol related disorders, to identify manifestations of the alcohol use

Tobacco use during pregnancy, childbirth, and the puerperium

- For documented use of any type of tobacco product during the pregnancy or postpartum, assign a code from subcategory O99.33 Smoking (tobacco) complicating pregnancy, childbirth, and the puerperium
- Assign a secondary code from category F17 Nicotine dependence, or code Z72.0 Tobacco use to identify the type of nicotine dependence

Drug use during pregnancy, childbirth, and the puerperium

- Codes from subcategory O99.32 Drug use complicating pregnancy, childbirth, and the puerperium should be assigned for any case in which the mother uses drugs during the pregnancy or postpartum period. This may involve illegal drugs or the inappropriate use or misuse of prescription drugs
- Assign secondary codes from categories F11-F16 and F18-F19 to identify manifestations of the drug use

Poisoning, Toxic Effects, Adverse Effects, and Underdosing in a Pregnant Patient

Sequencing rules for poisoning, toxic effects, adverse effects, and underdosing in pregnancy are as follows:

- A code from subcategory O9A.2 Injury, poisoning and certain other consequences of external causes complicating pregnancy, childbirth, and the puerperium is sequenced first
- The appropriate code for the injury, poisoning, toxic effect, adverse effect, or underdosing is sequenced second
- Additional codes are assigned to specify the condition(s) caused by the poisoning, toxic effect, adverse effect, or underdosing

Normal Delivery

Code O80 is assigned for a normal uncomplicated delivery. Guidelines are as follows:

Encounter for Full Term Uncomplicated Delivery

- Use code O80 for a full term uncomplicated delivery of a single, healthy infant without any antepartum, delivery, or postpartum complications during the delivery episode
- Code O80 is always assigned as the principal diagnosis
- Do not use code O80 if any other code from Chapter 15 is needed to describe a current complication of the antenatal, delivery, or perinatal period
- Additional codes from other chapters may be assigned with code O80 if the condition the code describes is not related to, or in any way associated with a complication of the pregnancy

Uncomplicated Delivery with Resolved Antepartum Complication

- Code O80 may be used if the patient had a complication at some point during the pregnancy, as long as the condition is not present at the time of admission for delivery

Outcome of Delivery for O80

- The only valid outcome of delivery code appropriate for use with code O80 is Z37.0 Single live birth

The Peripartum and Postpartum Periods

Peripartum is defined as the last month of pregnancy to five months postdelivery. Postpartum is defined as beginning immediately after delivery and continues for six weeks following delivery. Guidelines related to the peripartum and postpartum periods are as follows:

Complications

- A postpartum complication is any complication occurring within the 6-week period following delivery
- Pregnancy-related complications after the 6-week period may be reported with codes from Chapter 15 if the provider documents that the condition is pregnancy-related
- Pregnancy-associated cardiomyopathy, code O90.3, is unique in that it may be diagnosed in the third trimester, but may continue to progress for months after delivery. For this reason, it is considered a peripartum complication
- For documented pregnancy-associated cardiomyopathy, assign code O90.3 Peripartum cardiomyopathy only when the condition develops as a result of pregnancy in a patient who did not have pre-existing heart disease

Admission for Routine Postpartum Care following Delivery Outside Hospital

- Assign code Z39.0 Encounter for care and examination of mother immediately after delivery, when the mother delivers outside the hospital and is admitted only for routine postpartum care without any documented complications

Sequelae of Complication of Pregnancy, Childbirth, and the Puerperium

Code O94 Sequela of complication of pregnancy, childbirth, and the puerperium is assigned in cases when an initial complication of pregnancy develops sequelae that require care or treatment at a future date. Coding guidelines are as follows:

- Code O94 may be used at any time after the initial postpartum period
- Code O94 is sequenced following the code that describes the sequela of the complication

Termination of Pregnancy and Spontaneous Abortions

Abortion with liveborn fetus

- When an attempted termination of pregnancy results in a liveborn fetus, assign code Z33.2 Encounter for elective termination of pregnancy
- Assign a code from category Z37 Outcome of delivery as a secondary diagnosis

Retained Products of Conception Following an Abortion

- Assign code O03.4 Incomplete spontaneous abortion without complication or O07.4 Failed attempted termination of pregnancy without complication for subsequent encounters for retained products of conception following a spontaneous abortion or elective termination of pregnancy without complications
- Use these codes for subsequent encounters for retained products of conception even if the patient was discharged previously with a discharge diagnosis of complete abortion
- If the patient has a specific complication associated with the spontaneous abortion or elective termination of pregnancy in addition to retained products of conception, assign the appropriate complication in category O03 or O07 instead of code O03.4 or O07.4

Complications Leading to Abortion

- Chapter 15 codes may be used as additional codes to identify any documented complications of the pregnancy in conjunction with codes in categories O04 Complications following (induced) termination of pregnancy, O07 Failed attempted termination of pregnancy or O08 Complications following ectopic and molar pregnancy

Abuse in a Pregnant Patient

Suspected or confirmed abuse of a pregnant patient is reported as follows:

- A code from one of the following subcategories in Chapter 15 is sequenced first:
  - O9A.3 Physical abuse complicating pregnancy, childbirth, and the puerperium
  - O9A.4 Sexual abuse complicating pregnancy, childbirth, and the puerperium
  - O9A.5 Psychological abuse complicating pregnancy, childbirth, and the puerperium
- Assign secondary codes for any associated current injury resulting from the abuse

General Documentation Requirements

There are a number of general documentation requirements that are briefly reviewed here. They will be addressed in more detail in subsequent sections, and specific examples of the required documentation will be provided in the coding scenarios.

Trimester

Most codes for complications of pregnancy require identification of the trimester. The provider may document either the trimester or the weeks of gestation for complications occurring during pregnancy. If the weeks of pregnancy are documented, the coder must identify the trimester based on the ICD-10-CM definitions. This information is provided in coding note instructions at the beginning of Chapter 15. In addition, a supplementary code from category Z3A Weeks of gestation should be assigned to identify the specific week of gestation when documented.

Fetus

Some complications of pregnancy and childbirth occur more frequently in multiple gestation pregnancies than in single gestation pregnancies and these complications may affect one or more of the fetuses. To address this, 14 code categories and subcategories in ICD-10-CM now require identification of the fetus affected by the complication. When documenting these complications in multiple gestation pregnancies, the provider will clearly need to identify every fetus affected by each identified complication by assigning a number to the fetus. There are 7th character extensions that specifically identify each fetus up to five as Fetus 1, Fetus 2, Fetus 3, Fetus 4, and Fetus 5. For multiple gestations with more than five fetuses, the remaining fetuses are identified as "other fetus" by the seventh character extension 9. For single gestations, or multiple gestations in which the affected fetus has not been identified, the 7th character extension 0 is used to indicate that the fetus designation is not applicable or unspecified.

Combination Codes

Another documentation requirement relates to category O30 Multiple gestation. The code identifying the twin, triplet, quadruplet, or other specified multiple gestation includes the multiple gestation placenta status. These combination codes require documentation of the number of placentas and amniotic sacs for twin pregnancies as follows:

- O30.01- Twin pregnancy, monochorionic, monoamniotic
- O30.03- Twin pregnancy, monochorionic, diamniotic
- O30.04- Twin pregnancy, dichorionic, diamniotic

For triplet, quadruplet, and other multiple gestations, documentation must identify the placenta status:

- Two or more monochorionic fetuses
- Two or more monoamniotic fetuses
- Trichorionic/triamniotic (triplet pregnancy)
- Quadrachorionic/quadra-amniotic (quadruplet pregnancy)
- Number of chorions and amnions both equal to the number of fetuses (other multiple gestations)

There is also an unspecified group of codes in each of the multiple gestation subcategories to indicate that the number of placentas and amniotic sacs has not been documented, as well as codes to indicate that the number of placentas and amniotic sacs cannot be determined. When the provider cannot identify how many placentas and amniotic sacs are present, this should be documented to avoid assignment of an unspecified code.

Code-Specific Documentation Requirements

The next section presents some of the ICD-10-CM codes in Chapter 15 that have special documentation requirements. The focus is on frequently reported conditions that require additional or particular pieces of clinical documentation to assign the best code(s). Though not all of the codes with special documentation requirements are discussed, this section will provide a representative sample of the type of documentation elements required for complications of pregnancy, childbirth, and the puerperium. This section is organized by topic or groups of related topics.

Antepartum Hemorrhage, Abruptio Placentae, and Placenta Previa

Antepartum hemorrhage refers to any bleeding from the vagina beginning between 20-24 weeks gestation and term. The bleeding may have a benign obstetrical cause such as benign bloody show or it may indicate an obstetrical complication such as placenta previa or abruptio placentae.

Placenta previa is an obstetrical complication in which the placenta attaches low in the uterus, partially or totally obstructing the cervix and the opening to the birth canal. Complete placenta previa covers all of the cervical opening. Partial placenta previa covers part of the cervical opening. Marginal placenta previa lies right on the border of the cervix. A low-lying placenta is within 2 cm of the cervix, but not bordering it. Placenta previa can cause severe bleeding and other complications, and necessitates a cesarean delivery.

Abruptio placentae is an obstetrical complication in which the placenta separates from the wall of the uterus prior to delivery of the fetus. The separation may be apparent with bleeding from the vagina, or concealed if it occurs behind the wall of the uterus. Abruptio placentae can be life threatening to both the mother and fetus. Risk factors for developing the condition include trauma, hypertension, coagulation disorders, smoking, multiple gestation, multiparity, and infections.

There are three code categories for the three general placental complications and causes of antepartum hemorrhage. These include O44 Placenta previa; O45 Premature separation of placenta (abruptio placentae); and O46 Antepartum hemorrhage, not elsewhere classified. The codes are all specific to the trimester. Placenta previa codes are specified as with and without hemorrhage. Premature separation of the placenta may be coded as with coagulation defect (O45.0-), other (O45.8X-), or unspecified (O45.9-) premature separation. Category O46 reports antepartum hemorrhage, not elsewhere classified, which also includes a subcategory (046.0-) for antepartum hemorrhage with coagulation defect. Combination codes are provided for separation of placenta and antepartum hemorrhage that identify the condition with the specific type of coagulation defect, such as afibrinogenemia, disseminated intravascular coagulation, and other coagulation defect.

Coding and Documentation Requirements

Identify antepartum condition:

- Antepartum hemorrhage (not specified as with or due to abruptio placentae)
  - With coagulation defect:
    - Afibrinogenemia
    - Disseminated intravascular coagulation
    - Other coagulation defect
    - Unspecified coagulation defect
  - Other antepartum hemorrhage
  - Unspecified antepartum hemorrhage
- Placenta previa
  - Complete
    - With hemorrhage
    - Without hemorrhage/NOS

- Partial or Marginal
  - With hemorrhage
  - Without hemorrhage/NOS
- Low lying
  - With hemorrhage
  - Without hemorrhage/NOS

- Premature separation of placenta/abruptio placentae
  - With coagulation defect:
    - Afibrinogenemia
    - Disseminated intravascular coagulation
    - Other coagulation defect
    - Unspecified coagulation defect
  - Other premature separation of placenta
  - Unspecified premature separation of placenta

Identify trimester:

- First (less than 14 weeks Ø days)
- Second (14 weeks Ø days to less than 28 weeks Ø days)
- Third (28 weeks Ø days until delivery)
- Unspecified

ICD-1Ø-CM Code/Documentation	
O46.ØØ-	Antepartum hemorrhage with coagulation defect, unspecified
O46.Ø1-	Antepartum hemorrhage with afibrinogenemia
O46.Ø2-	Antepartum hemorrhage with disseminated intravascular coagulation
O46.Ø9-	Antepartum hemorrhage with other coagulation defect
O46.8X-	Other antepartum hemorrhage
O46.9-	Antepartum hemorrhage, unspecified
Note: Subcategory codes require a fifth or sixth character to identify the trimester.	
O45.ØØ-	Premature separation of placenta with coagulation defect, unspecified
O45.Ø1-	Premature separation of placenta with afibrinogenemia
O45.Ø2-	Premature separation of placenta with disseminated intravascular coagulation
O45.Ø9-	Premature separation of placenta with other coagulation defect
O45.8X-	Other premature separation of placenta
O45.9-	Premature separation of placenta, unspecified
Note: Subcategory codes require a fifth or sixth character to identify the trimester.	
O44.Ø-	Complete placenta previa NOS or without hemorrhage
O44.1-	Complete placenta previa with hemorrhage
O44.2-	Partial placenta previa without hemorrhage
O44.3-	Partial placenta previa with hemorrhage
O44.4-	Low lying placenta NOS or without hemorrhage
O44.5-	Low lying placenta with hemorrhage
Note: Subcategory codes require a fifth character to identify the trimester	

Note: Category O46 does not include threatened abortion or other conditions classified in category O2Ø nor does it include hemorrhage during labor and delivery (intrapartum hemorrhage) classified in category O67.

Documentation and Coding Example

Twenty-nine-year-old Caucasian female at **34 weeks gestation** with a history of placental abruption during previous pregnancy is admitted with **Grade 1 placental separation**. She is not in active labor. She is hemodynamically stable and fetal BPP WNL. A 16-gauge angiocath is placed in her left arm for infusion of LR. She is placed on cardiac and fetal monitors. Family allowed in to visit. Repeat US is ordered for this evening. Lab tests are ordered q 8 hours and include CBC w/ platelets and smear for schistocytes, electrolytes, PT, PTT, fibrinogen, D-dimer, FDP. She has been typed and crossmatched for PRBCs, platelets, and FFP. Critical care specialist (CCS) and hematology fellow have been contacted due to increased risk factor for DIC from placental abruption.

L&D Observation Day 2: Patient has a **rising DIC Score** with platelet count at <5Ø,ØØØ, D-dimer/FDP 3.Ø, Fibrinogen 1.Ø and PT < 4Ø % for a total score of 6. Decision made to perform emergency C-section under general anesthesia with transfer to SICU for recovery and treatment.

Post Delivery Note: Patient tolerated surgery very well and is under care of CCS and hematology in the SICU. Infant taken to NICU but is reported to be doing well without oxygen or respiratory support.

Post Op Day 1-CCS Note: Patient is extubated, alert and oriented. She is responding to FFP and platelet transfusions and has not shown signs of progressive organ involvement from DIC. She will remain in SICU for another 24 hours and if she continues to show stable bleeding times will consider transfer to OB floor so she can be with her infant.

OB Floor Notes: Patient transferred to OB unit post-op day 2, hemodynamically stable. Remainder of hospital stay of mother and infant unremarkable.

Discharge Diagnosis: **Emergency C-section for placental abruption complicated by DIC**

Diagnosis Code(s)

O45.Ø23	Premature separation of placenta with disseminated intravascular coagulation, third trimester
Z37.Ø	Single live birth

Coding Note(s)

A combination code is reported that identifies both the premature separation of the placenta and the specific type of coagulation defect. Antepartum hemorrhage due to coagulation defects is not reported additionally because there is an excludes note under O46 and it would only be reported if the patient had an antepartum hemorrhage due to coagulation defect without documentation of premature separation of the placenta.

Diabetes Mellitus (Pre-existing) in Pregnancy

Pre-existing diabetes mellitus is a significant complicating factor in pregnancy and requires careful management of nutrition and insulin or other diabetes medications during the pregnancy to keep blood sugar levels under control.

Subcategory codes in category O24 Diabetes mellitus in pregnancy, childbirth, and the puerperium provide information on the type of diabetes. There are specific codes for type 1, type 2, other pre-existing diabetes mellitus, unspecified pre-existing DM, and unspecified diabetes mellitus in pregnancy. Codes for pre-existing diabetes are also specific to the trimester, childbirth, or the puerperium. A secondary code is also required from category E08, E09, E10, E11, or E13 to identify further any manifestations or complications.

Coding and Documentation Requirements

Identify type of pre-existing diabetes mellitus:

- Diabetes mellitus Type 1
- Diabetes mellitus Type 2
- Other pre-existing type of diabetes, which includes:
  - Diabetes due to underlying conditions (such as congenital rubella, Cushing's syndrome, cystic fibrosis, malignant neoplasm, malnutrition, pancreatitis, and other diseases of the pancreas)
  - Drug or chemical induced diabetes
  - Other specified type, which includes:
    - Diabetes mellitus due to genetic defects of beta-cell function
    - Diabetes mellitus due to genetic defects of insulin action
    - Postpancreatectomy diabetes mellitus
    - Secondary diabetes mellitus NEC
- Unspecified type diabetes mellitus

Identify trimester:

- First (less than 14 weeks 0 days)
- Second (14 weeks 0 days to less than 28 weeks 0 days)
- Third (28 weeks 0 days until delivery)
- Unspecified

Use an additional code from the appropriate category (E08, E09, E10, E11, E13) to identify further any manifestations/complications:

- No complications
- Ketoacidosis
  - With coma
  - Without coma
- Kidney complications
  - Diabetic nephropathy
  - Diabetic chronic kidney disease
  - Other diabetic kidney complication
- Ophthalmic complications
  - Diabetic retinopathy
    - Mild nonproliferative
      - With macular edema
      - Without macular edema
    - Moderate nonproliferative
      - With macular edema
      - Without macular edema
    - Severe nonproliferative
      - With macular edema
      - Without macular edema
    - Proliferative
      - With macular edema
      - Without macular edema
      - With traction retinal detachment involving the macula
      - With traction retinal detachment not involving the macula
      - With combined traction retinal detachment and rhegmatogenous retinal detachment
    - Stable proliferative
    - Unspecified
      - With macular edema
      - Without macular edema
  - Diabetic cataract
  - Diabetic macular edema, resolved following treatment
  - Other diabetic ophthalmic complication
- Neurological complications
  - Diabetic amyotrophy
  - Diabetic autonomic (poly)neuropathy
  - Diabetic mononeuropathy
  - Diabetic polyneuropathy
  - Other diabetic neurological complication
  - Unspecified diabetic neuropathy
- Circulatory complications
  - Diabetic peripheral angiopathy
    - With gangrene
    - Without gangrene
  - Other specified circulatory complications
- Diabetic arthropathy
  - Neuropathic
  - Other
- Diabetic skin complications
  - Diabetic dermatitis
  - Foot ulcer
  - Other skin ulcer
  - Other skin complications
- Diabetic oral complications
  - Periodontal disease
  - Other oral complications
- Hyperglycemia
- Hyperosmolarity
  - with coma
  - without coma
- Hypoglycemia
  - With coma
  - Without coma
- Other specified complication
- Unspecified complication

ICD-10-CM Code/Documentation	
O24.011	Pre-existing type 1 diabetes mellitus, in pregnancy, first trimester
O24.012	Pre-existing type 1 diabetes mellitus, in pregnancy, second trimester
O24.013	Pre-existing type 1 diabetes mellitus, in pregnancy, third trimester
O24.019	Pre-existing type 1 diabetes mellitus, in pregnancy, unspecified trimester
O24.02	Pre-existing type 1 diabetes mellitus, in childbirth
O24.03	Pre-existing type 1 diabetes mellitus, in the puerperium
O24.111	Pre-existing type 2 diabetes mellitus, in pregnancy, first trimester
O24.112	Pre-existing type 2 diabetes mellitus, in pregnancy, second trimester
O24.113	Pre-existing type 2 diabetes mellitus, in pregnancy, third trimester
O24.119	Pre-existing type 2 diabetes mellitus, in pregnancy, unspecified trimester
O24.12	Pre-existing type 2 diabetes mellitus, in childbirth
O24.13	Pre-existing type 2 diabetes mellitus, in the puerperium
O24.311	Unspecified pre-existing diabetes mellitus in pregnancy, first trimester
O24.312	Unspecified pre-existing diabetes mellitus in pregnancy, second trimester
O24.313	Unspecified pre-existing diabetes mellitus in pregnancy, third trimester
O24.319	Unspecified pre-existing diabetes mellitus in pregnancy, unspecified trimester
O24.32	Unspecified pre-existing diabetes mellitus in childbirth
O24.33	Unspecified pre-existing diabetes mellitus in the puerperium
O24.811	Other pre-existing diabetes mellitus in pregnancy, first trimester
O24.812	Other pre-existing diabetes mellitus in pregnancy, second trimester
O24.813	Other pre-existing diabetes mellitus in pregnancy, third trimester
O24.819	Other pre-existing diabetes mellitus in pregnancy, unspecified trimester
O24.82	Other pre-existing diabetes mellitus in childbirth
O24.89	Other pre-existing diabetes mellitus in the puerperium

Documentation and Coding Example

Twenty-year-old Caucasian female at **35 weeks gestation** presents to high risk OB clinic for scheduled visit. PMH is significant **for IDDM, onset at age** 7. Her **diabetes was poorly controlled prior to this unplanned pregnancy and has remained poorly controlled during the pregnancy**. She experienced low BGL early in pregnancy and high levels in her second and third trimesters. Hemoglobin A1C has ranged from 7.8 to 10.4. She is using NPH and Novolog insulin. She states she has not felt well for several days and home BGL has been consistently elevated for the past two days. On examination, this is a thin, ill-appearing young woman. Temperature 99, HR 120, RR 20, BP 94/50. Strong ketotic breath odor, mucous membranes dry. Breath sounds clear. CBC shows no sign of infection. Urine positive for large amount of ketones, glucose, no WBC, casts, or bacteria present. Serum glucose 480 mg/dl.

Diagnosis: **Uncontrolled type 1 diabetes mellitus complicated by ketoacidosis.**

Plan: Admit under care of OB service for treatment of ketoacidosis and fetal monitoring.

Diagnosis Code(s)

O24.013	Pre-existing diabetes mellitus, type 1, in pregnancy, third trimester
E10.10	Type 1 diabetes mellitus with ketoacidosis without coma
Z3A.35	35 weeks gestation of pregnancy

Coding Note(s)

Uncontrolled diabetes is not an axis of classification for coding diabetes. When the diabetes is documented as uncontrolled, the specified type of diabetes is reported with hyperglycemia, which is listed under other specified complications. In this case, the type I diabetes with ketoacidosis means that the condition is already complicated by hyperglycemia, hyperketonemia, and metabolic acidosis. For this reason, code E10.65 Type 1 diabetes mellitus with hyperglycemia has not been reported in addition to E10.10.

Ectopic Pregnancy

An ectopic pregnancy occurs when a fertilized egg implants outside the uterus. The most common site of ectopic pregnancy is in one of the fallopian tubes, but implantation can also occur within an ovary, the abdominal cavity, or in the uterine cervix.

Ectopic pregnancy is classified in category O00. Codes are classified by site, laterality for tubal and ovarian sites, and whether or not there is a viable intrauterine pregnancy. There is an Excludes1 note for continuing pregnancy in multiple gestation after abortion of one fetus or more which is reported with codes in subcategories O31.1- or O31.3-. Ectopic pregnancies also include those that have ruptured.

Documentation and Coding Requirements

Identify site of ectopic pregnancy:

- Abdominal
- Ovarian
- Tubal
- Other specified site
- Unspecified ectopic pregnancy

Identify whether or not a viable intrauterine pregnancy is also present:

- With intrauterine pregnancy
- Without intrauterine pregnancy

Identify laterality for fallopian tube and ovarian ectopic sites:

- Left
- Right
- Unspecified

Use additional code from category O08 to identify any associated complications.

ICD-10-CM Code/Documentation	
O00.00	Abdominal pregnancy without intrauterine pregnancy
O00.01	Abdominal pregnancy with intrauterine pregnancy
O00.101	Right tubal pregnancy without intrauterine pregnancy
O00.102	Left tubal pregnancy without intrauterine pregnancy
O00.109	Unspecified tubal pregnancy without intrauterine pregnancy
O00.111	Right tubal pregnancy with intrauterine pregnancy
O00.112	Left tubal pregnancy with intrauterine pregnancy
O00.119	Unspecified tubal pregnancy with intrauterine pregnancy
O00.201	Right ovarian pregnancy without intrauterine pregnancy
O00.202	Left ovarian pregnancy without intrauterine pregnancy
O00.209	Unspecified ovarian pregnancy without intrauterine pregnancy
O00.211	Right ovarian pregnancy with intrauterine pregnancy
O00.212	Left ovarian pregnancy with intrauterine pregnancy
O00.219	Unspecified ovarian pregnancy with intrauterine pregnancy
O00.80	Other ectopic pregnancy without intrauterine pregnancy
O00.81	Other ectopic pregnancy with intrauterine pregnancy
O00.90	Unspecified ectopic pregnancy without intrauterine pregnancy
O00.91	Unspecified ectopic pregnancy with intrauterine pregnancy

Documentation and Coding Example

Thirty-three-year-old Hispanic female presents to OB/GYN with vaginal spotting and right lower abdominal pain. Patient initially called one week ago after a home pregnancy test was positive and was given an appointment 2 weeks out but she called back today and spoke to the triage nurse when she developed spotting and pain over the past 2 days. She is being seen emergently by the nurse-midwife. The patient is a G1 P1, who had an uncomplicated pregnancy with vaginal delivery at term 4 years ago. Her daughter is doing well. She states this is a planned pregnancy and she and her husband are excited. They have not yet told their daughter or other family members because she has just felt things were "not quite right" with the pregnancy. She admits to fatigue and increased urination but no nausea, vomiting, or food aversions which were early symptoms with her first pregnancy. T 98.8, P 76, R 12, BP 102/66, Ht. 66 inches, Wt. 133 lbs. On examination, this is a well-developed, well nourished, anxious young woman who looks her stated age. Color is pink, skin warm and dry. Heart rate regular without murmur, rubs, bruits. Extremities without evidence of clubbing. Breath sounds clear and equal bilaterally. Spine with normal curvature, no CVA tenderness is appreciated. Abdomen flat, bowel sounds present. Liver palpated at RCM, spleen is not palpated. No tenderness in upper quadrants but moderate tenderness in lower quadrants. External genitalia normal in appearance, no vaginal discharge noted. Speculum is easily inserted but there is pain when it is opened. Vaginal mucosa is dark red, cervix is closed with faint bluish discoloration consistent with pregnancy. Speculum was withdrawn and bimanual exam reveals CMT and fullness in the right adnexa. Left adnexa feels normal in size as does the uterus. Legs were brought out of stirrups and she remains resting on the examination table awaiting a vaginal US by the physician. Blood is drawn for quantitative beta hCG, CBC, PT, PTT and a comprehensive metabolic panel. They are sent to lab with request for stat analysis.

Attending OB/GYN note: Vaginal exam is consistent with the findings by midwife. Transvaginal US reveals a **normal size uterus without gestational sac or embryo present**. The left ovary and fallopian tube are normal size and shape. The right ovary is difficult to visualize due to swelling of the distal end of the right fallopian tube. A mass appears to be present in the tube but no bleeding or excess fluid is appreciated in the cul de sac or surrounding the right adnexa. Labs are reviewed and beta hCG level is 3850 mlU/mL, Hct. 38. Renal and hepatic functions, bleeding times WNL.

Impression: **Nonviable, right ectopic tubal pregnancy**. Patient and her husband are apprised of findings and offered condolences. Medical and surgical treatment plans are explained and discussed. Patient is an excellent candidate for methotrexate.

Plan: Administer Methotrexate 60 mg IM today. Patient to return to clinic in 4 days for repeat beta hCG and examination. She is advised to stop taking all vitamins or supplements that contain folic acid and she may take acetaminophen for pain. She should expect a decrease in abdominal pain and increase in vaginal spotting or bleeding over the next few days. If she experiences dizziness, fever, or pain that is not controlled by acetaminophen she should call immediately or go directly to the ED.

Diagnosis Code(s)

O00.101 Right tubal pregnancy without intrauterine pregnancy

Coding Note(s)

Tubal pregnancy that is not otherwise specified defaults to O00.10- for tubal pregnancy without intrauterine pregnancy. In this case, the physician has already documented a normal uterus without a gestational sac or embryo present.

Gestational Diabetes/Abnormal Glucose Tolerance in Pregnancy

Gestational diabetes is glucose intolerance during pregnancy. Hormones produced by the placenta block insulin receptors in the mother causing maternal blood glucose levels to rise. Gestational diabetes is diagnosed using glucose tolerance testing. Generally, an initial glucose tolerance test is performed. If the initial test is abnormal, usually considered to be a blood sugar level above 140 mg/dL or 7.8 mmol/L (although definitions of elevated blood sugar levels may vary by lab), a second glucose tolerance test is performed to make a diagnosis of gestational diabetes. It is possible to have an abnormal glucose tolerance test without a diagnosis of gestational diabetes.

Abnormal glucose tolerance test (O99.81-) is not synonymous with gestational diabetes. In addition, gestational diabetes reported with codes in subcategory O24.4 requires additional documentation related to whether the condition is being controlled by diet, oral hypoglycemics, or whether the patient requires insulin to control the condition.

Coding and Documentation Requirements

Identify the condition:

- Abnormal glucose complicating pregnancy, childbirth, and puerperium (O99.81-)
- Gestational diabetes (O24.4-)

Identify the maternal episode of care:

- Pregnancy
- Childbirth
- Puerperium

For gestational diabetes, specify method of control:

- Diet controlled
- Controlled by oral hypoglycemic drugs
- Insulin controlled
- Unspecified control

ICD-10-CM Code/Documentation	
O99.810	Abnormal glucose complicating pregnancy
O99.814	Abnormal glucose complicating childbirth
O99.815	Abnormal glucose complicating the puerperium
O24.410	Gestational diabetes mellitus in pregnancy, diet-controlled
O24.414	Gestational diabetes mellitus in pregnancy, insulin controlled
O24.415	Gestational diabetes mellitus in pregnancy, controlled by oral hypoglycemic drugs
O24.419	Gestational diabetes mellitus in pregnancy, unspecified control
O24.420	Gestational diabetes mellitus in childbirth, diet-controlled
O24.424	Gestational diabetes mellitus in childbirth, insulin controlled
O24.425	Gestational diabetes mellitus in childbirth, controlled by oral hypoglycemic drugs
O24.429	Gestational diabetes mellitus in childbirth, unspecified control
O24.430	Gestational diabetes mellitus in the puerperium, diet-controlled
O24.434	Gestational diabetes mellitus in the puerperium, insulin controlled
O24.435	Gestational diabetes mellitus in the puerperium, controlled by oral hypoglycemic drugs
O24.439	Gestational diabetes mellitus in the puerperium, unspecified control

Note: There are no codes for gestational diabetes or abnormal glucose for an unspecified episode of care. There must be clear documentation related to whether the condition is affecting the pregnancy, childbirth, or the puerperium.

Documentation and Coding Example

Patient is a 26-year-old G3 P2 Hispanic female at **33 weeks gestation** who presents to high risk OB clinic for follow-up appointment for **gestational diabetes**. Patient had an **abnormal glucose tolerance test 6 weeks ago** and has been followed by the dietician for nutritional counseling and home blood glucose monitoring. She struggled with compliance because she primarily eats rice and beans and was **started on insulin therapy 2 weeks ago**. Fasting BGL and postprandial levels have been WNL since beginning insulin therapy. On examination, this is a petite, young woman who is accompanied by her 5-year-old daughter and 3-year-old son. Wt.125 which is unchanged from last visit. HR 88, RR 14, BP 138/86. Gravid abdomen, single fetus in breech position. FHR 150. No edema noted in extremities. NST unremarkable, biophysical profile shows normal for GA fetus, adequate amniotic fluid. Patient will continue on **insulin therapy**.

Diagnosis Code(s)

O24.414	Gestational diabetes mellitus in pregnancy, insulin controlled
Z3A.33	33 weeks gestation of pregnancy

Coding Note(s)

The combination code identifies both the gestational diabetes mellitus in pregnancy and the insulin use, so only a single code is required.

Hydatidiform Mole

In molar pregnancy, also referred to as a hydatidiform mole or gestational trophoblastic disease, a non-viable fertilized egg implants in the uterus and forms a mass of chorionic villi tissue, as minute, elongated projections grow out from the chorion, the protective, nutritive membrane that attaches the new embryo growth to the uterus. A complete mole contains no fetal tissue and combines one duplicated or two unique sperm cells with an egg cell that does not contain maternal DNA, creating a 46XX or 46XY cell with only paternal DNA. This type of mole has no embryonic tissue but does have chorionic tissue, which increases the risk for a type of malignancy of the trophoblastic cells called choriocarcinoma. A partial mole contains some fetal tissue and combines an egg cell containing maternal DNA with one duplicated or two unique sperm cells yielding a 69XXX or 69XXY chromosomal complement cell (or in some cases, tetraploidy with more than 69 chromosomes) having both maternal and paternal DNA. This type of mole may contain both embryonic and chorionic tissue.

Molar pregnancy (category O01) is differentiated as classical or complete hydatidiform mole, incomplete or partial hydatidiform mole, and unspecified hydatidiform mole. There is an excludes note for chorioadenoma (destruens) and for hydatidiform mole documented as malignant, which are both reported with code D39.2 Neoplasm of uncertain behavior of placenta.

Coding and Documentation Requirements

Identify type of hydatidiform mole:

- Classical (complete)
- Incomplete and partial
- Unspecified, which includes:
  - Trophoblastic disease not otherwise specified
  - Vesicular mole not otherwise specified

ICD-10-CM Code/Documentation	
O01.0	Classical hydatidiform mole
O01.1	Incomplete and partial hydatidiform mole
O01.9	Hydatidiform mole unspecified

Documentation and Coding Example

Patient is a thirty-two-year-old Caucasian female referred to OB-GYN by her midwife after it was determined on US that she had a non-viable pregnancy. The patient and her husband have a 2 ½-year-old son and were actively trying to conceive a second child. Patient is a yoga instructor and strict vegetarian. First pregnancy uncomplicated although she gained only 15 lbs., with a midwife assisted home birth of a healthy 6 lb. infant at term. Patient states this pregnancy has felt different from the start, with severe nausea and vomiting resulting in a weight loss of 5 lbs. She feels weak and exhausted, notices that her hands shake all the time and her heart often feels like it is racing. Temperature 99, HR 98, RR 14, BP 138/80, Wt. 103 lbs. Ht. 64 inches. On examination, this is a well-groomed, thin, anxious appearing woman who looks younger than her stated age. Neck is supple, thyroid can be palpated and feels normal in size. Skin warm, dry to touch. HR regular, without gallop or rub. Breath sounds clear, equal bilaterally. Abdomen soft with active bowel sounds. Uterus can be palpated above the pubis, size consistent with a 12 to 14-week gestation, patient's dates indicate a pregnancy at only 7-8 weeks. US shows a complex uterine mass with cystic structure but no fetus or yolk sac. Two theca lutein cysts are present on the right ovary approximately 6 cm and 8 cm in size. Patient and her husband are advised that the US findings are quite consistent with **classical molar pregnancy** and a D & C is the recommended treatment. Patient and husband agree, OR is available tomorrow afternoon. Patient sent to OPS for pre-op blood work, chest x-ray, and anesthesia consult.

Pre Op Note: CBC shows mild anemia. PT, PTT, comprehensive metabolic panel all WNL. HCG and thyroxin levels are elevated. Chest x-ray negative.

Post Op Note: Abnormal tissue successfully evacuated with D & C under general anesthesia. Minimal bleeding. Tissue to pathology for identification. Patient discharged home in good condition with f/u appointment in 1 week. Pelvic rest until that time.

Office Visit Note: Patient is seen with her husband. She is recovering well. Nausea, vomiting, restlessness, tremors, and racing heart have all abated. She reports vaginal spotting x 2 days following procedure, now resolved. They are advised that pathology report showed an **androgenetic homozygous complete molar pregnancy**. She is scheduled for weekly blood draw to monitor HCG levels, advised to continue pelvic rest x 3 more weeks and return at that time for recheck and to discuss contraceptive methods.

Diagnosis Code(s)

O01.0 Classical hydatidiform mole

Coding Note(s)

Any complications following ectopic molar pregnancy such as genital tract and pelvic infection, delayed or excessive hemorrhage, embolism, shock, renal failure, metabolic disorders, damage to pelvic organs, other venous complications, cardiac arrest, sepsis, or urinary tract infection are reported separately with codes from category O08.

Hypertension Complicating Pregnancy, Childbirth and the Puerperium

Hypertension complicating pregnancy is classified based on whether the hypertension is pre-existing or pregnancy-induced. There are 6 categories for these conditions and additional subcategories within each category. All codes require documentation of the trimester. In order to describe the documentation requirements for hypertension complicating pregnancy, it is necessary to subdivide this section into codes covering pre-existing hypertension and codes covering gestational hypertension, pre-eclampsia, and eclampsia.

Pre-Existing Hypertension Complicating Pregnancy, Childbirth, Puerperium

Pre-existing hypertension in pregnancy may be either primary or secondary. Primary hypertension is sometimes referred to as essential hypertension, which is abnormally elevated blood pressure levels that have no particular underlying cause. Secondary hypertension refers to abnormally elevated blood pressure levels due to an underlying condition or cause. Pre-existing hypertension can be complicated by pre-eclampsia or eclampsia. Pre-eclampsia is hypertension (BP >140/90 mmHg) after the 20th week of gestation (and up to 6 weeks postpartum), with proteinuria. Pre-eclampsia may be considered severe with a BP >160/110 and additional symptoms such as edema and epigastric pain. Eclampsia is a life-threatening condition characterized by hypertension (BP >140/90 mmHg) after the 20th week of gestation (and up to 6 weeks postpartum), with proteinuria, and tonic-clonic (motor) seizures. Seizures are often preceded by headache, nausea, vomiting, and/or cortical blindness.

Hypertension is not differentiated as benign or malignant. It is classified in category O10 as pre-existing essential hypertension or pre-existing hypertensive heart and/or chronic kidney disease. There is also a category for pre-existing hypertension with pre-eclampsia (011). Hypertension complicated by pre-eclampsia requires an additional code from category O10 to identify the type of hypertension. An additional code is required from categories I11-I15 to identify the specified type of hypertensive heart and/or chronic kidney disease, or the specific type of secondary hypertension. No additional code is required for patients who have pre-existing essential hypertension.

Coding and Documentation Requirements

Identify pre-existing hypertension complicating pregnancy, childbirth, or the puerperium:

- Essential hypertension
- Hypertensive chronic kidney disease
- Hypertensive heart disease
- Hypertensive heart and chronic kidney disease
- Secondary hypertension
- Unspecified pre-existing hypertension

Identify complication as occurring during pregnancy, childbirth, puerperium:

- Pregnancy
  - First trimester (less than 14 weeks 0 days)
  - Second trimester (14 weeks 0 days to less than 28 weeks 0 days)
  - Third trimester (28 weeks 0 days until delivery)
  - Unspecified trimester
- Childbirth
- Puerperium

For pre-existing hypertension documented as hypertensive heart and/or hypertensive chronic kidney disease or secondary hypertension, assign an additional code from categories I11-I13 or I15 to identify the type of hypertension more specifically.

ICD-10-CM Code/Documentation	
O10.11-	Pre-existing hypertensive heart disease complicating pregnancy
O10.12	Pre-existing hypertensive heart disease complicating childbirth
O10.13	Pre-existing hypertensive heart disease complicating the puerperium
O10.01-	Pre-existing essential hypertension complicating pregnancy
O10.02	Pre-existing essential hypertension complicating childbirth
O10.03	Pre-existing essential hypertension complicating the puerperium
O10.21-	Pre-existing hypertensive chronic kidney disease complicating pregnancy
O10.22	Pre-existing hypertensive chronic kidney disease complicating childbirth
O10.23	Pre-existing hypertensive chronic kidney disease complicating the puerperium
O10.41-	Pre-existing secondary hypertension complicating pregnancy
O10.42	Pre-existing secondary hypertension complicating childbirth
O10.43	Pre-existing secondary hypertension complicating the puerperium
O10.31-	Pre-existing hypertensive heart and chronic kidney disease complicating pregnancy
O10.32	Pre-existing hypertensive heart and chronic kidney disease complicating childbirth
O10.33	Pre-existing hypertensive heart and chronic kidney disease complicating the puerperium
O11.1	Pre-existing hypertension with pre-eclampsia, first trimester
O11.2	Pre-existing hypertension with pre-eclampsia, second trimester
O11.3	Pre-existing hypertension with pre-eclampsia, third trimester
O11.9	Pre-existing hypertension with pre-eclampsia, unspecified trimester

Note: Codes from category O11 need a code from category O10 assigned in addition to identify the type of hypertension

Documentation and Coding Example

Antepartum Admission Note: Thirty-three-year-old Black female admitted to antepartum observation floor with **symptoms of pre-eclampsia at 30 weeks gestation**. Patient has a **3-year history of chronic hypertension well controlled with Tenormin**. She was switched to Aldomet when her pregnancy was identified and has been followed by both perinatology and cardiology for high risk pregnancy. Temperature 99, HR 72, RR 12, BP 152/100. Patient is a G1 P0 and states she and her husband were surprised when she became pregnant, having tried to conceive unsuccessfully for 10 years. They are thrilled to be having a baby and know that it is a boy. There is no evidence of IUGR on US and biophysical profiles have been WNL. Decision was made today at routine OB appointment to admit for monitoring of elevated BP, worsening edema, and protein in her urine. IV started in left arm and blood drawn for CBC, coagulation studies, comprehensive metabolic panel, type and hold. Magnesium sulfate infusion started. IM betamethasone also administered. Patient on bedrest, right side as much as tolerated.

Diagnosis: **Pregnancy at 30 weeks with pre-existing hypertension and superimposed pre-eclampsia**

Diagnosis Code(s)

O11.3	Pre-existing hypertension with pre-eclampsia, third trimester
O10.013	Pre-existing essential hypertension complicating pregnancy, third trimester
Z3A.30	30 weeks gestation of pregnancy

Coding Note(s)

There is no documentation of hypertensive heart or chronic kidney disease so the code for essential hypertension complicating pregnancy is reported as the additional code to identify the type of hypertension. When the weeks of gestation are documented, a code from category Z3A should be assigned.

Gestational Hypertension/Pre-Eclampsia/Eclampsia

Gestational hypertension, also called pregnancy-induced hypertension, is an arterial blood pressure >140/90 mmHg, without proteinuria (protein present in urine) in a pregnant woman without previously documented hypertension after 20 weeks gestation. Pre-eclampsia is hypertension (BP >140/90 mmHg) after the 20th week of gestation, and up to 6 weeks postpartum, with proteinuria. Pre-eclampsia may be considered severe with a BP >160/110 and additional symptoms such as edema and epigastric pain. In pre-eclampsia, the hypertension may be pre-existing or pregnancy-induced. Eclampsia is a life-threatening condition characterized by hypertension with a BP >140/90 mmHg after the 20th week of gestation, and up to 6 weeks postpartum, with proteinuria, and tonic-clonic (motor) seizures. Seizures are often preceded by headache, nausea, vomiting, and/or cortical blindness. In eclampsia, the hypertension may be pre-existing or pregnancy-induced.

Gestational hypertension is clarified as meaning pregnancy-induced hypertension. The category description for O13 also specifies that the gestational hypertension is without significant proteinuria, although if the diagnostic statement does not state that the condition is complicated by significant proteinuria, then this category is the default for gestational hypertension NOS. If the patient has gestational hypertension with significant proteinuria, the condition is classified as either mild to moderate pre-eclampsia (O14.0-), severe pre-eclampsia (O14.1-), or severe pre-eclampsia with hemolysis, elevated liver enzymes, and low platelet count (HELLP syndrome) (O14.2-). There is also a code for unspecified pre-eclampsia (O14.9). Eclampsia is reported with codes from category O15.

Coding and Documentation Requirements

Identify gestational hypertension, pre-eclampsia, or eclampsia:

- Gestational hypertension without significant proteinuria
- Pre-eclampsia
  - Mild to moderate
  - Severe
  - HELLP syndrome
  - Unspecified
- Eclampsia
- Unspecified maternal hypertension

Identify stage of pregnancy in which complication occurs:

- Pregnancy
- Childbirth/labor
- Puerperium

Identify trimester of pregnancy:

- First (less than 14 weeks 0 days)
- Second (14 weeks 0 days to less than 28 weeks 0 days)
- Third (28 weeks 0 days until delivery)
- Unspecified

ICD-10-CM Code/Documentation	
O13.1	Gestational [pregnancy-induced] hypertension without significant proteinuria, first trimester
O13.2	Gestational [pregnancy-induced] hypertension without significant proteinuria, second trimester
O13.3	Gestational [pregnancy-induced] hypertension without significant proteinuria, third trimester
O13.9	Gestational [pregnancy-induced] hypertension without significant proteinuria, unspecified trimester
O14.00	Mild to moderate pre-eclampsia, unspecified trimester
O14.02	Mild to moderate pre-eclampsia, second trimester
O14.03	Mild to moderate pre-eclampsia, third trimester
O14.04	Mild to moderate pre-eclampsia, complicating childbirth
O14.05	Mild to moderate pre-eclampsia, complicating the puerperium
O14.10	Severe pre-eclampsia, unspecified trimester
O14.12	Severe pre-eclampsia, second trimester
O14.13	Severe pre-eclampsia, third trimester
O14.14	Severe pre-eclampsia, complicating childbirth
O14.15	Severe pre-eclampsia, complicating the puerperium
O14.20	HELLP syndrome, unspecified trimester
O14.22	HELLP syndrome, second trimester
O14.23	HELLP syndrome, third trimester
O14.24	HELLP syndrome, complicating childbirth
O14.25	HELLP syndrome, complicating the puerperium
O15.00	Eclampsia complicating pregnancy, unspecified trimester
O15.02	Eclampsia complicating pregnancy, second trimester
O15.03	Eclampsia complicating pregnancy, third trimester
O15.1	Eclampsia complicating labor
O15.2	Eclampsia complicating the puerperium

Note: Codes are only available for pre-eclampsia and eclampsia in the second or third trimester in a patient without pre-existing hypertension. This is because these conditions do not occur in the first trimester.

Documentation and Coding Example

Twenty-seven-year-old Black female is seen in OB Clinic at **34 weeks gestation**. Patient is a G1P1 with a single gestation pregnancy that is now complicated by **gestational hypertension**. She is accompanied by her husband. Temperature 99, HR 70, RR 12, BP 150/96. Normal BP and urine protein until 4 weeks ago when she presented with BP 142/90 and 1+ protein on dipstick. Fetal ultrasound at that time showed normal fluid levels which have remained normal on subsequent US. BP has been monitored weekly by CNM/OB along with urine protein checks. On examination: PERRL, fundoscopic exam normal. Neck supple without lymphadenopathy, thyroid normal size/shape. She c/o mild nasal congestion which has been present throughout pregnancy. No history of allergies or respiratory problems. Breath sounds clear, equal bilaterally. HR regular without gallop or rub. Gravid abdomen, vertex presenting, not engaged. FHR 144. No hepatic tenderness. Reflexes are brisk, mild dependent edema noted in feet and ankles. Dipstick **urine is 2+ protein** and sample sent to lab for UA with Protein/Creatinine ratio. Blood drawn for CBC, comprehensive metabolic panel, coagulation studies. US reveals single female fetus with normal amniotic fluid levels. NST shows good variability with fetal activity. RTC in 1 week for BP check, US, and NST. Impression: **Moderate pre-eclampsia.** Patient is instructed on symptoms that need immediate attention and how to reach on call staff after clinic hours. She is advised that she will be seen in clinic 2 x week for monitoring and that she may be delivered early. RTC in 4 days.

Diagnosis Code(s)

O14.03	Mild to moderate pre-eclampsia, third trimester
Z3A.34	34 weeks gestation of pregnancy

Coding Note(s)

Gestational hypertension with significant proteinuria is coded as pre-eclampsia. The patient has both proteinuria and mild dependent edema, but the pre-eclampsia is specified as moderate not severe and so moderate pre-eclampsia is reported. Severe pre-eclampsia requires documentation of proteinuria and/or edema specified as severe.

Infection of Amniotic Sac/Membranes

An inflammation or infection of the amniotic cavity may involve the amniotic sac, which consists of a pair of membranes, the chorion and the amnion, known as the fetal membranes that exist during pregnancy between the developing fetus and the mother. When the pair of membranes that compose the amniotic sac is affected, the condition is referred to as chorioamnionitis, an inflammation of the chorion and the amnion. The chorion is the outermost membrane on the maternal side surrounding the embryo and contributing to the placenta's formation, and the amnion is the innermost membrane on the fetal side. Chorioamnionitis is usually caused by a bacterial infection. Bacteria can be introduced from the urogenital tract via vaginal examinations performed in late pregnancy and/or during labor. Symptoms may include maternal fever, uterine tenderness, and foul smelling vaginal discharge. Mild chorioamnionitis is characterized by infiltration of neutrophils in the chorionic plate. Moderate infection may involve necrosis and/or abscess of the subamniotic tissue or fetal membrane. With severe involvement, there may be vasculitis of the umbilical vessels and/or inflammation of the umbilical cord and connective tissue (funisitis).

An inflammation or infection of the amniotic cavity may also involve the placenta. Placentitis is an inflammation of the placenta, an organ that secretes hormones and provides nutrition, waste elimination, and gas exchange to the developing fetus. Placentitis may cause miscarriage, preterm labor, and/or placental retention post-delivery. TORCH infections are the most common cause of placentitis and include toxoplasmosis (T), other infections (O- coxsackievirus, varicella-Zoster virus, HIV, Parvovirus B19), Rubella (R), cytomegalovirus (C) and herpes simplex-2 (H).

There are specific codes for chorioamnionitis (O41.12-) and placentitis (O41.14-). Amnionitis and membranitis are reported with the code for chorioamnionitis.

Coding and Documentation Requirements

Identify site of infection of the amniotic sac and membranes:

- Chorioamnionitis
- Placentitis
- Unspecified site

Identify trimester:

- First (less than 14 weeks 0 days)
- Second (14 weeks 0 days to less than 28 weeks 0 days)
- Third (28 weeks 0 days until delivery)
- Unspecified

Identify fetus affected by complication:

- Fetus 1
- Fetus 2
- Fetus 3
- Fetus 4
- Fetus 5
- Other fetus
- Unspecified fetus/not applicable

ICD-10-CM Code/Documentation	
O41.101-	Infection of amniotic sac and membranes, unspecified, first trimester
O41.102-	Infection of amniotic sac and membranes, unspecified, second trimester
O41.103-	Infection of amniotic sac and membranes, unspecified, third trimester
O41.109-	Infection of amniotic sac and membranes, unspecified, unspecified trimester
O41.121-	Chorioamnionitis, first trimester
O41.122-	Chorioamnionitis, second trimester
O41.123-	Chorioamnionitis, third trimester
O41.129-	Chorioamnionitis, unspecified trimester
O41.141-	Placentitis, first trimester
O41.142-	Placentitis, second trimester
O41.143-	Placentitis, third trimester
O41.149-	Placentitis, unspecified trimester

Assign 7th character for fetus affected by infection of amniotic cavity:

- 1 for fetus 1
- 2 for fetus 2
- 3 for fetus 3
- 4 for fetus 4
- 5 for fetus 5
- 9 for other fetus
- 0 for unspecified fetus/not applicable

Documentation and Coding Example

Thirty-six-year-old female with **twin dichorionic, diamniotic gestation at 34 weeks** admitted to L&D with possible PROM. Patient is a G2 P0 who suffered a 2nd trimester loss with her first pregnancy 2 years ago due to **incompetent cervix**. She had a cerclage placed at 12 weeks and has been on bed rest for most of this pregnancy. Temperature 100.6, HR 88, RR 16 BP 120/70. On examination, this is an anxious woman, clean and well groomed. She states that she noticed some clear fluid on her underclothes yesterday but felt it was probably urine. This morning she awoke and felt a small gush of fluid when she got out of bed to use the BR. She called her doctor who ordered her to the hospital. She denies abdominal pain or contractions, urinary frequency or burning. Vaginal exam with sterile speculum reveals **fluid leaking from cervical os which is sutured closed.** Fluid sample sent to lab for leukocyte count, Gram stain, pH, glucose concentration, endotoxins, lactoferrin, and cytokines. US shows **male fetus (Fetus 1) in lower uterus, decreased amniotic fluid volume with particulate matter in the fluid.** Placenta appears to be on the posterior wall of the uterus and cannot be easily evaluated. **Female fetus (Fetus 2) is in upper uterus with adequate amniotic fluid and a normal appearing placenta located on the right side of the uterus.** BPP of each fetus is WNL. IV access established with 16-gauge angiocath in patients left forearm. LR infusing at 125 cc hour for hydration. Blood drawn for CBC, Chem panel, coagulation studies, Type and hold, CRP, Alpha 1-proteinase inhibitor, serum ferritin. She had a course of betamethasone at 28 weeks so it is presumed fetal lungs are mature.

Impression: **Premature rupture of membranes. Chorioamnionitis, male fetus**

Plan: Admit for monitoring and administration of antibiotics

13. Complications of Pregnancy/Childbirth

Diagnosis Code(s)

O42.913	Preterm premature rupture of membranes, unspecified as to length of time between rupture and onset of labor, third trimester
O41.1231	Chorioamnionitis, third trimester, fetus 1
O30.043	Twin pregnancy, dichorionic/diamniotic, third trimester
O34.33	Maternal care for incompetent cervix, third trimester
Z3A.34	34 weeks gestation of pregnancy

Coding Note(s)

Chorioamnionitis requires a 7th character extension to identify the fetus. In this scenario of a twin pregnancy, only the male fetus identified as fetus 1 is affected by the infection, so 7th character extension 1 is reported. Since the female fetus is not affected by the infection, no code is reported for fetus 2.

Infections of Genitourinary Tract in Pregnancy

Codes in category O23 Infections of the genitourinary tract in pregnancy, are specific to the antepartum period and the trimester must be specified. Codes from category O23 should not be used to report infections with a predominantly sexual mode of transmission, such as syphilis or gonorrhea. An additional code should be reported from category B95 or B96 to identify the organism. Codes are also specific to site. For genitourinary tract infections following delivery, a code from subcategory O86.1 Other infection of genital tract following delivery, or O86.2 Urinary tract infection following delivery, is reported. These codes are also site specific.

Coding and Documentation Requirements

Identify site for genitourinary tract infection during pregnancy (O23):

- Urinary tract
  - Kidney
  - Bladder
  - Urethra
  - Other parts of urinary tract
  - Unspecified infection of urinary tract
- Genital tract
  - Cervix
  - Ovary/tube (Salpingitis/Oophoritis)
  - Other part of genital tract
- Unspecified site of genitourinary tract

Identify trimester:

- First (less than 14 weeks 0 days)
- Second (14 weeks 0 days to less than 28 weeks 0 days)
- Third (28 weeks 0 days until delivery)
- Unspecified

Use additional code to identify organism (B95.-, B96.-).

Identify condition/site for genitourinary tract infection following delivery (O86.1-, O86.2-):

- Genital tract
  - Cervicitis/cervix
  - Endometritis/endometrium
  - Vaginitis/vagina
  - Other infection of genital tract
- Urinary tract
  - Bladder
  - Kidney
  - Other specified site
  - Unspecified site

Use additional code to identify organism (B95.-, B96.-).

ICD-10-CM Code/Documentation	
O23.0-	Infections of kidney in pregnancy
O23.1-	Infections of bladder in pregnancy
O23.2-	Infections of urethra in pregnancy
O23.3-	Infections of other parts of urinary tract in pregnancy
O23.4-	Unspecified infection of urinary tract in pregnancy
O23.51-	Infection of cervix in pregnancy
O23.52-	Salpingo-oophoritis in pregnancy
O23.59-	Infection of other part of genital tract in pregnancy
O23.9-	Unspecified genitourinary tract infection in pregnancy
Note: Subcategory codes require fifth or sixth characters to identify the trimester.	
O86.11	Cervicitis following delivery
O86.12	Endometritis following delivery
O86.13	Vaginitis following delivery
O86.19	Other infection of genital tract following delivery
O86.20	Urinary tract infection following delivery, unspecified
O86.21	Infection of kidney following delivery
O86.22	Infection of bladder following delivery
O86.29	Other urinary tract infection following delivery

Documentation and Coding Example

Patient is a 25-year-old Native American female referred to ED by her OB with c/o crampy lower abdominal pain x 2 days which has progressed to fever and back pain. She is a G3 P2 at **16 weeks gestation** and has a history of UTI with previous pregnancies. Temperature 100.4, HR 88, RR 16, BP 110/66. On examination, this is a thin, tired appearing woman who looks older than her stated age. Neck supple without lymphadenopathy. Throat, TMs clear. Mucous membranes pink, somewhat dry. HR regular without murmur or rubs. Breath sounds clear, equal bilaterally. Bilateral CVA tenderness. Abdomen soft with active BS. Spleen not palpated, liver palpated 1 cm below RCM. C/O suprapubic pain with palpation. FHR 156 by Doppler. Pelvic exam reveals red, mildly irritated external genitalia and vaginal vault. Cervix closed, no discharge noted. Urine specimen obtained by straight cath. Urine sent to lab for UA, C & S. Blood drawn for CBC, comprehensive metabolic panel, blood cultures. IV started in right arm with D5LR infusing. UA reveals WBC, casts, and large number of gram + bacteria. Patient started on IV antibiotics and admitted to medical floor.

Diagnosis: **Second trimester pregnancy complicated by acute pyelonephritis**.

Floor Note Day 2: **Urine culture positive for Staphylococcus saprophyticus** sensitive to Ciprofloxacin and Macrobid. Patient is afebrile, continues to have CVA tenderness more pronounced on right side and suprapubic discomfort. She will remain hospitalized for IV antibiotics. Urology consult requested due to history of previous UTIs during pregnancy to **R/O structural abnormalities**.

Urology Note: Patient seen for recurrent UTIs complicating a second trimester pregnancy. **Renal US obtained, shows no abnormalities**. Fever, CVA tenderness, suprapubic discomfort are resolving on antibiotics. Recommendation: Complete 7 days of IV Cipro and discharge patient on prophylactic Macrobid daily for the remainder of pregnancy.

Diagnosis Code(s)

O23.02	Infections of the kidney in pregnancy, second trimester
B95.7	Other staphylococcus as the cause of diseases classified elsewhere
Z3A.16	16 weeks gestation of pregnancy

Coding Note(s)

There is no code listed for Pregnancy, complicated by pyelonephritis. The subterm pyelitis is used to locate code O23.0-. Under O23.0 Infections of kidney in pregnancy in the tabular section is listed the alternate inclusion term 'Pyelonephritis in pregnancy'. Three codes are required, one for the infection of the kidney in pregnancy, one to identify the infectious organism, and a third to capture the weeks of gestation.

13. Complications of Pregnancy/Childbirth

Multiple Gestation

Multiple gestation refers to a pregnancy with more than one fetus. A twin pregnancy has two fetuses that may share a single placenta and amniotic sac, share a single placenta but have two amniotic sacs or each have a separate placenta and amniotic sac. A triplet pregnancy has three fetuses, two or more may share a placenta and/or amniotic sac. A quadruplet pregnancy has four fetuses, two or more may share a placenta and/or amniotic sac.

For multiple gestation pregnancies (O30), the number of fetuses is required along with documentation related to the number of placentas and the number of amniotic sacs. The code for conjoined twins is also listed in category O30.

Coding and Documentation Requirements

Identify multiple gestation and number of placenta/amniotic sacs as:

- Twin pregnancy
  - Conjoined twin pregnancy
  - One placenta/one amniotic sac (monochorionic/monoamniotic)
  - One placenta/two amniotic sacs (monochorionic/diamniotic)
  - Two placentae/two amniotic sacs (dichorionic/diamniotic)
  - Unable to determine number of placenta/amniotic sacs
  - Unspecified number of placenta/amniotic sacs
- Triplet pregnancy
  - Two or more monochorionic fetuses
  - Two or more monoamniotic fetuses
  - Trichorionic/triamniotic
  - Unable to determine number of placenta/amniotic sacs
  - Unspecified number of placenta/amniotic sacs
- Quadruplet pregnancy
  - Two or more monochorionic fetuses
  - Two or more monoamniotic fetuses
  - Quadrachorionic/quadra-amniotic
  - Unable to determine number of placenta/amniotic sacs
  - Unspecified number of placenta/amniotic sacs
- Other specified multiple gestation
  - Two or more monochorionic fetuses
  - Two or more monoamniotic fetuses
  - Number of chorions and amnions equal to the number of fetuses
  - Unable to determine number of placenta/amniotic sacs
  - Unspecified number of placenta/amniotic sacs
- Unspecified multiple gestation

Identify trimester:

- First (less than 14 weeks 0 days)
- Second (14 weeks 0 days to less than 28 weeks 0 days)
- Third (28 weeks 0 days until delivery)
- Unspecified

Twin Pregnancy

ICD-10-CM Code/Documentation	
O30.021	Conjoined twin pregnancy, first trimester
O30.022	Conjoined twin pregnancy, second trimester
O30.023	Conjoined twin pregnancy, third trimester
O30.029	Conjoined twin pregnancy, unspecified trimester
O30.011	Twin pregnancy, monochorionic/monoamniotic, first trimester
O30.012	Twin pregnancy, monochorionic/monoamniotic, second trimester
O30.013	Twin pregnancy, monochorionic/monoamniotic, third trimester
O30.019	Twin pregnancy, monochorionic/monoamniotic, unspecified trimester
O30.001	Twin pregnancy, unspecified number of placenta and unspecified number of amniotic sacs, first trimester
O30.002	Twin pregnancy, unspecified number of placenta and unspecified number of amniotic sacs, second trimester
O30.003	Twin pregnancy, unspecified number of placenta and unspecified number of amniotic sacs, third trimester
O30.009	Twin pregnancy, unspecified number of placenta and unspecified number of amniotic sacs, unspecified trimester
O30.031	Twin pregnancy, monochorionic/diamniotic, first trimester
O30.032	Twin pregnancy, monochorionic/diamniotic, second trimester
O30.033	Twin pregnancy, monochorionic/diamniotic, third trimester

O30.039	Twin pregnancy, monochorionic/diamniotic, unspecified trimester
O30.041	Twin pregnancy, dichorionic/diamniotic, first trimester
O30.042	Twin pregnancy, dichorionic/diamniotic, second trimester
O30.043	Twin pregnancy, dichorionic/diamniotic, third trimester
O30.049	Twin pregnancy, dichorionic/diamniotic, unspecified trimester
O30.091	Twin pregnancy, unable to determine number of placenta and number of amniotic sacs, first trimester
O30.092	Twin pregnancy, unable to determine number of placenta and number of amniotic sacs, second trimester
O30.093	Twin pregnancy, unable to determine number of placenta and number of amniotic sacs, third trimester
O30.099	Twin pregnancy, unable to determine number of placenta and number of amniotic sacs, unspecified trimester

Documentation and Coding Example

Patient is a 30-year-old Caucasian female who is accompanied by her husband for their first prenatal visit following a positive home pregnancy test. Patient had light vaginal bleeding and breast tenderness 4 weeks ago that she thought was her period. Her breasts have remained tender, she has had nausea without vomiting in the mornings and headaches in the afternoon and evenings. PMH is unremarkable. Patient is a legal secretary, husband is an attorney. Wt. 112 lbs. HR 70, RR 12, BP 102/60. PERRL, neck supple, thyroid gland smooth with slight fullness on right side. Mucous membranes, oral mucosa moist and pink, teeth in good repair. Breath sounds clear, equal bilaterally. HR regular without gallop or rub. Peripheral pulses strong, no edema noted. Breasts full, without masses. Abdomen soft, non-distended, bowel sounds present. FHR not found, patient assured this is quite normal. Pelvic exam shows normal external genitalia. Speculum easily inserted, pap smear obtained along with cultures for Chlamydia, GC, herpes, and HPV. Vaginal mucosa is deep red, cervix closed with bluish discoloration. Bimanual exam positive for gravid retroflexed uterus. Vaginal US reveals **a dichorionic/diamniotic twin gestation at 11-12 weeks**. Placentas are low lying but do not appear to cross the cervix. FHR strong. No abnormal findings. Patient and husband are congratulated. Copies of US are printed for them to keep. Prescription for prenatal vitamins written. Questions answered. Counseled in diet and exercise. RTC in 3 weeks. Sooner if problems arise.

Diagnosis Code(s)

O30.041	Twin pregnancy, dichorionic/diamniotic, first trimester
Z3A.11	11 weeks gestation of pregnancy

Coding Note(s)

Carefully select the code identifying the number of placentas and amniotic sacs and note that there is a differentiation between an unspecified number and the inability to determine the number. Weeks of gestation is documented at between 11 and 12 weeks, thus the code for 11 weeks is selected from category Z3A.

Other Conditions Related to Pregnancy

There are specific codes for maternal care predominantly related to pregnancy for conditions such as low weight gain, fatigue during pregnancy, herpes gestationis, and complications of anesthesia as well as many other conditions. It should be noted that codes in category O26 are specific to pregnancy and do not include the same conditions documented as occurring in childbirth or the puerperium. Specific codes for the following conditions in pregnancy include: low weight gain (O26.1-), retained intrauterine contraceptive device (O26.3), Herpes gestationis (O26.4-), subluxation of symphysis pubis (O26.7-), exhaustion and fatigue (O26.81), and pruritic urticarial papules and plaques of pregnancy (PUPPP) (O26.86-). Codes from category O29 Complications of anesthesia during pregnancy are also specific to pregnancy and do not include complications that occur in childbirth or the puerperium.

Coding and Documentation Requirements

Identify the specific complication of pregnancy:

- Anesthesia complication
  - Pulmonary
    - Aspiration pneumonitis
    - Pressure collapse of lung
    - Other pulmonary complication
  - Cardiac
    - Cardiac arrest
    - Cardiac failure
    - Other cardiac complication
  - Central nervous system
    - Cerebral anoxia
    - Other central nervous system complication
  - Toxic reaction to local anesthesia
  - Spinal and epidural anesthesia complication
    - Spinal/epidural induced headache
    - Other complication of spinal/epidural anesthesia
  - Failed or difficult intubation
  - Other complication of anesthesia
- Herpes gestationis
- Low weight gain
- Pregnancy related exhaustion and fatigue
- Pruritic urticarial papules and plaques of pregnancy
- Retained intrauterine contraceptive device
- Subluxation of symphysis pubis

For antepartum conditions, identify trimester:

- First (less than 14 weeks 0 days)
- Second (14 weeks 0 days to less than 28 weeks 0 days)
- Third (28 weeks 0 days until delivery)
- Unspecified

Complications of Anesthesia During Pregnancy

ICD-10-CM Code/Documentation	
O29.01-	Aspiration pneumonitis due to anesthesia during pregnancy
O29.02-	Pressure collapse of lung due to anesthesia during pregnancy
O29.09-	Other pulmonary complications of anesthesia during pregnancy
O29.11-	Cardiac arrest due to anesthesia during pregnancy
O29.12-	Cardiac failure due to anesthesia during pregnancy
O29.19-	Other cardiac complications of anesthesia during pregnancy
O29.21-	Cerebral anoxia due to anesthesia during pregnancy
O29.29-	Other central nervous system complications of anesthesia during pregnancy
O29.3X-	Toxic reaction to local anesthesia during pregnancy
O29.4-	Spinal and epidural anesthesia induced headache during pregnancy
O29.5X-	Other complications of spinal and epidural anesthesia during pregnancy
O29.6-	Failed or difficult intubation for anesthesia during pregnancy
O29.8-	Other complications of anesthesia during pregnancy
O29.9-	Unspecified complication of anesthesia during pregnancy
Note: Subcategory codes require fifth or sixth characters to identify the trimester	

Documentation and Coding Example

Anesthesiologist Note: Patient is a 31-year-old female who was admitted for traumatic fracture of right tibia and fibula requiring open reduction and internal fixation. Because she is **26 weeks pregnant** the procedure was performed using spinal anesthesia. A post-anesthesia evaluation was requested to evaluate for **post spinal headache/spinal fluid leak**. Patient is examined supine with 30-degree elevation in HOB. She states she has a history of migraine headaches and the pain she experienced when she tried to get up for crutch training was worse than migraine pain. She currently feels just a dull ache toward the top of her head and in the frontal area. With HOB at 45 degrees the headache begins to worsen and at 60 degrees it is unbearable. Headache decreases when HOB is lowered. Spinal column examined with patient lying on her side. There is a needle puncture site at L4 which is consistent with anesthesia record. No redness or drainage noted.

Impression: Post-spinal puncture headache.

Plan: Administer 1 liter LR w/500 mg caffeine sodium benzoate over 1 hour followed by 1 Liter of LR over 2 hours and re-evaluate.

Diagnosis Code(s)

O29.42 Spinal and epidural anesthesia induced headache during pregnancy, second trimester

Z3A.26 26 weeks gestation of pregnancy

Coding Note(s)

The anesthesiologist is evaluating and treating only the post-anesthesia spinal headache so that is the only code required for this episode of care.

Poor Fetal Growth

Poor fetal growth has many causes and determining the reason that the fetus has not reached its full growth potential is not always possible. Factors that affect fetal growth may be of fetal, placental, or maternal origin and include genetic or congenital anomalies, placental insufficiency, poor nutrition, or smoking.

The placenta is an organ that secretes hormones and provides nutrition, waste elimination, and oxygen exchange to the developing fetus. Placental insufficiency is a complication of pregnancy in which the fetus fails to receive adequate nutrition and/or oxygen because the placenta does not develop properly or becomes damaged during the pregnancy. Risk factors for placental insufficiency include maternal diabetes, hypertension, diseases that affect blood clotting, and smoking.

There is a subcategory for poor fetal growth specifically documented as due to known or suspected placental insufficiency. There is a separate subcategory for other known or suspected poor fetal growth. Because poor fetal growth is a complication that can affect one or more fetuses in a multiple gestation pregnancy, the codes for poor fetal growth require identification of the fetus(es) affected.

Coding and Documentation Requirements

Identify known or suspected poor fetal growth as due to:

- Suspected placental insufficiency
- Other known or suspected poor fetal growth (light-for-dates NOS)

Identify trimester:

- First (less than 14 weeks 0 days)
- Second (14 weeks 0 days to less than 28 weeks 0 days)
- Third (28 weeks 0 days until delivery)
- Unspecified

Identify fetus affected by complication:

- Fetus 1
- Fetus 2
- Fetus 3
- Fetus 4
- Fetus 5
- Other fetus
- Unspecified fetus/not applicable

ICD-10-CM Code/Documentation	
O36.511-	Maternal care for known or suspected placental insufficiency, first trimester
O36.512-	Maternal care for known or suspected placental insufficiency, second trimester
O36.513-	Maternal care for known or suspected placental insufficiency, third trimester
O36.519-	Maternal care for known or suspected placental insufficiency, unspecified trimester
O36.591-	Maternal care for other known or suspected poor fetal growth, first trimester
O36.592-	Maternal care for other known or suspected poor fetal growth, second trimester

ICD-10-CM Code/Documentation	
O36.593-	Maternal care for other known or suspected poor fetal growth, third trimester
O36.599-	Maternal care for other known or suspected poor fetal growth, unspecified trimester

Assign 7th character for fetus affected by poor fetal growth:

- 1 for fetus 1
- 2 for fetus 2
- 3 for fetus 3
- 4 for fetus 4
- 5 for fetus 5
- 9 for other fetus
- 0 for unspecified fetus/not applicable

Documentation and Coding Example

Patient is a 33-year-old primipara with a **triplet gestation** at **27 weeks** who presents for NST/BPP with perinatologist. Wt. 148, a 4 lb. wt. gain in 2 weeks. HR 88, RR 12. US verifies a triplet gestation with **Fetus 1 and Fetus 2 sharing a single placenta and separate amniotic sacs**. Fetus 1 is a 660-gram female with a crown to heel length of 31 cm. She is active with good FHR variability. Fetus 2 is a 720-gram female with a crown to heel length of 33 cm. She is also active with good FHR variability. Amniotic fluid is adequate. Placenta is high on the right side of the uterus. **Fetus 3 is a male, approximately 360 grams and 26.5 cm in length. There is very little amniotic fluid in the sac. Placenta is small in size**. FHR is 160 with no variability and very little fetal movement noted. Patient is scheduled for admission to antepartum unit for observation and monitoring. She is cautioned that the findings today are not favorable for Fetus 3 and delivery of all 3 babies may be necessary in the next day or two. Betamethasone IM is administered to stimulate fetal lung maturity. Patient's husband is here, questions answered. Perinatology fellow will accompany family to floor.

Impression: **Triplet gestation at 27 weeks with poor fetal growth, Fetus 3, due to placental insufficiency. Normal fetal growth for Fetus 1 and Fetus 2.**

Diagnosis Code(s)

O36.5123 Maternal care for known or suspected placental insufficiency, second trimester, fetus 3

O41.02X3 Oligohydramnios, second trimester, fetus 3

O30.112 Triplet pregnancy with two or more monochorionic fetuses

Z3A.27 27 weeks gestation of pregnancy

Coding Note(s)

The 7th character identifies the fetus affected by the condition or complication, not the number of fetuses affected. In a single gestation, the 7th character is always '0' for not applicable. The 7th character 0 would also be used for multiple gestations when the fetus affected is not specified. In this case, only one fetus is affected by the conditions and this fetus has been identified on the ultrasound as Fetus 3, so the codes for placental insufficiency and oligohydramnios are assigned the 7th character '3'. If more than one fetus were affected, the codes for each condition would be listed again for each identified fetus affected.

Rhesus/Other Isoimmunization

Isoimmunization of the red blood cells results when maternal antibodies cross the placenta and target fetal red blood cell antigens. This causes destruction of the fetal red blood cells and fetal anemia. Isoimmunization requires a sensitization event in the mother which is an initial exposure to the foreign red blood cell antigens. This usually occurs in a previous pregnancy during delivery when fetal red blood cells containing antigens that are not present in the mother cross into the mother's circulation causing the mother to develop antibodies to these foreign antigens. A subsequent pregnancy in which the fetus has the same foreign antigens can significantly increase the number of antibodies in the mother's red blood cells. The maternal antibodies may then cross the placenta and target and destroy the fetal red blood cells. While the condition primarily affects the fetus, additional maternal care is required to manage the hemolytic disease in the fetus. The most common type of incompatibility is anti-D, also known as Rh factor. However, there are other types of isoimmunization.

Isoimmunization is classified as anti-D [Rh] antibodies, also known as Rh incompatibility (O36.01-), other rhesus isoimmunization (O36.09-), anti-A sensitization (O36.11-), and other isoimmunization (O36.19-).

Coding and Documentation Requirements

Identify isoimmunization:

- Rhesus
  - Anti-D [Rh]
  - Other rhesus isoimmunization
- Anti-A sensitization
- Other isoimmunization

Identify trimester:

- First (less than 14 weeks 0 days)
- Second (14 weeks 0 days to less than 28 weeks 0 days)
- Third (28 weeks 0 days until delivery)
- Unspecified

Identify fetus affected by complication:

- Fetus 1
- Fetus 2
- Fetus 3
- Fetus 4
- Fetus 5
- Other fetus
- Unspecified fetus/not applicable

Maternal Isoimmunization

ICD-10-CM Code/Documentation	
O36.091-	Maternal care for other rhesus isoimmunization, first trimester
O36.092-	Maternal care for other rhesus isoimmunization, second trimester
O36.093-	Maternal care for other rhesus isoimmunization, third trimester
O36.099-	Maternal care for other rhesus isoimmunization, unspecified trimester
O36.011-	Maternal care for anti-D [Rh] antibodies, first trimester
O36.012-	Maternal care for anti-D [Rh] antibodies, second trimester
O36.013-	Maternal care for anti-D [Rh] antibodies, third trimester
O36.019-	Maternal care for anti-D [Rh] antibodies, unspecified trimester
O36.191-	Maternal care for other isoimmunization, first trimester
O36.192-	Maternal care for other isoimmunization, second trimester
O36.193-	Maternal care for other isoimmunization, third trimester
O36.199-	Maternal care for other isoimmunization, unspecified trimester
O36.111-	Maternal care for Anti-A sensitization, first trimester
O36.112-	Maternal care for Anti-A sensitization, second trimester
O36.113-	Maternal care for Anti-A sensitization, third trimester
O36.119-	Maternal care for Anti-A sensitization, unspecified trimester

Documentation and Coding Example

Thirty-one-year-old G4 P1 1 1 1 Black female is being followed for known **anti-U isoimmunization**. Patient has an eight-year-old daughter delivered via SVD at 38 weeks. Other obstetric history includes a spontaneous abortion at 14 weeks and a stillbirth at 32 weeks at which time the anti-U isoimmunization was identified. Anti-U serum titer has been monitored throughout the pregnancy. She is now at **30 weeks** and **anti-U serum titer is elevated at 1:1025**. She is seen today to discuss the results of her blood test. The need to monitor amniotic fluid bilirubin using serial amniocentesis so that hemolytic anemia in the fetus can be evaluated and treated if needed is also discussed. Her first amniocentesis is scheduled for tomorrow and amniocentesis will be repeated at 2-week intervals. She is advised that she may need to be delivered early depending on the results of the amniocentesis.

Diagnosis Code(s)

O36.1930 Maternal care for other isoimmunization, third trimester, fetus not applicable or unspecified

Z3A.30 30 weeks gestation of pregnancy

Coding Note(s)

Category O36 requires a 7th character extension for identification of the fetus, which only applies for multiple gestations. Since this is a single gestation, the 7th character extension is '0' which indicates that identification of the affected fetus is not applicable.

13. Complications of Pregnancy/Childbirth

Summary

Assigning the most specific codes for conditions and complications of pregnancy, childbirth, and the puerperium requires detail about the specific condition or complication. For example, patients with pre-existing diabetes mellitus must have the type of diabetes identified to capture the most specific code in Chapter 15. The severity of pre-eclampsia must be specified as mild, moderate, severe, or HELLP syndrome. Genitourinary tract infections occurring in pregnancy are specific to site. For conditions or complications that occur during pregnancy, trimester is an element of the majority of codes. For conditions and complications associated with multiple gestation that can affect one or more fetuses, the fetus experiencing the condition or complication must be identified. Current documentation analysis should include a review of all frequently encountered conditions and complications seen in pregnancy, childbirth, and the puerperium to ensure that documentation for these conditions and complications contains sufficient detail to code to the highest level of specificity.

Resources

Documentation checklists are available in Appendix A for the following condition(s):

- Gestational diabetes
- Multiple Gestation

Chapter 13 Quiz

1. Assignment of the most specific code for pre-existing essential hypertension (O10.0-) complicating pregnancy in Chapter 15 requires documentation of what information?
   a. Identification of the specific type of hypertension as benign or malignant
   b. Identification of the trimester
   c. Documentation of elevated blood pressure
   d. All of the above
2. A code from categories O35 or O36 is assigned only when the documentation indicates that the fetal condition is actually responsible for modifying the management of the mother. Which of the following would not support assignment of a code from these two categories?
   a. Performance of diagnostic studies
   b. Additional observation or special care of the mother
   c. Documentation that the patient is an elderly primigravida with an increased risk for chromosomal abnormality
   d. Termination of the pregnancy
3. Which of the following code categories does not require a 7th character extension to identify the fetus:
   a. O30 Multiple gestation
   b. O31 Complications specific to multiple gestation
   c. O40 Polyhydramnios
   d. O69 Labor and delivery complicated by umbilical cord complications
4. Documentation for a pregnant patient with gestational diabetes indicates that the condition is being controlled with diet and insulin. How is this coded?
   a. The code for diet-controlled gestational diabetes mellitus (O24.410) is assigned along with the code for long-term (current) use of insulin (Z79.4)
   b. Two codes from subcategory O24.4 are reported, one for diet-controlled gestational diabetes (O24.410) and one for insulin-controlled (O24.414)
   c. Only the code for the insulin-controlled gestational diabetes is reported (O24.414)
   d. The physician should be queried and the code assigned based on the response of the query
5. Documentation of peripartum cardiomyopathy is NOT reported with code O90.3 when:
   a. The condition complicates pregnancy in a patient with documented pre-existing heart disease
   b. The cardiomyopathy is diagnosed in the third trimester in a patient without pre-existing heart disease
   c. The condition develops as a result of pregnancy
   d. The condition is not diagnosed until the postpartum period
6. Assign codes for a triplet pregnancy, two monochorionic fetuses, with documented poor fetal growth due to placental insufficiency, second trimester, Fetus 2 and Fetus 3, and normal growth of Fetus 1.
   a. O30.112, O36.5122
   b. O30.112, O36.5120, O36.5122, O365123
   c. O30.112, O36.5122, O36.5123
   d. O30.112, O36.5129
7. What statement is true about antepartum hemorrhage with coagulation defects?
   a. A diagnosis documented as antepartum hemorrhage with afibrinogenemia is reported with the same code as premature separation of placenta with afibrinogenemia.
   b. Documentation of premature separation of placenta with disseminated intravascular coagulation and antepartum hemorrhage, requires two codes, one from category O46 and a second code from category O45.
   c. Documentation of premature separation of placenta with disseminated intravascular coagulation and antepartum hemorrhage is reported with a single code from category O46.
   d. Documentation of premature separation of placenta with disseminated intravascular coagulation and antepartum hemorrhage is reported with a single code from category O45.
8. What information is not required to assign the most specific code for infections of the amniotic sac and membranes?
   a. Trimester
   b. Infectious organism
   c. Fetus
   d. Identification of site as placenta or membranes/amnion
9. A pregnant patient, 12 weeks gestation, has pre-existing diabetes mellitus due to documented genetic defects of insulin action. What code would be the first-listed diagnosis?
   a. O24.111 Pre-existing diabetes mellitus, type 2, in pregnancy, first trimester
   b. O24.811 Other pre-existing diabetes mellitus in pregnancy, first trimester
   c. E13.9 Other specified diabetes mellitus without complications
   d. E11.9 Type 2 diabetes mellitus without complications
10. What information is required to assign the most specific code for pre-eclampsia?
   a. Trimester, Fetus, and Severity
   b. Fetus and Severity
   c. Trimester and Severity (mild, moderate, severe, HELLP)
   d. Laboratory results

See next page for answers and rationales.

Chapter-Specific Documentation Requirements

In this section, categories, subcategories, and subclassifications for some of the more frequently reported genitourinary diseases are reviewed. Valid codes are listed and documentation requirements are identified. The focus is on conditions with additional pieces of specific clinical documentation required in order to select the correct diagnostic code(s). Although not all codes with significant documentation requirements are discussed, this section will provide a representative sample of the type of additional documentation needed for genitourinary diseases. The section is organized alphabetically by the topic.

Absent, Scanty and Rare Menstruation

Amenorrhea is the clinical term for absence of menstruation for at least three menstrual periods in a row. Amenorrhea is most commonly caused by pregnancy but may also be due to problems with the reproductive organs or the glands that regulate hormone levels. In these cases, treatment of the underlying condition usually resolves the amenorrhea.

Primary amenorrhea is used to describe the condition in girls whose menstruation hasn't begun by the age of 16. Secondary amenorrhea is defined as the absence of menstrual periods for 6 months in a woman who had previously established regular menstrual periods.

Hypomenorrhea is the medical term used to describe unusually light menstrual flow. Women with hypomenorrhea have scanty periods or spotting during periods. There are various reasons responsible for this condition; one known cause is intrauterine adhesions after uterine surgery (e.g., myomectomy). Other causes of hypomenorrhea include hormonal imbalances (as in puberty or peri-menopause), uterine hypoplasia, long-term use of contraceptives, excessive stress, crash diets, and heavy exercise.

Oligomenorrhea describes infrequent menstruation in women with previously regular periods. Clinically, the diagnosis of oligomenorrhea is applied to women with menstrual periods occurring at intervals of greater than 35 days, with only four to nine periods in a year.

Although the practitioner may specifically diagnose either hypomenorrhea or oligomenorrhea in the medical documentation, hypomenorrhea is coded to oligomenorrhea.

Coding and Documentation Requirements

Identify the clinical condition:

- Amenorrhea
- Oligomenorrhea (includes hypomenorrhea)

Identify the type:

- Primary
- Secondary
- Unspecified

ICD-10-CM Code/Documentation	
N91.0	Primary amenorrhea
N91.1	Secondary amenorrhea
N91.2	Amenorrhea, unspecified
N91.3	Primary oligomenorrhea
N91.4	Secondary oligomenorrhea
N91.5	Oligomenorrhea, unspecified

Documentation and Coding Example

Twenty-one-year-old Caucasian female presents to OB-GYN with concerns about a **change in her menstrual flow.** Patient states her periods have always been regular with quite a heavy flow since they started at the age of 13. She has had a 75 lb. weight loss in the past year and while she was dieting she noticed her periods were sometimes **irregular but now they have become quite scanty** as well. Average length is just 2 days and she needs only a thin pad. She cannot insert a tampon because her vagina is too dry. Temp 98.4, Pulse 76, Resp 12, BP 110/68, Ht. 65 Wt. 132 lbs. On examination, this is a well-developed, well-nourished young woman. Neck supple without lymphadenopathy. Thyroid smooth, normal in size. Heart rate regular with a soft mid systolic ejection murmur which patient states she has had all of her life. Breath sounds clear, equal bilaterally. Breast exam is unremarkable. Abdomen is soft, flat with good muscle tone. Patient states she has been exercising with a personal trainer for the past 3 months. Pelvic exam is completely unremarkable. Impression: **Hypomenorrhea due to recent weight loss.**

Plan: Check FSH, LH, estrogen, prolactin, thyroid, and insulin levels just to r/o hormone etiology. Patient is congratulated on her weight loss and encouraged to continue with her exercise routine and healthy eating. She is advised that her current weight is appropriate for her height and bone structure and she should not attempt to lose more.

Diagnosis: **Secondary Oligomenorrhea/Hypomenorrhea.**

Diagnosis Code(s)

N91.4 Secondary oligomenorrhea

Coding Note(s)

Hypomenorrhea is indexed to direct the user to see oligomenorrhea. Since oligomenorrhea and hypomenorrhea are reported with the same code, and the status as secondary or primary is an axis of classification selected in the code title, a single diagnosis code is reported.

Cystitis

Cystitis, or inflammation of the bladder, is most often caused by a bacterial infection of the urinary tract. Cystitis may also result from a reaction to certain drugs, radiation therapy, irritants such as long-term use of a catheter, or as a complication of another illness. Documentation in the medical record needs to specify the type and cause of the cystitis and identify any infectious agent or organism, such as *E. coli.* Proper coding also requires documentation of cystitis as with or without hematuria.

Cystitis caused by certain specific infectious organisms are coded differently within the infectious disease chapter and are not included in the genitourinary chapter, so careful review of the documentation is needed to identify certain conditions such as candidal cystitis, chlamydial cystitis, diphtheritic cystitis, gonococcal cystitis, monilial cystitis, trichomonal cystitis, and tuberculous cystitis. Prostatocystitis is coded to N41.3 and not in category N30.

Coding and Documentation Requirements

Identify the type of cystitis:

- Acute
  - With hematuria
  - Without hematuria
- Chronic
  - Interstitial
    - » With hematuria
    - » Without hematuria
  - Other chronic
    - » With hematuria
    - » Without hematuria
- Irradiation
  - With hematuria
  - Without hematuria
- Trigonitis
  - With hematuria
  - Without hematuria
- Other specified type
  - With hematuria
  - Without hematuria
- Unspecified
  - With hematuria
  - Without hematuria

Use additional code to identify any infectious agent.

Note: Some types of cystitis are classified in Chapter 1 Infectious and Parasitic diseases. See Alphabetic Index when causative organism is documented to determine whether a code from category N30 should be assigned.

ICD-10-CM Code/Documentation	
N30.00	Acute cystitis without hematuria
N30.01	Acute cystitis with hematuria
N30.10	Interstitial cystitis (chronic) without hematuria
N30.11	Interstitial cystitis (chronic) with hematuria
N30.20	Other chronic cystitis without hematuria
N30.21	Other chronic cystitis with hematuria
N30.30	Trigonitis without hematuria
N30.31	Trigonitis with hematuria
N30.40	Irradiation cystitis without hematuria
N30.41	Irradiation cystitis with hematuria
N30.80	Other cystitis without hematuria
N30.81	Other cystitis with hematuria
N30.90	Cystitis, unspecified without hematuria
N30.91	Cystitis, unspecified with hematuria

Documentation and Coding Example

Twenty-nine-year-old Caucasian female is referred to Urology Clinic by her GYN for c/o ongoing urinary frequency, urgency, and pain. She was initially seen 3 months ago by her Internist for acute onset of symptoms and was prescribed Macrodantin for a UTI. Her symptoms improved but did not clear completely and she began to have pain with intercourse. She saw her GYN who diagnosed a yeast infection and prescribed Monostat. When her symptoms did not improve her GYN suggested she see a urologist. On examination, this is an anxious appearing, well-dressed woman who looks younger than her stated age. Voided UA was positive for blood, negative for protein, WBCs. Physical exam is unremarkable and informed consent obtained for cystoscopy. Patient positioned comfortably in dorsal lithotomy and cystoscope inserted without difficulty through the urethral meatus into the bladder. A patchy area of nonkeratinizing squamous metaplasia is easily identified at the trigone of the bladder by its glistening, fluffy white appearance. A biopsy is taken since patient does have hematuria. Remainder of the exam is unremarkable. Patient tolerated the procedure well and was interviewed after she had rested and gotten dressed. Advised patient she has **acute urethrotrigonitis** and biopsy should confirm that. Most appropriate treatment is Doxycycline 100 mg BID x 2 weeks for both she and her partner followed by Doxycycline 100 mg daily for 2 weeks for her. They should use a condom during intercourse for one month or abstain from intercourse altogether.

Diagnosis: **Hematuria due to acute urethrotrigonitis**

Diagnosis Code(s)

N30.31 Trigonitis with hematuria

Coding Note(s)

Urethrotrigonitis is listed as an included condition under the code for trigonitis, which includes both the acute and chronic forms of the disease. When coding cases of cystitis, an additional code is assigned for the infectious agent when it is identified in the medical record documentation.

Dysmenorrhea

Dysmenorrhea is the clinical term for menstrual cramps or painful menstruation. There are two types of dysmenorrhea: primary and secondary, which differ in age of onset and the severity of pain experienced. Primary dysmenorrhea is very common among adolescents with about 90% of adolescents reportedly suffering from the condition. Primary dysmenorrhea is cramping that is not associated with an identified underlying cause.

Secondary dysmenorrhea on the other hand, is menstrual pain associated with other diseases, such as pelvic infections, ovarian cysts, or endometriosis. Common causes of secondary dysmenorrhea include endometriosis, intrauterine devices, ovarian cysts, pelvic inflammatory disease, premenstrual syndrome or premenstrual dysmorphic disorder, tubo-ovarian abscess, and uterine leiomyoma or fibroids. Treatment for secondary dysmenorrhea depends on the underlying cause. Secondary dysmenorrhea is less common, affecting about 25% of women with dysmenorrhea.

Differentiating primary dysmenorrhea from secondary dysmenorrhea is essential for correct code assignment. Psychogenic dysmenorrhea is coded elsewhere.

Coding and Documentation Requirements

Identify type:

- Primary dysmenorrhea
- Secondary dysmenorrhea
- Unspecified

ICD-10-CM Code/Documentation	
N94.4	Primary dysmenorrhea
N94.5	Secondary dysmenorrhea
N94.6	Dysmenorrhea, unspecified

Documentation and Coding Example

Thirty-four-year-old Caucasian female presents to OB-GYN for her annual exam and has a new complaint of **menstrual cramps**. Patient has a **history of endometriosis**, diagnosed incidentally during an elective laparoscopic tubal ligation 2 years ago. She had no menstrual discomfort until now. The only change in her medical history is a benign cyst on her thyroid gland discovered by her PCP 8 months ago. Current medication is Tylenol for her pain. She did take meclizine and antibiotics for an ear infection with vertigo about 6 weeks ago. On examination, this is a tall, thin, attractive woman who looks her stated age. Neck supple, thyroid smooth with slight fullness on the left. Heart rate regular, breath sounds clear and equal. Breast exam is unremarkable. Abdomen soft, no pain with palpation. External genitalia normal. Speculum inserted without difficulty into vagina. Vaginal mucosa normal color, no discharge noted. Cervical os is closed. Cells collected for cytology and also HPV culture. Bimanual exam causes marked discomfort for patient. There is cervical motion tenderness and nodularity is appreciated in the cul de sac and around both ovaries. Rectal exam shows good sphincter tone but again marked discomfort during the exam.

Impression: **Dysmenorrhea due to endometriosis.**

Plan: Patient is given samples of Seasonique to take continuously for 3 months and advised to use ibuprofen instead of acetaminophen for pain. She will have blood drawn for CBC, ESR, and HCG to r/o infection, inflammation, or pregnancy. Return in 3 months for recheck, sooner if symptoms become worse.

Diagnosis: **Dysmenorrhea due to endometriosis.**

Diagnosis Code(s)

N94.5 Secondary dysmenorrhea

N80.9 Endometriosis, unspecified

Coding Note(s)

ICD-10-CM makes a distinction between primary and secondary dysmenorrhea. An additional code is assigned to report the endometriosis. Endometriosis is classified by site, but because the documentation does not describe the endometriosis or identify the site, the unspecified code must be assigned.

Hydronephrosis

Hydronephrosis is a condition in which the kidney's urine collecting system becomes dilated, usually due to an underlying illness or medical condition. In hydronephrosis, distention of the kidney with urine is caused by the backward pressure placed on the kidney when the flow of urine is obstructed. Obstruction or blockage is the most frequent cause of hydronephrosis, but the condition may also be congenital or occur as a response to pregnancy, or it may be caused by trauma, neoplastic disease, calculi, inflammatory processes, or surgical procedures. Documentation of the etiology is essential for code assignment.

Careful review of the medical record documentation is necessary to assign the correct code. For example, calculus of the kidney and ureter without hydronephrosis must be distinguished from cases with hydronephrosis. Other examples include congenital obstructive defects of the renal pelvis and ureter, and obstructive pyelonephritis. All of these conditions are coded differently.

Obstruction can occur anywhere from the urethral meatus to the calyceal infundibula and the physiological effects depend on the level of the obstruction, the extent of involvement, the patient's age at onset, and whether it is acute or chronic. Medical record documentation identifying the location of the obstruction is needed for code assignment. Hydronephrosis can also be unilateral involving just one kidney or bilateral involving both, although specific code selection does not require laterality.

Clinically, the term hydronephrosis describes dilation and swelling of the kidney, while the term hydroureter describes swelling of the ureter. These conditions, along with congenital hydronephrosis, are coded differently and therefore need to be clearly differentiated in the documentation.

Acquired hydronephrosis is a combination code that identifies the underlying medical condition causing the obstruction of urine and the resulting distension of the kidney.

Coding and Documentation Requirements

For acquired hydronephrosis, identify type of obstruction present:

- With infection
- With renal and ureteral calculous obstruction
- With ureteral stricture
- With ureteropelvic junction obstruction
- Other hydronephrosis

Unspecified hydronephrosis

ICD-10-CM Code/Documentation	
N13.0	Hydronephrosis with ureteropelvic junction obstruction
N13.1	Hydronephrosis with ureteral stricture, not elsewhere classified
N13.2	Hydronephrosis with renal and ureteral calculous obstruction
N13.30	Unspecified hydronephrosis
N13.39	Other hydronephrosis
N13.4	Hydroureter
N13.6	Pyonephrosis

Note: Pyonephrosis reports hydronephrosis/hydroureter with infection.

Documentation and Coding Example

Twenty-four-year-old male patient presents to ED with c/o worsening left flank pain with nausea and vomiting for the past 2 hours. PMH is significant for kidney stone at age 20 that resolved without intervention. Patient states he is a professional backup dancer for a well-known recording artist who performed locally this evening. On examination, this is a well-developed, well-nourished Black male who looks exhausted from recent physical exertion. Temp 99, Pulse 70, Resp 14, BP 102/66, O2 sat 99%. PERRL, neck supple. HR regular, breath sounds clear and equal. CVA tenderness present on left side with fullness detected in the kidney area. Abdomen soft with decreased bowel sounds. Liver and spleen not palpated. IV started in right forearm infusing LR. UA obtained and blood drawn for CBC, comprehensive metabolic panel. Medicated with MS and Phenergan with patient reporting decreased pain and nausea. Urology consult obtained and Spiral CT ordered. Patient is comfortable while waiting for CT scanner to be available.

Urology Note: Patient was examined after CT scan. He is resting comfortably after repeat IV morphine sulfate. Spiral CT shows a **stone in the left ureter with subsequent hydronephrosis of the left kidney**. Movement of the stone is noted from the time lapse of the scan with the **stone now mid-way between the kidney and bladder**. It should clear the ureter and enter the bladder in a few hours. Labs are unremarkable other than UA showing a slightly elevated pH and microscopic hematuria. Patient admitted to medical floor for continued IV hydration and pain management. Strain all urine and send all solid material to lab for analysis.

Diagnosis: **Unilateral hydronephrosis secondary to mid ureteral calculus**

Diagnosis Code(s)

N13.2 Hydronephrosis with renal and ureteral calculous obstruction

Coding Note(s)

A combination code reports both the hydronephrosis and the obstruction due to the ureteral calculus.

Male Infertility

Male infertility is defined as an inability to achieve pregnancy in a fertile female after one year of unprotected intercourse. The scope of male infertility is widespread. An estimated 15% of couples are considered infertile, with approximately 30%-40% due to male factors alone, and 20% due to a combination of female and male factors. The quality and the quantity of sperm greatly influence reproductive outcomes. Male infertility may be due to low or absent sperm production, immobile sperm, or blockages in the delivery of sperm. Other factors that can play a role in causing male infertility include illnesses, injuries, and chronic health problems.

Azoospermia describes a complete absence of sperm in the ejaculate, while hypospermatogenesis is abnormally decreased spermatozoa production. Because germ cells are precursors to spermatozoa, germ cell aplasia is often the cause of non-obstructive azoospermia.

Coding and Documentation Requirements

Identify the specific type and cause of infertility:

- Azoospermia
  - Due to extratesticular cause
    - Drug therapy
    - Infection
    - Obstruction of efferent ducts
    - Other extratesticular causes
    - Radiation
    - Systemic disease
  - Organic
- Oligospermia
  - Due to extratesticular cause
    - Drug therapy
    - Infection
    - Obstruction of efferent ducts
    - Other extratesticular causes
    - Radiation
    - Systemic disease
  - Organic
- Other male infertility
- Unspecified male infertility

For extratesticular causes, code also associated cause.

ICD-10-CM Code/Documentation	
N46.01	Organic azoospermia
N46.021	Azoospermia due to drug therapy
N46.022	Azoospermia due to infection
N46.023	Azoospermia due to obstruction of efferent ducts
N46.024	Azoospermia due to radiation
N46.025	Azoospermia due to systemic disease
N46.029	Azoospermia due to other extratesticular causes
N46.11	Organic oligospermia
N46.121	Oligospermia due to drug therapy
N46.122	Oligospermia due to infection
N46.123	Oligospermia due to obstruction of efferent ducts
N46.124	Oligospermia due to radiation
N46.125	Oligospermia due to systemic disease
N46.129	Oligospermia due to other extratesticular causes
N46.8	Other male infertility
N46.9	Male infertility, unspecified

Documentation and Coding Example

Fifty-two-year-old Caucasian male is referred to PMD for comprehensive physical as part of an infertility work up. Patient was able to father 3 healthy children with his first wife but his new wife has been unable to get pregnant despite unprotected intercourse x 8 months. His wife's work up has been benign thus far. Patient comes reluctantly to the appointment because he has an extremely busy work schedule. He travels in the continental US frequently and goes to Europe and/or Asia at least once a month. Accessibility is not a problem as his wife travels with him, nor does performance appear to be an issue. He states that he is able to maintain an erection, penetrate, and ejaculate. A recent semen analysis showed a very low sperm count but the sperm present in the ejaculate were healthy and motile.

Temp 97.6, Pulse 80, Resp 12, BP 142/90, Ht. 72 inches, Wt. 184 lbs. His Blackberry and phone vibrate every few minutes and although he does not answer them, he is clearly distracted by the interruptions and is anxious to get the exam over with. He had a company nurse draw blood and he provided a urine sample prior to this visit so lab results are available. His only medication is occasional OTC Tagamet and Tums for heartburn. On examination, this is a well-developed, well-nourished man who looks younger than his stated age. PERRL, neck supple without lymphadenopathy. Nares patent, mucous membranes moist and pink. Cranial nerves grossly intact. Pulses and reflexes normal in extremities. Heart rate regular without bruit, rub, murmur. Breath sounds clear, equal bilaterally. Abdomen soft, bowel sounds present. Liver palpated at 3 cm below RCM, spleen at 1 cm below LCM. No evidence of hernia, testicles smooth. Penis is circumcised without urethral drainage. Rectal exam shows good sphincter tone with a smooth, normal size prostate gland.

Patient allowed to dress and labs are reviewed with him seated in the consultation room. Of significance his FBGL is 125 and HgbA1C is 7.1. TSH is 5.8. Lipid and triglyceride levels are in high normal range but liver and renal function tests are mildly elevated. Patient admits to **smoking 2-3 cigarettes daily, cigars 1-2 x week**. His alcohol consumption includes 2-4 oz. of Scotch and 2-3 glasses of wine per day.

Impression: **Low sperm count due to underlying hypothyroid and insulin resistant diabetes Type II**.

Plan: Patient is given samples and a prescription for Synthroid 0.05 mg to take daily in the AM at least 30 minutes before breakfast. He is given samples and a prescription for Metformin 500 to be taken 2 x day with meals. He is advised to stop smoking, cut down on his alcohol consumption, and avoid taking Tagamet as all 3 of these can decrease sperm count. He is to repeat labs in 1 month and call at his convenience to discuss results. This note is electronically sent to his wife's infertility doctor. Further arrangements should be made with them for semen analysis.

Diagnosis: **Hypospermatogenesis due to systemic disease**.

Diagnosis Code(s)

N46.125	Oligospermia due to systemic disease
E11.69	Type 2 diabetes with other specified complication
E03.9	Hypothyroidism, unspecified
Z72.0	Tobacco use

Coding Note(s)

There is a specific code for infertility due to systemic disease; in this case, hypospermatogenesis, or oligospermia. Code(s) that specifically identify the systemic disease(s) present are coded additionally. The low sperm count is attributed to both hypothyroidism and type 2 diabetes. The type of hypothyroidism is not specified, and since there is no diabetes combination code specifically for reporting that occurring with infertility as a complication, the code for type 2 diabetes with other specific complication is assigned.

Redundant Prepuce and Phimosis

Phimosis is the inability of the prepuce or foreskin to be retracted behind the glans penis in uncircumcised males. This tightening of the foreskin may close the opening of the penis. Circumcision is the most common treatment to correct phimosis. In paraphimosis, the foreskin is retracted behind the crown of the penis which may cause entrapment of the penis, impairing blood flow.

Phimosis can be congenital or it may be due to infection. The symptoms of phimosis and paraphimosis are similar to other medical disorders, so clear documentation of the patient's condition is necessary. When the cause of the phimosis or paraphimosis is infection, the medical record documentation should also identify the infectious agent.

When balanitis (inflammation of the glans) and posthitis (inflammation of the foreskin) occur together, it is called balanoposthitis. Correct coding requires documentation clearly describing the patient's condition. Balanoposthitis is classified as a disorder of the prepuce and is reported within category N47 Disorders of prepuce, which provides specific codes for adherent prepuce of newborn, phimosis, paraphimosis, deficient foreskin, benign cyst, adhesions, and balanoposthitis. There is an additional code for other inflammatory disease of the prepuce and another code for other disorders (noninflammatory) of the prepuce.

Coding and Documentation Requirements

Identify type of prepuce disorder:

- Adherent prepuce, newborn
- Adhesions of prepuce and glans penis
- Balanoposthitis
- Benign cyst of prepuce
- Deficient foreskin
- Paraphimosis
- Phimosis
- Other disorders of prepuce
- Other inflammatory disease of prepuce

Use additional code as needed to identify any infectious agent.

ICD-10-CM Code/Documentation	
N47.0	Adherent prepuce, newborn
N47.1	Phimosis
N47.2	Paraphimosis
N47.3	Deficient foreskin
N47.4	Benign cyst of prepuce
N47.5	Adhesions of prepuce and glans penis
N47.6	Balanoposthitis

ICD-10-CM Code/Documentation	
N47.7	Other inflammatory diseases of prepuce
N47.8	Other disorders of prepuce

Documentation and Coding Example

Patient is an 18-month-old Hispanic male brought to ED by his grandmother and older sister. Parents are out of the country. Child is crying and appears uncomfortable. Through an interpreter, sister states her little brother woke this morning fussy and when she removed his diaper she saw that the tip of his penis was swollen. Child is seen immediately by the pediatric resident. On examination, the glans penis is red and swollen with an edematous, proximally retracted foreskin forming a circumferential constricting band. The penile shaft is soft and there is no evidence of necrosis in the glans or the shaft. EMLA cream is applied liberally to the penis, patient placed on monitors, and medicated with Demerol IM. Manual compression of the glans penis and foreskin x 10 minutes allows the foreskin to be easily reduced over the glans using gentle pressure. Patient monitored following procedure and discharged home in good condition. Family is given instructions for care/cleaning of uncircumcised penis and will follow up in Urology Clinic in one week.

Diagnosis: **Paraphimosis**.

Diagnosis Code(s)

N47.2 Paraphimosis

Salpingitis/Oophoritis

Salpingitis is an inflammation of the fallopian tubes and oophoritis is an inflammation of the ovaries. The two conditions are often seen in combination. Salpingitis and oophoritis are specified as acute or chronic. In chronic cases, the swelling and inflammation is often caused by a hydrosalpinx, which is the accumulation of fluid within the fallopian tube caused by a blockage at the distal end. The condition can affect one or both sides. Hydrosalpinx is an included condition for chronic cases.

ICD-10-CM provides separate codes for salpingitis alone and oophoritis alone. Conditions classified with salpingitis and/or oophoritis include:

- Abscess
  - Fallopian tube
  - Ovary
  - Tubo-ovarian
- Pyosalpinx
- Salpingo-oophoritis
- Tubo-ovarian inflammatory disease

An additional code is used to report the causative infectious organism(s), when it is identified.

Coding and Documentation Requirements

Identify the condition:

- Salpingitis alone
- Oophoritis alone
- Salpingitis and oophoritis

Identify the status of the condition:

- Acute
- Chronic
- Unspecified

ICD-10-CM Code/Documentation	
N70.01	Acute salpingitis
N70.02	Acute oophoritis
N70.03	Acute salpingitis and oophoritis
N70.11	Chronic salpingitis
N70.12	Chronic oophoritis
N70.13	Chronic salpingitis and oophoritis
N70.91	Salpingitis, unspecified
N70.92	Oophoritis, unspecified
N70.93	Salpingitis and oophoritis, unspecified

Documentation and Coding Example

Thirty-nine-year-old Caucasian female referred to radiology by her OB-GYN for pelvic ultrasound and possible hysterosalpingogram. Patient is a G1P1 who has been trying to conceive a second child for over a year without success. Her first child is 6 years old and conceived without difficulty. That pregnancy was uncomplicated with a spontaneous vaginal delivery. Her GYN exams are WNL with no history of PID or endometriosis. Husband's sperm quality is excellent. Informed consent obtained and pelvic US using vaginal probe shows a normal cervix and uterus, normal appearing ovary on the right but no visible tube. The view of the left ovary is somewhat obscured due to a large cylinder-shaped collection of fluid in the area of the left fallopian tube. Discussed findings with patient and decision made to proceed with HSG. Patient transferred to fluoroscopy suite where she is prepped and draped for the procedure. Catheter easily inserted through cervix into uterus and contrast injected. Uterine filling is normal, the right fallopian tube fills and spills contrast into the peritoneum within 5 minutes. The left fallopian tube has partial filling at the proximal end but appears large and bulbous past that area. Delayed films are obtained 15, 30, and 45 minutes post contrast injection and still show no dye spill from the distal end of the left fallopian tube.

Impression: **Hydrosalpinx of left fallopian tube**. Report and procedure note is electronically sent to referring physician. Results also discussed with patient who will follow up with her OB-GYN.

Diagnosis: **Hydrosalpinx**.

Diagnosis Code(s)

N70.11 Chronic salpingitis

Coding Note(s)

Hydrosalpinx is classified as an inclusion to subcategory N70.1-. Chronic salpingitis and oophoritis. Hydrosalpinx is indexed to code N70.11, specifically for chronic salpingitis.

Spermatocele

A spermatocele is a cyst on the epididymis usually filled with fluid and dead sperm cells. These spermatic cysts may occur alone or as multiple cysts. ICD-10-CM provides specific codes for spermatocele of the epididymis to identify the occurrence as single, multiple, or unspecified.

Coding and Documentation Requirements

Identify the occurrence of spermatocele:

- Multiple
- Single
- Unspecified

ICD-10-CM Code/Documentation	
N43.40	Spermatocele of epididymis, unspecified
N43.41	Spermatocele of epididymis, single
N43.42	Spermatocele of epididymis, multiple

Documentation and Coding Example

Twenty-three-year-old male presents to urologist concerned about a painless lump he discovered in his scrotum when he did a testicular self-exam. He has practiced TSE since the age of 17 when his brother-in-law was diagnosed with testicular cancer. Patient is a graduate student in International Relations and an elite cyclist on his college team. On examination, this is a muscular, but thin young man. He is very intense, extremely articulate, and able to provide a detailed health history on both himself and his family. On examination, the abdomen is very firm and muscular. He denies pain with palpation. There is no evidence of hernia in the inguinal area. Penis is circumcised, no urethral drainage. Scrotum has normal rugae. Left testicle is smooth and slightly higher than the right. The right testicle is also smooth with a soft, spherical, well circumscribed fullness in the epididymis at the superior aspect of the testicle. The area is positive to trans-illumination. Testicular ultrasound confirms that this is a **single spermatocele** located at the head of the epididymis on the right testicle. Patient is reassured that this is a benign cystic type of lesion and no treatment is necessary at this time. He should continue to do TSE and return if he has pain or the lump becomes larger.

Diagnosis: **Solitary spermatocele of epididymis**

Diagnosis Code(s)

N43.41 Spermatocele of epididymis, single

Urethral Stricture

Urethral strictures result from various causes and present a range of manifestations. Causes of urethral stricture include trauma, an adverse effect or complication from medical treatment, inflammatory or infectious processes, and malignancy. Urethral strictures may also be congenital.

Most urethral strictures are the result of trauma to the perineum, such as traumatic catheter placement or removal or a chronic indwelling Foley catheter. Postprocedural urethral stricture is classified at the end of the code block with other intraoperative and postprocedural complications and disorders of the genitourinary system.

Codes for urethral stricture capture the cause (postinfective, post-traumatic, postprocedural, other specified), gender, and for males, the site of the stricture as the meatus, bulbous urethra, membranous urethra, anterior urethra, overlapping sites, or unspecified site. For postinfective stricture, there are more specific codes for postinfective stricture due to the following organisms: schistosomiasis (B65.-, N29), gonorrhea (A54.01), syphilis (A52.76).

Coding and Documentation Requirements

Identify the cause of urethral stricture:

- Postinfective, NEC
- Postprocedural
- Post-traumatic
- Other specified cause
- Unspecified cause

Identify gender:

- Male
- Female

For males, identify the site of the stricture:

- Anterior urethra
- Bulbous urethra
- Meatus
- Membranous urethra
- Overlapping sites
- Unspecified

For female with post-traumatic stricture, identify cause:

- Due to childbirth
- Other specified trauma

ICD-10-CM Code/Documentation	
N35.010	Post-traumatic urethral stricture, male, meatal
N35.011	Post-traumatic bulbous urethral stricture
N35.012	Post-traumatic membranous urethral stricture
N35.013	Post-traumatic anterior urethral stricture
N35.014	Post-traumatic urethral stricture, male, unspecified
N35.016	Post-traumatic urethral stricture, male, overlapping sites
N35.021	Urethral stricture due to childbirth
N35.028	Other post-traumatic urethral stricture, female
N35.111	Postinfective urethral stricture, not elsewhere classified, male, meatal
N35.112	Postinfective bulbous urethral stricture, not elsewhere classified, male
N35.113	Postinfective membranous urethral stricture, not elsewhere classified
N35.114	Postinfective anterior urethral stricture, not elsewhere classified, male
N35.116	Postinfective urethral stricture, not elsewhere classified, male, overlapping sites
N35.119	Postinfective urethral stricture, not elsewhere classified, male, unspecified
N35.12	Postinfective urethral stricture, not elsewhere classified, female
N99.110	Postprocedural urethral stricture, male, meatal
N99.111	Postprocedural bulbous urethral stricture, male

ICD-10-CM Code/Documentation	
N99.112	Postprocedural membranous urethral stricture, male
N99.113	Postprocedural anterior bulbous urethral stricture, male
N99.114	Postprocedural urethral stricture, male, unspecified
N99.115	Postprocedural fossa navicularis urethral stricture
N99.116	Postprocedural urethral stricture, male, overlapping sites
N99.12	Postprocedural urethral stricture, female
N37	Urethral disorders in diseases classified elsewhere
N35.811	Other urethral stricture, male, meatal
N35.812	Other urethral bulbous stricture, male
N35.813	Other membranous urethral stricture, male
N35.814	Other anterior urethral stricture, male
N35.816	Other urethral stricture, male, overlapping sites
N35.819	Other urethral stricture, male, unspecified site
N35.82	Other urethral stricture, female
N35.911	Unspecified urethral stricture, male, meatal
N35.912	Unspecified bulbous urethral stricture, male
N35.913	Unspecified membranous urethral stricture, male
N35.914	Unspecified anterior urethral stricture, male
N35.916	Unspecified urethral stricture, male overlapping sites
N35.919	Unspecified urethral stricture, male, unspecified site
N35.92	Unspecified urethral stricture, female

Documentation and Coding Example

Patient is a thirty-four-year-old Hispanic female who presents for a second urethral dilatation. This healthy woman delivered her first child vaginally six months ago. The infant was over 10 lbs. with fetal distress which necessitated an emergency delivery using forceps. Patient sustained deep lacerations to the vagina, one of which extended close to the urethra. She was subsequently unable to void post-delivery and was straight cathed once and finally had a Foley placed for 24 hours. She mentioned to her OB at her postpartum checkup that she was having pain and urgency with voiding. Exam showed excellent healing of the vaginal mucosa without evidence of fistula and urine culture was negative. She was referred to urology where cystoscopic exam revealed **1 cm long urethral stricture, most likely due to catheterization following delivery**. The stricture was dilated using serial sounds and patient's urinary symptoms resolved. In the past 3 weeks, she has again noticed urinary urgency and frequency. She came into the office and was seen by the PA who found a PVR of 220 cc and sent a cathed urine specimen to the lab for culture which was negative at 72 hours. Procedure Note: Patient is prepped and draped in lithotomy position. The cystoscope inserted without difficulty through the urethral meatus and almost immediately encountered a **urethral stricture which is the same size as previously mentioned**. Cystoscope advanced into the bladder which appears normal and the scope removed. The urethra is dilated with serial sounds and cystoscope inserted again to visualize the urethra. Excellent dilatation achieved. Patient tolerated procedure well.

Diagnosis: **Urethral stricture, post-catheterization**

Diagnosis Code(s)

N99.12 Postprocedural urethral stricture, female

Coding Note(s)

Coding post-operative or postprocedural urethral stricture to the highest level of specificity available requires identification of the patient's gender. In a male, the anatomical position of the urethral stricture is also required. In females, the cause is reported as post-traumatic due to childbirth or other trauma, postinfective, and postprocedural. Postprocedural stricture has an inclusion term that specifies postcatheterization urethral stricture.

Vaginitis/Vulvovaginitis

Vaginitis describes an inflammation of the vagina while vulvovaginitis is inflammation or infection of the vulva and vagina together. Vulvovaginitis may be due to bacteria, yeast, virus, or other parasites, as well as sexually transmitted infections. Allergens, certain chemicals, and factors such as poor hygiene can also cause the condition. Vaginitis and vulvovaginitis are extremely common conditions with similar presentations, so clear documentation of the patient's condition, along with documentation of the etiology, is essential for correct code assignment.

Some types of cases are coded elsewhere. For instance, ICD-10-CM excludes cases of candidal, chlamydial, gonococcal, syphilitic, and tuberculous vaginitis/vulvitis/vulvovaginitis from the genitourinary chapter and provides separate classifications within the infectious disease chapter. Vaginitis and vulvovaginitis in other diseases, such as pinworm, requires documentation of the underlying disease first in order to assign the correct codes.

Separate codes for vaginitis and vulvitis are provided, and these conditions are subclassified as acute or subacute/chronic. Careful attention to the inclusions shows that inflammation/infection of both the vulva and the vagina together is coded to vaginitis and the default code for unspecified cases is acute.

Coding and Documentation Requirements

Identify site:

- Vaginitis (includes vaginitis with vulvitis)
- Vulvitis

Specify status:

- Acute
- Chronic (includes subacute)
- In diseases classified elsewhere

For acute and chronic types, use additional code to identify infectious agent.

Note: Vaginitis, vulvitis, and vulvovaginitis in diseases classified elsewhere is classified to subcategory N77.1 and site and status are not an axis of classification. The underlying disease should be coded first with attention to the specific causative types that are excluded and must be reported with a code in Chapter 1.

ICD-10-CM Code/Documentation	
N76.0	Acute vaginitis
N76.1	Subacute and chronic vaginitis
N76.2	Acute vulvitis
N76.3	Subacute and chronic vulvitis
N77.1	Vaginitis, vulvitis and vulvovaginitis in diseases classified elsewhere

Documentation and Coding Example

Twenty-year-old African American female presents to Student Health with c/o vaginal discharge, itching x two months, and pain with intercourse x one week. Patient is sexually active with one partner and uses oral contraceptives. Her symptoms began about a week after she returned from summer break. She states she was not sexually active during that time but she suspects her boyfriend was. On examination, the vulva appears mildly red but patient denies any vulvar symptoms. Speculum is inserted with some difficulty into the vagina due to extreme discomfort. The vaginal walls are pink but not erythematous. A frothy whitish-gray discharge adheres to the mucosal lining of the vagina. Sample of discharge placed on wet mount. Cervix is closed and without discharge. Bimanual exam elicits some cervical motion tenderness. The rest of the exam is WNL. Wet mount is positive for clue cells, negative for yeast buds, WBCs, or epithelial cells. Vaginal pH 5.5.

Impression: **Bacterial vaginitis.**

Plan: Clindamycin 2% cream, insert 1 applicator into vagina at bedtime x 7 days.

Diagnosis: **Bacterial vaginitis.**

Diagnosis Code(s)

N76.0 Acute vaginitis

B96.89 Other specified bacterial agents as the cause of disease classified elsewhere

Coding Note(s)

Acuity status is an axis of classification for this condition, which classifies bacterial vaginitis as acute vaginitis. Clue cells found on microscopic examination of vaginal wet mount preparations demonstrate bacterial vaginosis as clue cells are vaginal epithelial cells that have bacteria adhering to their surfaces. The code for bacteria, NEC causing disease classified elsewhere, B96.89, is also assigned.

Vesicoureteral Reflux

Vesicoureteral reflux is the abnormal flow of urine back up the ureters and is usually diagnosed in infants and children. Vesicoureteral reflux can be unilateral or bilateral and documentation of laterality is necessary for the most accurate code assignment. Vesicoureteral reflux can damage the kidneys. When this occurs, it is referred to as reflux nephropathy. Coding requires documentation indicating the presence or absence of damage to the kidneys caused by the reflux of urine. Codes for vesicoureteral reflux also capture the presence or absence of hydroureter. Vesicoureteral reflux with reflux nephropathy is not the same as reflux associated pyelonephritis and the two conditions are coded differently, so the two conditions must be clearly differentiated in the documentation.

Coding and Documentation Requirements

Identify the type/presentation of vesicoureteral reflux:

- With reflux nephropathy
  - With hydroureter
    - Bilateral
    - Unilateral
    - Unspecified
  - Without hydroureter
    - Bilateral
    - Unilateral
    - Unspecified
- Without reflux nephropathy
- Unspecified

ICD-10-CM Code/Documentation	
N13.70	Vesicoureteral-reflux, unspecified
N13.71	Vesicoureteral-reflux without reflux nephropathy
N13.721	Vesicoureteral-reflux with reflux nephropathy without hydroureter, unilateral
N13.722	Vesicoureteral-reflux with reflux nephropathy without hydroureter, bilateral
N13.729	Vesicoureteral-reflux with reflux nephropathy without hydroureter, unspecified
N13.731	Vesicoureteral-reflux with reflux nephropathy with hydroureter, unilateral
N13.732	Vesicoureteral-reflux with reflux nephropathy with hydroureter, bilateral
N13.739	Vesicoureteral-reflux with reflux nephropathy with hydroureter, unspecified

Documentation and Coding Example

Ten-year-old Caucasian female presents to Urology Clinic for annual exam. The patient is well known to our practice having been followed since the age of five when she presented with a UTI and subsequent work up revealed **vesicoureteral reflux with reflux nephropathy and hydroureter**. She had an ultrasound prior to this appointment that shows her condition to be stable, unchanged. Physical exam is unremarkable. Labs are significant for mildly elevated BUN and creatinine. Urine culture showed no growth of bacteria. She will continue to take daily Macrodantin and bring in a monthly clean catch voided urine for culture. RTC in 1 year, sooner if problems arise.

Diagnosis: **Vesicoureteral reflux with reflux nephropathy and hydroureter.**

Diagnosis Code(s)

N13.739 Vesicoureteral-reflux with reflux nephropathy with hydroureter, unspecified

Coding Note(s)

An unspecified code is assigned because the medical record documentation does not specify whether the patient's condition was affecting only one kidney or both.

Summary

Maintaining best practices in documentation of genitourinary disorders requires detailed information on the diagnosis and treatment of these conditions. Coders will find that some aspects of coding are streamlined thanks to an increased number of combination codes that identify both the (type of) disorder and its manifestation or status. For example, cystitis is now a combination code which bases the code selection on the type of cystitis and whether the patient has hematuria or not. The urinary section includes subchapters that classify each code into a code family, making it easier for coders to select the correct code. Many conditions affecting bilateral organs require code assignment that includes the side affected, such as ovarian cysts, torsion, prolapse, hernia, and acquired atrophy of ovaries and/or fallopian tubes, and testicular pain; or whether the condition affects only one side or both sides, such as vesicoureteral reflux.

The clinical terminology used to describe genitourinary disorders has been updated from that used previously in order to include advances in medical diagnosis and treatment for conditions. An example of this is erectile dysfunction following radiation therapy, interstitial seed therapy, or prostate ablative therapy. This, in turn, requires an understanding of specific coding terms as well as detailed documentation of the patient's condition.

Chapter 14 Quiz

1. What information is NOT required to code vesicoureteral reflux to the highest level of specificity?
   a. Documentation of the presence/absence of reflux nephropathy
   b. Documentation of unilateral vesicoureteral reflux as left or right
   c. Documentation of with or without hydroureter
   d. Documentation of laterality as unilateral or bilateral
2. Where is postprocedural urethral stricture classified?
   a. In the code block for urethral disorders in Chapter 14
   b. In a separate code block for intraoperative and postprocedural complications at the end of Chapter 14
   c. In Chapter 21 Factors Influencing Health Status and Contact with Health Services
   d. With infectious and parasitic diseases in Chapter 1
3. Which of the following statements is true regarding coding hydronephrosis and ureteral calculus?
   a. Dual coding is required to report hydronephrosis and ureteral calculus
   b. A combination code reports hydronephrosis with ureteral calculus
   c. A combination code reports hydronephrosis with ureteral calculus and the side affected
   d. Dual coding is required to report hydronephrosis by laterality and ureteral calculus by laterality
4. How is endometriosis classified?
   a. By site
   b. By etiology
   c. By site and laterality
   d. By both site and etiology
5. Coding post-traumatic urethral stricture to the highest level of specificity available requires identification of ____________________.
   a. The patient's gender
   b. The underlying cause
   c. The manifestation
   d. All of the above
6. When coding dysmenorrhea, what distinction is made for proper code selection?
   a. Site
   b. Etiology
   c. Type as primary or secondary
   d. With or without endometriosis
7. How is Chronic Kidney Disease (CKD) coded?
   a. Based on stage of severity
   b. Based on type
   c. Based on etiology
   d. Based on duration of the patient's chronic condition
8. The physician documents the patient's diagnosis as "subacute vaginitis." How is this coded?
   a. With the code for acute and subacute vaginitis
   b. With the code for chronic vaginitis
   c. With the code for subacute and chronic vaginitis
   d. With the code for unspecified vaginitis
9. According to the coding and sequencing guidelines for chronic kidney disease in a kidney transplant patient, which of the following is true?
   a. A kidney transplant status patient may still have some form of chronic kidney disease
   b. The presence of CKD alone does not constitute a transplant complication
   c. If the documentation does not clarify whether the CKD constitutes a transplant complication, the provider should be queried
   d. All of the above
10. What is the correct coding and sequencing for a patient diagnosed with hematuria and cystitis?
   a. A code for the type of cystitis is listed first, followed by a code for the hematuria
   b. A code for the hematuria is listed first, followed by the code for cystitis
   c. A combination code is assigned that includes the type of cystitis with hematuria
   d. A code for the underlying infection is listed first, followed by a code for the cystitis, and a code for the hematuria

See next page for answers and rationales.

Chapter 14 Answers and Rationales

1. What information is NOT required to code vesicoureteral reflux to the highest level of specificity?

   b. Documentation of unilateral vesicoureteral reflux as left or right

   Rationale: *While laterality is an element of coding vesicoureteral reflux, the codes only differentiate the condition as unilateral or bilateral. Unilateral vesicoureteral reflux does not need to be specified as right or left to assign the most specific code. Documentation of the presence or absence of reflux nephropathy and the presence or absence of hydroureter is needed to assign the most specific code.*

2. Where is postprocedural urethral stricture classified?

   b. In a separate code block for intraoperative and postprocedural complications at the end of Chapter 14

   Rationale: *ICD-10-CM has a separate code block at the end of Chapter 14 (N99) where all intraoperative and postprocedural complications from treatment of genitourinary disorders are classified.*

3. Which of the following statements is true regarding coding hydronephrosis and ureteral calculus?

   b. A combination code reports hydronephrosis with ureteral calculus

   Rationale: *Codes in category N13 Obstructive and reflux uropathy are combination codes which report hydronephrosis with ureteral stricture, with infection, and with renal and ureteral calculous obstruction. Separate codes are not required and laterality is not an axis of classification.*

4. How is endometriosis classified?

   a. By site

   Rationale: *Codes in category N80 Endometriosis specify endometriosis of the uterus, ovary, fallopian tube, pelvic peritoneum, rectovaginal septum and vagina, intestine, cutaneous scar, and other sites. Etiology and laterality are not components of coding endometriosis.*

5. Coding post-traumatic urethral stricture to the highest level of specificity available requires identification of ______________________.

   a. The patient's gender

   Rationale: *Identification of the patient's gender is required for code assignment because subcategory N35.0 Post-traumatic urethral stricture includes further subcategories of codes specifically for male types of post-traumatic urethral stricture and female causes of post-traumatic urethral stricture.*

6. When coding dysmenorrhea, what distinction is made for proper code selection?

   c. Type as primary or secondary

   Rationale: *Codes for dysmenorrhea (N94) specify primary type versus secondary type dysmenorrhea.*

7. How is Chronic Kidney Disease (CKD) coded?

   a. Based on stage of severity

   Rationale: *Chronic kidney disease is specified as stage 1-5.*

8. The physician documents the patient's diagnosis as "subacute vaginitis." How is this coded?

   c. With the code for subacute and chronic vaginitis

   Rationale: *Codes in category N76 Other inflammation of vagina and vulva specify cases of vaginitis as either acute (which is the default for unspecified cases), or as subacute and chronic together.*

9. According to the coding and sequencing guidelines for chronic kidney disease in a kidney transplant patient, which of the following is true?

   d. All of the above

   Rationale: *According to the ICD-10-CM Official Guidelines for Coding and Reporting Section I.C.14: patients who have undergone kidney transplant may still have some form of chronic kidney disease (CKD) because the kidney transplant may not fully restore kidney function. Therefore, the presence of CKD alone does not constitute a transplant complication. The guidelines further state that if the documentation is unclear as to whether the patient has a complication of the transplant, query the provider.*

10. What is the correct coding and sequencing for a patient diagnosed with hematuria and cystitis?

    c. A combination code is assigned that includes the type of cystitis with hematuria

    Rationale: *In the Tabular List, codes in category N30 for cystitis specify the type of cystitis as with or without hematuria in one combination code, so multiple codes are not needed.*

Chapter 15
DISEASES OF THE MUSCULOSKELETAL SYSTEM AND CONNECTIVE TISSUE

Introduction

Codes for diseases of the musculoskeletal system and connective tissue are found in Chapter 15 in ICD-10-CM. Like many of the other chapters, the documentation needed to code conditions of the musculoskeletal system accurately require specificity and detail. For example, conditions affecting the cervical spine now require identification of the level as occipito-atlanto-axial or high cervical region, mid-cervical region identified by level C3-4, C4-5, C5-6 or cervicothoracic region. Laterality is also included for most musculoskeletal and connective tissue conditions affecting the extremities. For some conditions only right and left is provided, but for other conditions that frequently affect both sides, codes for bilateral are listed. Although not a new documentation requirement, physicians will need to clearly document whether the condition being treated is an acute traumatic condition, in which case it is reported with an injury code from Chapter 19, or an old or chronic condition, in which case it is reported with a code from Chapter 15. Pathologic fractures are reported based upon the causation such as due to neoplastic or other disease, location as well as episode of care. While episode of care is often clearly evident from the nature of the visit, (i.e. a follow-up visit to evaluate healing of a pathological fracture) current documentation should be reviewed to ensure that the initial episode of care is clearly differentiated from subsequent visits for routine healing, delayed healing, malunion, or nonunion of these fractures. If the condition is a sequela of a pathological fracture, that information should also be clearly noted in the medical record as this is also captured with the code for the pathological fracture. Additionally, each visit must be specific in defining the fracture. No longer can the providers merely state the patient is being seen for follow-up of a tibia fracture.

A good way to begin an analysis of documentation and coding requirements for each chapter is to be familiar with the chapter sections and ICD-10-CM chapter blocks. A table containing this information is provided below.

ICD-10-CM Blocks	
M00-M02	Infectious Arthropathies
M05-M14	Inflammatory Polyarthropathies
M15-M19	Osteoarthritis
M20-M25	Other Joint Disorders
M26-M27	Dentofacial Anomalies [Including Malocclusion] and Other Disorders of Jaw
M30-M36	Systemic Connective Tissue Disorders
M40-M43	Deforming Dorsopathies
M45-M49	Spondylopathies
M50-M54	Other Dorsopathies
M60-M63	Disorders of Muscles
M65-M67	Disorders of Synovium and Tendon
M70-M79	Other Soft Tissue Disorders
M80-M85	Disorders of Bone Density and Structure
M86-M90	Other Osteopathies
M91-M94	Chondropathies
M95	Other Disorders of the Musculoskeletal System and Connective Tissue
M96	Intraoperative and Postprocedural Complications and Disorders of Musculoskeletal System, Not Elsewhere Classified
M99	Biomechanical Lesions, Not Elsewhere Classified

The categories of codes for the various diseases of the musculoskeletal system and connective tissues have expanded from previous systems to allow for more specific classification. For example, arthropathies and related disorders are classified based upon causation such as infection, inflammatory diseases or wear and tear arthritis as well as other disorders of the joint.

Coding Note(s)

There is single chapter level coding instruction in ICD-10-CM, which instructs the coder to use an external cause code, if applicable, to identify the cause of the musculoskeletal condition. The external cause code is sequenced after the code for the musculoskeletal condition.

Exclusions

There are only Excludes2 chapter level exclusions notes for Chapter 13.

Excludes1	Excludes2
None	Arthropathic psoriasis (L40.5-) Certain conditions originating in the perinatal period (P04-P96) Certain infectious and parasitic diseases (A00-B99) Compartment syndrome (traumatic) (T79.A-) Complications of pregnancy, childbirth, and the puerperium (O00-O9A) Congenital malformations, deformations and chromosomal abnormalities (Q00-Q99) Endocrine, nutritional and metabolic diseases (E00-E88) Injury, poisoning and certain other consequences of external causes (S00-T88) Neoplasms (C00-D49) Symptoms, signs, and abnormal clinical and laboratory findings, not elsewhere classified (R00-R94)

Chapter Guidelines

Chapter specific guidelines are provided for musculoskeletal system and connective tissue coding. In ICD-10-CM, guidelines are listed for pathological fractures as well as the following:

- Site and laterality
- Acute traumatic versus chronic or recurrent musculoskeletal conditions
- Coding of pathologic fractures
- Osteoporosis

Site and Laterality

Most codes in Chapter 13 have site and laterality designations.

Site

- Site represents either the bone, joint, or the muscle involved
- For some conditions where more than one bone, joint, or muscle is usually involved, such as osteoarthritis, there is a "multiple sites" code available
- For categories where no multiple site code is provided and more than one bone, joint, or muscle is involved, multiple codes should be used to indicate the different sites involved
- Bone Versus Joint – For certain conditions, the bone may be affected at the upper or lower end, (e.g., avascular necrosis of bone, M87; osteoporosis, M80-M81). Though the portion of the bone affected may be at the joint, the site designation will be the bone, not the joint

Laterality

- Most conditions involving the extremities require documentation of right or left in addition to the specific site
- If laterality is not documented, there are codes for unspecified side; however, unspecified codes particularly those defining laterality should be used only in rare circumstances.

Acute Traumatic Versus Chronic or Recurrent Musculoskeletal Conditions

Many musculoskeletal conditions are a result of a previous injury or trauma to a site, or are recurrent conditions. Musculoskeletal conditions are classified either in Chapter 13 Diseases of the Musculoskeletal System and Connective tissue or in Chapter 19 Injury, Poisoning, and Certain Other Consequences of External Causes as follows:

- Healed injury – Bone, joint, or muscle conditions that are a result of a healed injury are usually found in Chapter 13
- Recurrent condition – Recurrent bone, joint, or muscle conditions are usually found in Chapter 13
- Chronic or other recurrent conditions – Conditions are generally reported with a code from Chapter 13
- Current acute injury – Current, acute injuries are coded to the appropriate injury code in Chapter 19

If it is difficult to determine from the available documentation whether the condition should be reported with a code from Chapter 13 or Chapter 19, the provider should be queried.

Coding of Pathologic Fractures

ICD-10-CM contains chapter guidelines for reporting pathologic fractures. These guidelines are primarily defining the use of the 7th character extension to define the episode of care. It is important that these guidelines be understood before coding for pathologic and stress fractures. Guidelines for use of the 7th character extension for coding pathologic fractures in ICD-10-CM are as follows:

- Initial encounter for fracture – The 7th character 'A' for initial episode of care is used for as long as the patient is receiving active treatment for the pathologic fracture. Examples of active treatment are:
  - Surgical treatment
  - Emergency department encounter
  - Evaluation and continuing treatment by the same or different physician
- Subsequent encounter for fracture with routine healing – The 7th character 'D' is used for encounters after the patient has completed active treatment for the fracture and is receiving routine care for the fracture during the healing or recovery phase.
- Subsequent encounter for fracture with delayed healing – The 7th character 'G' for subsequent encounter for fracture with delayed healing is reported when the physician has documented that healing is delayed or is not occurring as rapidly as normally expected.
- Subsequent encounter for fracture with nonunion – The 7th character 'K' is reported when the physician has documented that there is nonunion of the fracture or that the fracture has failed to heal. This is a serious fracture complication that requires additional intervention and treatment by the physician.
- Subsequent encounter for fracture with malunion – The 7th character 'P' is reported when the fracture has healed in an abnormal or nonanatomic position. This is a serious fracture complication that requires additional intervention and treatment by the physician.
- Sequela – The 7th character 'S' is reported for complications or conditions that arise as a direct result of the pathological fracture, such as a leg length discrepancy following pathological fracture of the femur. The specific type of sequela is sequenced first followed by the pathological fracture code.

Care for complications of surgical treatment for pathological fracture repairs during the healing or recovery phase should be coded with the appropriate complication codes. See section I.C.19 of the Official Guidelines for information on coding of traumatic fractures.

Osteoporosis

Osteoporosis is a systemic condition, meaning that all bones of the musculoskeletal system are affected. Therefore, site is not a component of the codes under category M81 *Osteoporosis without current pathological fracture*. The site codes under M80 *Osteoporosis with current pathological fracture* identify the site of the fracture not the osteoporosis. Additional guidelines for osteoporosis are as follows:

- Osteoporosis without pathological fracture
  - Category M81 *Osteoporosis without current pathological fracture* is for use for patients with osteoporosis who do not currently have a pathological fracture due to the osteoporosis, even if they had a fracture in the past
  - For a patient with a history of osteoporosis fractures, status code Z87.31, *Personal history of osteoporosis fracture* should follow the code from M81
- Osteoporosis with current pathological fracture
  - Category M80 *Osteoporosis with current pathological fracture* is for patients who have a current pathologic fracture at the time of an encounter
  - The codes under M80 identify the site of the fracture
  - A code from category M80, not a traumatic fracture code, should be used for any patient with known osteoporosis who suffers a fracture, even if the patient had a minor fall or trauma, if that fall or trauma would not usually break a normal, healthy bone

General Documentation Requirements

When documenting diseases of the musculoskeletal system and connective tissue there are a number of general documentation requirements of which providers should be aware. The introduction and guidelines in the previous sections of this chapter identify some of the documentation requirements related to musculoskeletal and connective tissue diseases including more specific site designations and laterality. Documentation of episode of care is required for pathologic and stress fractures. The documentation must also clearly differentiate conditions that are acute traumatic conditions and those that are chronic or recurrent. Understanding documentation requirements for intraoperative and postprocedural complications will require a careful review of category M96 to ensure that the complication is described in sufficient detail to assign the most specific complication code. There are also combination codes that capture two or more related conditions, etiology and manifestations of certain conditions, or a disease process and common symptoms of the disease. Familiarity with the combination codes is needed to ensure that documentation is sufficient to capture any related conditions, both the etiology and manifestation, and/or any related symptoms for the condition being reported. A few examples of each of these general coding and documentation requirements are provided here. For those familiar with the former diagnosis system, ICD-10-CM has reclassified some conditions moving them into a different section. Such is the case of gout which was previously classified in Chapter 3 Endocrine, Nutritional, and Metabolic Diseases in ICD-9-CM but is now classified in Chapter 13 Diseases of the Musculoskeletal System and Connective Tissue.

Site

Site specificity is an important component of musculoskeletal system and connective tissue codes. Dorsopathies, which are conditions affecting the spine and intervertebral joints, provide a good example of site specificity. Codes for ankylosis (fusion) of the spine (M43.2-) are specific to the spine level and the ankylosis should be specified as affecting the occipito-atlanto-axial region, cervical region, cervicothoracic region, thoracic region, thoracolumbar region, lumbar region, lumbosacral region, or sacral and sacrococcygeal region.

Laterality

Laterality is required for the vast majority of musculoskeletal and connective tissue diseases and other conditions affecting the extremities. For example, trigger finger requires documentation of the specific finger (thumb, index finger, middle finger, ring finger, or little finger) and laterality (right, left). While there are also unspecified codes for unspecified finger and unspecified laterality, these codes should rarely be used because the affected finger and laterality should always be documented. Omission of this level of detail indicates to the health plan that the patient was not examined. An example of a condition where codes are available for bilateral conditions as well as for right and left is osteoarthritis of the hip (M16), knee (M17), and first carpometacarpal joints (M18). So, if a patient has primary arthritis of the knee, the physician must document both the condition and the site-specific location: right, left or bilateral. For osteoarthritis affecting other joints, there are codes for right and left but not for bilateral. If both joints of one of these sites is affected, two codes—one for the right and one for the left, are assigned.

Episode of Care

Documentation of episode of care is required for pathologic and stress fractures which include: fatigue fractures of the vertebra (M48.4), collapsed vertebra (M48.5-), osteoporosis with pathological fracture (M80.-), stress fracture (M84.3-), pathologic fracture not elsewhere classified (M84,.4-), pathological fracture in neoplastic disease (M84.5-), and pathologic fracture in other disease (M84.6-). For these conditions, a 7th character extension is required identifying the episode of care as:

A Initial encounter for fracture

D Subsequent encounter for fracture with routine healing

G Subsequent encounter for fracture with delayed healing

K Subsequent encounter for fracture with nonunion

P Subsequent encounter for fracture with malunion

S Sequela

The physician must clearly document the episode of care and for subsequent encounters must identify whether the healing is routine or delayed or whether it is complicated by nonunion or malunion. Documentation of the fracture type (stress, pathologic and cause), location (femur, humerus, etc.) and laterality must be documented for each encounter where the patient is being seen for the condition. Codes cannot be assigned based upon prior detailed documentation. Any conditions resulting from a previous pathological fracture must also be clearly documented as sequela so the appropriate pathological fracture sequela code can be assigned in addition to the condition being treated.

Acute Traumatic Versus Old or Chronic Conditions

Acute traumatic and old or chronic conditions must be clearly differentiated in the documentation. Acute traumatic conditions are reported with codes from Chapter 19 Injury, Poisoning and Certain Other Consequences of External Causes, while old or chronic conditions are reported with codes from Chapter 13. For example, an old bucket handle tear of the knee is reported with a code from subcategory M23.2 *Derangement of meniscus due to old tear or injury*, whereas an acute current bucket handle tear is reported with a code from subcategory S83.2 *Tear of meniscus, current injury*.

Intraoperative and Postprocedural Complications NEC

Many codes for intraoperative and postprocedural complications and disorders of the musculoskeletal system are found at the end of Chapter 13 in category M96. This category contains codes for conditions such as postlaminectomy syndrome, postradiation kyphosis and scoliosis, and pseudoarthrosis after surgical fusion or arthrodesis. It also contains codes for intraoperative hemorrhage and hematoma, accidental puncture or laceration, and postprocedural hemorrhage or hematoma of musculoskeletal system structures, which all require documentation of the procedure as a musculoskeletal procedure or a procedure on another body system.

Combination Codes

Combination codes may capture two or more related conditions, etiology and manifestations of certain conditions, or a disease process and common symptoms of the disease. Combination codes that capture two related conditions can be found in category M16 Osteoarthritis of the hip which defines the condition of osteoarthritis resulting from dysplasia (M16.2, M16.3-). An example of a combination code that captures a disease process and a common symptom of that disease is found in category M47 Spondylosis. Here codes are provided for spondylosis (disease process) with radiculopathy (symptom).

Code-Specific Documentation Requirements

In this section, ICD-10-CM code categories, subcategories, and subclassifications for some of the more frequently reported diseases of the musculoskeletal system and connective tissue are reviewed along with specific documentation requirements identified. The focus is on conditions with more specific clinical documentation requirements. Although not all codes with significant documentation requirements are discussed, this section will provide a representative sample of the type of additional documentation needed for diseases of the musculoskeletal system and connective tissue. The section is organized alphabetically by the ICD10-CM code category, subcategory, or subclassification depending on whether the documentation affects only a single code or an entire subcategory or category.

Contracture Tendon Sheath

A muscle contracture is a shortening of the muscle and/or tendon sheath which prevents normal movement and flexibility. Causes can include: prolonged immobilization, scarring (trauma, burns), paralysis (stroke, spinal cord injuries), ischemia (e.g., Volkmann's contracture), cerebral palsy, and degenerative diseases affecting the muscles (e.g., muscular dystrophy).

A muscle spasm is a sudden, involuntary contraction of a single muscle or a muscle group. This condition is usually benign and self-limiting. The contraction of the muscle is temporary. Causes include abnormal or malfunctioning nerve signals, muscle fatigue (overuse, exertion), dehydration, electrolyte imbalance, decreased blood supply, and certain medications.

In ICD-10-CM, tendon and muscle contractures and muscle spasms are found under the section of soft tissue disorders. Subcategory M62.4 Contracture of muscle contains the alternate term contracture of tendon sheath, so a code from this subcategory is reported for either diagnosis. Codes in this subcategory are specific to site and documentation of laterality is also required. Muscle spasm is found under subcategory M62.83 and is further subdivided by muscle spasm of the back calf and other. Documentation requirements and clinical documentation for muscle or tendon contracture follows.

Coding and Documentation Requirements

Identify the site of the muscle or tendon contracture:

- Upper extremity
  - Shoulder
  - Upper arm
  - Forearm
  - Hand
- Lower extremity
  - Thigh
  - Lower leg
  - Ankle/Foot
- Other site
- Multiple sites
- Unspecified site

For muscle/tendon contracture of extremity, identify laterality:

- Right
- Left
- Unspecified

ICD-10-CM Code/Documentation	
M62.40	Contracture of muscle unspecified site
M62.411	Contracture of muscle, right shoulder
M62.412	Contracture of muscle, left shoulder
M62.419	Contracture of muscle, unspecified shoulder
M62.421	Contracture of muscle, right upper arm
M62.422	Contracture of muscle, left upper arm
M62.429	Contracture of muscle, unspecified upper arm
M62.431	Contracture of muscle, right forearm

ICD-10-CM Code/Documentation	
M62.432	Contracture of muscle, left forearm
M62.439	Contracture of muscle, unspecified forearm
M62.441	Contracture of muscle, right hand
M62.442	Contracture of muscle, left hand
M62.449	Contracture of muscle, unspecified hand
M62.451	Contracture of muscle, right thigh
M62.452	Contracture of muscle, left thigh
M62.459	Contracture of muscle, unspecified thigh
M62.461	Contracture of muscle, right lower leg
M62.462	Contracture of muscle, left lower leg
M62.469	Contracture of muscle, unspecified lower leg
M62.471	Contracture of muscle, right ankle and foot
M62.472	Contracture of muscle, left ankle and foot
M62.479	Contracture of muscle, unspecified ankle and foot
M62.48	Contracture of muscle, other site
M62.49	Contracture of muscle, multiple sites

Documentation and Coding Example

Fourteen-year-old Black male presents to Orthopedic Clinic with an interesting **deformity to his right wrist**. He is right hand dominant. Patient and mother give a history of a skateboard accident 10 months ago where he slammed into a metal pole causing a **soft tissue injury to his right forearm. He developed an infected hematoma** that was incised and drained and ultimately healed. ROM to elbow is intact. He is able to supinate and pronate fully. There is a moderate amount of ulnar deviation in the right wrist, causing focal disability. He has difficulty performing a pincher grasp, holding utensils and is unable to hold a small half-filled water bottle for more than a minute. X-rays of elbow, forearm, wrist unremarkable.

Impression: **Contracture of right extensor carpi ulnaris tendon causing deformity and functional disability of the wrist and hand due to old soft tissue injury**.

Plan: Occupational Therapy evaluation and authorization for 12 visits if approved by patient's insurance company. RTC in one month.

Diagnosis Code(s)

M62.431	Contracture of muscle, right forearm
S56.501S	Unspecified injury of other extensor muscle, fascia and tendon at forearm level, sequela
V00.132S	Skateboarder colliding with stationary object, sequela

Coding Note(s)

The extensor carpi ulnaris muscle is a muscle in the forearm, so the code for contracture of the right forearm muscle is reported. Contracture of tendon is reported with the same code as contracture of muscle. Based upon the documentation, the tendon/muscle contracture is a sequela of a soft tissue injury so an injury code with 7th character 'S' should also be reported. Coding of sequela will be covered in Chapter 19 of this book. The external cause of the sequela (late effect) is specific to a skateboarder colliding with a stationary object.

Gouty Arthropathy

Gout is an arthritis-like condition caused by an accumulation of uric acid in the blood which leads to inflammation of the joints. Acute gout typically affects one joint. Chronic gout is characterized by repeated episodes of pain and inflammation in one or more joints. Following repeated episodes of gout, some individuals develop chronic tophaceous gout. This condition is characterized by solid deposits of monosodium urate (MSU) crystals, called tophi in the joints, cartilage, bones, and other areas of the body. In some cases, tophi break through the skin and appear as white or yellowish-white, chalky nodules on the skin.

Even though gout is often considered a metabolic disorder in its origins, ICD-10-CM classifies gout as a disease of the musculoskeletal system and connective tissue within two categories—M10 Gout and M1A Chronic gout. Gout may be due to toxic effects of lead or other drugs, renal impairment, other medical conditions, or an unknown cause (idiopathic). Category M10 includes gout due to any cause specified as acute gout, gout attack, gout flare, and other gout not specified as chronic. Subcategories identify the specific cause of the gout as idiopathic, lead-induced, drug-induced, due to renal impairment, due to other causes, or unspecified. Category M1A includes gout due to any cause specified as chronic.

Coding and Documentation Requirements

Identify type of gout:

- Chronic
- Other/unspecified, which includes:
  - Acute gout
  - Gout attack
  - Gout flare
  - Gout not otherwise specified
  - Podagra

Identify cause:

- Drug-induced
- Idiopathic
- Lead-induced
- Renal impairment
- Other secondary gout
- Unspecified

Identify site:

- Lower extremity
  - Ankle/foot
  - Hip
  - Knee
- Upper extremity
  - Elbow
  - Hand
  - Shoulder
  - Wrist

- Vertebrae
- Multiple sites
- Unspecified site

Identify laterality for extremities:

- Right
- Left
- Unspecified

For chronic gout, use a 7th character to identify any tophus:

- With tophus (1)
- Without tophus (0)

ICD-10-CM Code/Documentation	
M10.00	Idiopathic gout, unspecified site
M10.011	Idiopathic gout, right shoulder
M10.012	Idiopathic gout, left shoulder
M10.019	Idiopathic gout, unspecified shoulder
M10.021	Idiopathic gout, right elbow
M10.022	Idiopathic gout, left elbow
M10.029	Idiopathic gout, unspecified elbow
M10.031	Idiopathic gout, right wrist
M10.032	Idiopathic gout, left wrist
M10.039	Idiopathic gout, unspecified wrist
M10.041	Idiopathic gout, right hand
M10.042	Idiopathic gout, left hand
M10.049	Idiopathic gout, unspecified hand
M10.051	Idiopathic gout, right hip
M10.052	Idiopathic gout, left hip
M10.059	Idiopathic gout, unspecified hip
M10.061	Idiopathic gout, right knee
M10.062	Idiopathic gout, left knee
M10.069	Idiopathic gout, unspecified knee
M10.071	Idiopathic gout, right ankle and foot
M10.072	Idiopathic gout, left ankle and foot
M10.079	Idiopathic gout, unspecified ankle and foot
M10.08	Idiopathic gout, vertebrae
M10.09	Idiopathic gout, multiple sites

Documentation and Coding Example

Fifty-two-year-old Caucasian male presents to PMD with complaints of gout flare. PMH is significant for hypertension, seasonal allergies, and gout. Current medications include Lisinopril, Allopurinol, ASA, Enzyme CoQ10, Loratidine, and Nasonex spray. His only complaint is a **swollen great toe which he attributes to a gout flare**.

Temperature 97.4, HR 84, RR 14, BP 140/78, Wt. 189. On examination, this is a well-groomed, well-nourished male who looks his stated age. Skin is tan and he has a few scattered seborrheic keratoses lesions present on face and back. He is reminded to use sunscreen and a hat when outdoors. Peripheral pulses full. Right leg is unremarkable. Left knee and ankle normal. **Left great toe is red, swollen, and tender to touch**. He is advised to take OTC ibuprofen or naproxen for his toe pain and to avoid alcohol, limit meat for a few weeks. He will return in 1 week for a recheck of his great toe.

Diagnosis: **Primary gout with gout flare left great toe.**

Diagnosis Code(s)

M10.072 Idiopathic gout, left ankle and foot

Coding Note(s)

The patient has a history of gout and is being seen for a gout flare. The inclusion terms under M10 Gout includes gout flare. Reporting a code for chronic gout requires specific documentation of the gout as a chronic condition. In addition, if the patient has chronic gout and a gout flare, report only the code for the gout flare. There is an Excludes1 note indicating that chronic gout (category M1A) is never reported with acute gout (category M10).

Intervertebral Disc Disorders

Intervertebral disc disorders include conditions such as displacement, Schmorl's nodes, degenerative disc disease, intervertebral disc disorders, postlaminectomy syndrome, and other and unspecified disc disorders. Like spondylosis, several combination codes exist to define the disc disorder as well as associated symptoms of radiculopathy or myelopathy. Displacement of an intervertebral disc may also be referred to as ruptured or herniated intervertebral disc or herniated nucleus pulposus (HNP). This is because displacement occurs when the inner gel-like substance (nucleus pulposus) of the intervertebral disc bulges out from or herniates through the outer fibrous ring and into the spinal canal. The herniated or displaced nucleus pulposus may then press on spinal nerves causing pain or other sensory disturbances, such as tingling or numbness, as well as changes in motor function and reflexes.

In ICD-10-CM, category M50 contains codes for cervical disc disorders with sites specific to the high cervical region, midcervical region redefined for October 1, 2016 by disc space level (C4-C5, C5-C6, C6-C7), and cervicothoracic region. Category M51 contains codes for disc disorders of the thoracic, thoracolumbar, lumbar, and lumbosacral regions. In addition to codes specific to these sites, combination codes identify disc disorders as with myelopathy or with radiculopathy. There are also codes for other disc displacement, other disc degeneration, other cervical disc disorders, and unspecified disc disorders. Documentation must clearly describe the specific condition and any associated myelopathy or radiculopathy to ensure that the most specific code is assigned.

Coding and Documentation Requirements

Identify condition:

- Disc disorder
  - Identify symptom
    - » with myelopathy
    - » with radiculopathy
- Other disc displacement
- Other disc degeneration
- Other disc disorders
- Schmorl's nodes
- Unspecified disc disorder

Identify site:

- Cervical
  - Identify level
    - » High cervical (C2-C4)
    - » Mid-cervical (C4-5, C5-6, C6-7)
    - » Cervicothoracic (C7-T1)
- Thoracic region
- Thoracolumbar region (T10-L1)
- Lumbar region
- Lumbosacral region
- Unspecified site

Note: In ICD-10-CM, codes for "other" disc displacement, degeneration, disorder are used for the specified condition when there is no documentation of either myelopathy or radiculopathy. If disc displacement, degeneration, or disorder are documented as with myelopathy or with radiculopathy, the codes for disc disorder with myelopathy or disc disorder with radiculopathy are reported.

Cervical Intervertebral Disc Disorders

ICD-10-CM Code/Documentation	
M50.20	Other cervical disc displacement, unspecified cervical region
M50.21	Other cervical disc displacement, high cervical region
M50.220	Other cervical disc displacement, mid-cervical region, unspecified level
M50.221	Other cervical disc displacement at C4-C5 level
M50.222	Other cervical disc displacement at C5-C6 level
M50.223	Other cervical disc displacement at C6-C7 level
M50.23	Other cervical disc displacement, cervicothoracic region
M50.30	Other cervical disc degeneration, unspecified cervical region
M50.31	Other cervical disc degeneration, high cervical region
M50.320	Other cervical disc degeneration, mid-cervical region, unspecified level
M50.321	Other cervical disc degeneration at C4-C5 level
M50.322	Other cervical disc degeneration at C5-C6 level
M50.323	Other cervical disc degeneration at C6-C7 level
M50.33	Other cervical disc degeneration, cervicothoracic region
M50.00	Cervical disc disorder with myelopathy, unspecified cervical region
M50.01	Cervical disc disorder with myelopathy, high cervical region
M50.020	Cervical disc disorder with myelopathy, mid-cervical region, unspecified level
M50.021	Cervical disc disorder at C4-C5 level with myelopathy
M50.022	Cervical disc disorder at C5-C6 level with myelopathy
M50.023	Cervical disc disorder at C4-C5 level with myelopathy
M50.03	Cervical disc disorder with myelopathy, cervicothoracic region
M50.80	Other cervical disc disorders, unspecified cervical region
M50.81	Other cervical disc disorders, high cervical region
M50.820	Other cervical disc disorders, mid-cervical region, unspecified level
M50.821	Other cervical disc disorders at C4-C5 level
M50.822	Other cervical disc disorders at C5-C6 level
M50.823	Other cervical disc disorders at C6-C7 level
M50.83	Other cervical disc disorders, cervicothoracic region
M50.90	Cervical disc disorder, unspecified, unspecified cervical region
M50.91	Cervical disc disorder, unspecified, high cervical region
M50.920	Unspecified cervical disc disorder, mid-cervical region, unspecified level
M50.921	Unspecified cervical disc disorder at C4-C5 level
M50.922	Unspecified cervical disc disorder at C5-C6 level
M50.923	Unspecified cervical disc disorder at C6-C7 level
M50.93	Cervical disc disorder, unspecified, cervicothoracic region
M50.10	Cervical disc disorder with radiculopathy, unspecified cervical region
M50.11	Cervical disc disorder with radiculopathy, high cervical region
M50.120	Mid-cervical disc disorder, unspecified level
M50.121	Cervical disc disorder at C4-C5 level with radiculopathy
M50.122	Cervical disc disorder at C5-C6 level with radiculopathy
M50.123	Cervical disc disorder at C6-C7 level with radiculopathy
M50.13	Cervical disc disorder with radiculopathy, cervicothoracic region
M54.11	Radiculopathy, occipito-atlanto-axial cervical region
M54.12	Radiculopathy, cervical region
M54.13	Radiculopathy, cervicothoracic region

Documentation and Coding Example

Thirty-three-year-old Caucasian female is referred to Neurology Clinic by PMD for right arm pain and weakness. Patient is a NICU RN working 3-5 twelve-hour shifts/wk. primarily with premature infants. She can recall no injury to her neck or arm but simply awoke two weeks ago with a sharp pain that radiated through her shoulder, down her right arm to the tip of her thumb. She is left hand dominant. The pain is resolving but she continues to have weakness, numbness, and tingling in the arm. She treated her symptoms with rest, heat, and ibuprofen during 2 regularly scheduled days off and was able to return to work for her next scheduled shift. She was concerned about the residual weakness in her arm and called her PMD who ordered cervical spine films and an **MRI which showed disc displacement/protrusion at C5-C6**. He prescribed oral steroids and Tramadol for pain, Lunesta for sleep and referred her to Neurology. On examination, this is a moderately obese woman who looks her stated age. PERRL, there is stiffness and decreased ROM in her neck, cranial nerves grossly intact. Exam of left upper extremity is unremarkable with intact pulses, reflexes, ROM and strength. Exam of right arm is significant for moderate weakness in the right bicep muscle and wrist extensor muscles. Sensation to both dull and sharp stimuli is decreased along the anterior right arm beginning at shoulder to mid forearm level. Pincher grasp is weak on the right. Pulses are intact as are reflexes. MRI is reviewed with patient and she does indeed have a **small herniation of the disc at C5-C6 space which is most likely the cause of her current myelopathy**. She is advised to stop taking the Lunesta and Tramadol and is prescribed Celebrex and acetaminophen for pain. PT agrees to see her this afternoon for initial evaluation, possible soft cervical collar. She is cleared to work as long as she does not lift more than 10 lbs. RTC in 2 weeks for recheck.

Diagnosis Code(s)

M50.022 Cervical disc disorder at C5-C6 level with myelopathy

Coding Note(s)

To identify the correct code, instructions in the Alphabetic Index are followed. Under Displacement, intervertebral disc, with myelopathy there is an instruction, see Disorder, disc, cervical, with myelopathy. Code M50.022 is identified as the correct code for Disorder, disc, with myelopathy, C5-C6.

Limb pain

The cause of pain in a limb may not be readily evident. Often several conditions must be worked up and ruled out before a definitive diagnosis can be made. In the outpatient setting, conditions that are documented as possible or to be ruled-out cannot be listed as confirmed diagnoses. A non-specific symptom code is reported until the underlying cause of the pain has been diagnosed. Codes for limb pain refer to pain that is not located in the joint. There are more specific codes for joint pain. Limb pain would not be assigned if a known cause exists such as mononeuritis or neuralgia which would be reported with codes from the nervous system chapter. Limb pain is captured by codes in subcategory M79.6. The pain needs to be defined by the specific site and laterality. Details of documentation requirements are listed below.

Coding and Documentation Requirements

Identify site of pain:

- Upper extremity
  - Upper arm
  - Forearm
  - Hand
  - Finger(s)
  - Site not specified
- Lower extremity
  - Thigh
  - Lower leg
  - Foot
  - Toe(s)
  - Site not specified
- Unspecified limb

For upper and lower extremity, identify laterality

- Right
- Left
- Unspecified

There are codes for unspecified limb (not specified as upper or lower); unspecified arm (site not specified and not specified as right or left); unspecified leg (site not specified and laterality not specified). There are also codes for specified site but unspecified laterality for upper arm, forearm, hand, fingers, thigh, lower leg, foot, and toes. However, even though codes for unspecified limb and unspecified laterality are provided, they should be avoided as the specific limb affected and laterality should always be documented.

ICD-10-CM Code/Documentation	
Pain in Limb, Unspecified	
M79.601	Pain in right arm
M79.602	Pain in left arm
M79.603	Pain in arm, unspecified
M79.604	Pain in right leg
M79.605	Pain in left leg
M79.606	Pain in leg, unspecified
M79.609	Pain in unspecified limb
Pain in Upper Arm/Forearm/Hand/Fingers	
M79.621	Pain in right upper arm
M79.622	Pain in left upper arm
M79.629	Pain in unspecified upper arm
M79.631	Pain in right forearm
M79.632	Pain in left forearm
M79.639	Pain in unspecified forearm
M79.641	Pain in right hand
M79.642	Pain in left hand
M79.643	Pain in unspecified hand
M79.644	Pain in right finger(s)
M79.645	Pain in left finger(s)
M79.646	Pain in unspecified fingers
Pain in Thigh/Lower Leg/Foot/Toes	
M79.651	Pain in right thigh
M79.652	Pain in left thigh
M79.659	Pain in unspecified thigh
M79.661	Pain in right lower leg
M79.662	Pain in left lower leg
M79.669	Pain in unspecified lower leg
M79.671	Pain in right foot
M79.672	Pain in left foot
M79.673	Pain in unspecified foot
M79.674	Pain in right toe(s)
M79.675	Pain in left toes(s)
M79.676	Pain in unspecified toe(s)

Documentation and Coding Example

Twenty-five-year-old Hispanic male presents to Urgent Care Clinic with a four-day history of pain and swelling in left forearm. Patient is in good health and does not have a PMD, the last time he sought medical care was in college. He is employed full time developing computer software. He works from home most of the time, flying into the company's central office for a few days each month. His arm pain started on the last day of a 5-day trip to the central office. He can recall no injury although he did engage in daily, strenuous physical activities including ultimate Frisbee, volleyball, and basketball. Pain began as a dull ache in the inner arm midway between elbow and wrist. Upon returning home, he continues to experience a dull ache in the forearm which varies in intensity but is always present. He has applied ice to the area off and on for the past 2 days. This morning the remains achy so he seeks medical attention. On examination, this is a well-groomed, well nourished, somewhat anxious young man. T 98.5, P 60, R 12, BP 104/54, O2 Sat 99% on RA. Eyes clear, PERRLA. Nares patent, mucous membranes moist and pink, TMs normal. Neck supple without masses or lymphadenopathy. Cranial nerves grossly intact. Heart rate regular, breath sounds clear, equal bilaterally. Abdomen soft, nontender with active bowel sounds. No evidence of hernia, normal male genitalia. Examination of lower extremities is completely benign. Right upper extremity has normal strength, sensation and movement. Left upper arm has normal tone, strength, reflexes, sensation and circulation. The left elbow is unremarkable with normal ROM. The inner forearm is palpated. No mass or other signs of abnormality are noted other than the dull aching pain. Negative for Raynaud phenomena. Circulation and sensation intact through fingers. Supination and pronation exacerbates the pain as does fist clenching. X-ray of forearm is obtained and is negative for fracture.

Impression: **Pain left forearm of unknown etiology.**

Plan: Blood drawn for CBC w/diff, ESR, CRP, Quantitative Immunoglobulin levels, comprehensive metabolic panel. Results will be forwarded to Internal Medicine Department where he has an appointment scheduled in 3 days. He is fitted with a sling to be used PRN for comfort. He is advised to use ibuprofen for pain and to return to Urgent Care Clinic if symptoms worsen before his appointment with Internist.

Diagnosis Code(s)

M79.632 Pain in left forearm

Coding Note(s)

Pain of unknown etiology is specific to site and laterality.

Lumbago/Sciatica

Lumbago refers to non-specific pain in the lower back region. The condition is very common and may be acute, subacute, or chronic in nature. Lumbago is generally a symptom of benign musculoskeletal strain or sprain with no underlying disease or syndrome.

Sciatica is a set of symptoms characterized by pain, paresthesia (shock like pain in the arms and/or legs), and/or weakness in the low back, buttocks, or lower extremities. Symptoms result from compression of one or more spinal nerves (L4, L5, S1, S2, S3) that form the sciatic nerve (right and left branches). Causes can include herniated discs, spinal stenosis, pregnancy, injury or tumors.

In ICD-10-CM, there is a code for lumbago alone designated by the descriptor low back pain (M54.5). There are also codes for sciatica alone (M54.3-) and a combination code for lumbago with sciatica (M54.4-). Codes for sciatica require documentation of laterality to identify the side of the sciatic nerve pain.

Coding and Documentation Requirements

Identify the low back pain/sciatica:

- Low back pain
  - With sciatica
    - » Right side
    - » Left side
    - » Unspecified side
  - Without sciatica
- Sciatica
  - Right side
  - Left side
  - Unspecified side

ICD-10-CM Code/Documentation	
M54.5	Low back pain
M54.30	Sciatica, unspecified side
M54.31	Sciatica, right side
M54.32	Sciatica, left side
M54.40	Lumbago with sciatica, unspecified side
M54.41	Lumbago with sciatica, right side
M54.42	Lumbago with sciatica, left side

Documentation and Coding Example

Forty-two-year-old female presents to PMD with ongoing **sharp pain in her left buttocks radiating down the back of her left leg.** She states the pain began suddenly about 1 week ago as she was preparing and planting her Spring garden. She does not recall any specific injury only that she was hauling bags of soil and compost mix, bending a lot and on her knees weeding and planting. On examination, this is a very pleasant, quite tan, well developed, well-nourished woman who looks older than her stated age. She states she loves to be outdoors and never applies sunscreen, believing that sun exposure is healthy for her body. Cranial nerves grossly intact. Neurovascular exam of upper extremities is unremarkable. Thoracic spine is straight without swelling or tenderness to palpation. There is mild tenderness with palpation of her lumbar spine and moderate muscle spasm with deep palpation of her left buttocks. Forward bending elicits pain at the thoracolumbar junction. Leg lifts also elicit pain on the left. Patient states pain and stiffness is worse on rising in the morning, decreases when lying down and changes from sharp pain to dull ache when sitting. Patient declines x-ray of her spine as she believes radiation is harmful to her body. She declines prescriptions for pain medication, muscle relaxant, or NSAIDs. She is using topical arnica gel and an oral homeopathic for inflammation. She is agreeable to physical therapy for muscle flexibility and strengthening exercises. She is given a written prescription for PT because she would like to do some research and find a therapist who would be a good fit for her. RTC in 6 weeks, sooner if needed.

Impression: **Left sciatica with low back pain.**

Diagnosis Code(s)

M54.42 Lumbago with sciatica, left side

Coding Note(s)

There is a combination code for lumbago with sciatica is reported. Codes for sciatica and lumbago with sciatica are specific to the side of the sciatic pain. The physician has documented that the patient is experiencing left-sided sciatica.

Osteoarthritis

There are multiple codes in multiple code categories for osteoarthritis (M15, M16, M17, M18, and M19). These codes are to be used for osteoarthritis of extremity joints. Codes for osteoarthritis of the spine will be located in category M47. There are specific codes for primary and secondary arthritis with the codes for secondary arthritis being specific for post-traumatic osteoarthritis and other secondary osteoarthritis. It is important to note that there are also codes for post-traumatic arthritis, M12.5- that are not osteoarthritis. It is imperative that the documentation specifies whether the arthritis resulting from trauma is post-traumatic degenerative which is usually a result of trauma surrounding the joint such as following multiple ankle sprains vs. post-traumatic which is due to trauma involving the joint surface such as following a tibial pilon fracture. For secondary osteoarthritis of the hip there is also a specific code for osteoarthritis resulting from hip dysplasia. Codes for specific types of osteoarthritis require laterality (right, left). For the hip, knee and first CMC joint there are also bilateral codes. Codes for other secondary arthritis of the hip and knee must be specified as either bilateral or unilateral, but there are not specific codes for right and left. Unspecified osteoarthritis does not require any information on laterality. An additional category is available for polyosteoarthritis, category M15. This involved osteoarthritis of more than five joints and includes such disorders as Heberden's nodes and Bouchard's notes of the hands as well as primary generalized osteoarthritis. Bilateral osteoarthritis of a single joint should not be coded as polyosteoarthritis or generalized osteoarthritis.

Coding and documentation requirements for osteoarthritis are provided followed by a clinical example for osteoarthritis of the hip.

Coding and Documentation Requirements

Identify type of osteoarthritis:

- Primary
- Secondary
  - Post-traumatic
  - Resulting from hip dysplasia (hip only)
  - Other specified secondary osteoarthritis
  - Unspecified

Identify site:

- Hip
- Knee
- First carpometacarpal joint
- Shoulder
- Elbow
- Wrist
- Hand
- Ankle and foot

Identify laterality:

- Right
- Left
- Unspecified

Osteoarthritis of Hip

ICD-10-CM Code/Documentation	
M16.0	Bilateral primary osteoarthritis of hip
M16.10	Unilateral primary osteoarthritis, unspecified hip
M16.11	Unilateral primary osteoarthritis, right hip
M16.12	Unilateral primary osteoarthritis, left hip
M16.2	Bilateral osteoarthritis of hip resulting from hip dysplasia
M16.30	Unilateral osteoarthritis of hip resulting from hip dysplasia, unspecified hip
M16.31	Unilateral osteoarthritis of hip resulting from hip dysplasia, right hip
M16.32	Unilateral osteoarthritis of hip resulting from hip dysplasia, left hip
M16.4	Bilateral post-traumatic osteoarthritis of hip
M16.50	Unilateral post-traumatic osteoarthritis, unspecified hip
M16.51	Unilateral post-traumatic osteoarthritis, right hip
M16.52	Unilateral post-traumatic osteoarthritis, left hip
M16.6	Other bilateral secondary osteoarthritis of hip
M16.7	Other unilateral secondary osteoarthritis of hip
M16.9	Osteoarthritis of hip, unspecified

Documentation and Coding Example

Sixty-one-year-old Caucasian female is referred to orthopedic clinic by PMD for ongoing right hip pain and stiffness. Patient sustained a **soft tissue injury to her right hip and leg 6 years ago** in a bicycle accident. X-rays at the time showed no fracture and she was treated conservatively with rest, ice and ibuprofen. She was able to return to her usual active lifestyle within a few weeks but over the years she has noticed increased stiffness, especially in the morning and she is taking acetaminophen for pain 4-5 times a week. On examination, this is a trim, fit appearing woman who looks younger than her stated age. Gait is normal. There is no evidence of osteophytic changes to small joints. Patient denies fatigue, weight loss or fevers. Cranial nerves grossly intact, neuromuscular exam of upper extremities is unremarkable. Muscle strength equal in lower extremities, there is marked tenderness with palpation of the right hip, no swelling, muscle wasting or crepitus. X-ray obtained of bilateral hips for comparison. Left hip x-ray and exam is relatively benign. Radiograph of right hip is significant for sclerosis of the superior aspect of the acetabulum along with single Egger cyst. Findings are consistent with **post-traumatic osteoarthritis of the hip**. Treatment options discussed with patient and she prefers a conservative plan at this time. She is referred to physical therapy 3 x week for 4 weeks and advised to take Naproxen sodium 220 mg BID. RTC in one month for re-evaluation.

Diagnosis Code

M16.51 Unilateral post-traumatic osteoarthritis, right hip

Coding Note(s)

The ICD-10-CM code identifies the secondary osteoarthritis as post-traumatic and is also specific to site (hip) and laterality (right).

An external cause code is not required but if the documentation was sufficient on the circumstances of the accident an external cause code could also be reported to identify the cause of the post-traumatic osteoarthritis as a bicycle accident.

Osteoporosis

Osteoporosis is a systemic disease that affects previously constructed bone tissue. It is characterized by decreased bone density, weakness, and brittleness, making the bone more susceptible to fracture. Primary type 1 (postmenopausal) osteoporosis typically affects women after menopause. Primary type 2 (senile) osteoporosis is identified in both men and women after the age of 75. Secondary osteoporosis can occur in either sex and at any age. It arises from an underlying medical condition, prolonged immobilization or the use of certain drugs that affect mineral balance in the bones. With any type of osteoporosis, the most common bones affected are vertebrae, ribs, pelvis, and upper extremities. The condition is often asymptomatic until a fracture occurs.

In ICD-10-CM, there are two categories for osteoporosis. Codes from category M80 are reported for osteoporosis with a current pathological fracture and codes from M81 are reported for osteoporosis without a current pathological fracture. Osteoporosis with or without pathological fracture is then subclassified as age-related or other specified type, which includes drug-induced, disuse, idiopathic, post-oophorectomy, postsurgical malabsorption, and post-traumatic osteoporosis. There is no code for unspecified osteoporosis. If documentation does not identify a specific type or cause of osteoporosis, the Alphabetic Index directs to 'age-related'. If the osteoporosis is associated with a current fracture, the fracture site and laterality must be documented. In addition, osteoporosis codes with a current pathological fracture require a 7th character to identify the episode of care.

The applicable 7th character extensions for osteoporosis with pathological fracture are as follows:

A Initial encounter for fracture

D Subsequent encounter for fracture with routine healing

G Subsequent encounter for fracture with delayed healing

K Subsequent encounter for fracture with nonunion

P Subsequent encounter for fracture with malunion

S Sequela

Coding and Documentation Requirements

Identify osteoporosis as with or without current pathological fracture:

- With current pathological fracture
- Without current pathological fracture

Identify type/cause of osteoporosis:

- Age-related
- Localized
- Other

For osteoporosis with current pathological fracture, identify site of fracture:

- Shoulder
- Humerus
- Forearm
- Hand
- Femur
- Lower leg
- Ankle/foot
- Vertebra(e)
- Other site

Identify episode of care:

- Initial encounter
- Subsequent encounter
  - With routine healing
  - With delayed healing
  - With nonunion
  - With malunion
- Sequela

Senile/Age-Related Osteoporosis with Current Pathological Fracture of Forearm/Wrist

ICD-10-CM Code/Documentation	
M80.031-	Age related osteoporosis with current pathological fracture, right forearm
M80.032-	Age related osteoporosis with current pathological fracture, left forearm
M80.039-	Age related osteoporosis with current pathological fracture, unspecified forearm
Note: Requires 7th character to identify episode of care.	

Documentation and Coding Example

Fifty-nine-year-old Caucasian female returns to Orthopedic Clinic for a second postoperative visit. She is now five weeks S/P **fall at home** where she sustained a **fracture of the distal right radius.** She presented initially to the ED with pain, swelling and deformity of the right wrist and forearm with tenderness and swelling of the distal radius. Radiographs showed a **distal radial fracture and severe osteoporosis** of the radius and ulna. She underwent an ORIF that same day with application of soft cast/splint. She had a hard cast applied at her first PO visit 3 weeks ago. Patient states she is doing well and has no complaints. Bruising and swelling have subsided in her fingers and she has good ROM and neurovascular checks. She admits to mild pain, usually associated with over use, that is relieved with acetaminophen. X-ray in plaster shows the **fracture to be in good alignment with increased callus size when compared to previous film.** She is taking a Calcium supplement, Vitamin D 6000 units, Vitamin C 1000 mg daily and a multivitamin/mineral tablet. Patient is advised to continue with her present supplements. RTC in 3 weeks for x-ray out of plaster and application of splint. Patient is due for annual physical exam with her PCP in 3 months. She is advised to discuss having a DEXA scan to assess bone density since it has been 6 years since her last one and she has now entered menopause. Once they have those results she may need to consider more aggressive therapy for her osteoporosis.

Impression: **Healing distal radial fracture right forearm. Fracture due to postmenopausal osteoporosis**. S/P ORIF.

Diagnosis Code(s)

M80.031D Age related osteoporosis with current pathological fracture, right forearm, subsequent encounter for fracture with routine healing

W19.XXXD Unspecified fall, subsequent encounter

Coding Note(s)

Even though the fracture was sustained in a fall, ICD-10-CM coding guidelines state, "A code from category M80, not a traumatic fracture code, should be used for any patient with known osteoporosis who suffers a fracture, even if the patient had a minor fall or trauma, if that fall or trauma would not usually break a normal, healthy bone." An external cause code may be reported additionally to identify the pathological fracture as due to a fall. An unspecified fall is reported because the documentation does not provide any information on circumstances surrounding the fall, such as a fall due to tripping or a fall from one level to another. The 7th character D is assigned to identify this encounter as a subsequent visit for aftercare.

Radiculopathy

Neuritis is a general term for inflammation of a nerve or group of nerves. Symptoms will vary depending on the area of the body and the nerve(s) that are inflamed. Symptoms may include pain, tingling (paresthesia), weakness (paresis), numbness (hypoesthesia), paralysis, loss of reflexes, and muscle wasting. Causes can include injury, infection, disease, exposure to chemicals or toxins, and nutritional deficiencies.

Radiculitis is a term used to describe pain that radiates along the dermatome (sensory pathway) of a nerve or group of nerves and is caused by inflammation or irritation of the nerve root(s) near the spinal cord. Symptoms vary depending on the exact nerve root(s) affected, but can include pain with a sharp, stabbing, shooting or burning quality; tingling (paresthesia); numbness (hypoesthesia); weakness (paresis); loss of reflexes; and muscle wasting. Causes can include injury, anatomic abnormality (e.g., bone spur), degenerative disease, and bulging or ruptured intervertebral disc.

Neuralgia, neuritis, and radiculitis of unknown cause are reported with "not otherwise specified" codes. There are two subcategories, M54.1 Radiculopathy, which is specific to neuritis and radiculitis of a specific spinal level and M79.2 Neuralgia and neuritis unspecified.

Coding and Documentation Requirements

Identify site of neuritis/radiculitis:

- Occipito-atlanto-axial region
- Cervical region
- Cervicothoracic region
- Thoracic region
- Thoracolumbar region
- Lumbar region
- Lumbosacral region
- Sacral/sacrococcygeal region
- Unspecified site
  - Radiculitis
  - Neuritis/neuralgia

ICD-10-CM Code/Documentation	
M54.11	Radiculopathy, occipito-atlanto-axial region
M54.12	Radiculopathy, cervical region
M54.13	Radiculopathy, cervicothoracic region
M54.14	Radiculopathy, thoracic region
M54.15	Radiculopathy, thoracolumbar region
M54.18	Radiculopathy, lumbar region
M54.17	Radiculopathy, lumbosacral region
M54.10	Radiculopathy, site unspecified
M54.18	Radiculopathy, sacral and sacrococcygeal region
M79.2	Neuralgia and neuritis, unspecified

Documentation and Coding Example

Fifty-five-year-old Caucasian female presents to PMD with tingling and numbness in the labia/perineal area, right buttocks and back of right thigh X 2 months with weakness in the right leg for the past few days. Patient is divorced, her youngest son is living with his father and older son has moved out of state to attend school. She continues to work part time as an office assistant. She sits a lot for her job but is quite active outside of work. She regularly hikes and bikes, plays softball, bowls and swims. She can recall no injury or trauma to her back or legs, simply noticed tingling and numbness sitting on the seat of her bike one day. HT 70 inches, WT 138, T 99, P 66, R 14, BP 124/62. On examination, this is a pleasant, thin, athletic appearing woman who looks her stated age. Eyes clear, PERRLA. TMs normal, nares patent without drainage. Oral mucosa moist and pink. Neck supple without lymphadenopathy. Cranial nerves grossly intact. Upper extremities normal. HR regular without bruit, rub or murmur. Breath sounds clear and equal bilaterally. Abdomen soft with active bowel sounds. Last gynecological exam was 8 months ago and completely normal. LMP 14 days ago, periods are for the most part regular at an interval of 23-24 days. She is S/P left salpingectomy for ectopic pregnancy 15 years ago with tubal ligation on the right at the time of that surgery. Patient is sexually active with her boyfriend and reports no change in libido or diminished pleasure from intercourse. There have been no changes in her bowel or bladder habits. She has trouble discerning both sharp and dull sensation on the labia from the level of the urethral meatus through the perineum and anus, extending to the right buttocks and mid posterior right thigh. Tone is 5/5 on left leg, 4/5 on right with 3+ reflexes on left and 2+ on right. Mild, intermittent muscle fasciculation noted in right buttocks. No muscle atrophy, rigidity, resistance or tenderness noted in lower extremities. She has difficulty maintaining leg lift on right with very mild drift from midline. Gait is normal.

Impression: **Radiculitis, sacral region**.

Plan: MRI of lumbar spine and sacrum is scheduled. Patient is instructed to have fasting blood drawn for CBC w/diff, comprehensive metabolic panel, Thyroid panel, Lipid panel, Vitamin D3, Vitamin B panel. Follow up appointment in 1 week to review test results. Consider referral to neurologist for EMG at that time.

Diagnosis Code(s)

M54.18 Radiculopathy, sacral and sacrococcygeal region

Coding Note(s)

To identify radiculitis, instructions in the Alphabetic Index under radiculitis state to see radiculopathy. Under radiculopathy, the code is found based upon the location or causation. There is a specific code for radiculopathy of the sacral and sacrococcygeal region.

Rupture of Tendon, Nontraumatic

Nontraumatic ruptures of tendons occur most often in the elderly, particularly in patients with other risk factors such as corticosteroid use and/or use of certain antibiotics, particularly quinolones. Codes are specific to site, such as shoulder, upper arm, forearm, hand, thigh, lower leg, ankle and foot; and to action such as extensor, flexor, and other tendon. Because physicians may name the tendon, such as Achilles, and not the specific site and action such as lower leg flexor tendon, coders must become familiar with the muscles and tendons of the extremities and their action in order to assign the nontraumatic tendon rupture to the correct code. Muscles and tendon names are frequently based upon their action and location. Some of the terms related to muscles and tendons are listed below.

Abductor/Abduction – Abductor muscle(s) work to move a body part away from the midline (e.g., raising the arm).

Adductor/Adduction – Adductor muscle(s) work to bring a body part closer to the midline.

Circumduction – Circular or conical motion movement of a joint due to a composite action of flexion, abduction, extension and adduction in that order.

Dorsiflexion – Muscle(s) work to tip the upper surface of the foot (dorsum) toward the anterior leg, decreasing the angle between the foot and leg.

Elevation/Depression – Muscle(s) work to raise (elevate) a body part to a more superior level (shoulder shrug), then lower that body part to a more inferior position (depression).

Eversion/Inversion – Muscles work to obliquely rotate the foot along the medial side of the heel to the lateral side of the mid foot. With inversion, the sole of the foot is turned inward toward the opposite foot and in eversion, the sole of the foot is turned outward and away from the midline.

Extensor/Extension – An extensor muscle works to increase the angle between bones that converge at a joint. For example: straightening the elbow or knee and bending the wrist or spine backward. Muscles of the hand and foot often contain this function in their name (example: extensor digitorum).

Flexor/Flexion – A flexor muscle works to decrease the angle between bones that converge at a joint, for example bending the elbow or knee. Muscles of the hand and foot may contain this function in their name (example: flexor carpi radialis, flexor hallucis longus).

Insertion – Attachment of the muscle or tendon to the skeletal area that the muscle moves when it contracts. The location is usually more distal on the bone with greater mobility and less mass when compared to the muscle origin point.

Opposition – Special muscle action of the hand in which the carpal/metacarpal bones in the thumb and fingers allow them to come together at their fingertips.

Origin – Muscle origin is the fixed attachment of muscle to bone. The location is usually more proximal on the bone with greater stability and mass when compared to the muscle insertion site allowing the muscle to exert power when it contracts.

Plantar Flexion – Muscle(s) work to tip the lower surface of the foot (sole, plantar area) downward, increasing the angle between the foot and anterior leg.

Pronation/Supination – Special muscle action of the forearm in which the radius crosses over the ulna resulting in the dorsal surface of the hand turning forward or prone (pronation, palm down). When the radius uncrosses, the palmer surface of the hand returns to its normal supine forward position (supination, palm up).

Protraction/Retraction – Muscle(s) work to move a body part forward (protraction), for example hunching of shoulders, then backward (retraction) when shoulders are squared.

Rotation – A movement that occurs around the vertical or longitudinal axis moving the body part toward or away from the center axis. Lateral/external rotation moves the anterior surface away from the midline. Medial/internal rotation moves the anterior surface toward the midline of the body.

The table below identifies a number of specific muscles and tendons of the extremities, the location of the muscle (e.g., upper/lower extremity, upper/lower leg, upper/lower arm), a brief description of the muscle or tendon, the origin and insertion, and the action. When coding it is important to know the location of the rupture since many muscles/tendons cover multiple sites. The table is organized alphabetically by tendon/muscle. Following the table is a documentation and coding example.

Muscle/Tendon	Location	Origin (O)/Insertion (I)	Action
Abductor pollicis brevis	Wrist/Hand/Thumb	O: Transverse carpal ligament and the tubercle of the scaphoid bone or (occasionally) the tubercle of the trapezium I: Base of the proximal phalanx of the thumb	Abducts the thumb and with muscles of the thenar eminence, acts to oppose the thumb
Abductor pollicis longus (APL)	Forearm/Thumb/Hand/Wrist	O: Posterior radius, posterior ulna and interosseous membrane I: Base 1st metacarpal Combined with the extensor pollicis brevis makes the anatomic snuff box.	Abducts and extends thumb at CMC joint; assists wrist abduction (radial deviation)
Achilles tendon	Lower Leg	O: Joins the gastrocnemius and soleus muscles I: Calcaneus	Flexor tendon – plantar flexes foot
Anconeus	Elbow	O: Lateral epicondyle humerus I: Posterior olecranon	Extends forearm
Brachialis	Elbow	O: Distal ½ anterior humeral shaft I: Coronoid process and ulnar tuberosity	Flexes forearm
Biceps brachii	Shoulder/Upper Arm	Long Head: O: Supraglenoid tubercle of the scapula to join the biceps tendon, short head in the middle of the humerus forming the biceps muscle belly Short Head: O: Coracoid process at the top of the scapula I: Radial tuberosity Long head and short head join in the middle of the humerus forming the biceps muscle belly	Flexes elbow Supinates forearm Weakly assists shoulder with forward flexion (long head) Short head provides horizontal adduction to stabilize shoulder joint and resist dislocation. With elbow flexed becomes a powerful supinator
Common flexor tendon 1. Pronator teres 2. Flexor carpi radialis (FCR) 3. Palmaris longus 4. Flexor digitorum superficialis (sublimis) (FDS) 5. Flexor carpi ulnaris (FCU)	Forearm/Hand	Common flexor tendon formed by 5 muscles of the forearm. There are slight variations in the site of origin and insertion 1. O: Medial epicondyle humerus and coronoid process of the ulna. I: Mid-lateral surface radial shaft 2. O: Medial epicondyle humerus. I: Base of 2nd and 3rd metacarpal 3. O: Medial epicondyle humerus. I: Palmar aponeurosis and flexor retinaculum 4. O: Medial epicondyle humerus, coronoid process ulna and anterior oblique line of radius. I: shaft middle phalanx digits 2-5 5. O: Medial epicondyle of the humerus, olecranon and posterior border ulna I: Pisiform, hook of hamate and 5th metacarpal.	1. Pronator Teres-pronation of forearm; assists elbow flexion 2. FCR- flexion and abduction of wrist (radial deviation) 3. Palmaris longus-assists wrist flexion 4. FDS- flexion middle phalanx PIP joint digits 2-4; assists wrist flexion 5. FCU- flexes and adducts hand at the wrist
Coracobrachialis	Shoulder/Upper Arm	O: Coracoid process I: Midshaft of humerus	Adducts & flexes shoulder
Deltoid	Shoulder/Upper Arm	O: Lateral 1/3 of clavicle, acromion and spine of scapula I: Deltoid tuberosity of humerus Large triangular shaped muscle composed of three parts	Anterior-Flex & medially rotate shoulder; Middle-assist w/abduction of humerus at shoulder; Posterior-extend & laterally rotate humerus
Extensor carpi radialis longus (ECRL)	Forearm/Hand	O: Lateral epicondyle humerus I: Dorsal surface 2nd metacarpal	Extends and abducts wrist; active during fist clenching
Extensor (digitorum) communis (EDC)	Forearm/Wrist/Hand/Finger	O: Lateral epicondyle humerus terminates into 4 tendons in the hand I: On the lateral and dorsal surfaces of digits 2-5 (fingers)	Extends the metacarpophalangeal (MCP), proximal interphalangeal (PIP) and distal interphalangeal (DIP) joints of 2nd-5th fingers and wrist
Extensor digitorum longus (EDL)	Lower Leg/Ankle/Foot	O: Lateral condyle tibia, proximal 2/3 anterior fibula shaft and interosseous membrane I: Middle and distal phalanx toes 2-5	Extension lateral 4 digits at metatarsophalangeal joint; assists dorsiflexion of foot at ankle
Extensor hallicus longus (EHL)	Lower Leg/Ankle/Foot	O: Middle part anterior surface fibula and interosseous membrane I: Dorsal aspect base distal phalanx great toe	Extends great toe; assists dorsiflexion of foot at ankle; weak invertor

Muscle/Tendon	Location	Origin (O)/Insertion (I)	Action
Extensor pollicis brevis (EPB)	Wrist/Hand/Thumb	O: Distal radius (dorsal surface) and interosseous membrane I: Base proximal phalanx thumb Combined with the abductor pollicis longus makes the anatomic snuff box	Extends the thumb at metacarpophalangeal joint (MCPJ)
Extensor pollicis longus (EPL)	Wrist/Hand/Thumb	O: Dorsal surface of the ulna and interosseous membrane I: Base distal phalanx thumb	Extends distal phalanx thumb at IP joint; assists wrist abduction
Flexor digitorum longus (FDL)	Lower Leg/Ankle/Foot	O: Medial posterior tibia shaft I: Base distal phalanx digits 2-5	Flexes digits 2-5; plantar flex ankle; supports longitudinal arch of foot
Flexor digitorum profundus (FDP)	Forearm/Wrist/Hand	O: Proximal 1/3 anterior-medial surface ulna and interosseous membrane; in the hand splits into 4 tendons I: Base of the distal phalanx, digits 2-5 (fingers)	Flexes the distal phalanx, digits 2-5 (fingers)
Flexor hallucis longus (FHL)	Lower Leg/Ankle/Foot	O: Inferior 2/3 posterior fibula; inferior interosseous membrane I: Base distal phalanx great toe (hallux)	Flexes great toe at all joints; weakly plantar flexes ankle; supports medial longitudinal arches of foot
Flexor pollicis brevis (FPB)	Wrist/Hand/Thumb	O: Distal edge of the transverse carpal ligament and the tubercle of the trapezium I: Proximal phalanx of the thumb	Flexes the thumb at the metacarpophalangeal (MCPJ) and carpometacarpal (CMC) joint
Flexor pollicis longus (FPL)	Forearm/Wrist/Hand/ Thumb	O: Below the radial tuberosity on the anterior surface of the radius and interosseous membrane I: Base distal phalanx thumb	Flexes the thumb at the metacarpophalangeal (MCPJ) and interphalangeal (IPJ) joint
Hamstring	Upper Leg/Knee	Composed of three muscles 1. Semitendinosus O: Ischial tuberosity I: Anterior proximal tibial shaft Semimembranosus O: Ischial tuberosity I: Posterior medial tibial condyle 2. Biceps femoris O: Long head ischial tuberosity; short head linea aspera femoral shaft and lateral supracondylar line I: Head of fibula	1. Semitendinosus and Semimembranosus–Flexes leg at knee, when knee flexed medially rotates tibia; thigh extensor at hip joint; when hip & knee both flexed, extends trunk 2. Biceps femoris–Flexes leg and rotates laterally when knee flexed; extends thigh
Intrinsics of hand hypothenar 1. Abductor digiti minimi 2. Flexor digiti minimi brevis 3. Opponens digiti minimi	Wrist/Hand/Finger	1. O: Pisiform I: Medial side of base proximal phalanx 5th finger 2. O: Hook of hamate & flexor retinaculum I: Medial side of base proximal phalanx 5th finger 3. O: Hook of hamate and transverse carpal ligament I: Uulnar aspect shaft 5th metacarpal	1. Abducts 5th finger; assists flexion proximal phalanx 2. Flexes proximal phalanx 5th finger 3. Rotates the 5th metacarpal bone forward
Intrinsics of hand short 1. Dorsal interossei 1-4 2. Dorsal interossei 1-3 3. Lumbricals 1st & 2nd 4. Lumbricals 3rd & 4th	Wrist/Hand	1. O: Adjacent sides of 2 MC I: Bases of proximal phalanges; extensor expansions of 2-4 fingers 2. O: Palmar surface 2nd, 4th & 5th MC I: Bases of proximal phalanges; extensor expansions of 2nd, 4th & 5th fingers 3. O: Lateral two tendons of FDP I: Lateral sides of extensor expansion of 2nd-5th 4. O: Medial 3 tendons of FDP I: Lateral sides of extensor expansion of 2nd-5th	1. Abduct 2-4 fingers from axial line; acts w/ lumbricals to flex MCP jt and extend IP jt 2. Adduct 2nd, 4th, 5th fingers from axial line; assist lumbricals to flex MCP jt and extend IP jt; extensor expansions of 2nd-4th fingers 3. Flex MCP jt; extend IP joint 2-5 4. Flex MCP jt; extend IP joint 2-5

Muscle/Tendon	Location	Origin (O)/Insertion (I)	Action
Intrinsics of hand thenar 1. Abductor pollicis brevis 2. Adductor pollicis 3. Flexor pollicis brevis 4. Opponens pollicis	Wrist/Hand/Thumb	1. O: Flexor retinaculum & tubercle scaphoid & trapezium I: :Lateral side of base of proximal phalanx thumb 2. O: Oblique head base 2nd & 3rd MC, capitate, adjacent carpals and transverse head anterior surface shaft 3rd MC I: Medial side base of proximal phalanx thumb 3. O: Flexor retinaculum & tubercle scaphoid & trapezium I: Lateral side of base of proximal phalanx thumb 4. O: Transverse carpal ligament and the tubercle of the trapezium I: Lateral border shaft 1st metacarpal	1. Abducts thumb; helps w/opposition 2. Adducts thumb toward lateral border of palm 3. Flexes thumb 4. Rotates the thumb in opposition with fingers
Lumbricals (foot)	Foot	O: Lumbricals-flexor digitorum longus tendon I: Medial side base proximal phalanges 2-5	Assist in joint movement between metatarsals
Patellar tendon	Knee/Lower Leg	Connects the bottom of the patella to the top of the tibia The tendon is actually a ligament because it joins bone to bone	Works with the quadriceps tendon to bend and straighten the knee
Pectoralis major	Chest/Upper Arm	O: Clavicle, sternum, ribs 2-6 I: Upper shaft of humerus	Adducts, flexes, medially rotates humerus
Peroneus (fibularis) brevis	Lower Leg/Ankle/Foot	O: Distal 2/3 lateral shaft fibula I: Becomes a tendon midcalf that runs behind the lateral malleolus Inserts on tuberosity base 5th metatarsal	Eversion of foot; assists with plantar flexion of foot at ankle
Peroneus (fibularis) longus	Lower Leg/Ankle/Foot	O: Head and upper 2/3 lateral surface fibula I: Becomes a long tendon midcalf that runs behind the lateral malleolus and crosses obliquely on plantar surface of foot inserts on base 1st metatarsal and medial cuneiform	Eversion of foot; weak plantar flexion foot at ankle
Peroneus (fibularis) tertius	Lower Leg/Ankle/Foot	O: Inferior 1/3 anterior surface fibula and interosseous membrane I: Dorsum base 5th metatarsal	Dorsiflexes ankle and aids inversion of foot
Quadratus plantae	Foot	O: Calcaneus I: Flexor digitorum tendons	Assists flexor muscles
Quadriceps femoris	Upper Leg/Knee	Composed of four muscles: Rectus femoris O: Anterior inferior iliac spine and ilium superior to acetabulum I: Combines to form quadriceps tendon; inserts base of patella and tibial tuberosity via patellar ligament Vastus lateralis O: Greater trochanter and lateral aspect femoral shaft I: Lateral patella and tendon of rectus femoris Vastus medialis O: Intertrochanteric line and medial aspect femoral shaft I: Medial border of quadriceps tendon and medial aspect of patella; tibial tuberosity via patellar ligament Vastus intermedius: O: Anterior and lateral surface femoral shaft I: Posterior surface upper border of patella; tibial tuberosity via patellar ligament	Extends leg at knee joint; rectus femoris with iliopsoas helps flex thigh and stabilized hip joint
Quadriceps tendon	Upper Leg/Knee	Fibrous band of tissue that connects the quadriceps muscle of the anterior thigh to the patella (kneecap)	Holds the patella (kneecap) in the patellofemoral groove of the femur enabling it to act as a fulcrum and provide power to bend and straighten the knee

Muscle/Tendon	Location	Origin (O)/Insertion (I)	Action
Rotator cuff tendons: 1. Supraspinatus 2. Infraspinatus 3. Teres minor 4. Subscapularis	Shoulder/Upper Arm	Rotator cuff tendons are formed by 4 muscles of the shoulder/upper arm. They all originate from the scapula and insert (terminate) on the humerus: 1. O: Supraspinous fossa of scapula. I: Superior facet greater tuberosity humerus. 2. O: Infraspinous fossa of scapula. I: Middle facet greater tuberosity humerus. 3. O: Middle half of the lateral border of the scapula. I: Inferior facet greater tuberosity humerus 4. O: Subscapular fossa of scapula. I: Either the lesser tuberosity humerus or the humeral neck.	1. Initiates abduction of shoulder joint (completed by deltoid) 2. Externally rotates the arm; helps hold humeral head in glenoid cavity 3. Externally rotates the arm; helps hold humeral head in glenoid cavity 4. Internally rotates and adducts the humerus; helps hold humeral head in glenoid cavity
Tibialis anterior	Lower Leg/Ankle/Foot	O: Lateral condyle and superior half lateral tibia I: Base 1st metatarsal, plantar surface medial cuneiform	Dorsiflexion ankle, foot inversion at subtalar and midtarsal joints
Tibialis posterior	Lower Leg/Ankle/Foot	O: Interosseus membrane; posterior surface of tibia and fibula I: Tuberosity of tarsal navicula, cuneiform and cuboid and bases of 2nd, 3rd and 4th metatarsals	Plantar flexes ankle; inverts foot
Triceps	Shoulder/Upper Arm	Long head: O: Infraglenoid tubercle of scapula; Lateral head: O: Upper half of posterior surface shaft of humerus Medial head O: Lower half of posterior surface shaft of humerus I: Olecranon process Only muscle on the back of the arm	Extends elbow joint; long head can adduct humerus and extend it from flexed position; stabilizes shoulder joint

Except for nontraumatic tears of the rotator cuff which are captured in subcategory M75.1, codes for nontraumatic tendon tears are found in subcategories M66.2-M66.8 and are defined as spontaneous rupture.

Coding and Documentation Requirements

Identify rupture as not related to injury or trauma.

Identify site of nontraumatic tendon rupture:

- Upper extremity
  - Shoulder
  - Upper arm
  - Forearm
  - Hand
- Lower extremity
  - Thigh
  - Lower leg
  - Ankle/foot
- Other site
- Multiple sites
- Unspecified tendon

Identify action of tendon:

- Extensor
- Flexor
- Other

ICD-10-CM Code/Documentation	
M66.221	Spontaneous rupture of extensor tendons, right upper arm
M66.222	Spontaneous rupture of extensor tendons, left upper arm
M66.229	Spontaneous rupture of extensor tendons, unspecified upper arm
M66.311	Spontaneous rupture of flexor tendons, right shoulder
M66.312	Spontaneous rupture of flexor tendons, left shoulder
M66.319	Spontaneous rupture of flexor tendons, unspecified shoulder
M66.321	Spontaneous rupture of flexor tendons, right upper arm
M66.322	Spontaneous rupture of flexor tendons, left upper arm
M66.329	Spontaneous rupture of flexor tendons, left upper arm
M66.231	Spontaneous rupture of extensor tendons, right forearm
M66.232	Spontaneous rupture of extensor tendons, left forearm
M66.239	Spontaneous rupture of extensor tendons, unspecified forearm
M66.241	Spontaneous rupture of extensor tendons, right hand
M66.242	Spontaneous rupture of extensor tendons, left hand
M22.249	Spontaneous rupture of extensor tendons, unspecified hand
M66.331	Spontaneous rupture of flexor tendons, right forearm
M66.332	Spontaneous rupture of flexor tendons, left forearm
M66.339	Spontaneous rupture of flexor tendons, unspecified forearm
M66.341	Spontaneous rupture of flexor tendons, right hand
M66.342	Spontaneous rupture of flexor tendons, left hand
M66.349	Spontaneous rupture of flexor tendons, unspecified hand
M66.251	Spontaneous rupture of extensor tendons, right thigh

ICD-10-CM Code/Documentation	
M66.252	Spontaneous rupture of extensor tendons, left thigh
M66.259	Spontaneous rupture of extensor tendons, unspecified thigh
M66.261	Spontaneous rupture of extensor tendons, right lower leg
M66.262	Spontaneous rupture of extensor tendons, left lower leg
M66.269	Spontaneous rupture of extensor tendons, unspecified lower leg
M66.361	Spontaneous rupture flexor tendons, right lower leg
M66.362	Spontaneous rupture flexor tendons, left lower leg
M66.369	Spontaneous rupture flexor tendons, unspecified lower leg
M66.271	Spontaneous rupture of extensor tendons, right ankle and foot
M66.272	Spontaneous rupture of extensor tendons, left ankle and foot
M66.279	Spontaneous rupture of extensor tendons, unspecified ankle and foot
M66.371	Spontaneous rupture of flexor tendons, right ankle and foot
M66.372	Spontaneous rupture of flexor tendons, left ankle and foot
M66.379	Spontaneous rupture of flexor tendons, unspecified ankle and foot
M66.28	Spontaneous rupture of extensor tendons, other site
M66.29	Spontaneous rupture of extensor tendons, multiple sites
M66.351	Spontaneous rupture of flexor tendons, right thigh
M66.352	Spontaneous rupture of flexor tendons, left thigh
M66.359	Spontaneous rupture of flexor tendons, unspecified thigh
M66.38	Spontaneous rupture of flexor tendons, other site
M66.39	Spontaneous rupture of flexor tendons, multiple sites

Documentation and Coding Example

Eighty-one-year-old Caucasian female is brought into ED by EMS after she awoke this morning with bilateral ankle swelling and pain that prevented her from getting out of bed. Patient resides alone and is able to drive and care completely for herself. She was in her usual state of good health until approximately two weeks ago when she became acutely ill with fever, malaise, and cough. She is fastidious about obtaining an annual flu vaccine so she attributed her symptoms to a summer cold. When her cough became productive and was accompanied by wheezing, she visited her PMD who obtained a CXR which showed left lower lobe infiltrates and was subsequently prescribed Advair Inhaler BID, Levaquin 500 mg BID, and albuterol inhaler prn. She has been on these medications for 6 days and is just beginning to have some energy. She saw her PMD yesterday and a repeat CXR showed improvement. She noticed some stiffness in her right ankle last evening and dismissed it as simply muscle disuse but was dismayed this morning when both ankles were swollen and painful and she was unable to walk. She called her daughter who came right over and PMD advised transfer to ED by EMS. On examination, this is an anxious but pleasant octogenarian who looks younger than her stated age. She is alert and oriented x 3 and an excellent historian. T 96.1, P 80, R 18, BP 114/84 O2 Sat on RA is 96%. She states she is widowed x 20 years. Her husband was in the diplomatic service and they traveled extensively. After his death she become somewhat of a celebrity by authoring a series of books on cooking and culinary adventure. Travel immunizations are current and her last trip was 3 months ago to Belize. She swims and/or walks daily and has had no recent injuries that she can recall. Heart rate shows SR on monitor with occasional benign PVCs. No audible murmur, bruit, or rubs are appreciated. Breath sounds have scattered wheezes with slightly decreased sounds in the left base. Abdomen soft, non-distended. Cranial nerves grossly intact and upper extremities WNL. Hips and knees are without swelling or pain and ROM is intact. There is a moderate amount of circumferential swelling in each ankle. No redness, bruising, or discoloration noted. Unable to adequately palpate along the Achilles tendon due to swelling and discomfort but a gap may be present 3-4 cm above heel on the right. Neurovascular status of feet and toes is unremarkable. Passive ROM to ankles elicits considerable pain and she is unable to actively plantar flex. Thompson's sign is positive as is Homan's. Given her recent illness and immobility, venous Doppler study is performed and DVT is ruled out. **MRI of bilateral ankles was obtained which is significant for Achilles rupture 4.5 cm proximal to calcaneal insertion site on the right and 6 cm proximal on the left.** There is no evidence of pre-existing tendinopathy in either extremity.

Impression: **Non-traumatic bilateral Achilles tendon rupture** possibly due to fluoroquinolone and steroid use.

Plan: Discontinue Levaquin and Advair and admit to orthopedic service.

Diagnosis Code(s)

M66.361 Spontaneous rupture flexor tendons right lower leg

M66.362 Spontaneous rupture flexor tendons left lower leg

Coding Note(s)

Nontraumatic ruptures of the tendon are defined by their action, not the specific tendon. The Achilles tendon is a flexor tendon in the lower leg. Laterality is a component of the code and so separate codes for right and left are reported since there is not a bilateral code. The documentation states that the tendon ruptures are "possibly" due to the fluoroquinolone and steroid use. Because the qualifier "possibly" is used, this would not be coded as an adverse effect for the ED encounter; however, it may be appropriate to code the adverse effect if the discharge summary also lists these medications as the cause or possible cause of the tendon ruptures.

Scoliosis

Scoliosis is an abnormal sideways curvature in the spine. The condition may be congenital (present at birth) or develop later in life, usually around the time of puberty. Congenital scoliosis is usually caused by vertebral anomalies. Other causes can include neuromuscular disorders (cerebral palsy, spinal muscular atrophy), trauma, and certain syndromes (Marfan's, Prader-Willi). In the majority of cases, no cause can be found and the condition is termed idiopathic. Scoliosis can decrease lung capacity, place pressure on the heart and large blood vessels in the chest, and may restrict physical activity.

Codes for scoliosis are listed in category M41. Codes are classified as idiopathic, thoracogenic, neuromuscular, other secondary scoliosis, other forms of scoliosis, and unspecified scoliosis. Codes for idiopathic scoliosis are categorized based on age at diagnosis as infantile (from birth through age 4), juvenile (ages 5 through 9 years), and adolescent (ages 11 through 17 years). There is also a subcategory for other idiopathic scoliosis. In addition, the site of curvature must be documented as cervical, cervicothoracic, thoracic, thoracolumbar, lumbar, or lumbosacral. These codes are not reported for congenital scoliosis which is reported with a code from Chapter 17 Congenital Malformations, Deformations, and Chromosomal Abnormalities.

Coding and Documentation Requirements

Identify type of scoliosis:

- Idiopathic
  - Infantile
  - Juvenile
  - Adolescent
  - Other
- Secondary
  - Neuromuscular
  - Other
- Thoracogenic
- Other form
- Unspecified

Identify site:

- Cervical
- Cervicothoracic
- Thoracic
- Thoracolumbar
- Lumbar
- Lumbosacral
- Sacral/sacrococcygeal (only applies to infantile idiopathic scoliosis)
- Site unspecified

Idiopathic Scoliosis

ICD-1Ø-CM Code/Documentation	
Juvenile	
M41.112	Juvenile idiopathic scoliosis, cervical region
M41.113	Juvenile idiopathic scoliosis, cervicothoracic region
M41.114	Juvenile idiopathic scoliosis, thoracic region
M41.115	Juvenile idiopathic scoliosis, thoracolumbar region
M41.116	Juvenile idiopathic scoliosis, lumbar region
M41.117	Juvenile idiopathic scoliosis, lumbosacral region
M41.119	Juvenile idiopathic scoliosis, site unspecified
Adolescent	
M41.122	Adolescent idiopathic scoliosis, cervical region
M41.123	Adolescent idiopathic scoliosis, cervicothoracic region
M41.124	Adolescent idiopathic scoliosis, thoracic region
M41.125	Adolescent idiopathic scoliosis, thoracolumbar region
M41.126	Adolescent idiopathic scoliosis, lumbar region
M41.127	Adolescent idiopathic scoliosis, lumbosacral region
M41.129	Adolescent idiopathic scoliosis, site unspecified
Other	
M41.2Ø	Other idiopathic scoliosis, site unspecified
M41.22	Other idiopathic scoliosis, cervical region
M41.23	Other idiopathic scoliosis, cervicothoracic region
M41.24	Other idiopathic scoliosis, thoracic region
M41.25	Other idiopathic scoliosis, thoracolumbar region
M41.26	Other idiopathic scoliosis, lumbar region
M41.27	Other idiopathic scoliosis, lumbosacral region
Infantile	
M41.ØØ	Infantile idiopathic scoliosis, site unspecified
M41.Ø2	Infantile idiopathic scoliosis, cervical region
M41.Ø3	Infantile idiopathic scoliosis, cervicothoracic region
M41.Ø4	Infantile idiopathic scoliosis, thoracic region
M41.Ø5	Infantile idiopathic scoliosis, thoracolumbar region
M41.Ø6	Infantile idiopathic scoliosis, lumbar region
M41.Ø7	Infantile idiopathic scoliosis, lumbosacral region
M41.Ø8	Infantile idiopathic scoliosis, sacral and sacrococcygeal region

Documentation and Coding Example

Twelve-year-old Hispanic female is referred to Pediatric Orthopedic Clinic by PMD for suspected scoliosis. She was initially noted to have a **right thoracic curve of 7 degrees** during routine screening by her school nurse. Patient was subsequently seen by her **pediatrician who examined her and obtained x-rays that indeed supported the school screening results**. PMH is significant for allergies and asthma well controlled with Singulair 5 mg daily, Xopenex inhaler only occasionally for symptoms. She also uses topical hydrocortisone for eczema PRN. On examination, this is a thin but well-nourished adolescent female, developmentally a Tanner II-III. Upper and lower reflexes intact, abdominal reflex pattern normal. Right shoulder is rotated forward and medial border of right scapula protrudes posteriorly. Examination of lower extremities shows negative hamstring tightness and a 1 cm length discrepancy. No ataxia and negative Romberg. Radiographs viewed on computer with parent and patient and are significant for a **30 degree right thoracic curve**. Diagnosis and treatment options discussed and questions answered. Patient will be fitted with a brace to be worn 16 hours a day. RTC in 3 months for repeat x-rays and examination.

Diagnosis Code(s)

M41.124 Adolescent idiopathic scoliosis, thoracic region

Coding Note(s)

In order to assign the most specific code for idiopathic scoliosis, the age of the patient and the site of the curvature must be documented.

Spondylosis

Spondylosis is stiffening or fixation of the vertebral joint(s) with fibrous or bony union across the joint resulting from age or a disease process. Spondylosis affects the vertebrae, intervertebral disc, and soft tissues of the spine. The condition may be complicated by spinal cord dysfunction, also referred to as myelopathy, resulting from narrowing of the spinal column and compression of the spinal cord. Spondylosis may also cause radiculopathy which is a general term for pain resulting from compression of a nerve. There are a number of very similar terms for conditions affecting the spine. Do not confuse spondylosis with spondylosis which is a degenerative or developmental deficiency of a portion of the vertebra, commonly involving the pars interarticularis. Careful review of the documentation is required to ensure that the correct code is assigned.

Category M47 contains codes for spondylosis. This category includes conditions documented as arthrosis or osteoarthritis of the spine and degeneration of the facet joints. There are subcategories for anterior spinal artery compression syndromes (M47.01) and vertebral artery compression syndromes (M47.02). Combination codes exist for spondylosis with myelopathy (M47.1-) and with radiculopathy (M47.2-). Spondylosis without myelopathy or radiculopathy is reported with codes from subcategory (M47.81-). There is also a subcategory for other specified spondylosis (M47.89) and a single code for spondylosis unspecified (M47.9). Codes are specific to the following regions of the spine: occipito-atlanto-axial (occiput to 2nd cervical), cervical, cervicothoracic (6th cervical to 1st thoracic), thoracic, thoracolumbar (10th thoracic to 1st lumbar), lumbar, lumbosacral (5 lumbar and 5 sacral), and sacral/sacrococcygeal.

Coding and Documentation Requirements

Identify condition:

- Anterior spinal artery compression syndrome
- Vertebral artery compression syndrome
- Spondylosis
  - with myelopathy
  - with radiculopathy
  - without myelopathy or radiculopathy
  - Other specified type
  - Unspecified

Identify site:

- Occipito-atlanto-axial region
- Cervical region
- Cervicothoracic region
- Thoracic region
- Thoracolumbar region
- Lumbar region
- Lumbosacral region
- Sacral/sacrococcygeal region
- Unspecified site

ICD-10-CM Code/Documentation	
M47.016	Anterior spinal artery compression syndromes, lumbar region
M47.26	Other spondylosis with radiculopathy, lumbar region
M47.27	Other spondylosis with radiculopathy, lumbosacral region
M47.28	Other spondylosis with radiculopathy, sacral and sacrococcygeal region
M47.816	Spondylosis without myelopathy or radiculopathy, lumbar region
M47.817	Spondylosis without myelopathy or radiculopathy, lumbosacral region
M47.818	Spondylosis without myelopathy or radiculopathy, sacral and sacrococcygeal region
M47.896	Other spondylosis, lumbar region
M47.897	Other spondylosis, lumbosacral region
M47.898	Other spondylosis, sacral and sacrococcygeal region
M47.16	Other spondylosis with myelopathy, lumbar region

Documentation and Coding Example

Fifty-eight-year-old Caucasian male presents to Occupational Medicine for routine physical. Patient is a long-distance truck driver x 20 years. His only complaints are more frequent need to urinate and some mild low back pain and paresthesia in his left thigh. T 98.8, P 78, R 14, BP 138/88, Ht. 70 inches, Wt. 155 lbs. Vision is 20/30 with glasses. Hearing by audiometry is WNL. EKG shows NSR without ectopy. On examination PERRL, neck supple without lymphadenopathy. Nares patent, oral mucosa, pharynx moist and pink. Cranial nerves grossly intact. Neuromuscular exam of upper extremities unremarkable. Heart rate regular without bruit, rub, murmur. Breath sounds clear, equal bilaterally. Spinal column straight with mild tenderness in lumbar/sacral area. Abdomen soft, active bowel sounds. No evidence of hernia, testicles smooth. Circumcised penis is without discharge. Good sphincter tone on rectal exam, smooth, slightly enlarged prostate. Good ROM in lower extremities. Gait normal. Reflexes intact. Leg lifts do not produce pain. Sensation, both dull and sharp is reduced from lateral aspect to midline anterior of left thigh starting 4 cm below the hip ending 2 cm above the knee. He describes a prickling or tingling sensation at times over that entire area. Radiographs of spine obtained and reveal bony overgrowth on vertebral bodies L1-L4 and mild narrowing of the disc space. No disc protrusion is seen.

Impression: **Lumbar spondylosis with radiculopathy involving L1-L4.**

Plan: Occupational/Physical therapy evaluation and 12 treatments authorized. Risk management to evaluate his truck drivers seat for possible modifications after he is seen by OT/PT and recommendations are made. RTC in 4 weeks, sooner if symptoms worsen.

Diagnosis Code(s)

M47.26 Other spondylosis with radiculopathy, lumbar region

Coding Note(s)

There is a combination code that captures spondylosis, which is the disease process, and radiculopathy which is a common symptom of spondylosis.

Stress Fracture

A stress fracture is a small crack or break in a bone that arises from unusual or repeated force or overuse in an area of the body, most commonly the lower legs and feet. Symptoms include generalized pain and tenderness. When a stress fracture occurs in the lower extremity, pain and tenderness may increase with weight bearing. The pain may also be more pronounced at the beginning of exercise, decrease during the activity, and then increase again at the end of the workout.

There are specific codes for stress fractures of the pelvis and extremities as well as for stress fractures of the vertebrae. Stress fractures of the vertebrae are referred to as fatigue fractures with the alternate term stress fracture also listed. Fatigue fractures of the vertebrae are located in subcategory M48.4 and codes are specific to the region of the spine. There is also a subcategory (M48.5) for collapsed vertebra which may also be documented as wedging of vertebra. Codes for collapsed vertebra are not used to report fatigue fractures, pathological fractures due to neoplasm, osteoporosis or other pathological condition, or for traumatic fractures. Codes for stress fractures of other sites are located in subcategory M84.3 and codes are specific to site and also require documentation of laterality.

Coding and Documentation Requirements

For stress fracture of pelvis/extremity identify:

- Site
  - Lower extremity
    - » Femur
    - » Tibia
    - » Fibula
    - » Ankle
    - » Foot
    - » Toe(s)
  - Pelvis
  - Upper extremity
    - » Shoulder
    - » Humerus
    - » Radius
    - » Ulna
    - » Hand
    - » Finger(s)
- Laterality (not required for pelvis)
  - Right
  - Left
  - Unspecified
- Episode of care
  - Initial encounter
  - Subsequent encounter
    - » With routine healing
    - » With delayed healing
    - » With nonunion
    - » With malunion
  - Sequela

For fatigue fracture/collapsed vertebra, identify:

- Type
  - Fatigue fracture
  - Collapsed vertebra (wedging)
- Site/region of spine
  - Occipito-atlanto-axial region
  - Cervical
  - Cervicothoracic
  - Thoracic
  - Thoracolumbar
  - Lumbar
  - Lumbosacral
  - Sacral/sacrococcygeal
  - Unspecified site
- Episode of care
  - Initial encounter
  - Subsequent encounter
    - » With routine healing
    - » With delayed healing
  - Sequela

Stress Fracture Ankle/Foot/Toes

ICD-10-CM Code/Documentation	
M84.371-	Stress fracture, right ankle
M84.372-	Stress fracture, left ankle
M84.373-	Stress fracture, unspecified ankle
M84.374-	Stress fracture, right foot
M84.375-	Stress fracture, left foot
M84.376-	Stress fracture, unspecified foot
M84.377-	Stress fracture, right toe(s)
M84.378-	Stress fracture, left toe(s)
M84.379-	Stress fracture, unspecified toe(s)

Documentation and Coding Example

Patient is a twenty-eight-year-old Asian female who presents to Physiatrist with c/o right foot pain. She is well known to this practice as a member of a professional ballet company that we consult for. This petite, well nourished, graceful young woman is 3 months postdelivery of her first child. She retired from performing 2 years ago but has been teaching in the ballet school. She remained active during her pregnancy by taking ballet, Pilates, or yoga classes almost daily. She returned to teaching 2 months ago, usually assigned to upper level students 4 days a week. She noticed right mid-foot pain that radiated along the medial longitudinal arch one week after she returned to teaching. The pain increases with exercise and usually goes away with rest. For the past week she has noticed her shoes feel tight over that area but she has not noticed bruising or obvious swelling. On examination, there is mild dorsal foot swelling, pain with passive eversion and active inversion. Point tenderness is present at the mid medial arch and proximal to the dorsal portion of the navicular bone. X-ray obtained using a coned-down AP radiograph centered on the tarsal navicular which reveals a **small lateral fragment of the tarsal navicular bone**.

Impression: **Stress fracture of the right navicular**.

Plan: Walking boot x 6 weeks. Patient is advised to do non-weight bearing exercise only. RTC in 6 weeks for repeat x-ray and referral to PT.

Diagnosis Code(s)

M84.374A Stress fracture, right foot, initial encounter

Coding Note(s)

The tarsal navicular bone is one of the 7 tarsal bones of the foot. Under Fracture, traumatic, stress, tarsus in the Alphabetic Index, code M84.374- is identified as the correct code.

Summary

For the majority of connective tissue conditions and diseases of the musculoskeletal system specific documentation is required related to anatomic site and laterality. Episode of care is required for nontraumatic fractures (stress, pathologic and fractures related to osteoporosis). In addition, the need to clearly differentiate acute traumatic conditions from old or chronic conditions must be specified.

Resources

Documentation checklists are available in Appendix A for the following conditions:

- Gout
- Rheumatoid arthritis

Chapter 15 Quiz

1. What condition below does not require documentation of episode of care?
   a. Collapsed vertebra
   b. Fatigue fracture of vertebra
   c. Unspecified disorder of bone continuity
   d. Stress fracture of foot

2. The ED physician has documented that an 82-year-old patient with severe senile osteoporosis sustained a left hip fracture from a same level fall on a carpeted surface. What code is reported for the fracture?
   a. M80.052A Age-related osteoporosis with current pathological fracture, left femur, initial encounter
   b. M80.852A Other osteoporosis with current pathological fracture, left femur, initial visit
   c. S72.002A Fracture of unspecified part of neck of left femur, initial encounter for closed fracture
   d. S72.065A Nondisplaced articular fracture of head of left femur, initial encounter for closed fracture

3. Identify which condition affecting the musculoskeletal system would generally not be reported with a code from Chapter 13.
   a. Healed injury
   b. Recurrent bone, joint or muscle condition
   c. Chronic conditions
   d. Current acute injury

4. The physician has documented that the patient has idiopathic osteonecrosis of the right femoral head. Since this condition affects the joint, what site is reported?
   a. The site is the joint
   b. The site is the bone
   c. The site is a combination code for the joint and the bone
   d. Two sites are reported identifying the bone and the joint

5. What condition is not reported with a code from Chapter 13?
   a. Arthropathic psoriasis
   b. Drug-induced gout
   c. Adhesive capsulitis of the shoulder
   d. Nontraumatic compartment syndrome

6. What condition would be reported with a code from subcategory M48.5- Collapsed vertebra?
   a. Current injury due to fatigue fracture
   b. New pathological fracture of vertebra due to neoplasm
   c. Wedging of vertebra
   d. Traumatic vertebral fracture

7. What information is NOT required to assign the most specific code for idiopathic scoliosis?
   a. Age of the patient at onset of the condition
   b. Location of the curve
   c. Affected region of the spine
   d. The specific form of scoliosis

8. Codes for osteoporosis in category M80 are specific to site. What does the site designate?
   a. The site of the osteoporosis and fracture
   b. The site of the osteoporosis
   c. The site of the fracture
   d. None of the above

9. Code M61.371 Calcification and ossification of muscles associated with burns, right ankle and foot is an example of what type of code?
   a. An injury code
   b. A combination code
   c. An episode of care code
   d. None of the above

10. What descriptor is not an example of site specificity?
    a. Mid-cervical region
    b. Achilles tendon
    c. Synovium
    d. First carpometacarpal joints

11. What information must be documented to assign the most specific code in category M1A Chronic gout that is not required for codes in category M10 Gout?
    a. With or without tophus
    b. Site
    c. Laterality
    d. All of the above

See next page for answers and rationales.

Chapter 15 Answers and Rationales

1. What condition does not require documentation of episode of care?

   c. **Unspecified disorder of bone continuity**

   Rationale: *Collapsed vertebra (M48.5-), fatigue fracture of vertebra (M48.4), and stress fracture of foot (M84.37-) all require documentation of episode of care. Unspecified disorder of bone continuity, even though it is also classified in category M84, does not require documentation episode of care.*

2. The ED physician has documented that an 82-year-old patient with severe senile osteoporosis sustained a left hip fracture when he sustained a same level fall on a carpeted surface. What code is reported for the fracture?

   a. **M80.052A Age-related osteoporosis with current pathological fracture, left femur, initial encounter**

   Rationale: *A code from category M80, not a traumatic fracture code, should be used for any patient with known osteoporosis who suffers a fracture, even if the patient had a minor fall or trauma, if that fall or trauma would not usually break a normal, healthy bone. The physician has documented that the patient has senile osteoporosis which is a reported with the code for age-related osteoporosis.*

3. Identify which condition affecting the musculoskeletal system would generally not be reported with a code from Chapter 13.

   d. **Current acute injury**

   Rationale: *Chapter guidelines identify healed, recurrent injuries and chronic conditions affecting the musculoskeletal system as conditions that are usually reported with codes from Chapter 13. Current acute injuries are usually reported with codes from Chapter 19.*

4. The physician has documented that the patient has idiopathic osteonecrosis of the right femoral head. Since this condition affects the joint, what site is reported?

   b. **The site is the bone**

   Rationale: *Coding guidelines related to site state the following: For certain conditions, the bone may be affected at the upper or lower end, (e.g., avascular necrosis of bone, M87; osteoporosis, M80-M81). Though the portion of the bone affected may be at the joint, the site designation will be the bone, not the joint.*

5. What condition is not reported with a code from Chapter 13?

   a. **Arthropathic psoriasis**

   Rationale: *The chapter level Excludes2 note identifies arthropathic psoriasis (L40.5-) as a condition that is not reported with a code from Chapter 13.*

6. What condition would be reported with a code from subcategory M48.5- Collapsed vertebra?

   c. **Wedging of vertebra**

   Rationale: *Subcategory (M48.5) is reported for collapsed vertebra, which may also be documented as wedging of vertebra. Codes for collapsed vertebra are not used to report a current injury due to fatigue fracture, pathological fractures due to neoplasm, osteoporosis or other pathological condition, or for traumatic fractures.*

7. What information is NOT required to assign the most specific code for idiopathic scoliosis?

   d. **The specific form of scoliosis**

   Rationale: *Idiopathic scoliosis is a specific form of scoliosis. It identifies the condition as being of unknown cause. Other forms are thoracogenic, neuromuscular, other secondary and other specified forms. The age of the patient is required in order to correctly classify the condition as infantile, juvenile, or adolescent. The location of the curve must be identified which may be documented as involving the either by the vertebra (T5-T10) involved or the region of the spine (thoracic).*

8. Codes for osteoporosis in category M80 are specific to site. What does the site designate?

   c. **The site of the fracture**

   Rationale: *Osteoporosis is a systemic condition, meaning that all bones of the musculoskeletal system are affected. Therefore, site is not a component of the codes under category M81 Osteoporosis without current pathological fracture. The site codes under M80 Osteoporosis with current pathological fracture identify the site of the fracture not the osteoporosis.*

9. Code M61.371 Calcification and ossification of muscles associated with burns, right ankle and foot is an example of what type of code?

   b. **A combination code**

   Rationale: *This is an example of a combination code. It captures the disease, disorder or other condition which is calcification and ossification of the muscles and the cause or etiology of the condition which is the burn.*

10. What descriptor is not an example of site specificity?

    c. **Synovium**

    Rationale: *Synovium is a type of tissue in the joints not a specific site in the musculoskeletal system. The site would be a specific joint such as the shoulder, wrist, or knee.*

11. What information must be documented to assign the most specific code in category M1A Chronic gout that is not required for codes in category M10 Gout?

    a. **With or without tophus**

    Rationale: *A 7th character is required for chronic gout to identify the condition as with or without tophus.*

Chapter 16
CONGENITAL ANOMALIES

Introduction

Congenital anomalies are conditions that are present at birth. Congenital anomalies include both congenital malformations, such as spina bifida, atrial and ventricular septal heart defects, undescended testis, and chromosomal abnormalities such as trisomy 21 also known as Down syndrome. These conditions are coded in Chapter 16 Congenital Malformation, Deformations, and Chromosomal Abnormalities and are grouped together first by body system, followed by other congenital conditions such as syndromes affecting multiple systems, and chromosomal abnormalities not elsewhere classified.

Codes for congenital malformations, deformations, and chromosomal abnormalities require specific documentation related to these conditions. For example, codes for encephalocele are specific to site and must be documented as frontal, nasofrontal, occipital, or of other specific sites. Other conditions such as cleft lip and palate do not require documentation of the condition as complete or incomplete but do require specific documentation of the site of the opening in the palate as either the hard or soft palate, and the location of the cleft lip as unilateral, in the median, or bilateral.

Below is a table showing the 11 code blocks that make up Chapter 16:

ICD-10-CM Blocks	
Q00-Q07	Congenital Malformations of the Nervous System
Q10-Q18	Congenital Malformations of Eye, Ear, Face and Neck
Q20-Q28	Congenital Malformations of the Circulatory System
Q30-Q34	Congenital Malformations of the Respiratory System
Q35-Q37	Cleft Lip and Cleft Palate
Q38-Q45	Other Congenital Malformations of the Digestive System
Q50-Q56	Congenital Malformations of the Genital Organs
Q60-Q64	Congenital Malformations of the Urinary System
Q65-Q79	Congenital Malformations and Deformations of the Musculoskeletal System
Q80-Q89	Other Congenital Malformations
Q90-Q99	Chromosomal Abnormalities, Not Elsewhere Classified

Coding Note(s)

There is a chapter level note indicating that codes from Chapter 17 are not to be used on maternal or fetal records.

Exclusions

An Excludes2 note indicates that inborn errors of metabolism are not inherently included in codes from Chapter 17. Inborn errors of metabolism may occur at the same time and includes conditions such as classical phenylketonuria (PKU) (E70.0), albinism (E70.3-), congenital lactase deficiency (E73.0), and hereditary fructose intolerance (E74.12). If the patient has both types of conditions/diseases and it is clearly documented, codes for inborn errors of metabolism may be reported together with codes for congenital anomalies.

Excludes1	Excludes2
None	Inborn errors of metabolism (E70-E88)

Chapter Guidelines

When a malformation, deformation, or chromosomal abnormality is documented, the appropriate code from categories Q00-Q99 is assigned. Specific guidelines are as follows:

- A malformation, deformation, or chromosomal abnormality may be the principal or first-listed diagnosis or it may be a secondary diagnosis
- For the birth admission, the principal diagnosis is always a code from category Z38 Liveborn infants according to place of birth and type of delivery, followed by any applicable congenital anomaly codes in categories Q00-Q99
- When there is not a specific diagnosis for the malformation, deformation, or chromosomal abnormality, additional codes are assigned for any manifestations that are present
- When the code specifically identifies the malformation, deformation, or chromosomal abnormality, the following rules apply:
  - Manifestations that are an inherent component of the anomaly should not be coded separately
  - Additional codes may be reported for manifestations that are not an inherent component of the anomaly
- Codes from Chapter 17 may be used throughout the life of the patient
- If the congenital malformation or deformity has been corrected, a personal history code should be used to identify the history of the malformation or deformity
- Although present at birth the congenital malformation, deformation, or chromosomal abnormality may not be diagnosed until later in life and it is appropriate to assign a code from Chapter 17 when the physician documentation supports a diagnosis of a congenital anomaly

General Documentation Requirements

Documentation requirements for congenital malformations, deformations, and chromosomal abnormalities may involve site specificity. For example, there are specific codes for sacral spina bifida with and without hydrocephalus (Q05.3, Q05.8). Congenital absence, atresia, and stenosis of the small (Q41) and large (Q42) intestines provide another example of site specificity requiring documentation of the site as the duodenum, jejunum, ileum, other specified parts of the small intestine, rectum, anus, or other parts of the large intestine.

Another documentation requirement is laterality. For conditions classified in Chapter 17, this primarily involves identifying the condition as unilateral or bilateral for paired organs and structures, although congenital absence and reduction defects of the limbs also require documentation of right, left, or bilateral. Many similar conditions are assigned specific, separate codes instead of being covered together with one reportable code, such as specific codes for biliary atresia (Q44.2), congenital stenosis or stricture of the bile ducts (Q44.3), and choledochal cyst (Q44.4). The code for other congenital malformations of the bile ducts (Q44.5) includes accessory or duplicate hepatic duct, biliary duct, or cystic duct.

For congenital conditions, greater specificity often allows the severity of the condition to be captured. For example, the severity of hypospadias is captured by codes that identify the site of the malpositioned urethral opening as balanic, penile, penoscrotal, or perineal. Knowing where it manifests allows capture of the severity of this congenital malformation.

While in many cases the physician documentation will be sufficient to capture the most specific code, it is necessary for physicians and coders to review the documentation, even for many commonly treated conditions, to ensure that the documentation meets the requirements for reporting the code to the greatest degree of granularity.

Code-Specific Documentation Requirements

In this section, ICD-10-CM codes are listed and corresponding documentation requirements are identified. The focus is on conditions that require specific clinical documentation requirements in more than one axis. Although not all codes with significant documentation requirements are discussed, this section will provide a representative sample of the type of documentation needed for reporting congenital anomalies.

Cleft Palate and Cleft Lip

Cleft palate is a birth defect of the roof of the mouth characterized by a split or opening in the palate. The defect may involve the bony front portion of the palate, called the hard palate, the soft back portion of the palate, called the soft palate, or both the hard and soft palate. The defect in the palate may be complete or incomplete. A complete cleft palate involves both the soft and hard palate, and there may also be a gap in the maxilla. An incomplete cleft palate involves either the hard or soft palate but does not extend through both. It may present as an opening in the roof of the mouth, and most often involves only the soft palate. When cleft of the soft palate occurs (with or without the hard palate), the uvula is usually split, which occurs due to failure of fusion of the lateral palatine processes, the nasal septum, and/or the median palatine processes. Cleft palate may occur on one side (unilateral) or on both sides (bilateral).

Cleft lip is a birth defect of the upper lip that is characterized by a split, or gap, in the upper lip. The split may be only a small notch or it may extend into the nose and involve both the soft tissues and bone of the maxilla and nose. A cleft lip that does not extend into the nose may be referred to as an incomplete cleft lip, while one that extends into the nose may be referred to as a complete cleft clip. Cleft lip may affect one side or both sides. Because the palate and lip develop separately, these birth defects may occur alone or they may occur together.

Cleft palate and/or lip are classified first by whether they occur alone or together. For a cleft palate (Q35), the site of the defect is then identified. Instead of using the descriptors complete and incomplete, ICD-10-CM identifies the defect specifically as involving the hard palate, soft palate, or hard palate with soft palate. Complete and incomplete terminology is not used. There is also a code for cleft uvula. When cleft palate occurs alone, it is not classified as unilateral or bilateral. For cleft lip (Q36), the location defect is identified as bilateral, median, or unilateral. When the two defects occur together (Q37), the palate defect is identified first in the code description and must be documented as being in the hard, soft, or both hard and soft palate. The defect in the lip is then identified and must be documented as unilateral or bilateral.

Coding and Documentation Requirements

Identify condition:

- Cleft palate
- Cleft lip
- Cleft palate and cleft lip

For cleft palate without cleft lip identify site:

- Hard palate
- Soft palate
- Hard and soft palate
- Uvula
- Unspecified

For cleft lip without cleft palate identify site/laterality:

- Bilateral
- Median
- Unilateral

For cleft palate occurring with cleft lip, identify defect sites in combination:

- First for Cleft palate:
  - Hard palate
  - Soft palate
  - Hard and soft palate
  - Unspecified
- Together with Cleft lip:
  - Bilateral
  - Unilateral

ICD-1Ø-CM Code/Documentation	
Q35.1	Cleft hard palate
Q35.3	Cleft soft palate
Q35.5	Cleft hard palate with cleft soft palate
Q35.7	Cleft uvula
Q35.9	Cleft palate, unspecified
Q36.Ø	Cleft lip, bilateral
Q36.1	Cleft lip, median
Q36.9	Cleft lip, unilateral
Q37.Ø	Cleft hard palate with bilateral cleft lip
Q37.1	Cleft hard palate with unilateral cleft lip
Q37.2	Cleft soft palate with bilateral cleft lip
Q37.3	Cleft soft palate with unilateral cleft lip
Q37.4	Cleft hard and soft palate with bilateral cleft lip
Q37.5	Cleft hard and soft palate with unilateral cleft lip
Q37.8	Unspecified cleft palate with bilateral cleft lip
Q37.9	Unspecified cleft palate with unilateral cleft lip

Note: When cleft lip alone is unspecified as to site, Q36.9 for unilateral cleft lip is assigned.

Documentation and Coding Example

ENT Note: Patient is a newborn who was noted to have a **cleft palate** during routine exam in WBN. This healthy appearing Caucasian female was born via SVD seven hours ago to a G5 mother who had regular prenatal care with a midwife. Following the birth, mother attempted to breast feed but noticed the baby had trouble latching and had a poor suck. Infant has no dysmorphic facial features and is alert and active on exam. BW 345Ø grams, Length 5Ø cm. HC 34.5 cm. No defect in the lip is noted. There is a **V-shaped cleft of the hard and soft palates extending just to the uvula**. Patent nares. No ear deformities.

Impression: **Cleft hard palate with cleft soft palate**. Feeding specialist has already been in and is working with mother to pump and feed expressed breast milk. Met with parents to discuss findings and they appear comfortable with the infant and have supportive family to help them out. Mother had planned to leave the hospital within 12 hours of delivery but will stay until baby is stable and feeding well. Parents understand that surgery will be necessary but there is no urgency to it.

Plan: Continue feeding support with specialist. Newborn hearing exam prior to discharge. Genetic consult and work up. Patient may be discharged when pediatrician feels she is stable. Follow up with ENT in 2 weeks, sooner if there are any problems.

Diagnosis Code(s)

Q35.5 Cleft hard palate with cleft soft palate

Coding Note(s)

The site of the cleft palate is specifically identified in the code, and laterality is not reported for cleft palate alone.

Congenital Hydrocephalus

Congenital hydrocephalus is the excessive accumulation of cerebrospinal fluid (CSF) in the brain. Congenital hydrocephalus is a condition that is present at birth although it might not be diagnosed until later in infancy.

The ventricular system in the brain is made up of four ventricles connected by narrow passages. The ventricles are filled with CSF which is a clear fluid that surrounds the brain and spinal cord. Normally, CSF flows through the ventricles and then into cisterns which are closed spaces that serve as CSF reservoirs at the base of the brain. CSF bathes the surfaces of the brain and spinal cord and then is reabsorbed into the bloodstream. Any imbalance between production and absorption of CSF caused either by obstruction of CSF flow from one region of the brain to another, or by failure to reabsorb CSF, can cause an over-accumulation of CSF in the brain resulting in hydrocephalus.

Category QØ3 Congenital hydrocephalus contains four codes:

- Code QØ3.Ø Malformations of the aqueduct of Sylvius identifies one of the most common causes of congenital hydrocephalus, which is stenosis or narrowing of this small passage between the third and fourth ventricles in the middle of the brain.
- Code QØ3.1 Atresia of foramina of Magendie and Luschka, also called Dandy-Walker syndrome, is another common cause of obstructive internal hydrocephalus. An enlarged fourth ventricle and loss of the area between the two cerebellar hemispheres causes an increase in the fluid-filled spaces around the brain.
- There are also codes for other specified types of congenital hydrocephalus, QØ3.8, and unspecified congenital hydrocephalus, QØ3.9.

Careful attention must be paid to the documentation to ensure that the hydrocephalus is not associated with spina bifida or Arnold-Chiari syndrome Type II. Hydrocephalus with spina bifida is reported with codes QØ5.Ø-QØ5.4, and hydrocephalus associated with Arnold-Chiari syndrome Type II is reported with codes QØ7.Ø2 and QØ7.Ø3 (with both spina bifida and hydrocephalus).

Coding and Documentation Requirements

Identify the type of congenital hydrocephalus:

- Atresia of foramina of Magendie and Luschka (Dandy-Walker syndrome)
- Malformations of aqueduct of Sylvius
- Other specified type of congenital hydrocephalus
- Unspecified congenital hydrocephalus

ICD-1Ø-CM Code/Documentation	
QØ3.Ø	Malformations of aqueduct of Sylvius
QØ3.1	Atresia of foramina of Magendie and Luschka
QØ3.8	Other congenital hydrocephalus
QØ3.9	Congenital hydrocephalus, unspecified

Documentation and Coding Example

Seven-month-old male infant is brought to ED by mother with irritability and vomiting. Mother states she has been concerned about her child for a few months due to increasing head size and decreased muscle tone. She expressed her concerns to the pediatrician one month ago at his 6-month check-up but the doctor just dismissed them and said he was fine. T 98.8, P 100, R 16, BP 100/40, Wt. 17 lbs. HC 48 cm. On examination, this is fussy infant with a large head and poor neck muscle control. Anterior fontanelle open and bulging. Sutures are widely separated and he has a large network of veins over the scalp. PERRL with papilledema, downward pupil gaze, and nystagmus noted on exam. Cranial nerves grossly intact. Heart rate regular, breath sounds clear. Abdomen soft, round with active bowel sounds. Mother states infant appears hungry and will breast feed but vomits soon after eating. He has refused solid foods today. Pediatric Neurology called to see infant and orders a CT scan under sedation, admit to pediatric floor following the scan.

Pediatric Neurology Admit Note: CT scan shows **atresia of the foramen Magendie and Luschka with hydrocephalus in the fourth ventricle.** Pediatric neurosurgery has been called to consult for shunt insertion. Pre-operative labs have been drawn including CBC, coagulation studies, comprehensive metabolic panel. Patient is NPO and receiving IV fluids for hydration.

Diagnosis Code(s)

Q03.1 Atresia of foramina of Magendie and Luschka

Coding Note(s)

The congenital hydrocephalus is due to congenital absence of the two foramina (openings) in the fourth ventricle of the brain preventing the normal flow of CSF and causing accumulation of fluid in this region of the brain. There is a specific code for this condition, Q03.1 Atresia of foramina of Magendie and Luschka.

Down Syndrome

Normally each individual has 46 chromosomes – 23 from each parent. Some genetic anomalies are caused by an individual receiving an extra copy of a chromosome from one parent, so these individuals have 47 chromosomes. Down syndrome, now more commonly referred to as Trisomy 21, is caused by an additional copy of chromosome 21. There are three recognized genetic variations related to Trisomy 21 which include nonmosaicism, mosaicism, and translocation. The symptoms of the condition may vary significantly depending on the form of Trisomy 21.

Nonmosaicism – In nonmosaicism Down Syndrome, one of the gamete cells (either sperm or egg) which normally contain 23 chromosomes has an extra copy of Chromosome 21. The embryo then has 47 chromosomes. This is the most common form of Trisomy 21, occurring in 95 percent of individuals with this genetic condition. The maternal egg cell is responsible for this form of Down Syndrome about 88 percent of the time, the paternal sperm cell only about 8 percent of the time.

Mosaicism – In the mosaicism form of Down Syndrome, a nondisjunction event occurs on chromosome 21 during early cell division of normal gametes (egg or sperm cell with 23 chromosomes). This causes some cells to have 47 chromosomes and others to have the normal number of 46. This is an uncommon form of Trisomy 21, occurring in only 1-2 percent of all individuals identified with Down Syndrome.

Robertsonian Translocation – This form of Down Syndrome may also be referred to as Familial Down Syndrome and occurs in 2-3 percent of cases. It can come from either the paternal line or maternal line and is not associated with a maternal age defect. In a translocation, the long arm of Chromosome 21 attaches to another chromosome, most often Chromosome 14. The parent is phenotypically normal, but with normal disjunction it is possible for a gamete to be formed that has an extra 21st chromosome.

Coding and Documentation Requirements

Identify the form of Trisomy 21:

- Mosaicism
- Nonmosaicism
- Translocation
- Unspecified

ICD-10-CM Code/Documentation	
Q90.0	Trisomy 21, nonmosaicism (meiotic nondisjunction)
Q90.1	Trisomy 21, mosaicism (mitotic nondisjunction)
Q90.2	Trisomy 21, translocation
Q90.9	Down syndrome, unspecified

Documentation and Coding Example

Three-week-old Caucasian female is seen with her parents in genetic clinic to report on recent testing. Infant was observed to have some unusual features at birth, suggesting a genetic problem. Mother is age 27, father age 29 and this is their first child. Pregnancy was uncomplicated. Mothers AFP was WNL, prenatal ultrasounds were normal. The genetic history for both families is unremarkable. Infant is thriving despite having decreased muscle tone and poor suck. Mother has been assisted to pump and breast feed by a lactation consultant and infant is now getting most of her nutrition directly from the breast. Genetic tests confirm the infant has **Trisomy 21, mosaicism**. Patient has very few characteristics of Down Syndrome but of significance are small ears and mouth and some excess skin at the back of her neck. She had a cardiac echo prior to discharge because of a heart murmur and she does have a **small ASD** that will be monitored by Pediatric Cardiology. Parents are offered information on support groups and their questions are answered. We will remain in contact with the family for as long as they desire support and services.

Diagnosis Code(s)

Q90.1 Trisomy 21, mosaicism (mitotic nondisjunction)

Q21.1 Atrial septal defect

Coding Note(s)

Code Q90.1 specifically identifies the form of Trisomy 21 as mosaicism. Coding guidelines state that additional conditions that are not an inherent component of the anomaly should be reported. The atrial septal defect is a condition that is often associated with Trisomy 21 but is not an inherent component of the defect so code Q21.1 is assigned for the atrial septal defect additionally.

Encephalocele

An encephalocele is a rare disorder in which the bones of the skull do not close completely. This results in a bone gap through which cerebral spinal fluid, brain tissue, and the meninges (membrane that covers the brain) can protrude. This results in a sac-like malformation outside the skull. An encephalocele is a type of neural tube defect. The neural tube is the embryonic tissue that forms the brain, spinal cord, and the surrounding bones of the skull. An encephalocele may also be referred to by the following terms:

- Cephalocele
- Cerebral meningocele
- Cranial hydromeningocele
- Encephalocystocele
- Encephalomyelocele
- Hydroencephalocele
- Meningoencephalocele

Another term used to refer to an encephalocele is Type III Arnold-Chiari syndrome. Careful review of documentation for Arnold-Chiari syndrome is required because only Type III is reported with a code from category Q01 Encephalocele. Arnold-Chiari syndrome Type II is reported with codes from subcategory Q07.0-, which are also the default codes for Arnold-Chiari syndrome not otherwise specified. There is also a Type IV Arnold Chiari syndrome which is reported with code Q04.8 Other specified congenital malformations of the brain.

Codes for encephalocele are found in category Q01. There are specific codes for the most common encephalocele locations which include midline of the upper anterior part of the skull (frontal), the area between the forehead and the nose (nasofrontal), and the back of the skull (occipital or basal).

Coding and Documentation Requirements

Identify site of encephalocele:

- Frontal
- Nasofrontal
- Occipital
- Other specified site
- Unspecified site

ICD-10-CM Code/Documentation	
Q01.0	Frontal encephalocele
Q01.1	Nasofrontal encephalocele
Q01.2	Occipital encephalocele
Q01.8	Encephalocele of other sites
Q01.9	Encephalocele, unspecified

Documentation and Coding Example

Patient is a two-month-old Caucasian female scheduled for elective cranial surgery to close an **occipital encephalocele**. The defect was found on prenatal ultrasound at 28 weeks gestation. Mother did not have an elevated AFP level and amniocentesis revealed normal 46 XX chromosome pattern. Infant was delivered via elective C-section at 39 weeks and she had an unremarkable neonatal period. MRI imaging at 2 days of age, revealed a 2 x 2 cm rhombic roof encephalocele, caudal to the torcula, containing cerebral spinal fluid but no brain tissue. Patient had a normal neurological workup and because she was somewhat small for gestational age, the team decided to postpone surgery until she had gained weight and was thriving. Patient is now 8 lbs. 4 oz., up from a BW of 5 lbs. 13 oz. She is exclusively breast fed. On examination, this is an active, alert infant. Fontanelles are open and soft, **encephalocele is noted at base of skull as a soft cystic mass**. Heart rate regular, breath sounds clear and equal bilaterally. Abdomen soft and round with active bowel sounds. No hip click, diaper area clean. Patient is healthy and cleared for surgery. Note electronically sent to hospital, neurosurgeon and anesthesia.

Diagnosis Code(s)

Q01.2 Occipital encephalocele

Coding Note(s)

Code Q01.2 is specific for an occipital encephalocele, which might also be documented as basal encephalocele.

Gallbladder, Bile Ducts, and Liver Anomalies

Biliary atresia is a congenital condition characterized by a blockage in the bile ducts. The bile ducts carry bile from the liver to the gallbladder and a blockage of the ducts leads to liver damage which can be fatal if it is not treated. Congenital stenosis or stricture of the bile ducts is a narrowing of the ducts that impedes the flow of bile and can also cause liver damage. Choledochal cysts are cystic dilations of the bile ducts and may involve the intrahepatic and/or extrahepatic ducts.

Cystic liver disease is another condition that is believed to be congenital in origin. This type of liver disease is often benign, causing no symptoms and not requiring any treatment. The cause of simple liver cysts is not known. Adult polycystic liver disease is congenital and is usually associated with autosomal dominant polycystic kidney disease that is caused by genetic mutation of two genes, PKD1 and PKD2. The polycystic kidney disease (PKD) usually precedes the polycystic liver disease. While the PKD often results in kidney failure, liver failure is rarely seen due to polycystic liver disease.

Anomalies of the gallbladder include agenesis, aplasia, and hypoplasia. Agenesis, or absence of the gallbladder, is a rare anomaly and may be asymptomatic. Aplasia may also refer to congenital absence of the gallbladder or to defective development of the gallbladder, both of which are rare. Congenital hypoplasia, also a rare condition, refers to underdevelopment of the gallbladder.

There are specific codes for atresia of the bile ducts (Q44.2), congenital stenosis and stricture of the bile ducts (Q44.3), and choledochal cysts (Q44.4). There are also specific codes for cystic liver disease (Q44.6), and agenesis, aplasia and hypoplasia of the gallbladder (Q44.0). Codes for other specified anomalies of the gallbladder (Q44.1), bile ducts (Q44.5), and liver (Q44.7) are specific to each site. There are no codes for an unspecified anomaly of these organs.

Coding and Documentation Requirements

Identify condition by site:

- Bile ducts
  - Atresia
  - Choledochal cyst
  - Stenosis/stricture
  - Other congenital malformations, which includes:
    - » Accessory hepatic bile duct
    - » Bile duct duplication
    - » Cystic duct duplication
    - » Unspecified bile duct malformation
- Gallbladder
  - Agenesis/aplasia/hypoplasia
  - Other congenital malformations, which includes:
    - » Intrahepatic gallbladder
    - » Unspecified gallbladder malformation
- Liver
  - Cystic liver disease
  - Other congenital malformations, which includes:
    - » Accessory liver
    - » Alagille syndrome
    - » Congenital absence of liver
    - » Congenital hepatomegaly
    - » Unspecified liver malformation

ICD-10-CM Code/Documentation	
Q44.0	Agenesis, aplasia and hypoplasia of gallbladder
Q44.1	Other congenital malformation of gallbladder
Q44.2	Atresia of bile ducts
Q44.3	Congenital stenosis and stricture of bile ducts
Q44.4	Choledochal cyst
Q44.5	Other congenital malformations of bile ducts
Q44.6	Cystic disease of liver
Q44.7	Other congenital malformations of liver

Documentation and Coding Example

Four-week-old Asian female is referred to Pediatric Gastroenterology with new onset jaundice, irritability, and poor weight gain. Infant was born at 38 weeks, uncomplicated pregnancy and delivery, uneventful neonatal period. She was seen at 5 days of age and 14 days of age, was gaining weight and appeared to be doing well. Parents noticed mild jaundice a week ago that has gotten progressively worse with dark urine and grayish colored stools. Pediatrician ordered blood tests that revealed elevated bilirubin and LFTs. Abdominal x-ray significant for enlarged liver, spleen normal size. Liver was again noted to be enlarged on ultrasound and gallbladder could not be identified. She is scheduled for a HIDA scan in nuclear medicine tomorrow. On examination, this is an alert but fussy infant who is examined in her mother's arms. PERRL. Sclera and skin jaundiced. Skin is dry, muscle wasting is present. Nares patent with moist pink mucous membranes. Heart rate regular, breath sounds clear and equal. Abdomen is soft and round. Liver is palpated at 2 cm below the RCM, spleen at the LCM. Discussed possible causes of jaundice with parents, including a probable diagnosis of biliary atresia. Explained the HIDA test and its specificity for detecting that problem. Questions answered. They will return to clinic immediately following the HIDA scan tomorrow.

Peds GI Follow-up Note: HIDA scan showed no dye uptake by the gallbladder or flow into the intestine.

Diagnosis: **Congenital biliary atresia.**

Plan: Referral to Pediatric surgery for possible liver biopsy and/or exploratory laparotomy with operative cholangiogram.

Diagnosis Code(s)

Q44.2 Atresia of bile ducts

Coding Note(s)

Code Q44.2 is specific to congenital atresia of the bile ducts and does not include other congenital anomalies of the bile ducts, or the gallbladder. If they are also noted, separate codes would be reported for the specific conditions.

Hypospadias and Congenital Chordee

Hypospadias is a congenital anomaly in which the opening of the urethra is on the underside of the penis rather than being in its normal position at the tip of the penis. The condition varies in severity which is dependent upon the location of the urethral opening. The nearer the urethral opening is to the end or tip of the penis, the less severe the condition and the easier it is to treat.

Codes in category Q54 Hypospadias are specific to the site of the malpositioned urethral meatus (opening). Hypospadias is classified as follows:

Balanic hypospadias – The urethral meatus is near the tip on the underside of the glans penis; also referred to as glandular, or first-degree hypospadias. When the condition is described as coronal hypospadias, the urethral meatus is located in the coronal sulcus which is also reported with the code for balanic hypospadias and considered to be a first-degree hypospadias as well

Penile hypospadias – The urethral meatus is located on the underside of the penile shaft; also referred to as second-degree hypospadias

Penoscrotal hypospadias – The urethral meatus is located at the junction of the penis and scrotum; also referred to as third-degree hypospadias

Perineal hypospadias – The urethral meatus is located in the perineum near the anus. This is another form of third-degree hypospadias

Other hypospadias – Includes hypospadias due to intersex state

Unspecified hypospadias – Hypospadias without documentation of the site of the urethral meatus

Congenital chordee (Q54.4) is also classified in the hypospadias category. Congenital chordee refers to a downward bowing or curvature of the erect penis and is often associated with hypospadias. Code Q54.4 is also used to report congenital chordee without hypospadias.

Coding and Documentation Requirements

Identify condition:

- Hypospadias
- Congenital chordee

For hypospadias, identify site of urethral meatus:

- Balanic/glanular/coronal
- Penile
- Penoscrotal
- Perineal
- Other specified site
- Unspecified site

ICD-10-CM Code/Documentation	
Q54.0	Hypospadias, balanic
Q54.1	Hypospadias, penile
Q54.2	Hypospadias, penoscrotal
Q54.3	Hypospadias, perineal
Q54.8	Other hypospadias
Q54.9	Hypospadias, unspecified
Q54.4	Congenital chordee

Documentation and Coding Example

Patient is a one-month-old Caucasian male who is seen today in Pediatric Urology for **hypospadias**. Infant was born at 38 weeks gestation via repeat C-section. He voided in the delivery room and was noted to have an abnormal appearing foreskin and glans on initial newborn examination. Parents are of Jewish faith and it was very important for them to have their son circumcised within eight days of his birth. A pediatric urologist who is himself Jewish was called to examine the infant and meet with the family, their Mohel and Rabbi. Family was assured by their religious leaders that it was acceptable under these circumstances to have a urologist perform the circumcision in a hospital when the baby is older. On examination today, the infant is alert and active. Mother states he is breast feeding well, voiding and stooling. Abdomen is soft and round. Testes are descended bilaterally. The glans penis is spatulated with a prepuce cleft ventrally and a dorsally hooded foreskin. There is no chordee appreciated.

Impression: **Balanic hypospadias**.

Plan: Surgical repair when infant is 9-12 months or when he weighs at least 15 lbs.

Diagnosis Code(s)

Q54.0 Hypospadias, balanic

Coding Note(s)

The spatulated glans penis, ventral prepuce cleft, and dorsally hooded foreskin are commonly associated with balanic hypospadias and are not reported additionally.

Intestinal Atresia and Stenosis

Atresia of the small or large intestine refers to a complete obstruction of a portion of the intestine, while stenosis refers to a smaller than normal lumen with incomplete obstruction, often secondary to a diaphragm or web formation within the stenotic portion. This group of anomalies also includes congenital absence of a portion of the intestine.

Categories Q41 and Q42 contain codes for congenital absence, atresia, and stenosis of the small and large intestines respectively. For the small intestine, there are specific codes for the duodenum (Q41.0), jejunum (Q41.1), ileum (Q41.2), other specified parts of the small intestine (Q41.8), and unspecified part of small intestine (Q41.9). For the large intestine, there are specific codes for the rectum (Q42.0, Q42.1) and anus (Q42.2, Q42.3). The codes for these sites also require documentation of with or without fistula. When the condition affects other specified parts of the large intestine, code Q42.8 is reported and there is also a code for unspecified site in the large intestine (Q42.9).

Coding and Documentation Requirements

Identify site:

- Small intestine
  - Duodenum
  - Jejunum
  - Ileum
  - Other specified site
  - Unspecified site
- Large intestine
- Anus
  - With fistula
  - Without fistula
- Rectum
  - With fistula
  - Without fistula
- Other specified parts of the large intestine
- Unspecified part of the large intestine

ICD-10-CM Code/Documentation	
Q42.0	Congenital absence, atresia and stenosis of rectum with fistula
Q42.1	Congenital absence, atresia and stenosis of rectum without fistula
Q42.2	Congenital absence, atresia and stenosis of anus with fistula
Q42.3	Congenital absence, atresia and stenosis of anus without fistula
Q42.8	Congenital absence, atresia and stenosis of other specified parts of large intestine
Q42.9	Congenital absence, atresia and stenosis of large intestine, part unspecified
Q41.0	Congenital absence, atresia and stenosis of duodenum
Q41.1	Congenital absence, atresia and stenosis of jejunum
Q41.2	Congenital absence, atresia and stenosis of ileum
Q41.8	Congenital absence, atresia and stenosis of other specified parts of small intestine
Q41.9	Congenital absence, atresia and stenosis of small intestine, part unspecified

Documentation and Coding Example

Procedure Note: Four-day-old infant undergoes therapeutic endoscopy for **congenital duodenal stenosis**. This Hispanic male was noted to have a distended stomach and duodenum on prenatal ultrasound at 28 weeks while his mother was being monitored for polyhydramnios. Amniocentesis was performed and showed a normal 46 XY chromosome pattern. Mother's amniotic fluid level normalized by 36 weeks and the labor was induced at 40.5 weeks. She had a SVD, infant's Apgar scores were good and he went to NICU for monitoring. Initial abdominal x-ray showed dilated stomach and an air filled divided duodenum with very little bowel gas. He was stabilized with IV fluids and on day 2 he had a GI series with contrast that was significant for an **area of stenosis in the middle of the duodenum**. Case was discussed with Pediatric GI team and surgeons. Decision made to attempt an endoscopic repair in the OR under anesthesia and if unsuccessful the surgical team will perform an open laparotomy. The infant was brought to the OR, intubated, and under monitored anesthesia care the endoscope was passed easily into the stomach and then into the duodenum. A **mucosal diaphragm was then encountered which appeared to be the cause of the stenosis**. It was ablated with the laser and a balloon catheter was passed though the narrowed duodenum. The stenotic area was dilated successfully and the catheter was withdrawn. There was no bleeding and the endoscope was withdrawn. Patient went to the PACU in good condition.

Diagnosis: **Congenital stenosis of the duodenum**

Diagnosis Code(s)

Q41.0 Congenital absence, atresia and stenosis of duodenum

Coding Note(s)

There is a specific code for the congenital absence, atresia, and stenosis of the duodenum. A mucosal web or diaphragm is a common finding for the cause of atresia and stenosis of the duodenum and is not reported additionally.

Renal Agenesis / Dysgenesis

Renal agenesis is a condition in which one or both kidneys fail to develop. Unilateral renal agenesis is one of the more common congenital anomalies but is of relatively little concern as long as the single developed kidney is healthy. Bilateral renal agenesis is rare and is associated with Potter's syndrome which refers to additional malformations caused by low levels of amniotic fluid (oligohydramnios) that are a direct result of the bilateral renal agenesis. Additional malformations in Potter's syndrome include clubbed feet, pulmonary hypoplasia, and cranial anomalies that occur when there is not enough amniotic fluid to allow the fetus to develop normally. Potter's syndrome may also be referred to as Potter's sequence. Renal dysgenesis is a nonspecific term that refers to any form of abnormal development of the kidneys. Renal hypoplasia is a congenital condition in which one or both kidneys are smaller than normal but are normal in shape and retain some function.

Category Q60 Renal agenesis and other reduction defects of the kidney includes conditions documented as congenital absence or atrophy of the kidney and infantile atrophy of the kidney. There are specific codes for renal agenesis and renal hypoplasia, and also a code for Potter's syndrome. Renal agenesis and renal hypoplasia also require documentation indicating whether one (unilateral) or both (bilateral) kidneys are affected.

Coding and Documentation Requirements

Identify condition:

- Renal agenesis
- Renal hypoplasia
- Potter's syndrome

Identify laterality:

- Bilateral
- Unilateral
- Unspecified

Note: Potter's syndrome is always associated with bilateral renal agenesis, so documentation of laterality is not required.

ICD-10-CM Code/Documentation	
Q60.0	Renal agenesis, unilateral
Q60.1	Renal agenesis, bilateral
Q60.2	Renal agenesis, unspecified
Q60.3	Renal hypoplasia, unilateral
Q60.4	Renal hypoplasia, bilateral
Q60.5	Renal hypoplasia, unspecified
Q60.6	Potter's syndrome

Documentation and Coding Example

Twelve-year-old Caucasian female is seen in Pediatric Urology Clinic for ongoing monitoring and care of **solitary kidney**. This young lady was identified with a **solitary right kidney** during a prenatal ultrasound. Patient is a triplet, born at 31 weeks gestation, severely IUGR. She has had an unremarkable childhood with normal illnesses, and one UTI at age 3. She took prophylactic antibiotics for 5 years following that UTI. No repeat infections since discontinuing the antibiotics. Patient had an ultrasound prior to this appointment which is unchanged from previous scans. There is **agenesis of the left kidney** with an elongated left adrenal gland. Right kidney is slightly larger than normal but has remained stable in size with good renal blood flow. Comprehensive metabolic panel shows normal kidney function, UA negative for protein, RBC, WBC or cast cells. Blood pressure is WNL for age. Patient and her mother are knowledgeable of her condition. She is not playing contact sports but does like to dance. Mother expresses some concerns about Swing dancing because that can be quite physical. Mother is reassured that she should be fine doing that activity.

Impression: **Stable size and function of right kidney. Left renal agenesis.**

Plan: Continue to monitor yearly, more often if problems arise.

Diagnosis Code(s)

Q60.0 Renal agenesis, unilateral

Coding Note(s)

There is a specific code for unilateral renal agenesis. When there is only one kidney, it is common for it to be larger than normal, and since the physician has documented that it is stable in size and functioning well, no additional code is reported.

Undescended/Ectopic/Retractile Testes

An undescended testis, also called cryptorchidism, refers to a condition where one or both testes have not descended to their normal position within the scrotum. Undescended testes may be palpable or nonpalpable. Intraabdominal testis refers to an undescended testis that remains in the region of origin in the retroperitoneum or abdomen. An ectopic testis is a variant of an undescended testis where the testis lies outside the usual pathway of descent. An ectopic perineal testis is a condition that occurs when the testis descends but instead of descending into the scrotum, it lies in an abnormal position between the penoscrotal raphe and the genitofemoral fold. An inguinal testis is an undescended testicle found in the inguinal canal that has not moved down into the scrotum. In normally descended testicles, only the spermatic cord is located within the inguinal canal. A high scrotal testis can be located within the upper scrotum, but may glide back into the low inguinal canal. Retractile testis refers to the tendency of a descended testis to ascend into the upper part of the scrotum or into the inguinal canal.

Specific documentation is required for codes in category Q53 Undescended and ectopic testicle as there are different codes to identify abdominal vs. ectopic perineal undescended testis, as well as ectopic testicle. Location must also be further identified by laterality. Retractile testis is not classified together with ectopic and undescended testis. The code for retractile testis is in subcategory Q55.2- Other and unspecified congenital malformations of testis and scrotum.

Coding and Documentation Requirements

Identify condition:

- Ectopic testis
- Retractile testis
- Undescended testicle
  - Ectopic perineal testis
  - Intraabdominal
  - Inguinal
  - High scrotal
  - Unspecified undescended testicle

Identify laterality:

- Bilateral
- Unilateral
- Unspecified

Note: Laterality is not required for retractile testis.

ICD-10-CM Code/Documentation	
Q53.00	Ectopic testis, unspecified
Q53.01	Ectopic testis, unilateral
Q53.02	Ectopic testes, bilateral
Q53.10	Unspecified undescended testicle, unilateral
Q53.111	Unilateral intraabdominal testis
Q53.112	Unilateral inguinal testis
Q53.12	Ectopic perineal testis, unilateral
Q53.13	Unilateral high scrotal testis
Q53.20	Undescended testicle, unspecified, bilateral
Q53.211	Bilateral intraabdominal testes
Q53.212	Bilateral inguinal testes
Q53.22	Ectopic perineal testis, bilateral
Q53.23	Bilateral high scrotal testes
Q53.9	Undescended testicle, unspecified
Q55.22	Retractile testicles

Documentation and Coding Example

Six-week-old Black male is seen for well-baby check-up. This infant was born at 33 weeks, product of a twin gestation to a 42-year-old G4 P0. He had an excellent neonatal period, required supplemental O2 for one week but did not require intubation. Was weaned to an open crib at 2 weeks and was nipple feeding and gaining weight by 4 weeks. He and his sister have been home for one week. Weight 2450 kg, Length 44 cm, HC 31 cm. He is being fed expressed breast milk exclusively. On examination, this is a quiet but very alert infant. He has a narrow head, open sutures, and soft fontanelles. PERRL. Strong suck with patent nares. Heart rate regular, breath sounds clear and equal bilaterally. Abdomen soft and round. Liver and spleen are not palpated. Umbilicus without drainage. Hips without clicks. Penis uncircumcised, foreskin easily retracts. Left testicle is palpated in scrotum. Right testicle can be palpated in the inguinal canal and moved partially into the scrotum but retracts back when pressure is released.

Impression: Stable preemie. **Right undescended inguinal testicle.**

Plan: Refer to Peds Urology.

Diagnosis Code(s)

Q53.112 Unilateral inguinal testis

Coding Note(s)

The code for unilateral inguinal testis is reported because the documentation identifies that the right testicle is located within the inguinal canal, even though it can be temporarily manipulated into the upper scrotum.

Summary

Congenital malformations, deformations, and chromosomal abnormalities require precise documentation to assign the most specific code. This may include documentation with terms such as hypoplasia of the kidney rather than dysgenesis of the kidney. For paired organs, documentation should also specify whether one (unilateral) or both (bilateral) organs are affected. Some conditions require documentation regarding the characteristics of the congenital anomaly, such as hypospadias, which now requires identification of the location of the urethral opening. Other conditions, such as cleft palate and cleft lip, require an understanding of classification changes. Cleft palate and cleft lip are not designated as complete or incomplete. For cleft palate, the condition must be documented as affecting the hard and/or the soft palate and/or uvula. Physicians and coders should review current ICD-10-CM codes for conditions that are commonly seen for treatment in the physician's office so that documentation practices can be reviewed and any documentation deficiencies corrected.

Resources

The following documentation checklists are included in Appendix A:

- Undescended/Retractile Testes

Chapter 16 Quiz

1. Which of the following conditions is not reported with a code from Chapter 17 Congenital Malformations, Deformations, and Chromosomal Abnormalities?
   a. Potter's syndrome
   b. Albinism
   c. Biliary atresia
   d. Retractile testis
2. What additional information for a diagnosis of retractile testis is required to assign the most specific code?
   a. Unilateral/bilateral
   b. Abdominal/ectopic
   c. Right/left/bilateral
   d. None of the above
3. The physician has documented that the patient has Arnold-Chiari syndrome. Is this documentation specific enough to assign a diagnosis code?
   a. No, the physician must document the condition as Type II, Type III or Type IV
   b. No, this terminology is no longer used and the physician must be asked to document the condition as an encephalocele, hydrocephalus, or another specific central nervous system anomaly
   c. Yes, Arnold Chiari syndrome not otherwise specified is reported as Type II
   d. No, the condition must be more specifically identified as with or without spina bifida and/or hydrocephalus
4. What condition is not reported with a code from category Q60 Renal agenesis and other reduction defects of the kidney?
   a. Congenital absence of the kidney
   b. Polycystic kidney disease
   c. Infantile atrophy of the kidney
   d. Potter's syndrome
5. The physician has documented that a male infant has unilateral undescended testes. Does this documentation allow assignment of the most specific code for the condition?
   a. Yes, the only additional information captured for undescended testes is whether one (unilateral) or both (bilateral) testes are undescended and the physician has already documented the condition as unilateral
   b. No, the physician should have documented the condition as right or left
   c. No, a more specific code could be assigned if the physician had also documented the condition as ectopic, ectopic perineal, intraabdominal, inguinal, or high scrotal testis
   d. No, laterality is not a component of the code, but rather the site is a component of the code
6. What is the principal diagnosis on the inpatient facility claim for the birth admission of a newborn with a congenital anomaly?
   a. The principle diagnosis is dependent on whether there are other conditions complicating the birth or other aspects of the birth admission
   b. The principal diagnosis is always the congenital anomaly
   c. The congenital anomaly may be the principal diagnosis or a secondary diagnosis
   d. A code from category Z38 is reported as the principle diagnosis
7. What code is assigned for a patient with a congenital malformation who has had the condition surgically repaired or corrected earlier in life?
   a. The code for the congenital malformation continues to be reported throughout the patient's life
   b. A code identifying a personal history of the congenital malformation is reported
   c. No code is reported
   d. A code identifying a personal history of the congenital malformation is reported with a code from Chapter 17 to identify the specific condition that was corrected.
8. When an older child or an adult is diagnosed with a congenital anomaly that was not previously diagnosed in infancy, how is the condition coded?
   a. If the physician documentation supports a diagnosis of congenital anomaly, then the code for the congenital anomaly is assigned, at any time throughout the life of the patient
   b. Codes for congenital conditions can only be assigned in infancy, so a code is not assigned
   c. Codes for congenital conditions can only be assigned in infancy, so a code for an acquired condition is assigned
   d. None of the above
9. The physician has documented that the patient has a unilateral incomplete cleft palate. What code is assigned?
   a. Q35.1 Cleft hard palate
   b. Q35.3 Cleft soft palate
   c. Q35.5 Cleft hard palate with cleft soft palate
   d. Q35.9 Cleft palate, unspecified
10. The physician has documented that the patient has a first-degree hypospadias. What is another term for first-degree hypospadias?
    a. Balanic
    b. Glandular
    c. Coronal
    d. All of the above

See next page for answers and rationales.

Chapter 16 Answers and Rationales

1. Which of the following conditions is not reported with a code from Chapter 17 Congenital Malformations, Deformations, and Chromosomal Abnormalities?

   b. Albinism

   Rationale: *Albinism is classified as an inborn error of metabolism and is reported with codes from Chapter 4 Endocrine, Nutritional and Metabolic Diseases.*

2. What additional information for a diagnosis of retractile testis is required to assign the most specific code?

   d. None of the above

   Rationale: *There is a single code, Q55.22 for retractile testis so no additional information is required to assign the most specific code.*

3. The physician has documented that the patient has Arnold-Chiari syndrome. Is this documentation specific enough to assign a diagnosis code?

   c. Yes, Arnold Chiari syndrome not otherwise specified is reported as Type II

   Rationale: *A specific code can be assigned with only a documented diagnosis of Arnold Chiari syndrome. Code Q07.00 Arnold Chiari syndrome (Type II) without spina bifida or hydrocephalus is the default code for Arnold Chiari syndrome not otherwise specified.*

4. What condition is not reported with a code from category Q60 Renal agenesis and other reduction defects of the kidney?

   b. Polycystic kidney disease

   Rationale: *Polycystic kidney disease is classified in category Q61, Cystic kidney disease. All of the other conditions are classified in Category Q60.*

5. The physician has documented that a male infant has unilateral undescended testes. Does this documentation allow assignment of the most specific code for the condition?

   c. No, a more specific code could be assigned if the physician had also documented the condition as ectopic, ectopic perineal, intraabdominal, inguinal, or high scrotal testis

   Rationale: *The condition must be documented as unilateral/bilateral and the specific location of the undescended testis as intraabdominal, ectopic, ectopic perineal, inguinal, or high scrotal must also be specified in order to assign the most specific code. Documentation of unilateral undescended testis is reported with code Q53.10 Unspecified undescended testicle, unilateral.*

6. What is the principal diagnosis on the inpatient facility claim for the birth admission of a newborn with a congenital anomaly?

   d. A code from category Z38 is reported as the principle diagnosis

   Rationale: *The principle diagnosis for the birth admission of a liveborn infant is always a code from category Z38 Liveborn infant according to place of birth and type of delivery. Any conditions complicating the care of the newborn are reported as secondary diagnoses.*

7. What code is assigned for a patient with a congenital malformation who has had the condition surgically repaired or corrected earlier in life?

   b. A code identifying a personal history of the congenital malformation is reported

   Rationale: *Coding guidelines state that if the congenital malformation or deformity has been corrected, a personal history code should be used to identify the history of the malformation or deformity.*

8. When an older child or an adult is diagnosed with a congenital anomaly that was not previously diagnosed in infancy, how is the condition coded?

   a. If the physician documentation supports a diagnosis of congenital anomaly, then the code for the congenital anomaly is assigned, at any time throughout the life of the patient

   Rationale: *Although present at birth, the congenital malformation, deformation, or chromosomal abnormality may not be diagnosed until later in life and it is appropriate to assign a code from Chapter 17 when the physician documentation supports a diagnosis of a congenital anomaly.*

9. The physician has documented that the patient has a unilateral incomplete cleft palate. What code is assigned?

   d. Q35.9 Cleft palate, unspecified

   Rationale: *Cleft palate is not classified as unilateral/bilateral or complete/incomplete. There is no documentation related to whether the hard or soft palate is involved, so the nonspecific code Q35.9 Cleft palate, unspecified is assigned.*

10. The physician has documented that the patient has a first-degree hypospadias. What is another term for first-degree hypospadias?

    d. All of the above

    Rationale: *First degree hypospadias is an alternate term used to describe the least severe form of hypospadias in which the urethral opening is located on the head or glans of the penis, or the coronal sulcus. The terms balanic and glandular are synonymous and are used to describe hypospadias where the urethral meatus is located on the ventral glans penis. The urethral meatus is located in the coronal sulcus in coronal hypospadias which is reported with the same code as balanic hypospadias (Q54.0).*

Chapter 17
CERTAIN CONDITIONS ORIGINATING IN THE PERINATAL PERIOD

Introduction

Perinatal conditions are found in Chapter 17 and have their origin in the period beginning before birth and extending through the first 28 days after birth. These conditions must originate during this period even though for some conditions, morbidity may not manifest until later. Codes from this chapter are used only on the newborn medical record, never on the maternal medical record. As long as the documentation supports the origin of the condition during the perinatal period, codes for perinatal conditions may be reported throughout the life of the patient, as long as the condition persists. Examples of conditions included in this chapter are maternal conditions that have affected or are suspected to have affected the fetus or newborn, prematurity, light for dates, birth injuries, and other conditions originating in the perinatal period and affecting specific body systems. Below is a table of perinatal condition blocks for chapter 17.

ICD-10-CM Blocks	
P00-P04	Newborn Affected by Maternal Factors and by Complications of Pregnancy, Labor, and Delivery
P05-P08	Disorders of Newborn Related to Length of Gestation and Fetal Growth
P09	Abnormal Findings on Neonatal Screening
P10-P15	Birth Trauma
P19-P29	Respiratory and Cardiovascular Disorders Specific to the Perinatal Period
P35-P39	Infections Specific to the Perinatal Period
P50-P61	Hemorrhagic and Hematological Disorders of Newborn
P70-P74	Transitory Endocrine and Metabolic Disorders Specific to Newborn
P76-P78	Digestive System Disorders of Newborn
P80-P83	Conditions Involving the Integument and Temperature Regulation of Newborn
P84	Other Problems with Newborn
P90-P96	Other Disorders Originating in the Perinatal Period

Coding Note(s)

There are chapter level coding notes for perinatal conditions. The Includes note identifies the types of conditions reported with codes from chapter 16 as those that have their origin in the perinatal period, before birth through the first 28 days after birth, even if death or morbidity occurs later. There is also a note indicating that the codes from this chapter are to be used on newborn records only, never on maternal records.

Exclusions

There is a chapter level Excludes2 note that identifies other types of conditions that are not inherently included in this chapter, such as congenital malformations and deformations, which may also be present and should also be assigned, only if there is clear documentation that the patient has both. The table below identifies the other conditions, diseases, or abnormalities that are not inherently included in chapter 16:

Exclude1	Excludes2
None	Congenital malformations, deformations and chromosomal abnormalities (Q00-Q99)
None	Endocrine, nutritional and metabolic diseases (E00-E88)
None	Injury, poisoning and certain other consequences of external causes (S00-T88)
None	Neoplasms (C00-D49)
None	Tetanus neonatorum (A33)

Chapter Guidelines

Chapter specific guidelines begin with a definition of the perinatal period to ensure that these codes are only reported for conditions originating before birth through the 28th day following birth. Chapter specific guidelines are reviewed here and include:

- General perinatal rules
- Observation and evaluation of newborns for suspected conditions not found
- Coding additional perinatal diagnoses
- Prematurity and fetal growth retardation
- Low birth weight and immaturity status
- Bacterial sepsis of newborn
- Stillbirth

General Perinatal Rules

The general perinatal rules are as follows:

- Use of Chapter 16 codes:
  - Codes in Chapter 16 are never for use on the maternal record and codes from Chapter 15, the obstetric chapter, are never permitted on the newborn record
  - Chapter 16 codes may be used throughout the life of the patient if the condition is still present
- Principle diagnosis for birth record:

- When coding the birth episode in a newborn record, assign a code from category Z38 Liveborn infants according to place of birth and type of delivery, as the principle diagnosis
- A code from category Z38 is assigned on the newborn record only once, to a newborn at the time of birth
- If the newborn is transferred to another institution, a code from category Z38 should not be used at the receiving hospital
- A code from category Z38 is used only on the newborn record, not on the mother's record

- Use of codes from other chapters with codes from Chapter 16:
  - Codes from other chapters may be used with codes from Chapter 16 if the codes from the other chapters provide more specific detail
  - Codes for signs and symptoms may be assigned when a definitive diagnosis has not been established
  - If the reason for the encounter is a perinatal condition, the code from Chapter 16 should be sequenced first
- Use of Chapter 16 codes after the perinatal period:
  - If a condition originating in the perinatal period continues throughout the life of the patient, the perinatal code should continue to be used regardless of the patient's age
- Birth process or community acquired conditions:
  - If a newborn has a condition that may be either due to the birth process or community acquired, and the documentation does not indicate which it is, the default is due to the birth process and a code from Chapter 16 should be used.
  - If the condition is documented as community-acquired, a code from Chapter 16 should not be assigned
- Code all clinically significant conditions:
  - All clinically significant conditions noted on routine newborn examination should be coded. A condition is clinically significant if it requires any of the following:
    - » Clinical evaluation
    - » Therapeutic treatment
    - » Diagnostic procedures
    - » Extended length of hospital stay
    - » Increased nursing care and/or monitoring
    - » Has implications for future health care needs
  - The perinatal guidelines listed above for clinically significant conditions are the same as the general coding guidelines for "additional diagnoses", except for the final point regarding implications for future health care needs. Codes should be assigned for conditions that have been specified by the provider as having implications for future health care needs.

Observation and Evaluation of Newborns for Suspected Conditions Not Found

- When a healthy newborn is evaluated for a suspected condition that is determined after study not to be present, assign a code from category Z05 Observation and evaluation of newborns and infants for suspected conditions ruled out. Do not use category Z05 codes when the patient has signs or symptoms of a suspected problem; code the sign or symptom in such cases
- A code from category Z05 may also be assigned as a principal or first-listed code for readmissions or encounters when the code from category Z38 no longer applies
- Codes from category Z05 are for use only for healthy newborns and infants for which no condition after study is found to be present
- On a birth record, a code from category Z05 is to be used as a secondary code after the code from category Z38 Liveborn infants according to place of birth and type of delivery
- Codes in categories P00-P04 are for use when the listed maternal conditions are specified as the cause of confirmed or potential morbidity which has its origin in the perinatal period (before birth through the first 28 days after birth).

Coding Additional Perinatal Diagnoses

Guidelines for coding additional perinatal diagnoses are as follows:

- Assign codes for conditions that require treatment or further investigation, prolong the length of stay, or require additional resource utilization
- Assign codes for conditions that have been specified by the provider as having implications for future healthcare needs.

Note: This guideline should not be used for adult patients.

Prematurity and Fetal Growth Retardation

Providers utilize different criteria in determining prematurity. A code for prematurity should not be assigned unless specifically documented by the physician. Two code categories are provided in ICD-10-CM for reporting prematurity and fetal growth retardation:

- P05 Disorders of newborn related to slow fetal growth and fetal malnutrition
- P07 Disorders of newborn related to short gestation and low birth weight, not elsewhere classified

Guidelines for coding prematurity and fetal growth retardation documented by the physician are as follows:

- Assignment of codes in categories P05 and P07 should be based on the recorded birth weight and estimated gestational age
- Codes from category P05 and category P07 should not be assigned together
- When both the birth weight and gestational age are available, two codes from category P07 should be assigned, with the code for birth weight sequenced before the code for gestational age

Low Birth Weight and Immaturity Status

Codes for low birth weight and immaturity status are located in category P07 Disorders of newborn related to short gestation and low birth weight, not elsewhere classified. Codes from category P07 are for use for a child or adult who was premature or had a low birth weight as a newborn and this is affecting the patient's current health status. See also the chapter specific guidelines for

Chapter 21 Factors Influencing Health Status and Contact with Health Services.

Bacterial Sepsis of Newborn

Category P36 Bacterial sepsis of newborn, includes congenital sepsis. Guidelines are as follows:

- If the perinate is documented as having sepsis without documentation of congenital or community acquired, the default is congenital and a code from category P36 should be assigned
- If the P36 code includes the causal organism, an additional code from categories B95 or B96 should not be assigned
- If the P36 code does not include the causal organism, assign an additional code from category B96 Other bacterial agents as the cause of diseases classified elsewhere
- If applicable, use additional codes to identify severe sepsis (R65.2-) and any associated acute organ dysfunction

Stillbirth

Code P95 Stillbirth is only for use in institutions that maintain separate records for stillbirths. No other code should be used with code P95, which should not be used on the mother's record.

General Documentation Requirements

Code Specificity

Some codes for conditions originating in the perinatal period require site specificity and others specific documentation of the condition. An example of a condition requiring site specificity is subdural and cerebral hemorrhage due to birth trauma. Codes in category P10 Intracranial laceration and hemorrhage due to birth injury, are specific to the site of the laceration or hemorrhage and require documentation of the site as either subdural (P10.0), cerebral (P10.1), intraventricular (P10.2), subarachnoid (P10.4), or tentorial tear (P10.4). There is also a code for other specified intracranial lacerations and hemorrhages due to birth injury (P10.8) and a code for unspecified intracranial laceration and hemorrhage due to birth injury (P10.9). An example of required specificity related to a perinatal condition is found in feeding problems. Category P92 contains specific codes for the following feeding problems: slow feeding (P92.2), underfeeding (P92.3), overfeeding (P92.4), and neonatal difficulty feeding at breast (P92.5).

Combination Codes

Many conditions in ICD-10-CM have combination codes that may report two or more related conditions; the etiology and the manifestation of a disease or condition; or a condition and significant signs and symptoms related to that condition. For example, congenital pneumonia (P23) contains specific codes for the more common infections causing congenital pneumonia including chlamydia, staphylococcus, streptococcus B, Escherichia coli, and pseudomonas.

These and other coding and documentation requirements are discussed in more detail in the next section on code specific documentation.

Code-Specific Documentation Requirements

In this section some of the more frequently reported perinatal conditions are reviewed. The codes are listed and documentation requirements are identified. The focus is on conditions requiring additional clinical information for the condition's best code assignment. Although not all codes with significant documentation requirements are discussed, this section will provide a representative sample of the type of additional documentation needed for perinatal conditions. The section is organized by the specific condition or type of condition.

Congenital Pneumonia

Congenital pneumonia includes infective pneumonia acquired in utero or during birth. Pneumonia from an infection acquired after birth is not reported with this code, nor is aspiration pneumonia resulting from aspiration of meconium, amniotic fluid or mucus, or blood during birth, or from regurgitated milk after birth.

In ICD-10-CM, there are combination codes that identify some specific organisms and others that identify the general class of organism. Codes include congenital pneumonia due to a viral agent (P23.0), chlamydia (P23.1), staphylococcus (P23.2), streptococcus group B (P23.3), Escherichia coli (P23.4), Pseudomonas (P23.5), and other bacterial agents (P23.6). There are also codes for congenital pneumonia due to other organisms (P23.8) and unspecified congenital pneumonia (P23.9). An additional code should be reported from categories B95-B97 to identify the causative organism more specifically whenever it is documented and not available in the combination code, such as code P23.0, where the pneumonia is identified as due to a virus but does not specifically identify the organism.

Coding and Documentation Requirements

Identify congenital pneumonia as due to:

- Bacterial agent
  - Chlamydia
  - Escherichia coli
  - Pseudomonas
  - Staphylococcus
  - Streptococcus, group B
  - Other bacterial agents (use an additional code from category B95 or B96 to identify the organism)
  - Viral agent (use an additional code from category B97 to identify the organism)
- Other specified organisms
- Unspecified organism

ICD-10-CM Code/Documentation	
P23.0	Congenital pneumonia due to viral agent
P23.1	Congenital pneumonia due to Chlamydia
P23.2	Congenital pneumonia due to staphylococcus
P23.3	Congenital pneumonia due to streptococcus, group B
P23.4	Congenital pneumonia due to Escherichia coli
P23.5	Congenital pneumonia due to Pseudomonas
P23.6	Congenital pneumonia due to other bacterial agents
P23.8	Congenital pneumonia due to other organisms
P23.9	Congenital pneumonia, unspecified

Documentation and Coding Example

Twenty-six-day-old female infant is brought to ED by her parents with **eye drainage**, nasal congestion, and somewhat labored breathing. Born at term to a G3 P2 mother who elected to labor and deliver at home with a midwife. Infant was evaluated by pediatrician at 2 days of age and again 2 weeks ago and found to be well and thriving. Parents report eye drainage started about 1 week ago and nasal congestion a few days later. Older siblings have had URIs and parents thought infant had the same virus. When her breathing became labored today mother became concerned although she states infant's appetite has not changed and she is breast feeding normally. T 98.8, P 124, R 22, BP 50/38. Weight today is 9 lbs. 4 oz., an increase of 13 oz. since her 2-week checkup per mother. On examination, this is a mildly ill appearing female Asian infant. Fontanelles are soft and flat, sutures approximate. Eyes have moderate thick, white, purulent drainage. Nares have a small amount of white, thin secretions that can be easily removed with a bulb syringe. There is **bilateral otitis media** present. There is no lymphadenopathy. Mucous membranes moist, pink, posterior pharynx without exudate. Breath sounds have coarse scattered rales but good expansion of lungs and no wheezing noted. Capillary refill time is normal, color is pink, skin warm and dry. O2 Sat is 97% on RA. Chest x-ray obtained and shows bilateral interstitial infiltrates with hyperinflation of the alveoli. Conjunctival and nasopharyngeal smears obtained and **lab report is positive for chlamydial inclusions and elementary bodies on Giemsa stain**. Blood drawn for CBC, antichlamydial IgM titer, comprehensive metabolic panel. IV started in right ankle.

Diagnosis: **Congenital pneumonia due to Chlamydia, conjunctivitis, and bilateral otitis media.**

Plan: Infant will be admitted for antibiotic therapy. Parents are advised to see their PMDs to be tested and treated for Chlamydia infection.

Diagnosis Code(s)

P23.1	Congenital pneumonia due to Chlamydia
P39.1	Neonatal conjunctivitis and dacryocystitis
P39.8	Other specified infections specific to the perinatal period
H66.93	Otitis media, unspecified, bilateral

Coding Note(s)

The patient is 26 days old so even if the Chlamydial pneumonia had not been documented as congenital, the default for infections in an infant 28 days old or less is congenital. Pneumonia in an infant 28 days or less is only reported as a community acquired infection when it is specifically documented as community acquired. The conjunctivitis and bilateral otitis media are also reported as perinatal conditions because these infections have not been documented as being due to a community acquired infection. The organism is likely Chlamydia even though this is not documented because the conjunctivitis and otitis media are common symptoms of congenital Chlamydial infection.

Code P23.1 is a combination code identifying both the congenital pneumonia and the infectious organism. Code P39.1 identifies the neonatal conjunctivitis and this code lists as an alternate term neonatal chlamydial conjunctivitis. P39.8 is used to identify the neonatal otitis media and an additional code is assigned from Chapter 8 Diseases of the Ear and Mastoid Process to identify the condition specifically as bilateral otitis media. The unspecified otitis media code must be reported because the condition is not further identified as nonsuppurative or suppurative, acute, subacute, or chronic.

Feeding Problems in Newborn

Feeding problems are a common newborn condition. Classified along with feeding problems are vomiting and failure to thrive.

Category P92 contains specific codes for vomiting (bilious and other vomiting) and failure to thrive. Category 92 also contains codes for other feeding problems, such as slow feeding, underfeeding, overfeeding, and neonatal difficulty feeding at breast.

Coding and Documentation Requirements

Identify newborn condition:

- Failure to thrive
- Feeding problem
  - Difficulty feeding at breast
  - Overfeeding
  - Regurgitation and rumination
  - Slow feeding
  - Underfeeding
  - Other specified feeding problem
  - Unspecified feeding problem
- Vomiting
  - Bilious
  - Other vomiting

ICD-10-CM Code/Documentation	
P92.01	Bilious vomiting of newborn
P92.09	Other vomiting of newborn
P92.1	Regurgitation and rumination of newborn
P92.2	Slow feeding of newborn

ICD-10-CM Code/Documentation	
P92.3	Underfeeding of newborn
P92.4	Overfeeding of newborn
P92.5	Neonatal difficulty in feeding at breast
P92.6	Failure to thrive in newborn
P92.8	Other feeding problem of newborn
P92.9	Feeding problem of newborn, unspecified

Documentation and Coding Example

Three-week-old female is seen for weight check. Infant was born via SVD at 41 weeks to a G1, single, 16-year-old who lives with her mother and grandmother. Mother did not attempt to breast feed and the baby is being fed formula. At the 5-day newborn checkup infant was half a pound heavier than her BW. At her 2-week checkup the infant had gained another 2 lbs. Even though baby has gained weight mother states that she "throws up after every bottle" and her mother and grandmother insist that the baby be fed again because she has lost all her food.

Impression: **Overfeeding**.

Plan: Mother was counseled at length about feedings and a detailed feeding schedule was set up for mother to follow and a request was made for home visits by Public Health.

Diagnosis code(s)

P92.4 Overfeeding of newborn

Coding Note(s)

Even though the physician has documented that the infant vomits after feeding, this is not coded because it is a symptom of the overfeeding.

Neonatal Jaundice

Jaundice is caused by the alteration, dissolution, or destruction of red blood cells, also referred to as hemolysis. Perinatal jaundice may be due to a number of factors. One cause is maternal-fetal blood incompatibilities, such as Rh, ABO, or other blood group incompatibility. Jaundice resulting from maternal-fetal blood incompatibilities is also referred to as jaundice due to isoimmunization. Other causes include hereditary hemolytic anemias such as thalassemia and sickle cell disease, hemolysis due to bruising, drugs or toxins transmitted from the mother, infection, polycythemia, swallowed maternal blood, and prematurity as well as other conditions.

Category P55 contains codes for hemolytic disease and jaundice due to maternal fetal blood incompatibility (isoimmunization). Neonatal jaundice due to other causes is found in Category P58 Neonatal jaundice due to other excessive hemolysis and Category P59 Neonatal jaundice due to other and unspecified causes.

Detailed documentation is required to capture the most specific code for the perinatal jaundice. The coding and documentation requirements for perinatal jaundice are listed below.

Coding and Documentation Requirements

Identify neonatal jaundice as due to:

- Hemolytic disease
  - ABO isoimmunization
  - Rh isoimmunization
  - Other specified hemolytic disease
  - Unspecified hemolytic disease
- Other excessive hemolysis
  - Bleeding
  - Bruising
  - Drugs/toxins
    - Transmitted from mother
    - Given to newborn
  - Infection
  - Polycythemia
  - Swallowed maternal blood
  - Other specified excessive hemolysis
  - Unspecified excessive hemolysis
- Other and unspecified causes
  - Breast milk inhibitor
  - Hepatocellular damage
    - Inspissated bile syndrome
    - Other specified
    - Unspecified
  - Preterm delivery
  - Other specified causes
  - Unspecified cause

ICD-10-CM Code/Documentation	
P58.0	Neonatal jaundice due to bruising
P58.1	Neonatal jaundice due to bleeding
P58.2	Neonatal jaundice due to infection
P58.3	Neonatal jaundice due to polycythemia
P58.41	Neonatal jaundice due to drugs or toxins transmitted from mother
P58.42	Neonatal jaundice due to drugs or toxins given to newborn
P58.5	Neonatal jaundice due to swallowed maternal blood
P58.8	Neonatal jaundice due to other specified excessive hemolysis
P58.9	Neonatal jaundice due to excessive hemolysis, unspecified
P59.0	Neonatal jaundice associated with preterm delivery
P59.1	Inspissated bile syndrome
P59.20	Neonatal jaundice from unspecified hepatocellular damage
P59.29	Neonatal jaundice from other hepatocellular damage
P59.3	Neonatal jaundice from breast milk inhibitor
P59.8	Neonatal jaundice from other specific causes
P59.9	Neonatal jaundice, unspecified

Documentation and Coding Example

Birth admission. Day 1 follow-up. Patient is a 1-day-old **LGA male infant, BW 3940 grams who was born vaginally at 38 weeks.** He **presented face first and sustained massive soft tissue bruising of the head including the face and scalp.** Mother and **infant are struggling with breast feeding,** but mother has asked that he be given no supplements. **On examination, sclera is jaundiced, bruising masks signs of facial jaundice but mild jaundice is apparent on chest and abdomen.** Skin turgor is decreased, mucous membranes somewhat dry. No ABO incompatibilities, mother and infant both O+. Blood for bilirubin level drawn via heel stick and comes back at 8 mg/dl. Discussed with parents the **dehydration, jaundice, and elevated bilirubin due to bruising, and the need for hydration to treat both the dehydration and the jaundice.** Mother agrees reluctantly to supplement with D5W orally. Bilirubin will be rechecked in 8 hours if >12 mg/dl he will need to begin phototherapy.

Follow up Note: Bilirubin continues to elevate despite additional fluids. Level is now at 13.2 mg/dl and infant placed under phototherapy. Continue with breastfeeding q 2-3 hours, supplement with D5W 30 cc. orally between breastfeeds. Repeat bilirubin in 8 hours.

Diagnosis code(s)

Z38.00	Single live-born infant, delivered vaginally
P12.3	Bruising of scalp due to birth injury
P15.4	Birth injury to face
P08.1	Other heavy for gestational age newborn
P58.0	Neonatal jaundice due to bruising
P92.5	Neonatal difficulty in feeding at breast
P74.1	Dehydration of newborn
P03.1	Newborn (suspected to be) affected by other malpresentation, malposition and disproportion during labor and delivery

Coding Note(s)

The principal/first-listed diagnosis is the code for liveborn infant because this is a birth admission to the hospital. Other codes are listed secondarily.

The birth injury code is specific to bruising of the scalp, but another code must be used to identify the bruising of the face which is captured with a less specific code for birth injury of face. The physician has documented that the infant is large for gestational age (LGA). Even though the information under P08.1 states that this usually implies a birth weight of 4000 to 4499 grams, because the physician has documented LGA it is appropriate to assign code P08.1. The neonatal jaundice is specific to bruising, and there are also specific codes for difficulty feeding at breast and neonatal dehydration.

Omphalitis of the Newborn

Omphalitis of the newborn is an infection of the umbilical stump that typically presents as superficial cellulitis around the umbilicus that may spread to the entire abdominal wall, if untreated. The condition may be associated with mild hemorrhage.

There are two codes that identify omphalitis as with mild hemorrhage (P38.1) or without hemorrhage (P38.9). Omphalitis with mild hemorrhage must be clearly differentiated from massive or other umbilical hemorrhage not associated with infection as these conditions are reported with codes in category P51 Umbilical hemorrhage of newborn.

Coding and Documentation Requirements

Identify omphalitis:

- With mild hemorrhage
- Without hemorrhage

ICD-10-CM Code/Documentation	
P38.1	Omphalitis with mild hemorrhage
P38.9	Omphalitis without hemorrhage

Documentation and Coding Example

Nine-day-old male infant brought in by parents with a smelly, draining umbilical stump. He was born at term, delivered via SVD to a first time mother who has had a difficult time breast feeding. At his first newborn visit 6 days ago he showed signs of mild dehydration and weight loss. Lactation nurse worked with mother in clinic and reported some progress. The family has had a private lactation consultant assisting them at home. The consultant noticed new onset irritability and lethargy when she visited today and saw the umbilicus when she undressed him to try and stimulate him to feed. T 98.2, P 118, R 20, BP 54/38, Wt. 7 lbs. 4 oz. This is an increase of 4 oz. since last visit. On examination, he is alert but fussy. Fontanelles soft, flat with overriding sutures. Eyes without drainage, nares patent. TMs clear. Oral mucosa pink and moist. Breath sounds clear, equal bilaterally. Heart rate regular without murmur. Abdomen is round, the umbilical stump is still attached. There is **periumbilical edema, erythema, and bleeding noted.** There is thick, yellow, malodorous drainage oozing from the area. Parents state they are using baby wipes to clean the cord.

Impression: **Omphalitis with superficial periumbilical cellulitis and mild cord hemorrhage.**

Plan: Admit to Pediatrics and start IV antibiotics following collection of umbilical culture and blood culture for gram stain, anaerobic and aerobic organisms. Additional labs, CBC w/diff, platelets, CRP, ESR, electrolytes. abdominal x-ray to check for air in the intra-abdominal wall.

Diagnosis Code(s)

P38.1	Omphalitis with mild hemorrhage

Coding Note(s)

Superficial periumbilical cellulitis is a symptom of omphalitis and is not reported additionally. The infant has been followed for dehydration and weight loss, but these conditions have resolved as the infant has gained weight. The dehydration and weight loss are not listed as additional diagnoses for the ED visit and are not reported additionally. There is a combination code identifying both the omphalitis and the mild hemorrhage.

Septicemia [Sepsis] of Newborn

Codes in category P36 Bacterial sepsis of newborn, capture the sepsis and the causative organism for many of the more common types of sepsis affecting newborns. Specific codes are available for sepsis due to group B streptococcus, other and unspecified streptococci, Staphylococcus aureus, other and unspecified staphylococci, Escherichia coli, and anaerobes. There is also a code for other specified types of bacterial sepsis in the newborn which requires assignment of an additional code from category B96 to identify the organism. If the organism causing the perinatal sepsis is not identified, the code for unspecified bacterial sepsis must be assigned.

Coding and Documentation Requirements

Identify bacterial sepsis of newborn as due to:

- Anaerobes
- Escherichia coli
- Streptococcus
  - Group B
  - Other specified streptococci
  - Unspecified streptococci
- Staphylococcus
  - S. aureus
  - Other specified staphylococci
  - Unspecified staphylococci
- Other bacterial sepsis of newborn (use additional code from B96 to identify organism)
- Unspecified bacterial sepsis of newborn

ICD-10-CM Code/Documentation	
P36.0	Sepsis of newborn due to streptococcus, group B
P36.10	Sepsis of newborn due to unspecified streptococci
P36.19	Sepsis of newborn due to other streptococci
P36.2	Sepsis of newborn due to Staphylococcus aureus
P36.30	Sepsis of newborn due to unspecified staphylococci
P36.39	Sepsis of newborn due to other staphylococci
P36.4	Sepsis of newborn due to Escherichia coli
P36.5	Sepsis of newborn to anaerobes
P36.8	Other bacterial sepsis of newborn
P36.9	Bacterial sepsis of newborn, unspecified

Documentation and Coding Example

Five-day-old female infant brought to the ED by parents because of poor feeding, fast breathing, and bluish color around the mouth. Mother reports a vaginal delivery after 32 hours of labor, ruptured membranes x 20 hours and both internal and external fetal monitoring. Mother and infant were discharged 24 hours after delivery and infant was seen by pediatrician at 3 days of age and noted to have mild newborn jaundice. Parents were advised to keep her in filtered sunlight for periods during the day and feed her at least every 3 hours. Yesterday parents noticed infant was sleepy and had to be awakened for feedings. During the night she became increasingly lethargic, unable to latch onto the breast, suck nipple or pumped breast milk from a bottle. On examination, this is an acutely ill infant in obvious respiratory distress. RR 32 with grunting, nasal flaring, and generalized cyanosis. HR 160, BP 54/30. Color is pale, capillary refill time >5 seconds. Placed on supplemental oxygen via oxyhood, IV started in left lower extremity. Arterial blood gas drawn with additional blood for culture, CBC, and electrolytes. Urinary catheter inserted and urine sent to lab for culture. Chest x-ray obtained. Lumbar puncture performed and CSF sent to lab for culture. Blood culture positive for Streptococcus agalactiae.

Diagnosis: **Sepsis due to streptococcus, Group B.**

Diagnosis Code(s)

P36.0 Sepsis of newborn due to streptococcus, group B

Coding Note(s)

This is a 5-day-old infant so a sepsis code from the perinatal chapter is assigned rather than a septicemia or sepsis code from the infectious and parasitic diseases chapter. Severe sepsis is not reported because there is no documentation of septic shock or organ failure due to the sepsis.

Summary

Conditions that originate in the perinatal period are reported with codes from Chapter 16. The perinatal period is defined as the period before birth through 28 days after birth. Codes from this chapter may be used even if morbidity does not occur until later or is diagnosed after 28 days as long as the condition originated during the perinatal period. It is particularly important for physicians to document that the onset of a problem occurred during the perinatal period whenever this is the case. If this is not documented, a code from one of the other chapters must be reported. Coders and physicians providing care to newborns should review Chapter 16 in ICD-10-CM as well as the general and chapter-specific guidelines to ensure that documentation is sufficient to capture codes to the highest degree of specificity. There are also default rules in code assignment for conditions that occur due to the birth process versus community acquired conditions. When the documentation does not state the cause of the newborn condition as one or the other, the default is due to the birth process. Documentation of community acquired conditions should not be assigned a code from Chapter 16.

Resources

The following documentation checklists are included in Appendix A:

- Feeding problems of newborn
- Jaundice, neonatal

Chapter 17 Quiz

1. An infant whose mother had placenta previa does not show any specific signs or symptoms at birth of complications from this condition. However, the physician has documented suspected newborn complications due to the placenta previa. Is this condition reported on the newborn record and why?
   a. No, only confirmed diagnoses are reported
   b. No, if the physician had documented specific signs and symptoms those could be reported but no code is reported for suspected diagnoses
   c. Yes, a suspected perinatal condition that has implications for future healthcare needs is reported
   d. Yes, placenta previa is always harmful to the fetus and the newborn will eventually exhibit conditions caused by the placenta previa
2. Jaundice caused by maternal-fetal blood incompatibility is classified as:
   a. Hemolytic disease of newborn (P55)
   b. Neonatal jaundice due to other excessive hemolysis (P58)
   c. Neonatal jaundice from other and unspecified causes (P59)
   d. None of the above
3. What infectious disease documented as originating in the perinatal period is not reported with a code from Chapter 16?
   a. Sepsis due to Escherichia coli
   b. Pneumonia due to Chlamydia
   c. Pneumonia due to other bacterial agents
   d. Tetanus neonatorum
4. Identify the true statement:
   a. Codes from Chapter 16 may be reported on either the maternal or newborn record
   b. Codes from Chapter 16 may be reported on the maternal record when they are documented as affecting the fetus
   c. When a code from Chapter 16 is reported on the newborn record, the same code should be reported on the maternal record if the condition affected the fetus before birth
   d. Codes from Chapter 16 are for use on newborn records only, never on maternal records
5. Identify the false statement:
   a. Codes from other chapters may be used with codes from Chapter 16 if the codes from the other chapters provide more specific detail
   b. Codes for signs and symptoms may be assigned when a definitive diagnosis has not be established
   c. The only codes that may be reported on the newborn record from birth through the first 28 days after birth are codes from Chapter 16
   d. Codes from Chapter 16 may be reported if the reason for the encounter is a perinatal condition, even if the infant is more than 28 days old
6. A 26-day-old infant is admitted with a diagnosis of viral hepatitis. What code is reported?
   a. P35.3 Congenital viral hepatitis
   b. B19.9 Unspecified viral hepatitis without hepatic coma
   c. B17.9 Acute viral hepatitis, unspecified
   d. B18.9 Chronic viral hepatitis, unspecified
7. A 2-day-old infant is diagnosed with severe bacterial sepsis with septic shock due to Group B streptococcus. What code(s) are assigned?
   a. P36.0 Sepsis of newborn due to streptococcus, Group B
   b. P36.0 Sepsis of newborn due to streptococcus, Group B, B95.1 Streptococcus, group B, as the cause of diseases classified elsewhere
   c. P36.0 Sepsis of newborn due to streptococcus, Group B, R65.21 Severe sepsis with septic shock
   d. P36.0 Sepsis of newborn due to streptococcus, Group B, B95.1 Streptococcus, group B, as the cause of diseases classified elsewhere, R65.21 Severe sepsis with septic shock
8. The physician has documented that an 18-month-old toddler is being seen for current medical conditions related to prematurity. What code or category is used to identify the medical conditions as being related to prematurity?
   a. P03 Newborn (suspected to be) affected by other complications of labor and delivery
   b. P07 Disorders of newborn related to short gestation and low birth weight, not elsewhere classified
   c. P92.6 Failure to thrive in newborn
   d. R62.51 Failure to thrive (child)
9. What type of jaundice is NOT reported with a code from category P59 Neonatal jaundice from other and unspecified causes?
   a. Neonatal jaundice not otherwise specified
   b. Neonatal jaundice due to hereditary hemolytic anemias
   c. Neonatal jaundice due to hepatocellular damage
   d. Neonatal jaundice due to preterm delivery
10. How are metabolic disorders of the newborn that are documented as transitory reported?
    a. Transitory conditions are not reported
    b. With codes from categories E70-E88
    c. With codes from categories P70-P74
    d. With signs and symptoms codes

See next page for answers and rationales.

Chapter 17 Answer Key and Rationales

1. An infant whose mother had a placenta previa does not show any specific signs or symptoms at birth of complications from this condition. However, the physician has documented suspected newborn complications due to the placenta previa. Is this condition reported on the newborn record and why?

   c. **Yes, a suspected perinatal condition that has implications for future healthcare needs is reported**

   Rationale: *Coding guidelines for perinatal conditions state that a suspected perinatal condition that has implications for future healthcare needs is reported. Because the physician has documented suspected newborn complications due to the placenta previa, code P02.0 Newborn (suspected to be) affected by placenta previa is reported.*

2. Jaundice caused by maternal-fetal blood incompatibility is classified as:

   a. **Hemolytic disease of newborn (P55)**

   Rationale: *Jaundice caused by maternal-fetal blood incompatibility is classified in category P55 Hemolytic disease of the newborn. This can be verified by using the Alphabetic Index under Jaundice, newborn, due to isoimmunization. Isoimmunization refers to maternal-fetal blood type incompatibility. Jaundice is a symptom of the destruction of the red blood cells which is also referred to as hemolysis.*

3. What infectious disease documented as originating in the perinatal period is not reported with a code from Chapter 16?

   d. **Tetanus neonatorum**

   Rationale: *There is a chapter level Excludes2 note for tetanus neonatorum (A33) which indicates that the condition is not reported with a code in Chapter 16.*

4. Identify the true statement:

   d. **Codes from Chapter 16 are for use on newborn records only, never on maternal records**

   Rationale: *Instructions in the guidelines as well as instructions in the tabular list state that codes in Chapter 16 are for use on newborn records only, never on maternal records. A code from Chapter 15 Pregnancy, Childbirth and the Puerperium is reported on the maternal record for documented maternal conditions suspected of affecting the fetus or newborn.*

5. Identify the false statement:

   c. **The only codes that may be reported on the newborn record from birth through the first 28 days after birth are codes from Chapter 16.**

   Rationale: *Reporting codes from other chapters is allowed during the perinatal period. The chapter guidelines provide specific instructions for reporting codes from other chapters during the perinatal period. Codes from other chapters may be used with codes from Chapter 16 when they provide more specific detail. Signs and symptoms codes may also be reported when a definitive diagnosis has not been established. Codes from Chapter 16 may also be reported beyond 28 days as long as the condition originated in the perinatal period.*

6. A 26-day-old infant is admitted with a diagnosis of viral hepatitis. What code is reported?

   a. **P35.3 Congenital viral hepatitis**

   Rationale: *Chapter 16 coding guidelines state "If a newborn has a condition that may be either due to the birth process or community acquired, and the documentation does not indicate which it is, the default is to the birth process and the code from Chapter 16 should be used." Code P35.3 is the correct code.*

7. A 2-day-old infant is diagnosed with severe bacterial sepsis with septic shock due to Group B streptococcus. What code(s) are assigned?

   c. **P36.0 Sepsis of newborn due to streptococcus, Group B, R65.21 Severe sepsis with septic shock**

   Rationale: *Codes P36.0 and R65.21 are reported based on the following guidelines: 1) If the sepsis code includes the causal organism, an additional code from categories B95 or B96 should not be assigned. 2) If applicable, use additional codes to identify severe sepsis (R65.2-) and any associated acute organ dysfunction. The condition has been documented as severe bacterial sepsis and septic shock is classified as severe sepsis so the code for severe sepsis with septic shock is reported.*

8. The physician has documented that an 18-month-old toddler is being seen for current medical conditions related to prematurity. What code or category is used to identify the medical conditions as being related to prematurity?

   b. **P07 Disorders of newborn related to short gestation and low birth weight, not elsewhere classified**

   Rationale: *Chapter guidelines state codes from category P07 are for use for a child or adult who was premature or had a low birth weight as a newborn and this is affecting the patient's current health status.*

9. What type of jaundice is NOT reported with a code from category P59 Neonatal jaundice from other and unspecified causes?

   b. **Neonatal jaundice due to hereditary hemolytic anemias**

   Rationale: *Neonatal jaundice due to hereditary hemolytic anemias is reported with code P58.8 Neonatal jaundice due to other specified excessive hemolysis. All of the other types of neonatal jaundice are reported with a code from category P59.*

10. How are metabolic disorders of the newborn that are documented as transitory reported?

    c. **With codes from categories P70-P74**

    Rationale: *Code block P70-P74 contains codes for reporting transitory endocrine and metabolic disorders of the newborn.*

17. Conditions in the Perinatal Period

Chapter 18
SYMPTOMS, SIGNS, ILL-DEFINED CONDITIONS

Introduction

Codes for symptoms, signs, abnormal results of laboratory or other investigative procedures, and ill-defined conditions without a diagnosis classified elsewhere are classified in Chapter 18 Symptoms, Signs and Abnormal Clinical and Laboratory Findings, Not Elsewhere Classified. There are 7 code blocks that identify symptoms and signs for specific body systems followed by a code block for general symptoms and signs. Five code blocks report abnormal findings for laboratory tests, imaging and function studies, and tumor markers. Examples of signs and symptoms related to specific body systems include: shortness of breath (R06.02), epigastric pain (R10.13), cyanosis (R23.0), ataxia (R27.0), and dysuria (R30.0). Examples of general signs and symptoms include: fever (R50.9), chronic fatigue (R53.82), abnormal weight loss (R63.4), systemic inflammatory response syndrome (SIRS) of non-infectious origin (R65.1-), and severe sepsis (R65.2-). Examples of abnormal findings include: red blood cell abnormalities (R71.-), proteinuria (R80-), abnormal cytological findings in specimens from cervix uteri (R87.61-), and inconclusive mammogram (R92.2). Below is a table showing the blocks of Chapter 18:

ICD-10-CM Blocks	
R00-R09	Symptoms and Signs Involving the Circulatory and Respiratory Systems
R10-R19	Symptoms and Signs Involving the Digestive System and Abdomen
R20-R23	Symptoms and Signs Involving the Skin and Subcutaneous Tissue
R25-R29	Symptoms and Signs Involving the Nervous and Musculoskeletal Systems
R30-R39	Symptoms and Signs Involving the Genitourinary System
R40-R46	Symptoms and Signs Involving Cognition, Perception, Emotional State and Behavior
R47-R49	Symptoms and Signs Involving Speech and Voice
R50-R69	General Symptoms and Signs
R70-R79	Abnormal Findings on Examination of Blood, Without Diagnosis
R80-R82	Abnormal Findings on Examination of Urine, Without Diagnosis
R83-R89	Abnormal Findings on Examination of Other Body Fluids, Substances and Tissues, Without Diagnosis
R90-R94	Abnormal Findings on Diagnostic Imaging and in Function Studies Without Diagnosis
R97	Abnormal Tumor Markers
R99	Ill-Defined and Unknown Cause of Mortality

Coding Note(s)

Chapter level coding notes explain the types of conditions reported with codes for signs, symptoms, ill-defined conditions, and abnormal clinical and laboratory findings. Chapter 18 includes codes for:

- Symptoms, signs, abnormal results of clinical or other investigative procedures, and ill-defined conditions regarding which no diagnosis classifiable elsewhere is recorded
- Less well-defined conditions and symptoms that, without the necessary study of the case to establish a final diagnosis, point perhaps equally to two or more diseases or to two or more systems of the body
- Practically all categories in Chapter 18 could be designated as 'not otherwise specified', 'unknown etiology', or 'transient'. Residual subcategories numbered .8 are generally provided for other relevant symptoms that cannot be allocated elsewhere in the classification.

The conditions and signs or symptoms included in categories R00-R94 consist of the following:

1. Cases for which no more specific diagnosis can be made even after all the facts bearing on the case have been investigated;
2. Signs or symptoms existing at the time of initial encounter that proved to be transient and whose causes could not be determined;
3. Provisional diagnosis in a patient who failed to return for further investigation or care;
4. Cases referred elsewhere for investigation or treatment before the diagnosis was made;
5. Cases in which a more precise diagnosis was not available for any other reason;
6. Certain symptoms, for which supplementary information is provided, that represent important problems in medical care in their own right

Signs and symptoms that point rather definitely to a given diagnosis are not found in Chapter 18. Instead, they have been assigned to a category in other chapters of the classification. The Alphabetic Index should be consulted to determine which symptoms and signs are classified in Chapter 18 and which are allocated to other chapters.

Exclusions

The Excludes2 notes for Chapter 18 are listed below. There are no Excludes1 notes for Chapter 18:

Excludes1	Excludes2
None	Abnormal findings on antenatal screening of mother (O28.-)
	Certain conditions originating in the perinatal period (P04-P96)
	Signs and symptoms classified in the body system chapters
	Signs and symptoms of the breast (N63, N64.5)

Chapter Guidelines

In order to understand when it is appropriate to report codes for signs and symptoms, the *Official Guidelines* Sections II, III, and IV must be reviewed in addition to reviewing the Chapter Specific Guidelines in Section I. The Chapter Specific Guidelines are discussed first followed by the Section II, III and IV Guidelines.

Chapter Specific Guidelines

A number of chapter guidelines are written that cover the following:

- Use of symptom codes
- Use of a symptom code with a definitive diagnosis code
- Combination codes that include symptoms
- Repeated falls
- Coma scale
- Functional quadriplegia
- SIRS due to non-infectious process
- Death not otherwise specified (NOS)
- NIHSS Stroke Scale

Use of Symptom Codes

Codes that describe symptoms and signs are acceptable for reporting purposes when a related definitive diagnosis has not been established (confirmed) by the provider. For example, a common symptom that could be indicative of a number of conditions is abdominal pain. If the physician, has documented right upper quadrant abdominal pain and is in the process of investigating the cause of the pain, it is appropriate to report R10.11 Right upper quadrant pain until the physician has established and documented the specific cause of the pain, such as acute cholangitis.

Use of a Symptom Code with a Definitive Diagnosis Code

Assignment of a sign or symptom code with a definitive diagnosis code is dependent upon whether the symptom is routinely associated with the definitive diagnosis or disease process.

- When the sign or symptom is not routinely associated with the definitive diagnosis:
  - Codes for signs and symptoms may be reported in addition to a related definitive diagnosis, such as the various signs and symptoms associated with complex syndromes
  - The definitive diagnosis should be sequenced before the symptom code
- When the sign or symptom is routinely associated with the disease process:
  - Do no assign the sign or symptom code unless instructions for the category, subcategory, or code level classification state that the sign or symptom should be reported additionally

Combination Codes That Include Symptoms

ICD-10-CM contains a number of codes that identify both the definitive diagnosis and common symptoms of that diagnosis. When using one of these combination codes, an additional code should not be assigned for the symptom. For example, R18.8 Other ascites is not reported with the combination code K70.31 Alcoholic cirrhosis of the liver with ascites because code K70.31 identifies both the definitive diagnosis (alcoholic cirrhosis) and a common symptom of the condition (ascites).

Repeated Falls

ICD-10-CM provides a code for repeated falls (R29.6) and another code for history of falling (Z91.81) which are assigned as follows:

- R29.6 Repeated falls is for use for encounters when a patient has recently fallen and the reason for the fall is being investigated.
- Z91.81 History of falling is for use when a patient has fallen in the past and is at risk for future falls
- Both codes may be assigned together when the patient has had a recent fall that is being investigated and also has a history of falling

Coma Scale

The coma scale codes (R40.2-) are primarily for use by trauma registries, but they may be used in any setting where this information is collected. These codes are sequenced after the diagnosis code(s). The coma scale codes can be used in conjunction with traumatic brain injury codes, acute cerebrovascular disease, or sequelae of cerebrovascular disease codes. The coma scale may also be used to assess the status of the central nervous system for other nontrauma conditions, such as monitoring patients in the intensive care unit regardless of medical condition.

The coma scale consists of three elements, eye open (R40.21-), best verbal response (R40.22-), and best motor response (R40.23-). One code from each subcategory is needed to complete the coma scale. Individual scores for each element are as follows:

- Eyes open:
  - Never
  - To pain
  - To sound
  - Spontaneous
- Best verbal response:
  - None
  - Incomprehensible words
  - Inappropriate words
  - Confused conversation
  - Oriented

- Best motor response:
  - None
  - Extension
  - Abnormal flexion
  - Flexion withdrawal
  - Localizes pain
  - Obeys commands

A 7th character indicates when the scale was recorded. The 7th character should match for all three individual element codes.

At a minimum, the initial score documented on presentation at the facility should be reported. This may be a score from the emergency medicine technician (EMT) or ambulance, or from the emergency department. If desired, the facility may choose to capture multiple coma scale scores. The 7th character identifies the time/place as follows:

- 1 In the field (EMT/ambulance)
- 2 At arrival to emergency department
- 3 At hospital admission
- 4 24 hours or more after hospital admission
- 0 Unspecified time

When only the total Glasgow coma scale score is documented and not the individual element score(s), assign a code from R40.24- Glasgow coma scale, total score, also with the appropriate 7th character identifying the time/place the total scale was recorded:

- R40.241- Glasgow coma scale score 13-15
- R40.242- Glasgow coma scale score 9-12
- R40.243- Glasgow coma scale score 3-8
- R40.244- Other coma, without documented Glasgow coma scale score, or with partial score reported

Do not report codes for individual or total Glasgow coma scale scores for a sedated patient or a patient in a medically induced coma.

SIRS Due to Non-Infectious Process

Systemic inflammatory response syndrome (SIRS) can develop as a result of certain non-infectious disease processes, such as trauma, malignant neoplasm, or pancreatitis.

Sequencing of codes for SIRS documented with a noninfectious condition and no subsequent infection documented is as follows:

- The code for the underlying condition, such as an injury, is sequenced first
- A code from subcategory R65.1 is sequenced following the underlying, noninfectious condition
  - Assign R65.10 for SIRS of noninfectious origin without acute organ dysfunction
  - Assign R65.11 for SIRS of noninfectious origin with acute organ dysfunction
- Assign a code to identify the specific type of acute organ dysfunction associated with the SIRS of noninfectious origin when code R65.11 is assigned
- Query the provider if acute organ dysfunction is documented but it cannot be determined if the acute organ dysfunction is associated with the SIRS of noninfectious origin or due to another condition, such as acute organ dysfunction directly due to the trauma

Death, NOS

Code R99 Ill-defined and unknown cause of mortality is only for use in the very limited circumstance when a patient who has already died is brought into an emergency department or other healthcare facility and is pronounced dead upon arrival. It does not represent the discharge disposition of death.

NIHSS Stroke Scale

The National Institutes of Health stroke scale (NIHSS) codes (R29.7-) can be used in conjunction with acute stroke codes (I63) to identify the patient's neurological status and severity of the stroke. At a minimum, the initial score documented should be reported. A facility may choose to capture multiple stroke scale codes. The stroke scale codes should be sequenced after the acute stroke diagnosis code(s).

Note: See Section I.B.14 for information about medical record documentation that may be used for assignment of the NIHSS codes.

Section II, Section III, and Section IV Guidelines

Rules for reporting symptoms, signs, abnormal findings, and ill-defined conditions differ based on the place of service. Section II covers selection of the principle diagnosis for inpatient settings which includes all non-outpatient settings: acute care, short term care, long term care, and psychiatric hospitals; home health agencies, rehab facilities, and nursing homes as well as all levels of hospice service care. Section III covers reporting of additional diagnoses in inpatient settings with some specific guidelines related to abnormal findings and uncertain diagnoses. Section IV covers diagnostic coding and reporting for outpatient settings.

Section II – Selection of Principal Diagnosis (Inpatient Setting)

There are specific guidelines in this section related to reporting of symptoms, signs, and ill-defined conditions as the principal diagnosis. The circumstances of inpatient admission always govern the selection of principal diagnosis. Guidelines are as follows:

- Codes for symptoms, signs, and ill-defined conditions from Chapter 18 are not to be used as the principal diagnosis when a related definitive diagnosis has been established.
- If the diagnosis is uncertain and the documentation at the time of discharge is qualified as "probable", "suspected", "likely", "questionable", "possible", or "still to be ruled out", or other similar terms indicating uncertainty, code the condition as if it existed or were established. The bases for these guidelines are the diagnostic workup, arrangements for further workup or observation, and initial therapeutic approach that correspond most closely with the established diagnosis. This guideline only applies to inpatient admissions to short-term, acute, long-term care, and psychiatric hospitals.

Section III – Reporting Additional Diagnoses (Inpatient Setting)

There are specific guidelines in this section related to reporting symptoms, signs, and ill-defined conditions as additional diagnoses for inpatient settings including acute care, short term care, long term care, psychiatric hospitals, home health agencies, rehab facilities, and nursing homes as well as all levels of hospice service care. Guidelines are as follows:

- Abnormal findings (laboratory, x-ray, pathologic, and other diagnostic results) are not coded and reported unless the provider indicates their clinical significance. If the findings are outside the normal range and the attending provider has ordered other tests to evaluate the condition or prescribed treatment, it is appropriate to ask the provider whether the abnormal findings should be added. **Note:** This differs from the coding practices in the outpatient setting for coding encounters for diagnostic tests that have interpreted by a provider.
- If the diagnosis is uncertain and the documentation at the time of discharge is qualified as "probable", "suspected", "likely", "questionable", "possible", or "still to be ruled out" or other similar terms indicating uncertainty, code the condition as if it existed or were established. The bases for these guidelines are the diagnostic workup, arrangements for further workup or observation, and initial therapeutic approach that correspond most closely with the established diagnosis. This guideline only applies to short-term, acute, long-term care, and psychiatric hospitals.

Section IV – Diagnostic Coding and Reporting Guidelines for Outpatient Services

There are specific guidelines in this section related to reporting of symptoms and signs, uncertain diagnosis, and patients receiving diagnostic services only. These coding guidelines apply only to the outpatient setting which includes both hospital-based outpatient services and provider-based office visits. Guidelines in Section I, Conventions, general coding guidelines, and chapter specific guidelines should also be applied for outpatient services and office visits. Guidelines that apply to codes in Chapter 18 are as follows:

- Codes that describe symptoms and signs, as opposed to diagnoses, are acceptable for reporting purposes when a diagnosis has not be established (confirmed) by the provider. Chapter 18 of ICD-10-CM contains many, but not all, codes for symptoms.
- The first-listed diagnosis may be a symptom when a diagnosis has not been established (confirmed) by the physician.
- Do not code diagnoses documented as "probable", "suspected", "questionable", or "rule out", "working diagnosis" or other similar terms indicating uncertainty. Rather code the conditions(s) to the highest degree of certainty for that encounter/visit, such as symptoms, signs, abnormal test results, or other reason for the visit. **Note**: This guideline differs from the coding practices used by short-term, acute care, long-term care, and psychiatric hospitals.
- For patients receiving diagnostic services only during an encounter/visit, sequence first the diagnosis, condition, problem, or other reason for the encounter/visit shown in the medical record to be chiefly responsible for the outpatient services provided during the encounter/visit
- If a test is performed to evaluate a sign or symptom, it is appropriate to report the sign or symptom code describing the reason for the test.
- For outpatient encounters for diagnostic tests that have been interpreted by a physician, and the final report is available at the time of coding, code any confirmed or definitive diagnoses documented in the interpretation. Do not code related signs and symptoms as additional diagnoses. **Note**: This guideline differs from the coding practice in the hospital inpatient setting regarding abnormal findings on test results.

General Documentation Requirements

Like conditions classified in other chapters of ICD-10-CM, codes for signs, symptoms, and abnormal clinical and laboratory findings require specific documentation, such as:

- Site specificity and laterality for some signs and symptoms, such as localized swelling, mass, and lump of the upper and lower limbs (R22.3-, R22.4-)
- Further descriptions of some signs and symptoms, such as malaise and fatigue, which includes specific codes for neoplastic related fatigue (R53.0), and weakness (R53.1)
- Specific identification of certain test results, such as abnormalities of plasma proteins which includes specific codes for abnormality of albumin (R77.0), globulin (R77.1), and alpha-fetoprotein (R77.2)

Code-Specific Documentation Requirements

In this section, codes are listed and their documentation requirements are identified. The focus is on conditions with additional, specific clinical documentation requirements. Although not all codes with significant documentation requirements are discussed, this section will provide a representative sample of the type of additional documentation needed for codes classified in Chapter 18. The section is organized alphabetically by the topic or group of conditions.

Abnormal Involuntary Movements

Abnormal involuntary movements, such as shoulder shrug, head jerk, and tremor, may be documented during the work-up phase for a number of medical conditions. These signs or symptoms may be reported until a definitive diagnosis is made.

Category R25 Abnormal involuntary movements includes codes for abnormal head movements (R25.0), unspecified tremor (R25.1), cramp and spasm (R25.2), fasciculation (R25.3), other abnormal involuntary movements (R25.8), and unspecified abnormal involuntary movements (R25.9). Careful review of the documentation is required to ensure that the abnormal movements cannot be assigned a more specific code. For example, muscle spasms are not reported with code R25.2; a code from subcategory M62.83 Muscle spasm is assigned instead.

Coding and Documentation Requirements

Identify condition:

- Abnormal head movements
- Cramp/spasm
- Fasciculation (twitching)
- Tremor, unspecified
- Other abnormal involuntary movements
- Unspecified abnormal involuntary movements

ICD-10-CM Code/Documentation	
R25.0	Abnormal head movements
R25.1	Tremor, unspecified
R25.2	Cramp and spasm
R25.3	Fasciculation
R25.8	Other abnormal involuntary movements
R25.9	Unspecified abnormal involuntary movements

Documentation and Coding Example

Patient is a nine-year-old Hispanic female brought to clinic by her mother and older brother who are concerned about her **unusual blinking and head jerking**. This is the third time the child has come in this month and each time the examiner has not noticed any unusual movements. Today the brother has brought along his cell phone with video recordings of the movements. T 99, P 72, R 14, BP 110/64, Ht. 54 inches, Wt. 60 lbs. Patient is a quiet, cooperative little girl who seems anxious to please her mother and this examiner. She states she knows that she makes odd movements because people have pointed them out to her and lately they make fun of her. She tries very hard to control them especially at school or around new people. During this 5-minute chat with her, she has not had any involuntary movements. Her brother shares what he has captured on video and it is striking to see. **The patient has repetitive eye blinking for about 10 seconds. As that slows down, she twitches her left shoulder once and then jerks her head to the left side**. On the video she repeats the sequence twice before the video stops. On examination PERRL, neck supple without a few supraclavicular lymph nodes palpated. Mother states the child had a fever and sore throat about 6 weeks ago but recovered in a few days. Cranial nerves grossly intact. Heart rate regular without murmur, gallop, bruit or rub. Breath sounds clear, equal bilaterally. Abdomen soft with active BS. Liver and spleen not palpated. **At the end of the exam patient begins rapid eye blinking followed by a single shoulder twitch and head jerk**. She is able to gain control of the movements and does not repeat them a second time.

Impression: **Abnormal head and shoulder movements and eye blinking**, possibly due to transient tic disorder of childhood, Tourette Syndrome, or PANDAS.

Plan: Throat culture obtained to R/O strep infection, test blood for autoimmune disorders along with CBC, comprehensive metabolic panel. The mother and brother are asked to record the frequency with which these symptoms occur and to call if any new symptoms or concerns arise. Follow-up in two-weeks.

Diagnosis Code(s)

R25.0 Abnormal head movements

R25.8 Other abnormal involuntary movements

Coding Note(s)

Since this is an outpatient encounter, codes for the symptoms are assigned because the physician has not documented a definitive diagnosis. For outpatient services, uncertain diagnoses are not reported. The physician has documented that the abnormal movements are possibly due to new transient tic disorder, Tourette's syndrome, or PANDAS (Pediatric Autoimmune Neuropsychiatric Disorder Associated with Streptococcus), but the term "possibly due to" indicates that these are uncertain diagnoses. PANDAS is an autoimmune disorder that occurs following a strep infection when antibodies are created that attack both the streptococcal bacteria and body tissues. In the case of PANDAS, the antibodies attack the part of the brain that controls thought and movement. This can cause inflammation of the brain, leading to symptoms such as OCD, Tourette's, focusing problems, or other symptoms.

Abnormality of Gait/Difficulty Walking

Codes for difficulty walking and abnormal gait may be reported when the physician is working up the cause for these symptoms. It should be noted that difficulty walking is not classified in the musculoskeletal system, but is classified as a sign/symptom.

Codes for signs and symptoms related to walking and gait describe conditions more specifically as ataxic gait (R26.0), paralytic gait (R26.1), and unsteadiness on feet (R26.81). There are also codes for difficulty walking (R26.2), other specified abnormalities of gait and mobility (R26.89), and unspecified gait and mobility abnormalities (R26.9).

Coding and Documentation Requirements

Identify condition:

- Difficulty walking
- Gait abnormality
  - Ataxic gait
  - Paralytic gait
- Unsteadiness on feet
- Other abnormalities of gait and mobility
- Unspecified abnormalities of gait and mobility

ICD-10-CM Code/Documentation	
R26.0	Ataxic gait
R26.1	Paralytic gait
R26.2	Difficulty in walking, not elsewhere classified
R26.81	Unsteadiness on feet
R26.89	Other abnormalities of gait and mobility
R26.9	Unspecified abnormalities of gait and mobility

Documentation and Coding Example

Twenty-five-year-old Caucasian female is referred to neurology by PMD for poor muscle coordination in her lower body. Patient had been in her usual state of good health until 2 months ago when she noticed **problems with coordination particularly when walking which has led to stumbling and now frequent falls**. She can recall no illness, injury, or exposure to toxic chemicals but she does recall meeting some distant relatives of her mothers with this type of problem. On examination, this is a tired, thin, pleasant woman who looks older than her stated age. PERRL, cranial nerves are intact to face and upper extremities. Upper body muscle strength is normal with intact pulses and reflexes. Spine is straight, forward bending causes no pain but she has trouble adjusting her weight to maintain balance. Muscle tone and strength in lower extremities is decreased. Reflexes are brisk, pulses somewhat weak. When observed standing, patient moves her feet about 10 inches apart to maintain postural stability. She is unable to perform Romberg. When walking 25 feet, there is lateral deviation and unequal steps. She stumbles but does not fall.

Impression: **Ataxic gait, possibly due to hereditary ataxia.**

Plan: Lab tests including CBC, UA, comprehensive metabolic panel, Vitamin B12 and D3 levels. Will consider an MRI when lab tests are back. Patient will attempt to find out more regarding her relatives with this type of problem. Consider genetic w/u with or without that information.

Diagnosis Code(s)

R26.0	Ataxic gait
R29.6	Repeated falls

Coding Note(s)

Hereditary ataxia is not reported because it is an uncertain diagnosis and uncertain diagnoses are not reported in an outpatient setting. Code(s) for the highest degree of certainty for the encounter or visit should be assigned, including signs and symptoms. The physician has not diagnosed a definitive cause for the ataxic gait, so the symptom of ataxic gait is reported. The patient has also had repeated falls that are a significant symptom in their own right and so the code for repeated falls is also reported.

Alteration of Consciousness

Category R40 Somnolence, stupor and coma has specific codes for somnolence (R40.0), stupor (R40.1), persistent vegetative state (R40.3), and transient alteration of awareness (R40.4). In addition to these codes, subcategory R40.2 Coma has a code for unspecified coma (R40.20), but more importantly, it contains coma scale codes and Glasgow coma scale total scores. The coma scale codes and coma scale total scores are used primarily by trauma registries but may also be reported by emergency medical services, acute care facilities, and other providers and facilities wanting to capture this information.

In order to complete the coma scale, information must be collected on the following:

- Eye opening response
- Best verbal response
- Best motor response

Eye opening response is scored as follows:

- No eye opening response (1 point)
- Eye opening to pain only (not applied to face) (2 points)
- Eye opening to verbal stimuli, command, speech (3 points)
- Spontaneous – open with blinking at baseline (4 points)

Verbal response is scored as follows:

- No verbal response (1 point)
- Incomprehensible speech (2 points)
- Inappropriate words (3 points)
- Confused conversation, but able to answer questions (4 points)
- Oriented (5 points)

Motor response is scored as follows:

- No motor response (1 point)
- Extension response to pain (decerebrate posturing) (2 points)
- Flexion response to pain (decorticate posturing) (3 points)
- Withdraws in response to pain (flexion withdrawal) (4 points)
- Purposeful movement in response to painful stimulus (localizes pain) (5 points)
- Obeys commands for movement (6 points)

The scores for each of the three components are then added together to obtain the Glasgow Coma Scale (GCS) total score. The total score is used to determine the severity of the head injury which is as follows:

- Severe head injury – GCS total score 3-8
- Moderate head injury – GCS total score 9-12
- Mild head injury – GCS total score 13-15

Documentation and coding requirements below are provided for the Glasgow Coma Scale components and total score.

Coding and Documentation Requirements

Coma Scale – Use individual scores, if known. All three elements—eye opening, best verbal response, and best motor response must be known to use individual scores. If all three elements are not documented, but the Glasgow Coma Scale total score is documented, use the code for the total score.

Identify individual scores:

- Eyes open:
  - Never
  - To pain
  - To sound
  - Spontaneous
- Best verbal response:
  - None
  - Incomprehensible words
  - Inappropriate words
  - Confused conversation
  - Oriented
- Best motor response:
  - None

  - Extension
  - Abnormal flexion
  - Flexion withdrawal
  - Localizes pain
  - Obeys commands

Identify time/place of coma score obtained:

- In the field (EMT/ambulance)
- At arrival to emergency department
- At hospital admission
- 24 hours or more after hospital admission
- Unspecified time

-OR-

Identify Glasgow coma scale total score:

- Glasgow score 13-15
- Glasgow score 9-12
- Glasgow score 3-8
- Other coma, without documented Glasgow coma scale score, or with partial score reported

Identify time/place of coma scale total score obtained:

- In the field (EMT/ambulance)
- At arrival to emergency department
- At hospital admission
- 24 hours or more after hospital admission
- Unspecified time

ICD-10-CM Code/Documentation	
R40.0	Somnolence
R40.1	Stupor
R40.3	Persistent vegetative state
R40.4	Transient alteration of awareness
R40.20	Unspecified coma
Coma Scale, Eyes Open	
R40.211-	Coma scale, eyes open, never
R40.212-	Coma scale, eyes open, to pain
R40.213-	Coma scale, eyes open, to sound
R40.214-	Coma scale, eyes open, spontaneous
Coma Scale, Best Verbal Response	
R40.221-	Coma scale, best verbal response, none
R40.222-	Coma scale, best verbal response, incomprehensible words
R40.223-	Coma scale, best verbal response, inappropriate words
R40.224-	Coma scale, best verbal response, confused conversation
R40.225-	Coma scale, best verbal response, oriented
Coma Scale, Best Motor Response	
R40.231-	Coma scale, best motor response, none
R40.232-	Coma scale, best motor response, extension
R40.233-	Coma scale, best motor response, abnormal flexion
R40.234-	Coma scale, best motor response, flexion withdrawal
R40.235-	Coma scale, best motor response, localizes pain
R40.236-	Coma scale, best motor response, obeys commands
Glasgow Coma Scale, total score	
R40.241-	Glasgow coma scale score 13-15
R40.242-	Glasgow coma scale score 9-12
R40.243-	Glasgow coma scale score 3-8
R40.244-	Other coma, without documented Glasgow coma scale score, or with partial score reported

Note: A code from each coma scale subcategory is required to complete the coma scale and these codes should be used only when documentation is available for all three components (R40.21-, R40.22-, and R40.23-). Codes in subcategory R40.24 may be reported alone. Codes in all four of these subcategories require a 7th character to identify the site/time of the coma evaluation:

- 0 – Unspecified time
- 1 – In the field [EMT or ambulance]
- 2 – At arrival to emergency department
- 3 – At hospital admission
- 4 – 24 hours or more after hospital admission

Documentation and Coding Example

Sixteen-year-old Caucasian male transported to local ED via ambulance after he was found unresponsive at home by his mother. Patient has a fresh 4 cm x 5 cm hematoma on left temporal area. Mother states her son was surfing earlier in the day and was hit in the head by his board. He continued surfing for approximately 1 hour following the accident and drove himself home. He was alert and oriented all morning, only complaining of a headache, taking ibuprofen at 10 AM. He appeared to be sleeping at 1 PM when mother left to do errands and she was unable to arouse him when she returned 2 hours later. On examination, this is a well-developed, well-nourished, adolescent male. Temperature 97.4, HR 66, RR 12, BP 88/50. **Neurological examination reveals no spontaneous eye opening or response to verbal commands, there is withdrawal from painful stimuli. Score = 6 on Glasgow Coma Scale**. Call placed to Children's Hospital Trauma Center and life flight team dispatched. ETA 22 minutes. NSR on cardiac monitor. O2 saturation 92% by pulse oximetry, O2 started at 2 L/m via non-rebreather mask. HOB elevated 30%. IV line placed right forearm, LR infusing. Blood drawn for CBC, platelets, electrolytes, PT, PTT, type and hold and sent to lab. Bladder can be palpated above the pubic bone, Foley catheter placed without difficulty, 600 cc clear yellow urine returned.

Transport team note: Arrived in ED at 4:13 PM. Baseline lab tests all within normal limits. ABG drawn pH 7.32, pCO2 51, HCO3 25, pO2 88 %, SaO2 96 %. Patient intubated without difficulty, hand ventilated by RT. Transferred to life flight stretcher, on monitors, stable for transport. All consents obtained, parents following in private car. ETA Children's Hospital 17 minutes with neurosurgical team assembled and ready for patient. Uneventful helicopter transport. Patient taken directly from heliport to CT. Care assumed by neurosurgical team and radiology staff.

Code the Glasgow Coma Scale information only.

Diagnosis Code(s)

R40.2112 Coma scale, eyes open never, at arrival in emergency department

R40.2212 Coma scale, best verbal response, none, at arrival in emergency department

R40.2342 Coma scale, best motor response, flexion withdrawal, at arrival in emergency department

Reporting of the total score is not required since all three components are documented. If only the total score of 6 was reported it would be coded as follows:

R40.2432 Glasgow coma scale score 3-8, at arrival to emergency department

Coding Note(s)

Glasgow coma scale codes are reported additionally with fracture of skull (S02.-) and/or intracranial injury (S06.-) reported first.

Disturbance of Skin Sensation

Disturbance of skin sensation includes conditions such as anesthesia of skin, hypoesthesia of skin, paresthesia of skin, and hyperesthesia. Anesthesia of the skin is the complete loss of sensation in the skin. Hypoesthesia is decreased sensation. Paresthesia refers to abnormal sensation such as tingling or a "pins and needles" sensation. Hyperesthesia is exaggerated sensation or hypersensitivity to touch.

Codes in category R20 are specific for anesthesia of skin, hypoesthesia of skin, paresthesia of skin, and hyperesthesia. There are also codes for other specified disturbances of skin sensation and unspecified disturbances of skin sensation.

Coding and Documentation Requirements

Identify the skin sensation disturbance:

- Anesthesia of skin
- Hyperesthesia
- Hypoesthesia of skin
- Paresthesia of skin
- Other specified disturbances of skin sensation
- Unspecified disturbances of skin sensation

ICD-10-CM Code/Documentation	
R20.0	Anesthesia of skin
R20.1	Hypoesthesia of skin
R20.2	Paresthesia of skin
R20.3	Hyperesthesia
R20.8	Other disturbances of skin sensation
R20.9	Unspecified disturbances of skin sensation

Documentation and Coding Example

Twenty-eight-year-old Caucasian female presents to PMD with c/o tactile discomfort in her left thigh. She began to notice tingling and numbness approximately 3 months ago. Initially the discomfort was limited to a small area of the anterior thigh. The area of discomfort increased in size over the next few weeks and changed from numbness to hypersensitivity. She now finds it intolerable to have lightweight clothing touch her skin from left anterior mid-thigh to just above the knee cap. Heavier fabric is less bothersome but since it is summer with outdoor temperatures over 90 degrees, she finds herself either miserable from overheating in heavy pants and skirts or miserable from lightweight clothing brushing her thigh. She has tried over the counter topical anesthetic cream with some short-term relief but the hypersensitivity seemed to increase afterwards. She can recall no trauma to the leg or anything else that might have precipitated the condition.

On examination, this is a petite, thin, well groomed, young woman. Cranial nerves are grossly intact. Neck is supple and spine is straight. Forward bending elicits no discomfort in back or hips. Upper extremities have normal reflexes, pulses, and muscle strength. Lower extremities have no edema. Pulses, reflexes, and muscle strength all WNL. The right leg has normal sensation to dull/sharp stimulation from hip to toes. Left leg has normal sensation in all areas except for a strip down the anterior thigh beginning 6 cm below the inguinal crease and ending 1 cm above the center of the patella. The width of the area is 7.5 cm at mid-thigh and tapers to 2 cm at the distal and proximal ends.

Impression: **Hyperesthesia of the skin, unknown etiology**.

Plan: Tegretol 200 mg PO BID. Referral to neurologist for further workup.

Diagnosis Code(s)

R20.3 Hyperesthesia

Coding Note(s)

A symptom code must be reported because the physician has not identified the cause of the hyperesthesia. The patient is being referred to a specialist for further evaluation of the symptom.

Edema

Edema is an excessive accumulation of fluid in cells or intercellular tissues. The accumulation of fluid may be due to a number of causes, but it is also a significant symptom and when documented as such by the physician it may be reported as an additional diagnosis.

Category R60 Edema lists two specific codes, one for localized edema and another for generalized edema. There is also a code for unspecified edema.

Coding and Documentation Requirements

Identify extent of edema:

- Localized
- Generalized
- Unspecified

ICD-10-CM Code/Documentation	
R60.0	Localized edema
R60.1	Generalized edema
R60.9	Edema, unspecified

Documentation and Coding Example

Patient is a forty-seven-year-old Asian female who presents to Urgent Care Clinic with **edema of her left lower leg x 2 weeks**. Patient states she was in her usual state of good health, walking daily when she began to notice painless swelling around her left ankle. She could recall no injury and decided just to continue her normal routine. The swelling progressed toward her toes and then up to midcalf. At first the swelling seemed to decrease overnight but for the past four days the swelling is just as severe when she wakes in the morning. Yesterday her left knee felt a little stiff and this morning the swelling has clearly migrated upward to include the knee. T 98.8, P 74, R 12, BP 134/78, Wt. 111 lbs. On examination, this is a trim, athletic appearing woman who looks younger than her stated age. She states she is divorced, has no children and works as a food stylist for a syndicated TV show. Upper extremities show no signs of edema. Muscle tone and reflexes are WNL. There are no enlarged lymph nodes in her neck, axilla, or groin. Abdomen is soft with active bowel sounds. Liver is palpated 1 cm below the RCM, spleen 1 cm below the LCM. Breath sounds clear and heart rate regular without murmur. Examination of right lower extremity is completely benign. Pulses are intact, normal reflexes and muscle strength and no edema. The left lower extremity is normal from hip to right above the knee. The knee joint has marked swelling and crepitus with movement but patient denies pain. There is also no redness or increased warmth. The lower leg, including ankle, foot, and toes has pitting edema and decreased ROM of the ankle due to the swelling. The skin is intact with no signs of insect bites or stings, cuts, or bruising.

Impression: Perplexing presentation of **localized edema, unknown etiology**. Call placed to her PMD who would like to have a venous Doppler study done and labs drawn. Appointment scheduled for tomorrow in ultrasound for venous Doppler study and patient is sent to lab for blood draw. She will follow up with PMD.

Diagnosis Code(s)

R60.0 Localized edema

Coding Note(s)

The edema is limited to the left leg so the code for localized edema is reported.

Localized Swelling/Mass/Lump

Codes for localized swelling, mass, or lump are assigned when the documentation does not support a more specific diagnosis such as a sebaceous cyst, lipoma, or enlarged lymph node.

Subcategory R19.0 Intra-abdominal and pelvic swelling, mass or lump is specific to the intra-abdominal and pelvic regions and would not be reported for a superficial swelling, mass, or lump localized to the skin and subcutaneous tissue of the abdomen unless otherwise indicated in the Alphabetic Index. Category R22 reports localized swelling, mass, and lump of skin and subcutaneous tissue and codes are specific to site. While the category does indicate that these codes are for a swelling, mass, or lump in the skin and subcutaneous tissue, documentation of a chest mass without any further information is coded to R22.2. Documentation of the site as being in the skin or subcutaneous tissue is not required. However, if the mass were found on a diagnostic imaging study of the lung and was documented as being in the lung, code R91.8 Other nonspecific abnormal finding of lung field would be reported. Careful review of the documentation is needed to ensure that the most appropriate code is assigned.

Coding and Documentation Requirements

Identify site:

- Head
- Lower limb
  - Bilateral
  - Left
  - Right
  - Unspecified
- Neck
- Trunk
- Upper limb
  - Bilateral
  - Left
  - Right
  - Unspecified
- Unspecified site

ICD-10-CM Code/Documentation	
R19.00	Intra-abdominal and pelvic swelling, mass and lump, unspecified site
R19.01	Right upper quadrant abdominal swelling, mass and lump
R19.02	Left upper quadrant abdominal swelling, mass and lump
R19.03	Right lower quadrant abdominal swelling, mass and lump
R19.04	Left lower quadrant abdominal swelling, mass and lump
R19.05	Periumbilic swelling, mass or lump
R19.06	Epigastric swelling, mass or lump
R19.07	Generalized intra-abdominal and pelvic swelling, mass and lump
R19.09	Other intra-abdominal and pelvic swelling, mass and lump
R22.0	Localized swelling, mass and lump, head
R22.1	Localized swelling, mass and lump, neck
R22.2	Localized swelling, mass or lump, trunk
R22.30	Localized swelling, mass or lump, unspecified upper limb
R22.31	Localized swelling, mass and lump, right upper limb
R22.32	Localized swelling, mass and lump, left upper limb
R22.33	Localized swelling, mass and lump, upper limb, bilateral
R22.40	Localized swelling, mass and lump, unspecified lower limb
R22.41	Localized swelling, mass and lump, right lower limb
R22.42	Localized swelling, mass and lump, left lower limb
R22.43	Localized swelling, mass and lump, lower limb, bilateral
R22.9	Localized swelling, mass and lump, unspecified

Documentation and Coding Example

Forty-year-old Caucasian male presents to PMD with a **painless lump behind his right knee**. Patient can recall no trauma or injury to the area but simply noticed it one morning about two weeks ago in the shower. It appears to have increased in size over the last few days which causes him concern. Patient works as an accountant and was putting in long hours when he first noticed the lump. He states that with tax season over, he can finally take care of himself. On examination, this is a well-developed, well-nourished gentleman who looks somewhat older than his stated age. PERRL, neck supple without lymphadenopathy. Cranial nerves grossly intact. Upper extremities have normal pulses, reflexes, and muscle tone. Spine is straight. Forward bending elicits no pain or discomfort in back, hips, or legs. Heart rate regular, breath sounds clear. Abdomen soft and flat with liver palpated at 2 cm below the RCM and spleen at the LCM. No evidence of inguinal hernia, femoral pulses intact. Pulses, reflexes, and muscle strength WNL in lower extremities. **There is a soft superficial mass felt directly behind the right knee.** The mass measures 2 x 3 cm and is slightly mobile. Gentle and firm palpation around the knee joint does not cause pain or discomfort. The area is not red or warm to touch.

Plan: Will watch the area to see if the mass resolves on its own. May obtain a knee x-ray or biopsy, if mass doesn't resolve or continues to increase in size.

Diagnosis Code(s)

R22.41	Localized swelling, mass and lump, right lower limb

Coding Note(s)

The site of the lump/mass is reported as the right lower limb as a code specifically for the knee is not available.

Summary

Like definitive diagnoses from other chapters, the codes for symptoms, signs, abnormal results of laboratory and other investigative procedures, and ill-defined conditions require certain information in the documentation to assign the most specific code. Many physicians already provide sufficient documentation to capture the most specific codes, but a review of commonly reported signs and symptoms, abnormal test results for commonly performed tests, and other ill-defined conditions that are commonly documented in medical records for patients receiving diagnostic work-up is still required to ensure that documentation is sufficient to capture the most specific code.

Chapter 18 Quiz

1. Which of the following conditions is reported with a code from Chapter 18?
   a. Muscle spasm
   b. Breast lump
   c. Stupor
   d. All of the above
2. The physician has documented that the patient is being seen for repeated falls and is at risk for falling again and also has a history of falling. How is this reported?
   a. Only the code for repeated falls (R29.6) is reported
   b. Both the code for repeated falls (R29.6) and the code for history of falling (Z91.81) are reported.
   c. Only the code for history of falling (Z91.81) is reported
   d. Neither code is reported. The physician should document any injuries associated with the fall and the injuries should be reported.
3. Assignment of a sign or symptom code may be assigned with a definitive diagnosis code under what circumstances?
   a. When the sign or symptom is not routinely associated with the definitive diagnosis
   b. Whenever both a sign or symptom and a definitive diagnosis are documented
   c. When the sign or symptom is routinely associated with the disease process
   d. All of the above
4. What do the coding guidelines state for reporting uncertain diagnoses such as those documented as "probable" or "suspected" in the outpatient setting?
   a. Do not code the diagnoses documented as "probable" or "suspected". Instead code the condition(s) to the highest degree of specificity as documented in the medical record
   b. Code the sign/symptom as the first-listed diagnosis and all probable or suspected diagnoses as secondary codes
   c. Code any "probable" or "suspected" diagnoses that are currently being observed or worked up by the physician
   d. Code the "probable" or "suspected" diagnosis only if a diagnostic procedure has been performed
5. Coma scale codes may be used in conjunction with which of the following types of conditions?
   a. Traumatic brain injury codes
   b. Acute cerebrovascular disease
   c. Sequelae of cerebrovascular disease codes
   d. All of the above
6. The physician has seen the patient in his office and has documented that the patient has a chest mass. Can code R22.2 be reported for this diagnosis?
   a. No, the documentation must state that the mass is in the skin and subcutaneous tissue
   b. Yes, the default code for chest mass without any additional information is R22.2
   c. No, the physician must provide a more definitive diagnosis
   d. No, the physician must provide his/her impression of the type of mass, such as possible cyst or enlarged lymph node, so that these conditions can also be reported
7. A patient has come into the ED with a head injury and the physician has documented that the patient opens her eyes to sound; her attempts at conversation are confused; and she localizes pain. What information does this provide about her head injury?
   a. Her GCS total score is 12 and she has a moderate head injury
   b. Her GCS total core is 13 and she has a mild head injury
   c. Her GCS total score cannot be calculated for the information provided
   d. Her GCS score is 12 and she has a mild head injury
8. In the outpatient setting, codes that describe symptoms and signs are acceptable for reporting purposes under what circumstances?
   a. When the physician has documented signs and symptoms and has also documented a definitive diagnosis related to the signs and symptoms
   b. When a related definitive diagnosis has not been established (confirmed) by the provider at that encounter/visit.
   c. Whenever the physician documents a sign or symptom
   d. All of the above.
9. In the inpatient setting, the physician has documented abnormal laboratory findings. When should these abnormal findings be coded?
   a. Abnormal findings are always assigned a code
   b. Abnormal findings are never assigned a code
   c. Abnormal findings are reported if additional tests are ordered to further evaluate the abnormal finding
   d. Abnormal findings are coded and reported when the provider indicates their clinical significance
10. The chapter level note at the beginning of Chapter 18 identifies conditions and signs or symptoms that are reported with codes in categories R00-R94. Under which of the following circumstances would it NOT be appropriate to report a code from Chapter 18?
    a. Cases for which no more specific diagnosis can be made even after all the facts bearing on the case have been investigated
    b. Signs or symptoms existing at the time of initial encounter that proved to be transient and whose causes could not be determined.
    c. Cases referred elsewhere for treatment after a definitive diagnosis was made
    d. Certain symptoms for which supplementary information is provided that present important problems in medical care in their own right

See next page for answers and rationales.

Chapter 18 Answers and Rationales

1. Which of the following conditions is reported with a code from Chapter 18?

   c. **Stupor**

   Rationale: *Only stupor is reported with a code (R40.1) from Chapter 18. Muscle spasm (M62.83-) is reported with a code from Chapter 13 Diseases of the Musculoskeletal System and Connective Tissue and the excludes1 note at the beginning of Chapter 18 indicates that signs and symptoms of the breast (N63, N64.5) are not reported with codes from Chapter 18.*

2. The physician has documented that the patient is being seen for repeated falls and is at risk for falling again and also has a history of falling. How is this reported?

   b. **Both the code for repeated falls (R29.6) and the code for history of falling (Z91.81) are reported.**

   Rationale: *According the Chapter guidelines, both codes are reported when the patient is being seen for repeated falls and also has a history of falling.*

3. Assignment of a sign or symptom code may be assigned with a definitive diagnosis code under what circumstances?

   a. **When the sign or symptom is not routinely associated with the definitive diagnosis**

   Rationale: *According to the coding guidelines, a sign or symptom code should only be assigned if the sign or symptom is not routinely associated with the definitive diagnosis. A code for a sign or symptom that is routinely associated with the disease process is only assigned if the chapter, category, or subcategory instructions indicate that the sign or symptom should be coded additionally.*

4. What do the coding guidelines state for reporting of uncertain diagnoses such as those documented as "probable" or "suspected" in the outpatient setting?

   a. **Do not code the diagnoses documented as "probable" or "suspected". Instead code the conditions to the highest degree of specificity as documented in the medical record**

   Rationale: *While probable and suspected diagnoses may be reported in the inpatient setting, they are not reported in the outpatient setting. Instead, the condition is coded to the highest degree of specificity as documented in the medical record for that encounter or visit which may require reporting of a code for a sign, symptom, or abnormal test result.*

5. Coma scale codes may be used in conjunction with which of the following types of conditions?

   d. **All of the above**

   Rationale: *According to the chapter guidelines, coma scale codes may be used in conjunction with all of the listed conditions.*

6. The physician has seen the patient in his office and has documented that the patient has a chest mass. Can code R22.2 be reported for this diagnosis?

   b. **Yes, the default code for chest mass without any additional information is R22.2**

   Rationale: *Since no other information is available and there are no instructions in the Tabular List directing the coder to another code, the code identified in the Alphabetic Index is the correct code. In this case the Alphabetic Index directs the coder to R22.2 for a diagnosis of chest mass.*

7. A patient has come into the ED with a head injury and the physician has documented that the patient opens her eyes to sound, her attempts at conversation are confused, and she localizes pain. What information does this provide about her head injury?

   a. **Her GCS total score is 12 and she has a moderate head injury**

   Rationale: *Using the points assigned for each element of the GCS, 3 points for eyes open to sound, 4 points for confused conversation, and 5 points for localizing pain, her total GCS is 12, which corresponds to a moderate head injury.*

8. In the outpatient setting, codes that describe symptoms and signs are acceptable for reporting purposes under what circumstances?

   b. **When a related definitive diagnosis has not been established (confirmed) by the provider at that encounter/visit.**

   Rationale: *Only established (confirmed) diagnoses should be reported. If the physician has not established a diagnosis related to the signs and symptoms, a code or codes for the signs and symptoms is assigned.*

9. In the inpatient setting, the physician has documented abnormal laboratory findings. When should these abnormal findings be coded?

   d. **Abnormal findings are coded and reported when the provider indicates their clinical significance**

   Rationale: *Coding guidelines state "Abnormal findings" (laboratory, x-ray, pathologic, and other diagnostic results) are not coded and reported unless the provider indicates their clinical significance. If the findings are outside the normal range and the attending provider has ordered other tests to evaluate the condition or prescribed treatment, it is appropriate to ask the provider whether the abnormal findings should be added.* ***Note:*** *This differs from the coding practices in the outpatient setting for coding encounters for diagnostic tests that have been interpreted by a provider.*

10. The chapter level note at the beginning of Chapter 18 identifies conditions and signs or symptoms that are reported with codes in categories R00-R94. Under which of the following circumstances would it NOT be appropriate to report a code from Chapter 18?

    c. **Cases referred elsewhere for treatment after a definitive diagnosis was made**

    Rationale: *When a case is referred elsewhere for treatment after a definitive diagnosis is made, the code for the definitive diagnosis is assigned, not a code for the signs or symptoms that initially prompted the encounter. However, a sign or symptom code may be reported when the case is referred elsewhere for investigation and treatment BEFORE a definitive diagnosis has been established.*

Chapter 19

INJURY, POISONING, AND CERTAIN OTHER CONSEQUENCES OF EXTERNAL CAUSES

Introduction

Codes for injury, poisoning and certain other consequences of external causes are found in Chapter 19. Coding to the highest level of specificity for injuries requires extensive documentation. Documentation for injuries now requires more detailed information related to the type of injury, the specific location, and laterality to name a few. The requirements necessary for documentation of fractures discussed in Chapter 15 Musculoskeletal System is true for the majority of injuries in Chapter 19. In addition to the codes for injuries, Chapter 19 also includes a separate section for codes for burns, corrosions and frostbite. These, like the injury codes are classified first by location then by type and severity. The codes for adverse effects, poisoning, underdosing, and toxicity are combination codes that capture both the drug and the external cause. Finally, codes for consequences of external cause which includes complications due to past surgery or trauma are included in this chapter.

The majority of the codes related to injury, poisoning and certain complications also require the use of a 7th character to identify the episode of care. While episode of care is required only for some code categories in other chapters, the vast majority of codes in Chapter 19 require identification of the episode of care. One thing to note about episode of care codes is that there is no 7th character for "episode of care not otherwise specified." Documentation must clearly identify the visit as the initial encounter, subsequent encounter, or sequela. The term 'initial encounter' is somewhat misleading as it actually refers to the period of time when the patient is receiving active treatment for the condition. Examples of encounters that would be for active treatment include: emergency department encounter, surgical treatment, and evaluation and continuing treatment by the same or a different physician. Active treatment is based upon whether the patient is undergoing active treatment not whether the provider is seeing the patient for the first time. Active treatment should not be confused with ongoing management of the condition during the healing phase.

Injuries and poisoning should also have documentation of the external cause of injury. This is particularly important in the inpatient acute care setting for trauma registry purposes. External cause coding and documentation requirements will be reviewed in Chapter 2Ø. However, because the external cause is integral to complete coding and documentation for injury and poisoning, a brief review of the types of information captured by these codes is included here. External cause codes identify the following:

- Cause of injury (such as fall, auto accident, gunshot wound)
- Place of occurrence (such as home, school, work, highway, park, wilderness area)
- Activity (such as shoveling snow, swimming, showering/bathing)
- External cause status (civilian activity done for pay/income, military activity, volunteer activity, hobby, leisure, student)

The documentation and coding examples in this chapter include external cause, place of occurrence, activity and external cause status. These have also been coded in the examples but will be covered more thoroughly in Chapter 2Ø.

Organization of Injury Codes

Injury codes are organized first by body area and then by type of injury. The code blocks are listed below. When reviewing the injury code blocks it is helpful to remember that the second character identifies the body area. For example, all injuries related to the foot and ankle will have a second character of 9 (S90-S99).

ICD-1Ø-CM Blocks	
SØØ-SØ9	Injuries to the Head
S1Ø-S19	Injuries to the Neck
S2Ø-S29	Injuries to the Thorax
S3Ø-S39	Injuries to the Abdomen, Lower Back, Lumbar Spine, Pelvis, and External Genitals
S4Ø-S49	Injuries to the Shoulder and Upper Arm
S5Ø-S59	Injuries to the Elbow and Forearm
S6Ø-S69	Injuries to the Wrist, Hand and Fingers
S7Ø-S79	Injuries to the Hip and Thigh
S8Ø-S89	Injuries to the Knee and Lower Leg
S9Ø-S99	Injuries to the Ankle and Foot
TØ7	Injuries Involving Multiple Body Regions
T14	Injury of Unspecified Body Region
T15-T19	Effects of Foreign Body Entering Through Natural Orifice
T2Ø-T25	Burns and Corrosions of External Body Surface, Specified by Site
T26-T28	Burns and Corrosions Confined to Eye and Internal Organs
T3Ø-T32	Burns and Corrosions of Multiple and Unspecified Body Regions
T33-T34	Frostbite
T36-T5Ø	Poisoning by, Adverse Effects of and Underdosing of Drugs, Medicaments and Biological Substances
T51-T65	Toxic Effects of Substances Chiefly Nonmedicinal as to Source
T66-T78	Other and Unspecified Effects of External Causes
T79	Certain Early Complications of Trauma
T8Ø-T88	Complications of Surgical and Medical Care, Not Elsewhere Classified

Coding Notes

In ICD-10-CM, there are some important coding notes and instructions at the beginning of the chapter. The first note references the need to use secondary codes from Chapter 20 External Causes of Morbidity, to indicate cause of injury. Some codes in Chapter 19, such as codes for toxic effects of drugs and chemicals, include the external cause and do not require an additional external cause code for the intent. The second note is a 'use additional code' instruction to identify any retained foreign body, if applicable (Z18.-).

There are no instructions at the beginning of Chapter 19 related to coding of multiple injuries. Instead, coding instructions related to multiple injuries are now provided in the guidelines. There are also no instructions for coding late effects of injuries. In ICD-10-CM late effects are considered sequelae. Instructions related to coding of sequelae are also found in the guidelines. One thing to note is that codes for sequelae of injuries are reported with the same code as the injury with a 7th character 'S' to identify that the encounter/treatment is for a sequela of the injury.

Exclusions

Chapter 19 in ICD-10-CM lists trauma diagnoses that are excluded from the injury and poisoning chapter.

Excludes 1	Excludes2
Birth trauma (P10-P15) Obstetric trauma (O10-O71)	None

Chapter Guidelines

There are detailed guidelines for the majority of the sections in Chapter 19. The guideline topics are listed below with detailed information on each of these guidelines to follow.

- Application of 7th characters
- Coding of injuries
- Coding of traumatic fractures
- Coding of burns and corrosions
- Adverse effects, poisoning, underdosing, and toxic effects
- Adult and child abuse, neglect, and other maltreatment
- Complications of care

Application of 7th Characters

Most categories in the injury and poisoning chapter require assignment of a 7th character to codes to identify the episode of care. For most categories, there are three 7th character values to select from: 'A' for initial encounter; 'D' for subsequent encounter; and 'S' for sequela. Categories for fractures are an exception with fractures having six to sixteen 7th character values. The 7th character value for fractures is necessary to capture additional information about the fracture, including whether it is open or closed and whether the healing phase is routine or complicated by delayed healing, nonunion, or malunion. Detailed guidelines are provided related to selection of the 7th character value. Related guidelines and some examples of encounters representative of the three episode of care 7th character values found in the majority of categories are as follows:

A Initial encounter. Initial encounter is defined as the period when the patient is receiving active treatment for the injury, poisoning, or other consequences of an external cause. An 'A' may be assigned on more than one claim. For example, if a patient is seen in the emergency department (ED) for a head injury that is first evaluated by the ED physician who requests a CT scan, which is read by a radiologist and a consultation by a neurologist, the 7th character 'A' is used by all three physicians and also reported on the ED claim. If the patient required admission to an acute care hospital, the 7th character 'A' would be reported for the entire acute care hospital stay because the 7th character extension 'A' is used for the entire period that the patient receives active treatment for the injury.

D Subsequent encounter. This is an encounter after the active phase of treatment and when the patient is receiving routine care for the injury or poisoning during the period of healing or recovery. Unlike aftercare following medical or surgical services for other conditions which are reported with codes from Chapter 21 Factors Influencing Health Status and Contact with Health Services (Z00-Z99), aftercare for injuries and poisonings is captured by the 7th character 'D'. For example, a patient with an ankle sprain may return to the office to have joint stability re-evaluated to ensure that the injury is healing properly. In this case, the 7th character 'D' would be assigned.

S Sequela. The 7th character extension 'S' is assigned for complications or conditions that arise as a direct result of an injury. An example of a sequela is a scar resulting from a burn.

Coding of Injuries

General coding and sequencing guidelines for injuries are as follows:

- Separate codes are required for each injury unless a combination code is provided, in which case the combination code should be used
- The code for unspecified multiple injuries (T07) should not be assigned in the inpatient setting unless more specific information about the injuries is not available. This would be an extremely rare occurrence
- Traumatic injury codes (S00-T14.9) are not used to report normal, healing surgical wounds or complications of surgical wounds
- Sequencing of injury codes
  - The most serious injury as determined by the provider and the focus of treatment based on the provider's documentation is sequenced first
  - Superficial injuries such as abrasions or contusions are not coded when associated with more severe injuries of the same site. For example, a closed fracture sustained in a fall with contusions at the fracture site would require coding of the fracture only. The contusions are considered superficial injuries and would not be coded.

- Determining the primary injury for injuries that occur with damage to nerves and blood vessels
  - When a primary injury occurs with minor damage to nerves and/or blood vessels, the primary injury is sequenced first followed by additional codes for injuries to nerves and spinal cord and/or codes for injuries to blood vessels
  - When the primary injury is to a blood vessel or nerves, the blood vessel or nerve injury is sequenced first

Coding of Traumatic Fractures

The overall principles for coding traumatic fractures are the same as for other injuries but more expansive. Guidelines are as follows:

- A fracture not indicated as open or closed is coded as closed
- A fracture not indicated as displaced or nondisplaced is coded as displaced
- Multiple fractures:
  - When there are multiple fractures, a separate code is required for each specified fracture site in accordance with instructions provided at the category and subcategory level and the level of detail documented in the medical record.
  - Multiple fractures are sequenced in accordance with the severity of the fracture as documented by the provider. The provider should be asked to list fracture diagnoses in order of severity
- Initial versus subsequent encounter for fractures and assignment of 7th character extensions:
  - Initial encounter – 7th character extensions A, B, C
    - Use an initial encounter 7th character extension when the patient is receiving active treatment for the fracture, which includes emergency department encounter, surgical treatment, and evaluation and continuing (ongoing) treatment by the same or a different physician. Active treatment is based upon whether the patient is undergoing active treatment not whether the provider is seeing the patient for the first time.
    - Use initial encounter 7th character extensions for individuals who delayed seeking treatment for the fracture or delayed seeking treatment for a nonunion
  - Subsequent encounter – 7th character extensions D, E, F, G, H, J, K, M, N, P, Q, R
    - Use a subsequent encounter 7th character extension when the patient has completed active treatment of the fracture and is receiving routine care for the fracture during the healing or recovery phase
    - Routine aftercare for the fracture includes: cast change or removal, an x-ray to check healing status of a fracture, removal of external or internal fixation device, medication adjustment, other follow-up visits for fracture aftercare
    - Aftercare Z codes are not used for aftercare of traumatic fractures
- Complications of fractures:
  - Any complications of surgical treatment for fracture repairs during the healing or recovery phase should be coded with the appropriate complication code
  - Delayed healing, nonunion, and malunion are reported with the appropriate 7th character extensions for subsequent care as follows:
    - Delayed healing – G, H, J
    - Nonunion – K, M, N
    - Malunion – P, Q, R
    - Assign the appropriate 7th character for initial visit not subsequent encounter for a patient with a nonunion/malunion who delayed seeking treatment and is being evaluated for the first time.
- Fractures in a patient with known osteoporosis:
  - Do not use a traumatic fracture code for a patient with known osteoporosis who suffers a fracture even when the fracture occurs after a minor fall or trauma if that fall or trauma would not normally break a normal, healthy bone
  - A code from category M80 Osteoporosis with current pathological fracture, should be reported in the above described instance
- Other nontraumatic fractures are reported with codes from Chapter 13 Diseases of the Musculoskeletal System and Connective Tissue:
  - Fatigue fracture of vertebrae (M48.4)
  - Stress fracture (M84.3)
  - Pathological fracture, not elsewhere classified (M84.4)
  - Pathological fracture in neoplastic disease (M84.5)
  - Pathological fracture in other disease (M84.6)
  - Atypical femoral fracture (M84.7)

Coding of Burns and Corrosions

Burns are classified first by type, thermal or corrosion burns, and then by depth and extent. Corrosions are burns due to chemicals. Thermal burns are burns that come from a heat source but exclude sunburns. Examples of heat sources include fire, hot appliance, electricity, and radiation.

The guidelines are the same for both corrosions and thermal burns with one exception—corrosions require identification of the chemical substance. The chemical substance that caused the corrosion is the first listed diagnosis. The chemical substance is found in the Table of Drugs and Chemicals. Codes for drugs and chemicals are combination codes that identify the substance and the external cause or intent, so an external cause of injury code is not required. However, codes should be assigned for the place of occurrence, activity, and external cause status. Guidelines for the use of the external cause codes can be found in Chapter 20 External Causes of Morbidity. The correct code for an accidental corrosion is found in the column for poisoning, accidental (unintentional).

Classification of Current Burns

Current corrosions and thermal burns are classified by:

- Depth
  - First degree (erythema)
  - Second degree (blistering)
  - Third degree (full thickness involvement)
- Extent
  - Total body surface burned
  - Total body surface with third degree burns
- Agent
  - Corrosive (T-code)
    - » Acids
    - » Alkalines
    - » Caustics
    - » Chemicals
  - Thermal (except sunburn) (X-code)
    - » Electricity
    - » Flame
    - » Heat (gas, liquid, or object)
    - » Radiation
    - » Steam

The agent can be found in the Table of Drugs and Chemicals for corrosions and in the Alphabetic Index to External Causes for thermal burns.

Note: Burns of the eye and internal organs are classified by site but not by degree.

Sequencing of Burn Codes

Coding Guidelines for burns, related conditions, and complications of burns are as follows:

- Sequencing of multiple burns and/or burn injuries with related conditions:
  - Multiple external burns only. When more than one external burn is present, the first listed diagnosis code is the code that reflects the highest degree burn
  - Internal and external burns. The circumstances of the admission or encounter govern the selection of the principle or first-listed diagnosis
  - Burn injuries and other related conditions such as smoke inhalation or respiratory failure. The circumstances of the admission or encounter govern the selection of the principal or first-listed diagnosis
- Assign separate codes for each burn site
- Burns of the same anatomic site
  - Classify burns of the same anatomic site and on the same side but of different degrees to the subcategory identifying the highest degree recorded in the diagnosis (e.g., for second and third degree burns of right thigh, assign only code T24.311-)
- Burns of unspecified site
  - Codes from category T30 Burn and corrosion, body region unspecified, is extremely vague and should rarely be used
- Classifying burns and corrosions by extent of body surface area involved:
  - A code from category T31 Burns classified according to extent of body surface involved, or T32 Corrosions classified according to extent of body surface involved, may be reported as the first listed diagnosis when:
    - » The site of the burn is not specified
    - » There is a need for additional information on the extent of the burns
  - Codes from category T31 should be used whenever possible to:
    - » Provide data for evaluating burn mortality, such as that needed by burn units
    - » When there is mention of a third-degree burn involving 20% or more of body surface
  - Rule of nines - Extent of body surface for categories T31 and T32 are governed by the rule of nines as follows:
    - » Head and neck – 9%
    - » Each arm – 9%
    - » Each leg – 18%
    - » Anterior trunk – 18%
    - » Posterior trunk – 18%
    - » Genitalia – 1%

    Note: Providers may modify these percentages for infants and children who have larger heads than adults and for adults with large buttocks, thighs, and abdomens when those regions are burned.
- Non-healing and infected burns:
  - Non-healing burns are coded as acute burns with 7th character extension 'A'
  - Necrosis of burned skin is coded as a non-healing burn
  - Infected burns require use of an additional code for the infection
- Late effects/sequelae of burns:
  - Sequelae are reported using a burn or corrosion code with the 7th character 'S'
  - Both a code for a current burn or corrosion code and a code for sequela may be assigned on the same record. It is possible for a patient to receive treatment for a current burn and treatment for sequela because corrosions and burns do not heal at the same rate.
- External cause codes are reported additionally for burns and corrosions to:
  - Identify the source and intent of the burn (X-code) or corrosion (T-code)
  - Place of occurrence
  - Activity
  - External cause status

Adverse Effects, Poisoning, Underdosing, and Toxic Effects

Codes for adverse effects, poisoning, underdosing, and toxic effects are combination codes that include both the substance taken and the intent. No additional external cause code is reported with these codes.

Locating the correct code for the drug, medicament, other biological substance, or nonmedicinal substance is done as follows:

- Use the Table of Drugs and Chemicals to find the correct drug or other substance
- Identify the condition:
  - Poisoning (includes toxic effect)
    - » Accidental
    - » Intentional self-harm
    - » Assault
    - » Undetermined
  - Adverse effect
  - Underdosing

    Note: For toxic effect of substances chiefly nonmedicinal as to source (T51-T65), when no intent is indicated, code to accidental. Undetermined intent is only for use when there is specific documentation to indicate that the intent of the toxic effect cannot be determined
- Refer to the Tabular list to verify code selection
- Use as many codes as necessary to describe completely all drugs, medicinal, biological, or other substances responsible for the adverse effect, poisoning, underdosing, or toxic effect
- If a single causative agent has resulted in more than one adverse effect, poisoning, underdosing, or toxic effect list the code for the causative agent only once
- If two or more drugs or other substances are responsible for the adverse effect, poisoning, underdosing, or toxic effect, assign a code for each one individually unless a combination code is available

Toxicity due to drugs or other substances is classified in ICD-10-CM as:

- Adverse effect
- Poisoning
- Underdosing
- Toxic Effect

Guidelines and sequencing of adverse effect, poisoning, underdosing, and toxic effects are as follows:

- Adverse effect
  - Defined as a drug or other substance that has been correctly prescribed and properly administered
  - Sequencing of codes for adverse effect:
    - » In I.C.19.e.5(a) it states, "assign the appropriate code for the nature of the adverse effect followed by the appropriate code for the adverse effect of the drug (T36-T50)"
    - » There is also an instruction in the Tabular List for the code block T36-T50 that states, "Code first, for adverse effects, the nature of the adverse effect"
- Poisoning
  - Defined as the improper use of a drug or other substance which includes:
    - » Overdose
    - » Wrong substance given or taken
    - » Wrong route of administration
    - » Nonprescribed drug taken with correctly prescribed and properly administered drug
    - » Interaction of drugs and alcohol
  - Sequencing of codes for poisoning:
    - » The appropriate poisoning code(s) which includes the intent (T36-T50) is sequenced first
    - » The code(s) that specify the manifestation(s) of the poisoning are listed as additional code(s)
- Underdosing
  - Defined as taking less of a medication than is prescribed by the provider or the manufacturer's instructions. Discontinuing the use of a prescribed medication on the patient's own initiative, not directed by the patient's provider, is also classified as underdosing
  - Sequencing of codes for underdosing:
    - » Underdosing codes are never assigned as the principal or first-listed code
    - » Assign the code for the relapse or exacerbation of the medical condition for which the drug is prescribed as the principal or first-listed code
    - » Assign the code for the underdosing as an additional code
    - » Assign an additional code for noncompliance, if known (Z91.12-, Z91.13-, and Z91.14-) to capture intent
    - » Assign an additional code for complication of care, if known (Y63.8-, Y63.9) to capture intent
- Toxic effects
  - Defined as ingesting or coming in contact with a harmful substance that is chiefly non-medicinal as to source
  - Use for toxic effect of substances chiefly nonmedicinal as to source (T51-T65)
  - Toxic effects are captured with poisoning codes and have an associated intent (accidental, intentional self-harm, assault, undetermined)
    - » When no intent is indicated, code to accidental
    - » Undetermined intent is only for use when there is specific documentation to indicate that the intent of the toxic effect cannot be determined
  - The appropriate toxic effect code, which includes the intent (T51-T65), is sequenced first
  - The code(s) that specify the manifestation(s) of the toxic effect are listed as additional code(s).

Adult and Child Abuse, Neglect, and Other Maltreatment

If the documentation in the health record indicates that there is known or suspected neglect or abuse of a child or adult, a code from category T74 Adult and child abuse, neglect and other maltreatment, confirmed; or T76 Adult and child abuse, neglect and other maltreatment, suspected is assigned as the first-listed diagnosis. Additional code(s) are reported to capture mental health conditions or injuries resulting from the confirmed or suspected abuse or neglect. The Guidelines are below.

- Confirmed abuse or neglect codes are reported with external cause and perpetrator codes which are sequenced as follows:
  - A code from category T74 Adult and child abuse, neglect and other maltreatment, confirmed, is sequenced first
  - Codes for mental health conditions or injuries resulting from the abuse or neglect are coded additionally
  - An external cause code from the assault section (X92-Y08) is reported
  - A perpetrator code from category Y07 is reported when the perpetrator is known
- Suspected abuse or neglect codes are reported as follows:
  - A code from category T76 Adult and child abuse, neglect and other maltreatment, suspected, is sequenced first
  - Codes for mental health conditions or injuries resulting from the abuse or neglect are coded additionally
  - No external cause codes or perpetrator are reported when the abuse or neglect is documented as suspected
  - If suspected abuse or neglect is ruled out during the encounter, do not report a code from category T76. Report one of the following codes instead:
    - » Z04.71 Encounter for examination and observation following alleged physical adult abuse, ruled out
    - » Z04.72 Encounter for examination and observation following alleged physical child abuse, ruled out
  - If suspected rape or sexual abuse is ruled out during the encounter, do not report a code from category T76. Report one of the following codes instead:
    - » Z04.41 Encounter for examination and observation following alleged adult rape
    - » Z04.42 Encounter for examination and observation following alleged child rape
  - If suspected forced sexual exploitation or forced labor exploitation is ruled out during the encounter, do not report a code from category T76. Report one of the following codes instead:
    - » Z04.81 Encounter for examination and observation of victim following forced sexual exploitation
    - » Z04.82 Encounter for examination and observation of victim following forced labor exploitation

Complications of Care

Complications of surgical and medical care, not elsewhere classified are reported with codes from categories T80-T88. However, intraoperative and post-procedural complications are reported with codes from the body system chapters. For example, ventilator associated pneumonia is considered a procedural or post-procedural complication and is reported with code J95.851 Ventilator associated pneumonia, from Chapter 10 Diseases of the Respiratory System.

Complication of care code assignment is based on the provider's documentation of the relationship between the condition and the care or procedure. Not all conditions that occur following medical or surgical treatment are classified as complications. Only those conditions for which the provider has documented a cause-and-effect relationship between the care and the complication should be classified as complications of care. If the documentation is unclear, query the provider.

Some complications of care codes include the external cause in the code. These codes include the nature of the complication as well as the type of procedure that caused the complication. An additional external cause code indicating the type of procedure is not necessary for these codes.

Pain due to medical devices, implants, or grafts require two codes, one from the T-codes to identify the device causing the pain, such as T84.84-, Pain due to internal orthopedic prosthetic devices, implants and grafts, and one from category G89 to identify acute or chronic pain due to presence of the device, implant, or graft.

Transplant complications are reported with codes from category T86. These codes should be used for both complications and rejection of transplanted organs. A transplant complication code is assigned only when the complication affects the function of the transplanted organ. Two codes are required to describe a transplant complication, one from category T86 and a secondary code that identifies the specific complication.

Patients who have undergone a kidney transplant may still have some form of chronic kidney disease (CKD) because the transplant may not fully restore kidney function. CKD is not considered to be a transplant complication unless the provider documents a transplant complication such as transplant failure or rejection. If the documentation is unclear, the provider should be queried. Other complications (other than CKD) that affect function of the kidney are assigned a code from subcategory T86.1 Complications of transplanted kidney, and a secondary code that identifies the complication.

General Documentation Requirements

There are some specific documentation requirements for injuries, poisonings, and other consequences of external causes. In this section, we will discuss fracture classification systems, 7th character extensions for fractures, and laterality. It is important to note that because the 7th character extension defines the episode of care as well as whether the fracture was open or closed the level of detail (fracture level, type, open vs closed) must be documented for every encounter. The codes cannot be determined based upon previous documentation.

Fracture Classification Systems

Some of the most important documentation requirements for injuries relate to fractures. Some fractures such as surgical neck fractures of the humerus, physeal fractures, and open fractures of the long bones are coded using specific classification systems. Three of these classification systems are discussed here and they include:

- Neer classification for fracture of the proximal or upper end of the humerus
- Gustilo classification for open fracture of the long bones
- Salter-Harris classification for physeal fractures

Neer Classification

Fractures of the proximal or upper end of the humerus are classified using the Neer system. The proximal humerus is divided into four parts, the humeral head, greater tubercle, lesser tubercle, and diaphysis or shaft. These four parts are separated by epiphyseal lines, also called growth plates, when the bones are still growing during the developmental years. The surgical neck is at the narrowest aspect of the humerus just below the tubercles. When the proximal humerus is fractured, it typically occurs at the surgical neck and along one or more of the three epiphyseal lines. The proximal humerus may fracture into 2, 3, or 4 parts at the surgical neck which is why surgical neck fractures are designated as 2-part, 3-part or 4-part fractures.

The classification of the fracture is based upon the number of fragments and whether there is separation or angulation of the fragments. A fracture part is considered displaced if it is angulated more than 45° or displaced greater than 1 cm. A fracture that is not displaced <1cm **and** angulated < 45° regardless of how many pieces is considered a one-part fracture. All other Neer classifications are based upon the total number of fractures and the number of fractures that are displaced or angulated. For example, a 2-part fracture can be 2-4 parts with one of those parts being displaced **or** angulated. A three-part fracture can be 3-4 parts with two of the parts being displaced or angulated

Gustilo Classification

The Gustilo classification applies to open fractures of the long bones including the humerus, radius, ulna, femur, tibia, and fibula. The Gustilo open fracture classification groups open fractures into three main categories designated as Type I, Type II, and Type III with Type III injuries being further divided into Type IIIA, Type IIIB, and Type IIIC subcategories. The categories are defined by three characteristics which include:

- Mechanism of injury
- Extent of soft tissue damage
- Degree of bone injury or involvement

In order to assign the correct code for open fractures of the long bones, the specific characteristics for each type must be understood. The specific characteristics are as follows:

Type I

- Wound < 1 cm
- Minimal soft tissue damage
- Wound bed is clean
- Typically, low-energy type injury
- Fracture type is typically one of the following:
  - Simple transverse
  - Short oblique
  - Minimally comminuted

Type II

- Wound > 1 cm
- Moderate soft tissue damage/crush injury
- Moderate wound bed contamination
- Typically, low-energy type injury
- Fracture type is typically one of the following:
  - Simple transverse
  - Short oblique
  - Mildly comminuted

Type III

- Wound > 1 cm
- Extensive soft tissue damage
- Typically, a high-energy type injury
- Highly unstable fractures often with multiple bone fragments
- Injury patterns resulting in fractures that are always classified to this category include:
  - Open segmental fracture regardless of wound size
  - Diaphyseal fractures with segmental bone loss
  - Open fractures with any type of vascular involvement
  - Farmyard injuries or severely contaminated open fractures
  - High velocity gunshot wound
  - Fracture caused by crushing force from fast moving vehicle
  - Open fractures with delayed treatment (over 8 hours)

Type IIIA

- Wound <10cm with crushed tissue and contamination
- Adequate soft tissue coverage of open wound
- No local or distant flap coverage required
- Fracture may be open segmental or severely comminuted and still be subclassified as Type IIIA

Type IIIB

- Wound >10cm with crushed tissue, massive contamination and extensive soft tissue loss
- Local or distant flap coverage required
- Wound bed contamination requiring serial irrigation and debridement to clean the open fracture site

Type IIIC

- Major arterial injury requiring repair regardless of size of wound
- Extensive repair usually requiring the skills of a vascular surgeon is required for limb salvage
- Fractures classified using the Mangled Extremity Severity Score
- Often results in amputation

Providers should be encouraged to identify the Gustilo type in documentation related to fractures of the long bones, but in the absence of documentation of a specific type of fracture, the coder may be able to determine the correct code assignment using the descriptions above. However, the correct classification should also be verified by the physician.

Salter-Harris Classification

Physeal fractures may also be referred to as Salter-Harris fractures or traumatic epiphyseal separations. These fractures occur along the epiphyseal (growth) plates in bones that have not reached their full maturity and in which the plates are still open and filled with cartilaginous tissue. They are listed in the alphabetic index under the main term 'fracture' traumatic and then by site under the term 'physeal'.

Salter-Harris fractures are classified into 9 types. Documentation as to type is required to assign the most specific code. Types I-IV have specific codes for most sites. Types V-IX are reported under other physeal fracture. If no type is specified, the Salter-Harris fracture is reported with an unspecified code.

Types I-IV are the most common types of physeal injuries and have the following characteristics:

- Type I – Epiphyseal separation with displacement of the epiphysis from the metaphysis at the physis
- Type II – Fracture through the physis and a portion of the metaphysis without fracture of the epiphysis
- Type III – Fracture through the physis and epiphysis which damages the reproductive layer of the physis
- Type IV – Fracture through the metaphysis, physis, and epiphysis causing damage to the reproductive layer of the physis

Types V-IX are less common types of physeal injuries, which are determined as follows:

- Type V – A crush or compression injuring involving the physis without fracture of the metaphysis or epiphysis
- Type VI – A rare injury involving perichondral structures
- Type VII – An isolated injury of the epiphyseal plate
- Type VIII – An isolated injury to the metaphysis with potential complications related to endochondral ossification
- Type IX – An injury to the periosteum that may interfere with membranous growth

7th Character Extensions for Fractures

7th character extensions are used capture the episode of care for most injuries, poisonings, and other consequences of external causes. Fractures require 7th character extensions, but these extensions differ from those used for other types of injuries. The 7th character fracture extensions capture the following:

- Episode of care
- The status of the fracture as open or closed
  - The Gustilo classification for open fractures of the long bones
- Healing status of the fracture for subsequent encounters:
  - Routine healing
  - Delayed healing
  - Malunion
  - Nonunion

The applicable 7th character extensions for most fractures are as follows:

A Initial encounter for closed fracture

B Initial encounter for open fracture

D Subsequent encounter for fracture with routine healing

G Subsequent encounter for fracture with delayed healing

K Subsequent encounter for fracture with nonunion

P Subsequent encounter for fracture with malunion

S Sequela

The applicable 7th character extensions for fractures of the shafts of the long bones are as follows:

A Initial encounter for closed fracture

B Initial encounter for open fracture type I or II or open fracture NOS

C Initial encounter for open fracture type IIIA, IIIB, or IIIC

D Subsequent encounter for closed fracture with routine healing

E Subsequent encounter for open fracture type I or II with routine healing

F Subsequent encounter for open fracture type IIIA, IIIB, or IIIC with routine healing

G Subsequent encounter for closed fracture with delayed healing

H Subsequent encounter for open fracture type I or II with delayed healing

J Subsequent encounter for open fracture type IIIA, IIIB, or IIIC with delayed healing

K Subsequent encounter for closed fracture with nonunion

M Subsequent encounter for open fracture type I or II with nonunion

N Subsequent encounter for open fracture type IIIA, IIIB, or IIIC with nonunion

P Subsequent encounter for closed fracture with malunion

Q Subsequent encounter for open fracture type I or II with malunion

R Subsequent encounter for open fracture type IIIA, IIIB, or IIIC with malunion

S Sequela

Laterality

The vast majority of injuries to paired organs and the extremities require documentation of the organ or extremity as the right or left. In addition, some injuries such as open wounds of the thorax, require documentation of the site as the right back wall, left back wall, right front wall or left front wall. For open wounds of the abdominal wall, documentation must identify the site as right upper quadrant, left upper quadrant, epigastric region, right lower quadrant, or left lower quadrant.

Injury and Poisoning Documentation Requirements

In this section, some of the more frequently reported injury, poisoning, and other consequences of external causes code categories, subcategories, and subclassifications are reviewed and the documentation requirements are identified. The focus is on frequently reported conditions with specific clinical documentation requirements. Even though not all codes with significant documentation requirements are discussed, this section will provide a representative sample of the type of documentation required for injury, poisoning, and other consequences of external causes. The section is organized alphabetically by the code category, subcategory, or subclassification depending on whether the documentation affects only a single code or an entire subcategory or category. If injuries of multiple areas are reviewed such as fractures, the sections will then be further organized by anatomic order based upon the ICD-10-CM categories.

Burns

Burns are classified first as chemical or thermal burns and then by depth and extent. Chemical burns are classified as corrosions and thermal burns are classified as burns. A toxic effect code provides more information on the type of agent that caused the corrosion or burn and on the intent (accidental, intentional self-harm, assault, undetermined). Burns of the same local site but of different degrees are coded to the highest degree documented. Non-healing burns are coded as acute burns. Necrosis of burned skin is coded as non-healing burn.

Coding and Documentation Requirements

Identify type of burn:

- Corrosion, which includes burns due to
  - Acids
  - Alkalines
  - Caustics
  - Chemicals
- Thermal (except sunburn), which includes burns due to
  - Electricity
  - Flame
  - Heat (gas, liquid, or object)
  - Radiation
  - Steam

Identify site:

- External – See ICD-10-CM book for sites
- Eye and adnexa only
  - Eyelid and periocular area
  - Cornea and conjunctival sac
  - Resulting in rupture and destruction of eyeball
  - Other specified parts of eye/adnexa
  - Unspecified part of eye
- Internal – See ICD-10-CM book for sites

Identify laterality:

- Right
- Left
- Unspecified

Identify depth:

- First degree-erythema
- Second degree-blisters, epidermal loss
- Third degree-full thickness skin loss, deep necrosis of underlying tissue
- Unspecified degree

Identify extent of total body surface area (TBSA):

- Less than 10%
- 10-19%
  - With 0-9% third degree
  - With 10-19% third degree
- 20-29%
  - With 0-9% third degree
  - With 10-19% third degree
  - With 20-29% third degree
- 30-39%
  - With 0-9% third degree
  - With 10-19% third degree
  - With 20-29% third degree
  - With 30-39% third degree
- 40-49%
  - With 0-9% third degree
  - With 10-19% third degree
  - With 20-29% third degree
  - With 30-39% third degree
  - With 40-49% third degree
- 50-59%
  - With 0-9% third degree
  - With 10-19% third degree
  - With 20-29% third degree
  - With 30-39% third degree
  - With 40-49% third degree
  - With 50-59% third degree
- 60-69%
  - With 0-9% third degree
  - With 10-19% third degree
  - With 20-29% third degree
  - With 30-39% third degree
  - With 40-49% third degree
  - With 50-59% third degree
  - With 60-69% third degree
- 70-79%
  - With 0-9% third degree
  - With 10-19% third degree
  - With 20-29% third degree
  - With 30-39% third degree
  - With 40-49% third degree
  - With 50-59% third degree
  - With 60-69% third degree
  - With 70-79% third degree
- 80-89%
  - With 0-9% third degree
  - With 10-19% third degree
  - With 20-29% third degree
  - With 30-39% third degree
  - With 40-49% third degree
  - With 50-59% third degree
  - With 60-69% third degree
  - With 70-79% third degree
  - With 80-89% third degree
-

- More than 90%
  - With 0-9% third degree
  - With 10-19% third degree
  - With 20-29% third degree
  - With 30-39% third degree
  - With 40-49% third degree
  - With 50-59% third degree
  - With 60-69% third degree
  - With 70-79% third degree
  - With 80-89% third degree
  - With more than 90% third degree

Identify agent and intent:

- Agent (corrosion) – See code range T51-T65 in ICD-10-CM for agents
- Intent
  - Accidental (unintentional)
  - Intentional self-harm
  - Assault
  - Undetermined

Example 1

Corrosion, First Degree, Fingers Not Including Thumb

ICD-10-CM Code/Documentation	
T23.521-	Corrosion of first degree of single right finger (nail) except thumb
T23.522-	Corrosion of first degree of single left finger (nail) except thumb
T23.529-	Corrosion of first degree of unspecified single finger (nail) except thumb
T23.531-	Corrosion of first degree of multiple right fingers (nail) not including thumb
T23.532-	Corrosion of first degree of multiple left fingers (nail) not including thumb
T23.539-	Corrosion of first degree of unspecified multiple fingers (nail) not including thumb

Note: Only the burn codes are listed in the table above. Additional codes are required to identify the chemical and intent (external cause). See scenario below for an example.

Documentation and Coding Example

Patient is a sixty-eight your old gentleman who presents to ED with intense pain in the tips of his **right index and middle fingers**. He states he attended a decorative glass workshop at the local **Adult Education Center** earlier in the day and was handling **dilute hydrofluoric acid that spilled** but he believed he had cleaned it up without contaminating himself. He looked up symptoms of chemical burns on the internet when the pain began and decided it would be best to have it checked out. On examination, this is a small, thin, immaculately groomed Asian male who looks younger than his stated age. He states he is a retired mathematics professor and enjoys studying art. No significant PMH, he takes OTC vitamins and nutritional supplements for recently diagnosed macular degeneration. Temperature 98.6, HR 66, RR 12, BP 120/70. **The tips of the index and middle fingers on the right hand have small white patches measuring <0.25 cm with surrounding erythema.** The pain is most pronounced in that area and he describes it as deep and throbbing. Calcium gluconate 2.5 % gel applied to area and blood is drawn for CBC and serum electrolytes including stat magnesium, calcium, and potassium. X-ray of right index and middle fingers also obtained to check bone integrity. Pain has decreased substantially with application of topical calcium gluconate. X-ray shows no bone damage. Serum electrolytes are WNL.

Impression: **Grade I Hydrofluoric acid burn to tips of two fingers,** no systemic involvement. Discharged with index and middle fingers immersed in 2.5 % Calcium gluconate gel covered with vinyl glove. He is instructed to limit use of hand and to keep glove in place x 24 hours. He is given a follow up appointment tomorrow in burn clinic.

Diagnosis Code(s)

T54.2X1A	Toxic effect of corrosive acids and acid-like substances, accidental (unintentional), initial encounter
T23.531A	Corrosion of first degree of multiple right fingers (nail) not including thumb, initial encounter
T32.0	Corrosions involving less than 10% of body surface
Y92.218	Other school as place of occurrence of external cause
Y93.D9	Activity, other, involving arts and handicrafts
Y99.8	Other external cause status

Coding Note(s)

Corrosions are chemical burns that require identification of the chemical substance and the chemical substance is the first listed diagnosis. The chemical substance is found in the Table of Drugs and Chemicals. The correct code for an accidental corrosion is found in the column for poisoning, accidental (unintentional). Codes for drugs and chemicals are combination codes that identify the substance and the external cause or intent, so an additional external cause of injury code to identify the intent is not required. However, for the initial encounter only, codes should be assigned for the place of occurrence, activity, and external cause status when documented.

Example 2

Second Degree Burn of Lower Leg

ICD-10-CM Code/Documentation	
T24.231-	Burn of second degree of right lower leg
T24.232-	Burn of second degree of left lower leg
T24.239-	Burn of second degree of unspecified lower leg

Documentation and Coding Example

Twenty-eight-year-old male presents to ED with a **burn injury to lower left leg.** Patient states he was **deep frying a turkey in his backyard of his condominium when the fryer was bumped and hot oil spilled out onto his leg.** On examination, this is a mildly obese Caucasian male who looks somewhat older than his stated age. He is wearing short pants and the injury is easily visualized. The **burn extends from just below the knee** to just above the ankle. The skin is intact, red appearing, with area of blistering over anterior aspect of lower leg and patchy areas of white over the remaining burned region. Patient denies much pain. Peripheral pulses present via Doppler. Temperature 97.4, HR 104, RR 16, BP 136/66. IV placed in left forearm, Lactated Ringers infusing. Blood drawn for CBC, electrolytes. Regional burn center agrees to accept patient, request wounds be covered with TransCyte if available, Xeroform gauze if not. Arrangement made for EMS ground transport. Wound dressed with Xeroform gauze. Transferred to transport stretcher, cardiac monitor shows NSR, pulse oximeter 99 % on 2 L O2 via nasal cannula. Report to EMS crew. Stable for 60-minute drive to burn center.

Impression: **Second degree burn anterior aspect lower leg. TBSA 5%.**

Diagnosis Code(s)

T24.232A	Burn of second degree of left lower leg, initial encounter
T31.0	Burns involving less than 10% of body surface
X10.2XXA	Contact with fats and cooking oils, initial encounter
Y92.038	Other place in apartment as the place of occurrence of the external cause
Y93.G9	Activity, other involving cooking and grilling
Y99.8	Other external cause status

Dislocation of Acromioclavicular Joint

In ICD-10-CM, AC joint dislocation is a subcategory under category S43, Dislocation and sprain of joints and ligaments of shoulder girdle. In subcategory S43.1 Subluxation and dislocation of AC joint, injuries are specific to type, subluxation, or dislocation, and dislocation is further differentiated by the amount and the direction of the displacement. It may be difficult to translate the physician documentation into the correct code for AC joint subluxation and dislocation because the commonly used Allman and Tossy classification for injuries identified as Type I-III, and the Rockwood modification that added Types IV-VI, do not correlate exactly with the ICD-10-CM code descriptions.

Subluxation is an incomplete dislocation and may be described as a sprain or separation of the joint. There is only one subcategory for subluxation of the AC joint (S43.11-). Dislocation codes are reported when there is a complete dislocation of joint. Complete dislocation is further differentiated by the amount of displacement and the direction of the displacement of the AC joint structures. The six types of injuries described by the Allman-Tossy-Rockwood classification are as follows:

- Type I – Sprain of AC ligament only
- Type II – Injury to AC ligament and joint capsule with disrupted but intact coracoacromial ligament. Vertical subluxation of clavicle
- Type III – Disruption of AC ligament, joint capsule, and coracoacromial ligament. Complete AC joint dislocation with clavicle displaced superiorly and complete loss of contact between the clavicle and acromion. The coracoclavicular interspace is 25%-100% greater than the normal shoulder
- Type IV – Disruption of AC ligament, joint capsule, and coracoacromial ligament. Complete AC joint dislocation with clavicle displaced posteriorly into or through the trapezius muscle
- Type V - Disruption of AC ligament, joint capsule, and coracoacromial ligament. Complete AC joint dislocation with extreme superior elevation of the clavicle (100%-300%). Complete detachment of deltoid and trapezius from the distal clavicle
- Type VI - Disruption of AC ligament, joint capsule, and coracoacromial ligament. Complete AC joint dislocation with clavicle displaced inferior to acromion and coracoid process

Correlation between Allman-Tossy-Rockwood classification and ICD-10-CM codes are as follows:

- Type I – Report a code from subcategory S43.5- Sprain of acromioclavicular joint
- Type II – Report a code from subcategory S43.11 Subluxation of AC joint
- Type III – Report a code from subcategory S43.10 Unspecified dislocation of AC joint. Even though the code description is for an unspecified dislocation, it is also used to report other specified dislocations that do not fall into one of the other subcategories. Since a Type III dislocation results in superior displacement, but the coracoclavicular interspace is less than 100% when compared to the normal shoulder, no other AC joint dislocation applies
- Type IV – Report a code from subcategory S43.15 Posterior dislocation of AC joint
- Type V – Report either a code from subcategory S43.12 Dislocation of AC joint, 100%-200% displacement or subcategory S43.13 Dislocation of AC joint, greater than 200% displacement. If the amount of displacement as compared to the normal shoulder is not specified, query the physician
- Type VI – Report a code from subcategory S43.14 Inferior dislocation of AC joint.

Coding and Documentation Requirements

Identify type of AC joint injury:

- Sprain
- Subluxation
- Dislocation
  - 100%-200% (superior) displacement
  - 200% (superior) displacement
  - Inferior
  - Posterior
  - Unspecified

Identify laterality:

- Right
- Left

- Unspecified

Identify episode of care:

- Initial encounter
- Subsequent encounter
- Sequela

Note: There is no 7th character to classify an open subluxation/dislocation nor is there a separate code. If documented as an open dislocation a code from category S41.-Open wound of shoulder must also be added.

ICD-10-CM Code/Documentation	
S43.101-	Unspecified dislocation of right acromioclavicular joint
S43.102-	Unspecified dislocation of left acromioclavicular joint
S43.109-	Unspecified dislocation of unspecified acromioclavicular joint
S43.111-	Subluxation of right acromioclavicular joint
S43.112-	Subluxation of left acromioclavicular joint
S43.119-	Subluxation of unspecified acromioclavicular joint
S43.121-	Dislocation of right acromioclavicular joint, 100%-200% displacement
S43.122-	Dislocation of left acromioclavicular joint, 100%-200% displacement
S43.129-	Dislocation of unspecified acromioclavicular joint, 100%-200% displacement
S43.131-	Dislocation of right acromioclavicular joint, greater than 200% displacement
S43.132-	Dislocation of left acromioclavicular joint, greater than 200% displacement
S43.139-	Dislocation of unspecified acromioclavicular joint, greater than 200% displacement
S43.141-	Inferior dislocation of right acromioclavicular joint
S43.142-	Inferior dislocation of left acromioclavicular joint
S43.149-	Inferior dislocation of unspecified acromioclavicular joint
S43.151-	Posterior dislocation of right acromioclavicular joint
S43.152-	Posterior dislocation of left acromioclavicular joint
S43.159-	Posterior dislocation of unspecified acromioclavicular joint
S43.50-	Sprain of unspecified acromioclavicular joint
S43.51-	Sprain of right acromioclavicular joint
S43.52-	Sprain of left acromioclavicular joint

Documentation and Coding Example

Twenty-three-year-old Black male **employed as a gardener** on a private estate presents to Urgent Care Clinic with a right shoulder injury sustained about 6 hours ago. He reports that he **fell approximately 5 feet off a ladder while trimming hedges**, landing on his outstretched right arm and hand. He describes a "popping" feeling in the shoulder followed by numbness in the arm and hand. He was able to move the extremity after a few minutes and the numbness subsided in approximately one hour, but the shoulder has continued to feel loose all day. PMH includes asthma for which he takes Singulair, Advair daily and Albuterol when needed and TB treated with INH seven years ago. On examination, this is a soft spoken, slightly built, thin young man. Temperature 97.4, HR 62, RR 14, BP 116/70. Alert and oriented x 3, PERRL, patient denies striking head, neck, or back in the fall. Heart rate regular without murmur, breath sounds have a few expiratory wheezes but otherwise clear and equal bilaterally. Left upper extremity is normal in appearance. Right clavicle has slight prominence but otherwise normal contour, there is no shoulder sag. Moderate point tenderness is localized over the AC joint which can be easily manipulated out of position. There are no obvious neurovascular deficits. X-rays obtained including AP and lateral views of shoulder, lateral projection of scapula and weight bearing view (AP projection w/15 lb. weight). No fractures visible and no obvious dislocation of clavicle or humerus.

Impression: **Subluxation of right acromioclavicular joint.** Treatment: Patient is fitted with a sling which can be worn for comfort. He is instructed to ice shoulder x 20 minutes, 3-4 x day and may continue with exercise/activity as tolerated. He is prescribed Ibuprofen 600 mg TID for pain. He will F/U with PMD in one week with possible referral to orthopedist and/or physical therapy for strengthening exercises if the right shoulder joint continues to feel loose.

Diagnosis Code(s)

S43.111A	Subluxation of right acromioclavicular joint, initial encounter
W11.XXXA	Fall on and from ladder, initial encounter
Y92.017	Garden or yard in single-family (private) house as the place of occurrence of the external cause
Y93.H2	Activity, gardening and landscaping
Y99.0	Civilian activity for income or pay

Coding Note(s)

Documentation of a Type II AC joint injury or partial dislocation would be reported with the code for subluxation.

Fracture of Skull

Fractures of the skull are captured with codes from subcategories S02.0- Fracture of vault of skull and S02.1- Fracture of base of skull (unspecified site of base of skull, fracture of the occiput or occipital condyle, orbital roof, and other specified fractures of the base of the skull which includes anterior, middle, or posterior fossa, sphenoid bone, temporal bone, and ethmoid and frontal sinus). Fractures of the orbital floor are reported in category S02.3- while orbital wall fractures are coded to S02.8-. A 7th character extension identifies the fracture as open or closed and identifies the episode of care. A second code from category S06 is required to capture any intracranial injury with or without loss of consciousness. Intracranial injury codes are much more specific as to the type of injury. In addition, when there is a loss of consciousness, the codes are much more specific as to the period of time and to the outcome—including survival with or without return to previous conscious level for loss of consciousness greater than 24 hours, or death due to intracranial injury or other cause prior to regaining consciousness. In addition to the fracture and intracranial injury codes, one or more supplementary codes may be required to capture elements of any documented coma using the Glasgow coma scale classification.

Coding and Documentation Requirements

Identify skull fracture site:

- Vault of skull, which includes
  - Frontal bone
  - Parietal bone

- Base of skull, which includes
  - Anterior fossa
  - Ethmoid sinus
  - Frontal sinus
  - Middle fossa
  - Occipital bone
  - Posterior fossa
  - Sphenoid bone
  - Temporal bone
- Orbital floor
- Orbital roof
- Orbital wall
  - Lateral
  - Medial

Identify laterality

- Right
- Left
- Unspecified side

Identify fracture as:

- Closed
- Open

Identify episode of care:

- Initial
- Subsequent
  - With routine fracture healing
  - With delayed fracture healing
  - With nonunion of fracture
- Sequela

Identify nature of any intracranial injury:

- Concussion
- Cerebral edema, which includes
  - Diffuse edema
  - Focal edema
- Contusion/laceration
  - Brainstem
  - Cerebellum
  - Cerebrum
    - » Right
    - » Left
    - » Unspecified site
- Diffuse traumatic brain injury
- Focal traumatic brain injury
- Hemorrhage
  - Intracranial
    - » Brainstem
    - » Cerebellum
    - » Cerebrum, left
    - » Cerebrum, right
    - » Cerebrum, unspecified
  - Epidural (extradural)
  - Subarachnoid
  - Subdural
- Other specified intracranial injury
  - Internal carotid artery, intracranial portion
    - » Left
    - » Right
  - Other specified intracranial injury
- Unspecified intracranial injury

Identify any loss of consciousness:

- No loss of consciousness
- 30 minutes or less
- 31 minutes to 59 minutes
- 1 hour to 5 hours 59 minutes
- 6 hours to 24 hours
- Greater than 24 hours
  - With return to pre-existing conscious level
  - Without return to pre-existing conscious level
- Any duration with death prior to regaining consciousness
  - Death due to brain injury
  - Death due to other cause
- Unspecified duration

Episode of care:

- Initial
- Subsequent
- Sequela

Coma Scale reporting requires the use of individual scores, if known. All three elements—eye opening, verbal response, and motor response must be known to use individual scores. If all three elements are not known, but Glasgow coma scale is documented, use the Glasgow coma scale total score.

Identify individual scores:

- Eyes open
  - Never
  - To pain
  - To sound
  - Spontaneous
- Best verbal response
  - None
  - Incomprehensible words
  - Inappropriate words
  - Confused conversation
  - Oriented
- Best motor response
  - None
  - Extension
  - Abnormal flexion
  - Flexion withdrawal
  - Localizes pain
  - Obeys commands

Identify Glasgow coma scale total score:

- Glasgow score 13-15
- Glasgow score 9-12
- Glasgow score 3-8

Identify time/place of coma score obtained:

- In the field (EMT/ambulance)
- At arrival in emergency department
- At hospital admission
- 24 hours or more after hospital admission
- Unspecified time

OR

- Other coma without documented Glasgow coma scale score or with partial score reported

Closed Fracture of Skull with Cerebral Edema

ICD-1Ø-CM Code/Documentation	
Fracture Skull Vault	
SØ2.ØXXA	Fracture of vault of skull, initial encounter for closed fracture
Traumatic Cerebral Edema/Loss of Consciousness	
SØ6.1XØA	Traumatic cerebral edema without loss of consciousness, initial encounter
SØ6.1X1A	Traumatic cerebral edema with loss of consciousness ≤ 3Ø min, initial encounter
SØ6.1X2A	Traumatic cerebral edema with loss of consciousness 31 min to 59 min, initial encounter
SØ6.1X3A	Traumatic cerebral edema with loss of consciousness 1 hr. to 5 hrs. 59 min, initial encounter
SØ6.1X4A	Traumatic cerebral edema with loss of consciousness 6 hours to 24 hours, initial encounter
SØ6.1X5A	Traumatic cerebral edema with loss of consciousness greater than 24 hours with return to pre-existing conscious level, initial encounter
SØ6.1X6A	Traumatic cerebral edema with loss of consciousness greater than 24 hours without return to pre-existing conscious level with patient surviving, initial encounter
SØ6.1X7A	Traumatic cerebral edema with loss of consciousness of any duration with death due to brain injury prior to regaining consciousness
SØ6.1X8A	Traumatic cerebral edema with loss of consciousness of any duration with death due to other cause prior to regaining consciousness
SØ6.1x9A	Traumatic cerebral edema with loss of consciousness of unspecified duration, initial encounter

Note 1: An initial encounter for an open fracture of vault of skull without mention of intracranial injury is reported with the same codes listed above except that the 7th character extension 'A' is replaced with a 'B' for initial encounter for open fracture.

Note 2: The 7th character 'A' for codes in category S06 indicates only that this is the initial encounter, not whether or not the injury is open or closed.

Closed Fracture of Skull with Cerebral Laceration/Contusion/Loss of Consciousness

ICD-1Ø-CM Code/Documentation	
Fracture Skull Vault	
SØ2.ØXXA	Fracture of vault of skull, initial encounter for closed fracture
Contusion/Laceration/Loss of Consciousness, Unspecified Duration	
SØ6.319A	Contusion and laceration of right cerebrum with loss of consciousness of unspecified duration, initial encounter
SØ6.329A	Contusion and laceration of left cerebrum with loss of consciousness of unspecified duration, initial encounter
SØ6.339A	Contusion and laceration of unspecified cerebrum with loss of consciousness of unspecified duration, initial encounter
Contusion/Laceration/Without Loss of Consciousness	
SØ6.31ØA	Contusion and laceration of right cerebrum without loss of consciousness, initial encounter
SØ6.32ØA	Contusion and laceration of left cerebrum without loss of consciousness, initial encounter
SØ6.33ØA	Contusion and laceration of unspecified cerebrum without loss of consciousness, initial encounter
Contusion/Laceration/Loss of Consciousness Under 1 Hour	
SØ6.311A	Contusion and laceration of right cerebrum with loss of consciousness ≤ 3Ø min, initial encounter
SØ6.312A	Contusion and laceration of right cerebrum with loss of consciousness 31 min to 59 min, initial encounter
SØ6.321A	Contusion and laceration of left cerebrum with loss of consciousness ≤ 3Ø min, initial encounter
SØ6.322A	Contusion and laceration of left cerebrum with loss of consciousness 31 min to 59 min, initial encounter
SØ6.331A	Contusion and laceration of unspecified cerebrum with loss of consciousness ≤ 3Ø min, initial encounter
SØ6.332A	Contusion and laceration of unspecified cerebrum with loss of consciousness 31 min to 59 min, initial encounter
Contusion/Laceration/Loss of Consciousness 1-24 Hours	
SØ6.313A	Contusion and laceration of right cerebrum with loss of consciousness 1 hr. to 5 hrs. 59 min, initial encounter
SØ6.314A	Contusion and laceration of right cerebrum with loss of consciousness 6 hrs. to 24 hrs., initial encounter
SØ6.323A	Contusion and laceration of left cerebrum with loss of consciousness 1 hr. to 5 hrs. 59 min, initial encounter
SØ6.324A	Contusion and laceration of left cerebrum with loss of consciousness 6 hrs. to 24 hrs., initial encounter
SØ6.333A	Contusion and laceration of unspecified cerebrum with loss of consciousness 1 hr. to 5 hrs. 59 min, initial encounter
SØ6.334A	Contusion and laceration of unspecified cerebrum with loss of consciousness 6 hrs. to 24 hrs., initial encounter

Contusion/Laceration/Loss of Consciousness, More Than 24 Hours	
S06.315A	Contusion and laceration of right cerebrum with loss of consciousness greater than 24 hours with return to pre-existing conscious level, initial encounter
S06.325A	Contusion and laceration of left cerebrum with loss of consciousness greater than 24 hours with return to pre-existing conscious level, initial encounter
S06.335A	Contusion and laceration of unspecified cerebrum with loss of consciousness greater than 24 hours with return to pre-existing conscious level, initial encounter
S06.316A	Contusion and laceration of right cerebrum with loss of consciousness greater than 24 hours without return to pre-existing conscious level with patient surviving, initial encounter
S06.326A	Contusion and laceration of left cerebrum with loss of consciousness greater than 24 hours without return to pre-existing conscious level with patient surviving, initial encounter
S06.336A	Contusion and laceration of unspecified cerebrum with loss of consciousness greater than 24 hours without return to pre-existing conscious level with patient surviving, initial encounter

Note 1: An initial encounter for an open fracture of vault of skull with cerebral laceration and contusion is reported with the same codes listed above except that the 7th character extension 'A' is replaced with a 'B' for initial encounter for open fracture.

Note 2: The 7th character 'A' for codes in category S06 indicates only that this is the initial encounter, not whether or not the injury is open or closed.

Note 3: There are additional contusion and laceration codes that reflect death either due to the brain injury or other brain injury. These codes are:

S06.017A Contusion and laceration of right cerebrum with loss of consciousness of any duration with death due to brain injury prior to regaining consciousness, initial encounter

S06.018A Contusion and laceration of right cerebrum with loss of consciousness of any duration with death due to other cause prior to regaining consciousness, initial encounter

S06.027A Contusion and laceration of left cerebrum with loss of consciousness of any duration with death due to brain injury prior to regaining consciousness, initial encounter

S06.028A Contusion and laceration of left cerebrum with loss of consciousness of any duration with death due to other cause prior to regaining consciousness, initial encounter

S06.037A Contusion and laceration of unspecified cerebrum with loss of consciousness of any duration with death due to brain injury prior to regaining consciousness, initial encounter

S06.038A Contusion and laceration of unspecified cerebrum with loss of consciousness of any duration with death due to other cause prior to regaining consciousness, initial encounter

Closed Fracture of Skull with Subarachnoid, Subdural, and Extradural Hemorrhage

ICD-10-CM Code/Documentation	
Fracture Skull Vault	
S02.0XXA	Fracture of vault of skull, initial encounter for closed fracture
Hemorrhage/Loss of Consciousness, Unspecified Duration	
S06.4X9A	Epidural hemorrhage with loss of consciousness of unspecified duration, initial encounter
S06.5X9A	Traumatic subdural hemorrhage with loss of consciousness of unspecified duration, initial encounter
S06.6X9A	Traumatic subarachnoid hemorrhage with loss of consciousness of unspecified duration, initial encounter
Hemorrhage/Without Loss of Consciousness	
S06.4X0A	Epidural hemorrhage without loss of consciousness, initial encounter
S06.5X0A	Traumatic subdural hemorrhage without loss of consciousness, initial encounter
S06.6X0A	Traumatic subarachnoid hemorrhage without loss of consciousness, initial encounter
Hemorrhage/Loss of Consciousness ≤ 30 Minutes	
S06.4X1A	Epidural hemorrhage with loss of consciousness ≤ 30 min, initial encounter
S06.5X1A	Traumatic subdural hemorrhage with loss of consciousness ≤ 30 min, initial encounter
S06.6X1A	Traumatic subarachnoid hemorrhage with loss of consciousness ≤ 30 min, initial encounter
Hemorrhage/Loss of Consciousness, 31-59 Minutes	
S06.4X2A	Epidural hemorrhage with loss of consciousness 31 min to 59 min, initial encounter
S06.5X2A	Traumatic subdural hemorrhage with loss of consciousness 31 min to 59 min, initial encounter
S06.6X2A	Traumatic subarachnoid hemorrhage with loss of consciousness 31 min to 59 min, initial encounter
Hemorrhage/Loss of Consciousness, 1 Hr - 5 Hrs. 59 Min	
S06.4X3A	Epidural hemorrhage with loss of consciousness 1 hr. to 5 hrs. 59 min, initial encounter
S06.5X3A	Traumatic subdural hemorrhage with loss of consciousness 1 hr. to 5 hrs. 59 min, initial encounter
S06.6X3A	Traumatic subarachnoid hemorrhage with loss of consciousness 1 hr. to 5 hrs. 59 min, initial encounter
Hemorrhage/Loss of Consciousness, 6-24 Hours	
S06.4X4A	Epidural hemorrhage with loss of consciousness 6 hrs. to 24 hrs., initial encounter
S06.5X4A	Traumatic subdural hemorrhage with loss of consciousness 6 hrs. to 24 hrs., initial encounter
S06.6X4A	Traumatic subarachnoid hemorrhage with loss of consciousness 6 hrs. to 24 hrs., initial encounter

Hemorrhage/Loss of Consciousness, More Than 24 Hours	
S06.4X5A	Epidural hemorrhage with loss of consciousness greater than 24 hours with return to pre-existing conscious level, initial encounter
S06.5X5A	Traumatic subdural hemorrhage with loss of consciousness greater than 24 hours with return to pre-existing conscious level, initial encounter
S06.6X5A	Traumatic subarachnoid hemorrhage with loss of consciousness greater than 24 hours with return to pre-existing conscious level, initial encounter
S06.4X6A	Epidural hemorrhage with loss of consciousness greater than 24 hours without return to pre-existing conscious level with patient surviving, initial encounter
S06.5X6A	Traumatic subdural hemorrhage with loss of consciousness greater than 24 hours without return to pre-existing conscious level with patient surviving, initial encounter
S06.6X6A	Traumatic subarachnoid hemorrhage with loss of consciousness greater than 24 hours without return to pre-existing conscious level with patient surviving, initial encounter

Note 1: An initial encounter for an open fracture of vault of skull with subarachnoid, subdural, and extradural hemorrhage is reported with the same codes listed above except that the 7th character extension 'A' is replaced with a 'B' for initial encounter for open fracture.

Note 2: The 7th character 'A' for codes in category S06 indicates only that this is the initial encounter, not whether or not the injury is open or closed.

Note 3: There are ICD-10-CM epidural hemorrhage, traumatic subarachnoid hemorrhage, and traumatic subdural hemorrhage codes that reflect death either due to the brain injury or other brain injury. These codes are:

S06.4X7A Epidural hemorrhage with loss of consciousness of any duration with death due to brain injury prior to regaining consciousness, initial encounter

S06.4X8A Epidural hemorrhage with loss of consciousness of any duration with death due to other cause prior to regaining consciousness, initial encounter

S06.5X7A Traumatic subdural hemorrhage with loss of consciousness of any duration with death due to brain injury prior to regaining consciousness, initial encounter

S06.5X8A Traumatic subdural hemorrhage with loss of consciousness of any duration with death due to other cause prior to regaining consciousness, initial encounter

S06.6X7A Traumatic subarachnoid hemorrhage with loss of consciousness of any duration with death due to brain injury prior to regaining consciousness, initial encounter

S06.6X8A Traumatic subarachnoid hemorrhage with loss of consciousness of any duration with death due to other cause prior to regaining consciousness, initial encounter

Documentation and Coding Example

Sixteen-year-old Caucasian male transported to local ED via ambulance after he was found unresponsive at home by his mother. Patient has a fresh **4 cm x 5 cm hematoma on left temporal area**. Mother states her son was **surfing** earlier in the day and was hit in the head by his board. He continued surfing for approximately 1 hour following the accident and drove himself home. He was alert and oriented all morning, only complaining of a headache, taking ibuprofen at 10 AM. He **appeared to be sleeping at 1 PM when mother left to do errands and she was unable to arouse him when she returned 2 hours later**. On examination, this is a well-developed, well-nourished, adolescent male. Temperature 97.4, HR 66, RR 12, BP 88/50. **Neurological examination reveals no spontaneous eye opening or response to verbal commands, there is withdrawal from painful stimuli. Score = 6 on Glasgow Coma Scale**. Call placed to Children's Hospital Trauma Center and life flight team dispatched. ETA 22 minutes. NSR on cardiac monitor. O2 saturation 92% by pulse oximetry, O2 started at 2 L/m via non-rebreather mask. HOB elevated 30%. IV line placed right forearm, LR infusing. Blood drawn for CBC, platelets, electrolytes, PT, PTT, type and hold and sent to lab. Bladder can be palpated above the pubic bone, Foley catheter placed without difficulty, 600 cc clear yellow urine returned.

Transport Team Note: Arrived in ED at 4:13 PM. Baseline lab tests all within normal limits. ABG drawn pH 7.32, pCO2 51, HCO3 25, pO2 88 %, SaO2 96 %. Patient intubated without difficulty, hand ventilated by RT. Transferred to life flight stretcher, on monitors, stable for transport. All consents obtained, parents following in private car. ETA Children's Hospital 17 minutes with neurosurgical team assembled and ready for patient. Uneventful helicopter transport. Patient taken directly from heliport to CT. Care assumed by neurosurgical team and radiology staff.

Neurosurgical Note: CT scan reveals a linear fracture of the left parietal bone with large subdural hematoma. Patient taken to OR at 6:15 PM where a craniotomy was performed under general anesthesia. Hematoma evacuated and patient taken to Neurosurgical ICU with arterial line, CVP line, ICP catheter. Mannitol drip, prophylactic antibiotics, and anti-seizure medications.

Neurosurgical ICU Note: Patient arrived in unit at 9:50 PM. VSS stable on monitors. CVP, ICP pressures WNL. Patient comfortably sedated, taking spontaneous breaths on ventilator. Parents in to visit. **Opens eyes to parents' voices, localizes painful stimuli, unable to vocalize due to intubation, Glasgow coma scale=9**. Continued progress throughout night, extubated at 6 AM. Alert, recognizes parents, oriented to person only, last memory he has is surfing.

Discharge Note: Patient made an excellent physical recovery from surgery and is discharged on post-op day 5, wound staples removed prior to discharge. He has no residual weakness or visual deficits. He still has no memory of the time between surfing and waking up in the ICU. Patient weaned from anti-seizure medications with normal EEG. He is discharged without medications and will be seen in Neurosurgical Clinic in 2 days.

Discharge diagnosis:

- Linear skull fracture, left parietal bone
- Large subdural hematoma
- Total duration of loss of consciousness estimated at 6-7 hours

Diagnosis Code(s)

Note: Codes are for inpatient services at 2nd facility

S06.5X4A	Traumatic subdural hemorrhage with loss of consciousness 6 hours to 24 hours, initial encounter
S02.0XXA	Fracture of vault of skull, initial encounter for closed fracture
R40.2134	Coma scale, eyes open to sound, 24 hours or more after hospital admission
R40.2214	Coma scale, best verbal response, none, 24 hours or more after hospital admission
R40.2354	Coma scale, best motor response, localizes pain, 24 hours or more after hospital admission
W21.89XA	Striking against or struck by other sports equipment, initial encounter
Y92.832	Beach as the place of occurrence of the external cause
Y93.18	Activity, surfing, windsurfing and boogie boarding
Y99.8	Other external cause status

Coding Note(s)

In ICD-10-CM, there is a sequencing note indicating that the intracranial injury is coded first. Glasgow coma scale codes are reported additionally with the fracture of skull (S02.-) and/or intracranial injury (S06.-) reported first. Both facilities and all physicians and ancillary service providers will report skull fracture codes with 7th character 'A' for initial episode of care because the services described above are related to the acute phase of the injury. The patient has a hematoma but no open wound of the head is documented, so the skull fracture is classified as a closed fracture which is also captured by the 7th character 'A'. The traumatic subdural hemorrhage is also reported with 7th character 'A'. There is documentation related to each element of the coma scale so each of the three components are coded rather than assigning the code for the Glasgow coma scale total score from subcategory R40.24. If only the total score had been reported, code R40.242 Glasgow coma scale score 9-12 would be assigned instead of the individual coma scores for eyes open, best verbal response, and best motor response.

Fracture of Cervical Vertebra with Spinal Cord Injury

Fractures of the cervical vertebra or other parts of the neck are reported with codes from category S12. If the fracture is associated with a cervical spinal cord injury, a code from category S14 is also required, and the code from category S14 is listed first. Fracture and spinal cord injury codes require the specific level of the fracture (C1, C2, C3, C4, C5, C6, C7). Associated spinal cord injuries require documentation of the type and extent of the injury to include incomplete lesion, Brown-Séquard syndrome, and a subcategory for other specified incomplete lesion.

Coding and Documentation Requirements

Fracture of cervical spine

Identify level/site of cervical spine fracture:

- C1
- C2
- C3
- C4
- C5
- C6
- C7

Identify type of fracture:

- For C1
  - Burst fracture
    - » Stable
    - » Unstable
  - » Posterior arch
  - » Lateral mass
  - » Other specified fracture
  - » Unspecified fracture
- For C2
  - Dens fracture
    - » Type II anterior displaced
    - » Type II posterior displaced
    - » Type II nondisplaced
    - » Other displaced
    - » Other nondisplaced
  - Traumatic spondylolisthesis
    - » Type III
    - » Other specified traumatic spondylolisthesis
    - » Unspecified traumatic spondylolisthesis
  - Other specified fracture
  - Unspecified fracture
- For C3-C7
  - Traumatic spondylolisthesis
    - » Type III
    - » Other specified traumatic spondylolisthesis
    - » Unspecified traumatic spondylolisthesis
  - Other specified fracture
  - Unspecified fracture

Identify fracture as nondisplaced or displaced as needed:

- Displaced
- Nondisplaced

Note: Some specific types of fractures are by definition either nondisplaced or displaced so this qualifier is not always required.

Identify fracture as:

- Closed
- Open

Identify episode of care:

- Initial
- Subsequent
  - With routine healing of fracture
  - With delayed healing of fracture
  - With nonunion of fracture
- Sequela

Spinal Cord Injury (if present)

Identify type of spinal cord injury:

- Anterior cord syndrome
- Brown-Séquard syndrome
- Central cord syndrome
- Complete lesion of cord
- Concussion/edema
- Other specified incomplete lesion of spinal cord
- Unspecified spinal cord injury

Identify highest level of cervical spinal cord injury:

- C1
- C2
- C3
- C4
- C5
- C6
- C7
- C8
- Unspecified level

Identify episode of care:

- Initial
- Subsequent
- Sequela

C5 Fracture with Spinal Cord Injury

ICD-10-CM Code/Documentation	
C5 Vertebral Fracture	
S12.400A	Unspecified displaced fracture of fifth cervical vertebrae, initial encounter for closed fracture
S12.401A	Unspecified nondisplaced fracture of fifth cervical vertebra, initial encounter for closed fracture
S12.430A	Unspecified traumatic displaced spondylolisthesis of fifth cervical vertebra, initial encounter for closed fracture
S12.431A	Unspecified traumatic nondisplaced spondylolisthesis of fifth cervical vertebra, initial encounter for closed fracture
S12.44xA	Type III traumatic spondylolisthesis of fifth cervical vertebra, initial encounter for closed fracture
S12.450A	Other traumatic displaced spondylolisthesis of fifth cervical vertebra, initial encounter for closed fracture

ICD-10-CM Code/Documentation	
S12.451A	Other traumatic nondisplaced spondylolisthesis of fifth cervical vertebra, initial encounter for closed fracture
S12.490A	Other displaced fracture of fifth cervical vertebra, initial encounter for closed fracture
S12.491A	Other nondisplaced fracture of fifth cervical vertebra, initial encounter for closed fracture
C5 Spinal Cord Injury	
S14.105A	Unspecified injury at C5 level of cervical spinal cord, initial encounter
C5 Vertebral Fracture	
S12.400A	Unspecified displaced fracture of fifth cervical vertebrae, initial encounter for closed fracture
S12.401A	Unspecified nondisplaced fracture of fifth cervical vertebra, initial encounter for closed fracture
S12.430A	Unspecified traumatic displaced spondylolisthesis of fifth cervical vertebra, initial encounter for closed fracture
S12.431A	Unspecified traumatic nondisplaced spondylolisthesis of fifth cervical vertebra, initial encounter for closed fracture
S12.44xA	Type III traumatic spondylolisthesis of fifth cervical vertebra, initial encounter for closed fracture
S12.450A	Other traumatic displaced spondylolisthesis of fifth cervical vertebra, initial encounter for closed fracture
S12.451A	Other traumatic nondisplaced spondylolisthesis of fifth cervical vertebra, initial encounter for closed fracture
S12.490A	Other displaced fracture of fifth cervical vertebra, initial encounter for closed fracture
S12.491A	Other nondisplaced fracture of fifth cervical vertebra, initial encounter for closed fracture
C5 Spinal Cord Injury	
S14.115A	Complete lesion at C5 level of cervical spinal cord, initial encounter
S12.451A	Other traumatic nondisplaced spondylolisthesis of fifth cervical vertebra, initial encounter for closed fracture
S12.490A	Other displaced fracture of fifth cervical vertebra, initial encounter for closed fracture
S12.491A	Other nondisplaced fracture of fifth cervical vertebra, initial encounter for closed fracture
C5 Spinal Cord Injury	
S14.135A	Anterior cord syndrome at C5 level of cervical spinal cord, initial encounter
C5 Vertebral Fracture	
S12.400A	Unspecified displaced fracture of fifth cervical vertebrae, initial encounter for closed fracture
S12.401A	Unspecified nondisplaced fracture of fifth cervical vertebra, initial encounter for closed fracture
S12.430A	Unspecified traumatic displaced spondylolisthesis of fifth cervical vertebra, initial encounter for closed fracture
S12.431A	Unspecified traumatic nondisplaced spondylolisthesis of fifth cervical vertebra, initial encounter for closed fracture
S12.44xA	Type III traumatic spondylolisthesis of fifth cervical vertebra, initial encounter for closed fracture
S12.450A	Other traumatic displaced spondylolisthesis of fifth cervical vertebra, initial encounter for closed fracture

ICD-10-CM Code/Documentation	
S12.451A	Other traumatic nondisplaced spondylolisthesis of fifth cervical vertebra, initial encounter for closed fracture
S12.490A	Other displaced fracture of fifth cervical vertebra, initial encounter for closed fracture
S12.491A	Other nondisplaced fracture of fifth cervical vertebra, initial encounter for closed fracture
C5 Spinal Cord Injury	
S14.125A	Central cord syndrome at C5 level of cervical spinal cord, initial encounter
C5 Vertebral Fracture	
S12.400A	Unspecified displaced fracture of fifth cervical vertebrae, initial encounter for closed fracture
S12.401A	Unspecified nondisplaced fracture of fifth cervical vertebra, initial encounter for closed fracture
S12.430A	Unspecified traumatic displaced spondylolisthesis of fifth cervical vertebra, initial encounter for closed fracture
S12.431A	Unspecified traumatic nondisplaced spondylolisthesis of fifth cervical vertebra, initial encounter for closed fracture
S12.44xA	Type III traumatic spondylolisthesis of fifth cervical vertebra, initial encounter for closed fracture
S12.450A	Other traumatic displaced spondylolisthesis of fifth cervical vertebra, initial encounter for closed fracture
S12.451A	Other traumatic nondisplaced spondylolisthesis of fifth cervical vertebra, initial encounter for closed fracture
S12.490A	Other displaced fracture of fifth cervical vertebra, initial encounter for closed fracture
S12.491A	Other nondisplaced fracture of fifth cervical vertebra, initial encounter for closed fracture
C5 Spinal Cord Injury	
S14.0XXA	Concussion and edema of cervical spinal cord, initial encounter
S14.145A	Brown-Séquard syndrome at C5 level of spinal cord, initial encounter
S14.155A	Other incomplete lesion at C5 level of spinal cord, initial encounter

Documentation and Coding Example

Patient is a thirty-eight-year-old Hispanic female brought to ED following **MVA**. Patient was an **unrestrained passenger** in the rear seat of a **car struck head on by another car at a high rate** of speed. She was completely ejected and found semi-conscious with no spontaneous movement on the pavement approximately 50 feet from the **crash site on I-15**. IV started in left antecubital, C-spine immobilized, placed on backboard and transported via ambulance to ED. On examination, this is a mildly obese, middle-aged female. She has **abrasions and contusions on face, upper right shoulder, and right thoracic region of back** consistent with sliding on asphalt. Patient **opens her eyes on command and can state her name**. She is able to recall being in a car accident, is not able to provide any medical history. Vocal quality is weak and breathless. PERRL. HR 50, RR 20, BP 84/50. O2 Sat. 93% on O2 4 L/m via mask. Color pale, skin diaphoretic. Breath sounds clear, shallow. Apical pulse irregular, peripheral pulses weak. SR on monitor with frequent PVCs. Abdomen soft, non-distended with poor tone. Bedside US reveals no free fluid in peritoneum. Foley catheter placed and returns clear yellow urine. Patient has no sensory awareness from shoulders down and no spontaneous muscle movement. She does complain of pain in her face, jaw, and neck. Findings are consistent with traumatic injury to the neck and spinal cord.

C-spine x-ray reveals a fracture of C5 with small fragment anteriorly and angulation of C5-C6 with displacement of C5 posteriorly. Neurosurgical team assembled and ready to assume care. CT reveals severe axial loading with propulsion of a teardrop bone fragment anteriorly and larger portion of the bone resting posterior against the spinal cord. MRI is consistent with soft tissue injury both anterior and posterior to the spinal cord. Patient is taken to surgery for decompression of spinal cord and stabilization of fracture.

Surgical ICU Note: Patient admitted from OR following decompression laminectomy, intubated, on ventilator, neck immobilized with hard cervical collar. Arterial line patent left wrist, peripheral IV lines in left antecubital and right hand. Abrasions cleaned in OR are covered with Xeroform gauze. There is no voluntary muscle movement and flaccid muscle tone from shoulders to toes. **Weaned from ventilator** on day four.

Step Down Unit Note: Transferred 5 days with one peripheral IV line. Patient has very flat affect, she reportedly lost all family members in the accident. Reflexes are consistent with a **complete spinal cord injury** at C5. She is able to perform a very weak shoulder shrug bilaterally but has no sensation or movement below that level. Patient receiving PT, OT, and ST.

Diagnosis Code(s)

S14.115A	Complete lesion at C5 level of cervical spinal cord, initial encounter
S12.490A	Other displaced fracture of fifth cervical vertebrae, initial encounter for closed fracture
S00.81XA	Abrasion of other part of head, initial encounter
S00.83XA	Contusion of other part of head, initial encounter
S20.221A	Contusion of right back wall of thorax, initial encounter
S20.411A	Abrasion of right back wall of thorax, initial encounter
S40.011A	Contusion of right shoulder, initial encounter
S40.211A	Abrasion of right shoulder, initial encounter
V43.62XA	Car passenger injured in collision with other type car in traffic accident, initial encounter
Y92.411	Interstate highway as the place of occurrence of the external cause

Coding Note(s)

There is a note under category S14 to code also any transient paralysis (R29.5). Code R29.5 would not be reported as the patient has sustained an injury resulting in permanent paralysis.

Fracture of Dorsal (Thoracic) Vertebra

Similar to cervical spine fractures both the level of the fracture and the type of fracture must be specified. In addition, the fracture must be documented as open or closed and the episode of care must be known. For follow-up care, healing must be documented as routine, delayed, or with nonunion.

Coding and Documentation Requirements

Identify level of vertebral fracture:

- T1
- T2
- T3
- T4
- T5-T6
- T7-T8
- T9-T10
- T11-T12

Identify type of fracture:

- Burst
  - Stable
  - Unstable
- Wedge compression
- Other specified type of fracture
- Unspecified type of fracture

Identify fracture:

- Closed
- Open

Identify episode of care:

- Initial
- Subsequent
  - With routine healing of fracture
  - With delayed healing of fracture
  - With nonunion of fracture
- Sequela

Fracture of T11-T12 Vertebra

ICD-10-CM Code/Documentation	
Closed fracture	
S22.080A	Wedge compression fracture of T11-T12 vertebra, initial encounter for closed fracture
S22.081A	Stable burst fracture of T11-T12 vertebra, initial encounter for closed fracture
S22.082A	Unstable burst fracture of T11-T12 vertebra, initial encounter for closed fracture
S22.088A	Other fracture of T11-T12 vertebra, initial encounter for closed fracture
S22.089A	Unspecified fracture of T11-T12 vertebra, initial encounter for closed fracture
Open fracture	
S22.080B	Wedge compression fracture of T11-T12 vertebra, initial encounter for open fracture
S22.081B	Stable burst fracture of T11-T12 vertebra, initial encounter for open fracture
S22.082B	Unstable burst fracture of T11-T12 vertebra, initial encounter for open fracture
S22.088B	Other fracture of T11-T12 vertebra, initial encounter for open fracture
S22.089V	Unspecified fracture of T11-T12 vertebra, initial encounter for open fracture

Documentation and Coding Example

Thirty-nine-year-old male presents to ED with c/o moderate to severe pain in his back after falling approximately 15 feet from a boulder while **rock climbing**. Accident occurred approximately 2 hours ago. Patient is a well-developed, well-nourished male who looks younger than his stated age. He is muscular and very tan. He states he is a professional guide leading hiking tours and rock climbing expeditions. The accident today occurred in his **leisure time** on a familiar rock face and was witnessed by friends. As he descended from the top of the rock, his equipment malfunctioned and he dropped rapidly, landing with a hard jolt upright on both legs. He felt an immediate sharp pain in the mid back which is relieved somewhat by lying flat. He denies pain in his hips, knees, or ankles and was able to hike approximately ½ mile to a vehicle. On examination: Temperature 99 degrees, HR 72, RR 12, BP 114/60. Skin warm, slightly diaphoretic, outdoor temperature is in upper 80s. O2 saturation on RA 96%. PERRL, oriented x 3. No cervical spine tenderness and cranial nerves are grossly intact. Motor and sensory function is intact to upper extremities. Breath sounds clear and equal bilaterally, HR regular, no murmur or muffling of heart sounds appreciated. No visual deformities to spine but there is exquisite tenderness with muscle guarding at level of T10 to L4. There is no sign of crepitus. He has limited ROM when attempting flexion, extension, and rotation of spine due to pain. There are no neurological deficits in lower extremities. IV started in left forearm, D5 LR infusing. Medicated for pain with MS 2 mg IV push with good relief. AP and lateral spine x-rays reveal a possible **wedge compression fracture at T12**. CT confirms wedge compression fracture involving the anterior column at T12. Orthopedic consult obtained. Patient fitted with TLSO brace and discharged home with oral narcotic pain medication and instructions to schedule a follow-up in orthopedic clinic in 1 week.

Diagnosis Code(s)

S22.080A	Wedge compression fracture of T11-T12 vertebra, initial encounter for closed fracture
W17.89XA	Other fall from one level to another, initial encounter
Y93.31	Activity, mountain climbing, rock climbing, and wall climbing
Y92.838	Other recreation area as place of occurrence of the external cause
Y99.8	Other external cause status

Coding Note(s)

Y99.8 Other external cause status which includes leisure activity, is used instead of Y99.0 Civilian activity done for income or pay because even though the patient works as a guide on rock climbing expeditions, he incurred this injury during his leisure time not while he was working.

19. Injury/Poisoning of External Causes

Fracture of Humerus, Surgical Neck

Fractures of the upper end of the humerus are classified as surgical neck fractures, greater tuberosity fractures, lesser tuberosity fractures, torus fractures, other specified fractures of the upper end of the humerus, and unspecified fractures. Surgical neck fractures of the proximal or upper end of the humerus are further classified using the Neer system. The proximal humerus is divided into four parts—the humeral head, greater tubercle, lesser tubercle, and diaphysis or shaft. These four parts are separated by epiphyseal lines, also called growth plates which were present when the bones were still growing during the developmental years. The surgical neck is at the narrowest aspect of the humerus just below the tubercles. When the proximal humerus is fractured, it typically occurs at the surgical neck and along one or more of the three epiphyseal lines. The proximal humerus may fracture into 2, 3, or 4 parts at the surgical neck which is why surgical neck fractures are designated as 2-part, 3-part, or 4-part fractures.

The classification of the fracture is based upon the number of fragments and whether there is separation or angulation of the fragments. A fracture part is considered displaced if it is angulated more than 45° or displaced greater than 1 cm. A fracture that is not displaced <1cm **and** angulated < 45° regardless of how many pieces is considered a one-part fracture. All other Neer classifications are based upon the total number of fractures and the number of fractures that are displaced or angulated. For example, a 2-part fracture can be 2-4 parts with one of those parts being displaced **or** angulated. A three-part fracture can be 3-4 parts with two of the parts being displaced or angulated.

Coding and Documentation Requirements

Identify site/type:

- Greater tuberosity
- Lesser tuberosity
- Surgical neck
  - 2-part
  - 3-part
  - 4-part
  - Unspecified type surgical neck fracture
- Torus fracture
- Other specified site, which includes
  - Anatomical neck
  - Articular head
- Unspecified site/type fracture of upper end of humerus

Identify fracture status:

- Displaced
- Nondisplaced

Note: Some fracture types are by definition displaced or nondisplaced and codes for these types of fractures do not require documentation as displaced/nondisplaced.

Identify laterality:

- Right
- Left
- Unspecified

Identify fracture as:

- Closed
- Open

Identify episode of care:

- Initial encounter
- Subsequent encounter
  - With routine healing
  - With delayed healing
  - With nonunion
  - With malunion
- Sequela

Surgical Neck Fracture, Initial Encounter, Open and Closed Fractures

ICD-10-CM Code/Documentation	
Closed Fracture	
Unspecified Surgical Neck Fracture	
S42.211A	Unspecified displaced fracture of surgical neck of right humerus, initial encounter for closed fracture
S42.212A	Unspecified displaced fracture of surgical neck of left humerus, initial encounter for closed fracture
S42.213A	Unspecified displaced fracture of surgical neck of unspecified humerus, initial encounter for closed fracture
S42.214A	Unspecified nondisplaced fracture of surgical neck of right humerus, initial encounter for closed fracture
S42.215A	Unspecified nondisplaced fracture of surgical neck of left humerus, initial encounter for closed fracture
S42.216A	Unspecified nondisplaced fracture of surgical neck of unspecified humerus, initial encounter for closed fracture
2-Part Fracture	
S42.221A	2-part displaced fracture of surgical neck of right humerus, initial encounter for closed fracture
S42.222A	2-part displaced fracture of surgical neck of left humerus, initial encounter for closed fracture
S42.223A	2-part displaced fracture of surgical neck of unspecified humerus, initial encounter for closed fracture
S42.224A	2-part nondisplaced fracture of surgical neck of right humerus, initial encounter for closed fracture
S42.225A	2-part nondisplaced fracture of surgical neck of left humerus, initial encounter for closed fracture
S42.226A	2-part nondisplaced fracture of surgical neck of unspecified humerus, initial encounter for closed fracture
3-Part Fracture	
S42.231A	3-part fracture of surgical neck of right humerus, initial encounter for closed fracture
S42.232A	3-part fracture of surgical neck of left humerus, initial encounter for closed fracture

ICD-10-CM Code/Documentation	
S42.239A	3-part fracture of surgical neck of unspecified humerus, initial encounter for closed fracture
4-Part Fracture	
S42.241A	4-part fracture of surgical neck of right humerus, initial encounter for closed fracture
S42.242A	4-part fracture of surgical neck of left humerus, initial encounter for closed fracture
S42.249A	4-part fracture of surgical neck of unspecified humerus, initial encounter for closed fracture
Open Fracture	
Unspecified Fracture	
S42.211B	Unspecified displaced fracture of surgical neck of right humerus, initial encounter for open fracture
S42.212B	Unspecified displaced fracture of surgical neck of left humerus, initial encounter for open fracture
S42.213B	Unspecified displaced fracture of surgical neck of unspecified humerus, initial encounter for open fracture
S42.214B	Unspecified nondisplaced fracture of surgical neck of right humerus, initial encounter for open fracture
S42.215B	Unspecified nondisplaced fracture of surgical neck of left humerus, initial encounter for open fracture
S42.216B	Unspecified nondisplaced fracture of surgical neck of unspecified humerus, initial encounter for open fracture
2-Part Fracture	
S42.221B	2-part displaced fracture of surgical neck of right humerus, initial encounter for open fracture
S42.222B	2-part displaced fracture of surgical neck of left humerus, initial encounter for open fracture
S42.223B	2-part displaced fracture of surgical neck of unspecified humerus, initial encounter for open fracture
S42.224B	2-part nondisplaced fracture of surgical neck of right humerus, initial encounter for open fracture
S42.225B	2-part nondisplaced fracture of surgical neck of left humerus, initial encounter for open fracture
S42.226B	2-part nondisplaced fracture of surgical neck of unspecified humerus, initial encounter for open fracture
3-Part Fracture	
S42.231B	3-part fracture of surgical neck of right humerus, initial encounter for open fracture
S42.232B	3-part fracture of surgical neck of left humerus, initial encounter for open fracture
S42.239B	3-part fracture of surgical neck of unspecified humerus, initial encounter for open fracture
4-Part Fracture	
S42.241B	4-part fracture of surgical neck of right humerus, initial encounter for open fracture
S42.242B	4-part fracture of surgical neck of left humerus, initial encounter for open fracture
S42.249B	4-part fracture of surgical neck of unspecified humerus, initial encounter for open fracture

Documentation and Coding Example

Patient is a ninety-three-year-old Chinese female who comes reluctantly to ED accompanied by her family to evaluate an **injury to her left arm**. Patient speaks only Mandarin and her grandson serves as translator. Patient lives alone and is in overall good health. Grandson states the patient tripped over a box at home the day before, falling onto her left arm but was able to get up off the floor and go about her normal routine. Patient has immobilized her own arm by using a scarf to keep it tight to her body. HR 60, RR 12, BP 90/62. On examination, this is a very thin, frail appearing elderly woman. PERRL, neck supple. Right upper extremity is normal appearing with intact sensation and ROM. **Left arm has ecchymosis extending the length of the arm, through the shoulder and 6-8 cm into the chest wall. Tenderness and swelling are appreciated in the upper arm and shoulder.** No crepitus appreciated in arm or chest. Sensation intact to deltoid muscle and distally to fingers. ROM intact in fingers, wrist but decreased due to pain in elbow and shoulder. Breath sounds clear and equal bilaterally, HR regular, abdomen soft, non-tender. Lower extremities have good strength and ROM. Blood drawn for CBC, electrolytes, coagulation studies. Neer trauma series obtained for left upper extremity including AP and lateral films in scapular plane and axillary views with results consistent for a 3-part (possibly 4-part) fracture of the proximal humerus. AP and lateral chest films to R/O rib/chest trauma are WNL. CT shows a 3-part fracture. Patient evaluated by orthopedic service and decision made with family to treat with immobilization as an outpatient. Immobilizer applied, patient refuses a prescription for pain medication. She will be re-evaluated in orthopedic clinic in 2 days, if fracture remains stable she can begin PT.

Diagnosis Code(s)

S42.232A	3-part fracture of surgical neck of left humerus, initial encounter for closed fracture
W18.09XA	Striking against other object with subsequent fall, initial encounter
Y92.009	Unspecified place in unspecified non-institutional (private) residence as the place of occurrence of the external cause

Coding Note(s)

While the documentation does not specifically indicate that the fracture is closed, from the documentation it is evident that there is no open injury at the fracture site. In addition, when a fracture is not documented as open or closed the default is closed.

19. Injury/Poisoning of External Causes

Fracture Radius/Ulna Shaft

Fractures of the radius and ulna are classified by the type of fracture, such as greenstick, transverse, or oblique, then by whether the fracture is displaced or nondisplaced, and lastly by which arm (right, left) is involved. The 7th character captures whether the fracture is open or closed and for open fractures the 7th character also captures the Gustilo classification. When both the radius and ulna are fractured, two codes are assigned as there are no combination codes for fractures of the radius and ulna together. There are however combination codes for specific fracture patterns that include a fracture of the radius with an associated subluxation or dislocation of the distal radioulnar joint (Galeazzi) as well as for a Monteggia fracture pattern which is a fracture of the ulnar shaft with a dislocation of the radial head. Because these are combination codes defining both the fracture and dislocation, a separate dislocation code would not also be assigned.

Coding and Documentation Requirements

Radial shaft fractures

Identify type of radial shaft fracture:

- Bent bone
- Comminuted
- Galeazzi's fracture
- Greenstick
- Oblique
- Segmental
- Spiral
- Transverse
- Other specified type of radial shaft fracture
- Unspecified

Identify fracture status:

- Displaced
- Nondisplaced

Note: Some fracture types are by definition displaced or nondisplaced and codes for these types of fractures do not require documentation as displaced/nondisplaced.

Identify laterality:

- Right
- Left
- Unspecified

Identify fracture as:

- Closed
- Open
  - Gustilo Type I, II or open, but not otherwise specified (NOS)
  - Gustilo Type IIIA, IIIB, IIIC

Identify episode of care:

- Initial encounter
- Subsequent encounter
  - With routine healing
  - With delayed healing
  - With nonunion
  - With malunion
- Sequela

Ulnar shaft fractures

Identify type of ulnar shaft fracture:

- Bent bone
- Comminuted
- Greenstick
- Monteggia's fracture
- Oblique
- Segmental
- Spiral
- Transverse
- Other specified type of radial shaft fracture
- Unspecified

Identify fracture status:

- Displaced
- Nondisplaced

Note: Some fracture types are by definition displaced or nondisplaced and codes for these types of fractures do not require documentation as displaced/nondisplaced.

Identify laterality:

- Right
- Left
- Unspecified

Identify fracture as:

- Closed
- Open
  - Gustilo Type I, II or open but not otherwise specified (NOS)
  - Gustilo Type IIIA, IIIB, IIIC

Identify episode of care:

- Initial encounter
- Subsequent encounter
  - » With routine healing
  - » With delayed healing
  - » With nonunion
  - » With malunion
- Sequela

Closed Fracture of Radius and/or Ulna

ICD-10-CM Code/Documentation	
Unspecified Forearm Fracture	
S52.90xA	Unspecified fracture of unspecified forearm, initial encounter for closed fracture
S52.91xA	Unspecified fracture of right forearm, initial encounter for closed fracture
S52.92xA	Unspecified fracture of left forearm, initial encounter for closed fracture

ICD-10-CM Code/Documentation	
Radius Shaft	
Unspecified Fracture	
S52.301A	Unspecified fracture of shaft of right radius, initial encounter for closed fracture
S52.302A	Unspecified fracture of shaft of left radius, initial encounter for closed fracture
S52.309A	Unspecified fracture of shaft of unspecified radius, initial encounter for closed fracture
Greenstick Fracture	
S52.311A	Greenstick fracture of shaft of radius, right arm, initial encounter for closed fracture
S52.312A	Greenstick fracture of shaft of radius, left arm, initial encounter for closed fracture
S52.319A	Greenstick fracture of shaft of radius, unspecified arm, initial encounter for closed fracture
Transverse Fracture	
S52.321A	Displaced transverse fracture of shaft of right radius, initial encounter for closed fracture
S52.322A	Displaced transverse fracture of shaft of left radius, initial encounter for closed fracture
S52.323A	Displaced transverse fracture of shaft of unspecified radius, initial encounter for closed fracture
S52.324A	Nondisplaced transverse fracture of shaft of right radius, initial encounter for closed fracture
S52.325A	Nondisplaced transverse fracture of shaft of left radius, initial encounter for closed fracture
S52.326A	Nondisplaced transverse fracture of shaft of unspecified radius, initial encounter for closed fracture
Oblique Fracture	
S52.331A	Displaced oblique fracture of shaft of right radius, initial encounter for closed fracture
S52.332A	Displaced oblique fracture of shaft of left radius, initial encounter for closed fracture
S52.333A	Displaced oblique fracture of shaft of unspecified radius, initial encounter for closed fracture
S52.334A	Nondisplaced oblique fracture of shaft of right radius, initial encounter for closed fracture
S52.335A	Nondisplaced oblique fracture of shaft of left radius, initial encounter for closed fracture
S52.336A	Nondisplaced oblique fracture of shaft of unspecified radius, initial encounter for closed fracture
Spiral Fracture	
S52.341A	Displaced spiral fracture of shaft of radius, right arm, initial encounter for closed fracture
S52.342A	Displaced spiral fracture of shaft of radius, left arm, initial encounter for closed fracture
S52.343A	Displaced spiral fracture of shaft of radius, unspecified arm, initial encounter for closed fracture

ICD-10-CM Code/Documentation	
S52.344A	Nondisplaced spiral fracture of shaft of radius, right arm, initial encounter for closed fracture
S52.345A	Nondisplaced spiral fracture of shaft of radius, left arm, initial encounter for closed fracture
S52.346A	Nondisplaced spiral fracture of shaft of radius, unspecified arm, initial encounter for closed fracture
Comminuted Fracture	
S52.351A	Displaced comminuted fracture of shaft of radius, right arm, initial encounter for closed fracture
S52.352A	Displaced comminuted fracture of shaft of radius, left arm, initial encounter for closed fracture
S52.353A	Displaced comminuted fracture of shaft of radius, unspecified arm, initial encounter for closed fracture
S52.354A	Nondisplaced comminuted fracture of shaft of radius, right arm, initial encounter for closed fracture
S52.355A	Nondisplaced comminuted fracture of shaft of radius, left arm, initial encounter for closed fracture
S52.356A	Nondisplaced comminuted fracture of shaft of radius, unspecified arm, initial encounter for closed fracture
Segmental Fracture	
S52.361A	Displaced segmental fracture of shaft of radius, right arm, initial encounter for closed fracture
S52.362A	Displaced segmental fracture of shaft of radius, left arm, initial encounter for closed fracture
S52.363A	Displaced segmental fracture of shaft of radius, unspecified arm, initial encounter for closed fracture
S52.364A	Nondisplaced segmental fracture of shaft of radius, right arm, initial encounter for closed fracture
S52.365A	Nondisplaced segmental fracture of shaft of radius, left arm, initial encounter for closed fracture
S52.366A	Nondisplaced segmental fracture of shaft of radius, unspecified arm, initial encounter for closed fracture
Bent Bone	
S52.381A	Bent bone of right radius, initial encounter for closed fracture
S52.382A	Bent bone of left radius, initial encounter for closed fracture
S52.389A	Bent bone of unspecified radius, initial encounter for closed fracture
Other Fracture	
S52.391A	Other fracture of shaft of radius, right arm, initial encounter for closed fracture
S52.392A	Other fracture of shaft of radius, left arm, initial encounter for closed fracture
S52.399A	Other fracture of shaft of radius, unspecified arm, initial encounter for closed fracture
Galeazzi's	
S52.371A	Galeazzi's fracture of right radius, initial encounter for closed fracture
S52.372A	Galeazzi's fracture of left radius, initial encounter for closed fracture
S52.379A	Galeazzi's fracture of unspecified radius, initial encounter for closed fracture

ICD-10-CM Code/Documentation	
Ulna Shaft	
Unspecified Fracture	
S52.201A	Unspecified fracture of shaft of right ulna, initial encounter for closed fracture
S52.202A	Unspecified fracture of shaft of left ulna, initial encounter for closed fracture
S52.209A	Unspecified fracture of shaft of unspecified ulna, initial encounter for closed fracture
Greenstick Fracture	
S52.211A	Greenstick fracture of shaft of right ulna, initial encounter for closed fracture
S52.212A	Greenstick fracture of shaft of left ulna, initial encounter for closed fracture
S52.219A	Greenstick fracture of shaft of unspecified ulna, initial encounter for closed fracture
Transverse Fracture	
S52.221A	Displaced transverse fracture of shaft of right ulna, initial encounter for closed fracture
S52.222A	Displaced transverse fracture of shaft of left ulna, initial encounter for closed fracture
S52.223A	Displaced transverse fracture of shaft of unspecified ulna, initial encounter for closed fracture
S52.224A	Nondisplaced transverse fracture of shaft of right ulna, initial encounter for closed fracture
S52.225A	Nondisplaced transverse fracture of shaft of left ulna, initial encounter for closed fracture
S52.226A	Nondisplaced transverse fracture of shaft of unspecified ulna, initial encounter for closed fracture
Oblique Fracture	
S52.231A	Displaced oblique fracture of shaft of right ulna, initial encounter for closed fracture
S52.232A	Displaced oblique fracture of shaft of left ulna, initial encounter for closed fracture
S52.233A	Displaced oblique fracture of shaft of unspecified ulna, initial encounter for closed fracture
S52.234A	Nondisplaced oblique fracture of shaft of right ulna, initial encounter for closed fracture
S52.235A	Nondisplaced oblique fracture of shaft of left ulna, initial encounter for closed fracture
S52.236A	Nondisplaced oblique fracture of shaft of unspecified ulna, initial encounter for closed fracture
Spiral Fracture	
S52.241A	Displaced spiral fracture of shaft of ulna, right arm, initial encounter for closed fracture
S52.242A	Displaced spiral fracture of shaft of ulna, left arm, initial encounter for closed fracture
S52.243A	Displaced spiral fracture of shaft of ulna, unspecified arm, initial encounter for closed fracture
S52.244A	Nondisplaced spiral fracture of shaft of ulna, right arm, initial encounter for closed fracture

ICD-10-CM Code/Documentation	
S52.245A	Nondisplaced spiral fracture of shaft of ulna, left arm, initial encounter for closed fracture
S52.246A	Nondisplaced spiral fracture of shaft of ulna, unspecified arm, initial encounter for closed fracture
Comminuted Fracture	
S52.251A	Displaced comminuted fracture of shaft of ulna, right arm, initial encounter for closed fracture
S52.252A	Displaced comminuted fracture of shaft of ulna, left arm, initial encounter for closed fracture
S52.253A	Displaced comminuted fracture of shaft of ulna, unspecified arm, initial encounter for closed fracture
S52.254A	Nondisplaced comminuted fracture of shaft of ulna, right arm, initial encounter for closed fracture
S52.255A	Nondisplaced comminuted fracture of shaft of ulna, left arm, initial encounter for closed fracture
S52.256A	Nondisplaced comminuted fracture of shaft of ulna, unspecified arm, initial encounter for closed fracture
Segmental Fracture	
S52.261A	Displaced segmental fracture of shaft of ulna, right arm, initial encounter for closed fracture
S52.262A	Displaced segmental fracture of shaft of ulna, left arm, initial encounter for closed fracture
S52.263A	Displaced segmental fracture of shaft of ulna, unspecified arm, initial encounter for closed fracture
S52.264A	Nondisplaced segmental fracture of shaft of ulna, right arm, initial encounter for closed fracture
S52.265A	Nondisplaced segmental fracture of shaft of ulna, left arm, initial encounter for closed fracture
S52.266A	Nondisplaced segmental fracture of shaft of ulna, unspecified arm, initial encounter for closed fracture
Bent Bone	
S52.281A	Bent bone of right ulna, initial encounter for closed fracture
S52.282A	Bent bone of left ulna, initial encounter for closed fracture
S52.283A	Bent bone of unspecified ulna, initial encounter for closed fracture
Other Fracture	
S52.291A	Other fracture of shaft of right ulna, initial encounter for closed fracture
S52.292A	Other fracture of shaft of left ulna, initial encounter for closed fracture
S52.299A	Other fracture of shaft of unspecified ulna, initial encounter for closed fracture
Note: There are no combined codes for fracture of shaft of radius with ulna. Two codes, one from subcategory S52.2- Fracture of shaft of ulna and one from subcategory S52.3- Fracture of shaft of radius, are required to capture fractures of the radius with the ulna.	
Monteggia's	
S52.271A	Monteggia's fracture of right ulna, initial encounter for closed fracture
S52.272A	Monteggia's fracture of left ulna, initial encounter for closed fracture
S52.279A	Monteggia's fracture of unspecified ulna, initial encounter for closed fracture

Note 1: The initial encounter for an open fracture is reported with the same codes listed above except that the 7th character extension 'A' is replaced with a 'B' or 'C' as follows:

B Initial encounter for open fracture type I or II or not otherwise specified (NOS)

C Initial encounter for open fracture type IIIA, IIIB, or IIIC

Note 2: Monteggia's fracture is classified as a fracture of the ulnar shaft (upper region of ulnar shaft).

Note 3: Galeazzi's fracture is classified as a fracture of the radial shaft (lower region of radial shaft).

Documentation and Coding Example

Ten-year-old Caucasian female brought to ED by parent with bilateral forearm injuries. Child was on a **school sponsored picnic to a local public park when she fell from a rope swing,** landing on outstretched arms. Accident occurred approximately 15 minutes ago. She is ambulatory, pale and diaphoretic, crying but cooperative with her arms braced against her body. There is obvious deformity of both forearms with patient c/o severe pain in the area of deformity and also some numbness in forearm and hand on the right. Placed on monitors, HR 104, RR 18, BP 76/40, O2 saturation on RA 94%. AP and lateral films of both upper extremities obtained. The most serious fracture appears to be in the **right arm with a closed, displaced comminuted fracture of the radius and a nondisplaced oblique fracture of the ulna, both at midshaft level. Left arm has a closed, displaced Galeazzi type fracture of the lower radius with dislocation of the ulna at the wrist**. Orthopedics called to evaluate patient. Decision made after discussion with parents to attempt closed reduction with conscious sedation/MAC in ED. Anesthesiologist here, IV started in right foot. O2 started at 2 L/m via NC. Patient comfortably sedated with Versed, Propofol, and Fentanyl. All fractures easily reduced. Soft cast/splints applied. X-rays show satisfactory alignment of all bones. Patient tolerated procedure well, monitored x 1 hour by anesthesia and cleared for discharge home. Appointment made for orthopedic clinic visit in 5 days. Alignment will be evaluated with repeat x-rays, possible hard cast placement if alignment remains satisfactory.

Diagnosis Code(s)

S52.351A Displaced comminuted fracture of shaft of right radius, initial encounter for closed fracture

S52.234A Nondisplaced oblique fracture of shaft of right ulna, initial encounter for closed fracture

S52.372A Galeazzi's fracture of left radius, initial encounter for closed fracture

W09.1XXA Fall from playground swing, initial encounter

Y92.830 Pubic park as place of occurrence of the external cause

Coding Note(s)

Galeazzi's fracture by definition involves fracture of lower shaft of radius with radioulnar joint dislocation so the dislocation is not coded separately.

Fracture of Carpal Bones

Fractures of the carpal bones require documentation of the specific carpal bone fractured. For fractures of the navicular and hamate bones, additional information is required related to the site of the fracture.

Coding and Documentation Requirements

Identify site:

- Capitate (os magnum)
- Hamate (unciform)
  - Body
  - Hook process
- Lunate
- Navicular (scaphoid)
  - Distal pole
  - Middle third (waist)
  - Proximal third
  - Unspecified
- Pisiform
- Trapezoid (smaller multangular)
- Trapezium (larger multangular)
- Triquetrum (cuneiform)
- Other and unspecified carpal bone fracture

Identify fracture status:

- Displaced
- Nondisplaced

Identify laterality:

- Right
- Left
- Unspecified

Identify fracture as:

- Closed
- Open

Identify episode of care:

- Initial encounter
- Subsequent encounter
  - With routine healing
  - With delayed healing
  - With nonunion
  - With malunion
- Sequela

Fracture of Carpal Navicula (Scaphoid) Bone

ICD-10-CM Code/Documentation	
Unspecified site navicular bone	
S62.001-	Unspecified fracture of navicular [scaphoid] bone of right wrist
S62.002-	Unspecified fracture of navicular [scaphoid] bone of left wrist

19. Injury/Poisoning of External Causes

ICD-10-CM Code/Documentation	
S62.009-	Unspecified fracture of navicular [scaphoid] bone of unspecified wrist
Distal pole	
S62.011-	Displaced fracture of distal pole of navicular [scaphoid] bone of right wrist
S62.012-	Displaced fracture of distal pole of navicular [scaphoid] bone of left wrist
S62.013-	Displaced fracture of distal pole of navicular [scaphoid] bone of unspecified wrist
S62.014-	Nondisplaced fracture of distal pole of navicular [scaphoid] bone of right wrist
S62.015-	Nondisplaced fracture of distal pole of navicular [scaphoid] bone of left wrist
S62.016-	Nondisplaced fracture of distal pole of navicular [scaphoid] bone of unspecified wrist
Middle third	
S62.021-	Displaced fracture of middle third of navicular [scaphoid] bone of right wrist
S62.022-	Displaced fracture of middle third of navicular [scaphoid] bone of left wrist
S62.023-	Displaced fracture of middle third of navicular [scaphoid] bone of unspecified wrist
S62.024-	Nondisplaced fracture of middle third of navicular [scaphoid] bone of right wrist
S62.025-	Nondisplaced fracture of middle third of navicular [scaphoid] bone of left wrist
S62.026-	Nondisplaced fracture of middle third of navicular [scaphoid] bone of unspecified wrist
Proximal third	
S62.031-	Displaced fracture of proximal third of navicular [scaphoid] bone of right wrist
S62.032-	Displaced fracture of proximal third of navicular [scaphoid] bone of left wrist
S62.033-	Displaced fracture of proximal third of navicular [scaphoid] bone of unspecified wrist
S62.034-	Nondisplaced fracture of proximal third of navicular [scaphoid] bone of right wrist
S62.035-	Nondisplaced fracture of proximal third of navicular [scaphoid] bone of left wrist
S62.036-	Nondisplaced fracture of proximal third of navicular [scaphoid] bone of unspecified wrist

Note: For initial encounter for closed fracture, use 7th character 'A'; for initial encounter for open fracture, use 7th character 'B'. The Gustilo classification for open fractures does not apply to carpal bone fractures.

Documentation and Coding Example

Thirty-two-year-old Black male presents to Urgent Care clinic with c/o pain, swelling in left wrist x 2 weeks. Patient injured his hand when he **slipped and fell on an icy public sidewalk.** Patient did not seek medical care for the injury until today because he has been traveling. On examination, there is swelling at the base of left thumb with marked tenderness when palpated. Patient describes the pain as deep and aching. Grip is weaker on the left. X-ray of left hand and wrist reveals a **closed, nondisplaced, vertical fracture through the proximal pole carpal navicular.** Telephone consult with orthopedist on-call. Fracture will be treated conservatively with short arm, thumb spica cast. Patient is given the name and contact number for consulting orthopedist with instructions to see him in 2 weeks for re-evaluation. Patient is cautioned that this type of fracture has a high risk of avascular necrosis, especially given the delay with diagnosis and treatment.

Diagnosis Code(s)

S62.035A	Nondisplaced fracture of proximal third of navicular [scaphoid] bone of left wrist, initial encounter for closed fracture
W00.0XXA	Fall on same level due to ice and snow
Y92.480	Sidewalk as place of occurrence of external cause

Coding Note(s)

The place of occurrence in the scenario is a public sidewalk. There is a specific code for sidewalk as the place of occurrence of the external cause.

Fracture of Metacarpal Bones

There are two subcategories for fractures of the metacarpal bones, S62.2 Fracture of first metacarpal bone (thumb), and S62.3 Fracture of other and unspecified metacarpal bone. For fractures of the first metacarpal bone, codes are then classified by general site as the base, shaft, or neck. Fractures of the base of the metacarpal bone of the thumb include specific codes for Bennett's fractures and Rolando's fractures as well as a code for other fracture of the base of the first metacarpal. The 6th character captures displaced/nondisplaced status of the fracture and laterality. Fractures of other and unspecified metacarpal bones are specific to general site (base, shaft, neck), the specific metacarpal bone fractured (second, third, fourth, fifth), displaced/nondisplaced status of the fracture, and laterality.

Coding and Documentation Requirements

Identify metacarpal bone fractured:

- First metacarpal (thumb)
- Other metacarpal bone
  - Second
  - Third
  - Fourth
  - Fifth

For thumb, identify fracture site/type:

- Base
  - Bennett's fracture
  - Rolando's fracture
  - Other fracture of base
- Neck
- Shaft
- Unspecified site/type

For other metacarpal bones (second, third, fourth, fifth), identify fracture site:

- Base

- Neck
- Shaft
- Other fracture
- Unspecified fracture

Identify fracture status:

- Displaced
- Nondisplaced

Identify laterality:

- Right
- Left
- Unspecified

Identify fracture as:

- Closed
- Open

Identify episode of care:

- Initial encounter
- Subsequent encounter
  - With routine healing
  - With delayed healing
  - With nonunion
  - With malunion
- Sequela

Fracture Base of First Metacarpal (Thumb)

ICD-10-CM Code/Documentation	
Closed Fracture	
Unspecified Fracture	
S62.201A	Unspecified fracture of first metacarpal bone, right hand, initial encounter for closed fracture
S62.202A	Unspecified fracture of first metacarpal bone, left hand, initial encounter for closed fracture
S62.209A	Unspecified fracture of first metacarpal bone, unspecified hand, initial encounter for closed fracture
Bennett's Fracture	
S62.211A	Bennett's fracture, right hand, initial encounter for closed fracture
S62.212A	Bennett's fracture, left hand, initial encounter for closed fracture
S62.213A	Bennett's fracture, unspecified hand, initial encounter for closed fracture
Rolando's Fracture	
S62.221A	Displaced Rolando's fracture right hand, initial encounter for closed fracture
S62.222A	Displaced Rolando's fracture left hand, initial encounter for closed fracture
S62.223A	Displaced Rolando's fracture unspecified hand, initial encounter for closed fracture
S62.224A	Nondisplaced Rolando's fracture right hand, initial encounter for closed fracture
S62.225A	Nondisplaced Rolando's fracture left hand, initial encounter for closed fracture
S62.226A	Nondisplaced Rolando's fracture unspecified hand, initial encounter for closed fracture
Other Displaced Fracture	
S62.231A	Other displaced fracture base of first metacarpal bone, right hand, initial encounter for closed fracture
S62.232A	Other displaced fracture base of first metacarpal bone, left hand, initial encounter for closed fracture
S62.233A	Other displaced fracture base of first metacarpal bone, unspecified hand, initial encounter for closed fracture
S62.234A	Other nondisplaced fracture base of first metacarpal bone, right hand, initial encounter for closed fracture
S62.235A	Other nondisplaced fracture base of first metacarpal bone, left hand, initial encounter for closed fracture
S62.236A	Other nondisplaced fracture base of first metacarpal bone, unspecified hand, initial encounter for closed fracture
Open Fracture	
Unspecified Fracture	
S62.201B	Unspecified fracture of first metacarpal bone, right hand, initial encounter for open fracture
S62.202B	Unspecified fracture of first metacarpal bone, left hand, initial encounter for open fracture
S62.209B	Unspecified fracture of first metacarpal bone, unspecified hand, initial encounter for open fracture
Bennett's Fracture	
S62.211B	Bennett's fracture, right hand, initial encounter for open fracture
S62.212B	Bennett's fracture, left hand, initial encounter for open fracture
S62.213B	Bennett's fracture, unspecified hand, initial encounter for open fracture
Rolando's Fracture	
S62.221B	Displaced Rolando's fracture right hand, initial encounter for open fracture
S62.222B	Displaced Rolando's fracture left hand, initial encounter for open fracture
S62.223B	Displaced Rolando's fracture unspecified hand, initial encounter for open fracture
S62.224B	Nondisplaced Rolando's fracture, right hand, initial encounter for open fracture
S62.225B	Nondisplaced Rolando's fracture, left hand, initial encounter for open fracture
S62.226B	Nondisplaced Rolando's fracture, unspecified hand, initial encounter for open fracture
Other Displaced Fracture	
S62.231B	Other displaced fracture base of first metacarpal bone, right hand, initial encounter for open fracture
S62.232B	Other displaced fracture base of first metacarpal bone, left hand, initial encounter for open fracture
S62.233B	Other displaced fracture base of first metacarpal bone, unspecified hand, initial encounter for open fracture
S62.234B	Other nondisplaced fracture base of first metacarpal bone, right hand, initial encounter for open fracture

ICD-10-CM Code/Documentation	
S62.235B	Other nondisplaced fracture base of first metacarpal bone, left hand, initial encounter for open fracture
S62.236B	Other nondisplaced fracture base of first metacarpal bone, unspecified hand, initial encounter for open fracture

Documentation and Coding Example

Twenty-two-year-old construction worker arrives in ED with an open wound to his right hand. This well-developed, well-nourished Caucasian male states he was working outdoors on a private home remodeling job when a piece of equipment fell from the roof. He reacted by placing his hand up to shield his head with the tool striking his hand and causing the injury. On examination, there is visual deformity toward the base of the **right thumb. An opening in the skin, 3 cm long x 1 cm deep** with minimal bleeding and easily approximated skin edges is present. There are no boney fragments visible through the open skin. Wound irrigated with dilute betadine/H2O and gauze dressing applied. Pt taken to x-ray for AP, lateral, and Robert's view of right hand. Films show a **comminuted intraarticular fracture in three fragments including the metacarpal shaft, dorsal metacarpal base, and volar metacarpal base**. Care turned over to orthopedic service and patient taken to OR for further exploration, debridement of wound, reduction of **displaced fragments**, and pin fixation of fracture and antibiotic coverage.

Final diagnosis: **Open Rolando's fracture, right thumb**

Diagnosis Code(s)

S62.221B Displaced Rolando's fracture, right hand, initial encounter for open fracture

W20.8XXA Other cause of strike by thrown, projected or falling object, initial encounter

Y93.H3 Activity, building and construction

Y99.0 Civilian activity done for income or pay

Coding Note(s)

Open fractures include any fracture that has direct communication with the external environment. The open wound may be caused by the fracture penetrating the skin or the traumatic event may have resulted in an open wound with an underlying fracture. The presence of an open wound with a fracture does not necessarily mean there is an open fracture. Provider documentation must clearly support the relationship of the wound and the fracture. The description of the fracture fragments as including the metacarpal shaft, dorsal metacarpal base, and volar metacarpal base might lead one to believe that this type of fracture would be coded as S62.291 Other fracture of first metacarpal bone, right hand. However, a Rolando's fracture is a comminuted intraarticular fracture of the base of the 1st metacarpal in a Y or T configuration resulting in an extension into the shaft as well as base. There is a specific code for a Rolando's fracture of the thumb. The status of the fracture as open or closed is captured by the 7th character, which in this case is 'B' for initial encounter for open fracture.

Fracture of Pelvis

Codes are specific as to site and laterality. Documentation is also required regarding characteristics of the fracture, including whether the fracture is closed or open, and whether it is displaced or nondisplaced. The specific characteristics of the fracture will vary depending on the site of the fracture. For example, fractures of the ilium and ischium must be described as avulsion or another specified type in order to assign the most specific code. Fractures that disrupt the pelvic ring must be documented as stable or unstable. Documentation for fractures of the acetabulum requires additional detail on the specific area of involvement such as the anterior wall, dome or posterior column.

Coding and Documentation Requirements

Identify fracture site/type:

- Acetabulum
  - Anterior column (iliopubic)
  - Anterior wall
  - Dome
  - Medial wall
  - Posterior column (ilioischial)
  - Posterior wall
  - Transverse
    - » Alone (without associated posterior wall fracture)
    - » With associated posterior wall fracture
  - Other specified acetabular fracture
  - Unspecified acetabular fracture
- Ilium
  - Avulsion
  - Other specified fracture of ilium
  - Unspecified fracture ilium
- Ischium
  - Avulsion
  - Other specified fracture of ischium
  - Unspecified fracture of ischium
- Pubis
  - Superior rim
  - Other specified fracture of pubis
  - Unspecified fracture of pubis
- Multiple fractures of pelvis
  - With disruption of pelvic circle
    - » Stable
    - » Unstable
  - Without disruption of pelvic circle
- Other specified site of pelvis
- Unspecified site of pelvis

Identify fracture status:

- Displaced
- Nondisplaced

Identify laterality:

- Right
- Left
- Unspecified

Identify fracture as:

- Closed
- Open

Identify episode of care:

- Initial encounter
- Subsequent encounter
  - With routine healing
  - With delayed healing
  - With nonunion
- Sequela

Transverse Fracture of Acetabulum with Associated Posterior Wall Fracture

ICD-10-CM Code/Documentation	
S32.461-	Displaced associated transverse-posterior fracture of right acetabulum
S32.462-	Displaced associated transverse-posterior fracture of left acetabulum
S32.463-	Displaced associated transverse-posterior fracture of unspecified acetabulum
S32.464-	Nondisplaced associated transverse-posterior fracture of right acetabulum
S32.465-	Nondisplaced associated transverse-posterior fracture of left acetabulum
S32.466-	Nondisplaced associated transverse-posterior fracture of unspecified acetabulum

Note: The ICD-10-CM codes in the table above are listed with a dash in the 7th character position to indicate that a 7th character is required for the episode of care.

Documentation and Coding Example

ED Note: Patient is a 53-year-old female involved in a **pedestrian vs. van accident.** Patient was crossing the street in a marked crosswalk when she was struck by a van making a left turn. The van struck the patient on her **right side** with the impact propelling her into the air landing approximately 10 feet away on the pavement. She is complaining of pain in her right hip. On examination, this is a well-developed, well-nourished female who is alert and oriented x 3. HR 94, RR 16, BP 150/86. O2 saturation 97 % on oxygen at 2 L/m via NC. PERRL. Breath sounds clear, equal bilaterally. HR regular without murmur or muffling. No abdominal or flank tenderness, bladder is not palpated. There is bruising over the right hip area with visual limb length inequality. Bedside US reveals no free fluid in peritoneum. Foley catheter placed with some difficulty due to hip pain and deformity. Urine returned is dark yellow, dipstick negative for blood. Blood drawn for CBC, electrolytes, PT, PTT, type and hold. EKG obtained. AP and oblique views of pelvis reveal a transverse-posterior wall fracture of the right acetabulum. CT scan of pelvis and abdomen R/O intra-abdominal organ injury and enhanced 3D reconstruction shows a **nondisplaced transverse acetabular fracture with an associated moderately displaced posterior wall fracture on the right.** Care of patient is assumed by orthopedic team as patient awaits transfer to OR.

Diagnosis Code(s)

S32.461A	Displaced associated transverse-posterior fracture of right acetabulum, initial encounter for closed fracture
V03.10XA	Pedestrian on foot injured in collision with car, pick-up truck or van in traffic accident, initial encounter
Y92.410	Unspecified street and highway as the place of occurrence of the external cause

Coding Note(s)

The documentation does not indicate whether the fracture is open or closed, so it is coded to closed. Because the posterior wall fracture is moderately displaced, the fracture is coded as displaced even though the transverse component of the fracture is nondisplaced.

Fracture of Femoral Neck

Category S72 Fracture of femur contains six subcategories: S72.0 Fracture of head and neck of femur; S72.1 Pertrochanteric fracture (fracture line passes through trochanter); S72.2 Subtrochanteric fracture (transverse fracture just below the lesser trochanter); S72.3 Fracture of shaft of femur; S72.4 Fracture of lower end of femur; S72.8 Other fracture of femur; S72.9 Unspecified fracture of femur. Fractures in most of these 4th digit subcategories are further subclassified with additional information related to fracture site and/or fracture configuration/type, such as transverse, oblique, or comminuted. Fractures of the head, neck, pertrochanteric, and subtrochanteric regions are detailed here.

Coding and Documentation Requirements

Identify site of femoral fracture:

- Neck
  - Base of neck
  - Epiphysis
  - Intracapsular, unspecified
    - » Includes subcapital
  - Midcervical
  - Other specified site
  - Unspecified part
- Head
  - Articular
  - Other specified site
  - Unspecified part
- Pertrochanteric
  - Apophyseal
  - Greater trochanter
  - Intertrochanteric

  - Lesser trochanter
  - Unspecified trochanteric site
- Subtrochanteric

Identify fracture status:

- Displaced
- Nondisplaced

Identify laterality:

- Right
- Left
- Unspecified

Identify fracture as:

- Closed
- Open Gustilo classification
  - Type I or II, or open NOS
  - Type IIIA, IIIB, or IIIC

Identify episode of care:

- Initial
- Subsequent with
  - Delayed healing
  - Malunion
  - Nonunion
  - Routine healing
- Sequela

Fractures of the femoral head and neck, pertrochanteric and subtrochanteric region require 7th characters which should be assigned as follows:

A Initial encounter for closed fracture

B Initial encounter for open fracture type I or II, or open fracture NOS

C Initial encounter for open fracture type IIIA, IIIB, or IIIC

D Subsequent encounter for closed fracture with routine healing

E Subsequent encounter for open fracture type I or II with routine healing

F Subsequent encounter for open fracture type IIIA, IIIB, or IIIC with routine healing

G Subsequent encounter for closed fracture with delayed healing

H Subsequent encounter for open fracture type I or II with delayed healing

J Subsequent encounter for open fracture type IIIA, IIIB, or IIIC with delayed healing

K Subsequent encounter for closed fracture with nonunion

M Subsequent encounter for open fracture type I or II with nonunion

N Subsequent encounter for open fracture type IIIA, IIIB, or IIIC with nonunion

P Subsequent encounter for closed fracture with malunion

Q Subsequent encounter for open fracture type I or II with malunion

R Subsequent encounter for open fracture type IIIA, IIIB, or IIIC with malunion

S Sequela

Fracture Femoral Head and Neck

ICD-10-CM Code/Documentation	
Neck, unspecified	
S72.001-	Fracture of unspecified part of neck of right femur
S72.002-	Fracture of unspecified part of neck of left femur
S72.009-	Fracture of unspecified part of neck of unspecified femur
Intracapsular	
S72.011-	Unspecified intracapsular fracture right femur
S72.012-	Unspecified intracapsular fracture left femur
S72.019-	Unspecified intracapsular fracture unspecified femur
Proximal Epiphysis Fracture/Separation	
S72.021-	Displaced fracture of epiphysis (separation) (upper) of right femur
S72.022-	Displaced fracture of epiphysis (separation) (upper) of left femur
S72.023-	Displaced fracture of epiphysis (separation) (upper) of unspecified femur
S72.024-	Nondisplaced fracture of epiphysis (separation) (upper) of right femur
S72.025-	Nondisplaced fracture of epiphysis (separation) (upper) of left femur
S72.026-	Nondisplaced fracture of epiphysis (separation) (upper) of unspecified femur
Midcervical Fracture	
S72.031-	Displaced midcervical fracture of right femur
S72.032-	Displaced midcervical fracture of left femur
S72.033-	Displaced midcervical fracture of unspecified femur
S72.034-	Nondisplaced midcervical fracture of right femur
S72.035-	Nondisplaced midcervical fracture of left femur
S72.036-	Nondisplaced midcervical fracture of unspecified femur
Basilar Neck fracture	
S72.041-	Displaced fracture of base of neck of right femur
S72.042-	Displaced fracture of base of neck of left femur
S72.043-	Displaced fracture of base of neck of unspecified femur
S72.044-	Nondisplaced fracture of base of neck of right femur
S72.045-	Nondisplaced fracture of base of neck of left femur
S72.046-	Nondisplaced fracture of base of neck of unspecified femur
Femoral Head Fractures	
S72.051-	Unspecified fracture of head of right femur
S72.052-	Unspecified fracture of head of left femur
S72.059-	Unspecified fracture of head of unspecified femur
S72.061-	Displaced articular fracture of head of right femur
S72.062-	Displaced articular fracture of head of left femur
S72.063-	Displaced articular fracture of head of unspecified femur
S72.064-	Nondisplaced articular fracture of head of right femur

Trochanteric Fractures	
S72.101-	Unspecified trochanteric fracture of right femur
S72.102-	Unspecified trochanteric fracture of left femur
S72.109-	Unspecified trochanteric fracture of unspecified femur
S72.111-	Displaced fracture of greater trochanter of right femur
S72.112-	Displaced fracture of greater trochanter of left femur
S72.113-	Displaced fracture of greater trochanter of unspecified femur
S72.114-	Nondisplaced fracture of greater trochanter of right femur
S72.115-	Nondisplaced fracture of greater trochanter of left femur
S72.116-	Nondisplaced fracture of greater trochanter of unspecified femur
S72.121-	Displaced fracture of lesser trochanter of right femur
S72.122-	Displaced fracture of lesser trochanter of left femur
S72.123-	Displaced fracture of lesser trochanter of unspecified femur
S72.124-	Nondisplaced fracture of lesser trochanter of right femur
S72.125-	Nondisplaced fracture of lesser trochanter of left femur
S72.126-	Nondisplaced fracture of lesser trochanter of unspecified femur
Apophyseal Fracture	
S72.131-	Displaced apophyseal fracture of right femur
S72.132-	Displaced apophyseal fracture of left femur
S72.133-	Displaced apophyseal fracture of unspecified femur
S72.134-	Nondisplaced apophyseal fracture of right femur
S72.135-	Nondisplaced apophyseal fracture of left femur
S72.136-	Nondisplaced apophyseal fracture of unspecified femur
Intertrochanteric Fracture	
S72.141-	Displaced intertrochanteric fracture of right femur
S72.142-	Displaced intertrochanteric fracture of left femur
S72.143-	Displaced intertrochanteric fracture of unspecified femur
S72.144-	Nondisplaced intertrochanteric fracture of right femur
S72.145-	Nondisplaced intertrochanteric fracture of left femur
S72.146-	Nondisplaced intertrochanteric fracture of unspecified femur
Subtrochanteric Fracture	
S72.21X-	Displaced subtrochanteric fracture of right femur
S72.22X-	Displaced subtrochanteric fracture of left femur
S72.23X-	Displaced subtrochanteric fracture of unspecified femur
S72.24X-	Nondisplaced subtrochanteric fracture of right femur
S72.25X-	Nondisplaced subtrochanteric fracture of left femur
S72.26X-	Nondisplaced subtrochanteric fracture of unspecified femur

Documentation and Coding Example

ED Note: This 64-year-old woman arrives in ED via ambulance with a probable hip fracture sustained in a **hard fall onto her right hip**. She states she was in the **kitchen of her apartment on a step ladder getting a large metal bowl from an upper shelf**, was startled by a loud noise outside, lost her balance, and fell. Her right leg is shortened in length and externally rotated. There is swelling and tenderness in the area of the right hip/upper femur with redness and very faint ecchymosis. She complains of pain with the slightest manipulation. No neurovascular compromise to the extremity. Temperature 97.8, HR 84, RR 14, BP 150/82. Pulse oximetry shows O2 saturation of 94% on RA, patient was brought in on oxygen, 2 L/m via NC but is now refusing to use it. NSR with occasional benign PVCs on monitor. Alert and oriented x 3, PERRL, there is a small opacity suggestive of a cataract in her right eye which patient confirms and states she is under care of ophthalmologist. Medical history is remarkable only for osteopenia treated with calcium and Vitamin D supplements, appendectomy in her 30's and an episode of acute diverticulitis 20 years ago. Patient is married, no children. Both she and her husband are retired. IV started in left forearm, blood drawn for CBC, electrolytes, PT, PTT, Type and hold. Medicated with MS 2mg IV prior to obtaining AP and lateral x-rays of right hip which reveal a **closed, nondisplaced intertrochanteric fracture of the right femur**. Orthopedic service called to examine patient and ordered her NPO, transferred to floor with Bucks traction while waiting for OR to become available. No beds available on floor at present time. Patient transferred to ED holding area.

Diagnosis Code(s)

S72.144A	Nondisplaced intertrochanteric fracture of right femur, initial encounter for closed fracture
W11.XXXA	Fall on and from ladder, initial encounter
Y92.030	Kitchen in apartment as the place of occurrence of the external cause
Y93.G1	Activity, food preparation and clean up
Y99.8	Other external cause status

Coding Note(s)

There are codes for osteoporosis with related pathological fractures, which are listed with Osteopathies and Chrondropathies (M80-M94) in Chapter 18 Diseases of the Musculoskeletal System and Connective Tissue. Although the patient has a history of osteopenia there is no documented osteoporosis, nor is the fracture documented to be pathological in nature. Documentation indicates that the fracture is due to the fall. Therefore, the fracture is reported with a code for a traumatic fracture rather than a code for a pathological fracture.

Fracture of Tibia and Fibula (Upper End/Shaft)

Fractures of the tibia and fibula require separate codes for each of the fractures to allow for more accurate reporting of the specific location and type of fracture. Like fractures of the radius and ulna, in ICD-10CM there are no combination codes for fractures of the tibia and fibula.

Coding and Documentation Requirements

Identify lower leg bone:

- Tibia
- Fibula

Identify site/type:

- Tibia, upper end
  - Condylar
    - » Lateral

    - » Medial
    - » Bicondylar (includes tibial plateau NOS)
  - Tibial spine
  - Torus
  - Tuberosity
  - Other specified site
  - Unspecified site upper end
- Tibial shaft
  - Comminuted
  - Oblique
  - Segmental
  - Spiral
  - Transverse
  - Other specified site
  - Unspecified
- Fibular shaft
  - Comminuted
  - Oblique
  - Segmental
  - Spiral
  - Transverse
  - Other
  - Unspecified

Identify fracture status:

- Displaced
- Nondisplaced

Identify laterality:

- Right
- Left
- Unspecified

Identify as closed/open:

- Closed
- Open Gustilo classification
  - Type I or II, or open NOS
  - Type IIIA, IIIB, or IIIC

Identify episode of care:

- Initial
- Subsequent with
  - Delayed healing
  - Malunion
  - Nonunion
  - Routine healing
- Sequela

Fractures of the upper end or shaft of the tibia and fibula require 7th characters which should be assigned as follows:

A Initial encounter for closed fracture

B Initial encounter for open fracture type I or II, or open fracture NOS

C Initial encounter for open fracture type IIIA, IIIB, or IIIC

D Subsequent encounter for closed fracture with routine healing

E Subsequent encounter for open fracture type I or II with routine healing

F Subsequent encounter for open fracture type IIIA, IIIB, or IIIC with routine healing

G Subsequent encounter for closed fracture with delayed healing

H Subsequent encounter for open fracture type I or II with delayed healing

J Subsequent encounter for open fracture type IIIA, IIIB, or IIIC with delayed healing

K Subsequent encounter for closed fracture with nonunion

M Subsequent encounter for open fracture type I or II with nonunion

N Subsequent encounter for open fracture type IIIA, IIIB, or IIIC with nonunion

P Subsequent encounter for closed fracture with malunion

Q Subsequent encounter for open fracture type I or II with malunion

R Subsequent encounter for open fracture type IIIA, IIIB, or IIIC with malunion

S Sequela

Note: Torus fractures are closed fractures by definition and valid 7th characters include only: A, D, G, K, P, or S.

Fracture of Upper End of Tibia/Fibula

ICD-10-CM Code/Documentation	
Unspecified Fracture	
S82.101-	Unspecified fracture of upper end of right tibia
S82.102-	Unspecified fracture of upper end of left tibia
S82.109-	Unspecified fracture of upper end of unspecified tibia
Tibial Spine Fracture	
S82.111-	Displaced fracture of right tibial spine
S82.112-	Displaced fracture of left tibial spine
S82.113-	Displaced fracture of unspecified tibial spine
S82.114-	Nondisplaced fracture of right tibial spine
S82.115-	Nondisplaced fracture of left tibial spine
S82.116-	Nondisplaced fracture of unspecified tibial spine
Condylar Fracture	
Lateral Condyle Fracture	
S82.121-	Displaced fracture of lateral condyle of right tibia
S82.122-	Displaced fracture of lateral condyle of left tibia
S82.123-	Displaced fracture of lateral condyle of unspecified tibia
S82.124-	Nondisplaced fracture of lateral condyle of right tibia
S82.125-	Nondisplaced fracture of lateral condyle of left tibia
S82.126-	Nondisplaced fracture of lateral condyle of unspecified tibia

Medial Condyle Fracture	
S82.131-	Displaced fracture of medial condyle of right tibia
S82.132-	Displaced fracture of medial condyle of left tibia
S82.133-	Displaced fracture of medial condyle of unspecified tibia
S82.134-	Nondisplaced fracture of medial condyle of right tibia
S82.135-	Nondisplaced fracture of medial condyle of left tibia
S82.136-	Nondisplaced fracture of medial condyle of unspecified tibia
Bicondylar Fracture	
S82.141-	Displaced bicondylar fracture of right tibia
S82.142-	Displaced bicondylar fracture of left tibia
S82.143-	Displaced bicondylar fracture of unspecified tibia
S82.144-	Nondisplaced bicondylar fracture of right tibia
S82.145-	Nondisplaced bicondylar fracture of left tibia
S82.146-	Nondisplaced bicondylar fracture of unspecified tibia
Tibial Tuberosity Fracture	
S82.151-	Displaced fracture of right tibial tuberosity
S82.152-	Displaced fracture of left tibial tuberosity
S82.153-	Displaced fracture of unspecified tibial tuberosity
S82.154-	Nondisplaced fracture of right tibial tuberosity
S82.155-	Nondisplaced fracture of left tibial tuberosity
S82.156-	Nondisplaced fracture of unspecified tibial tuberosity
Other Fracture	
S82.191-	Other fracture upper end of right tibia
S82.192-	Other fracture upper end of left tibia
S82.199-	Other fracture upper end of unspecified tibia
Torus	
S82.161-	Torus fracture upper end of right tibia
S82.162-	Torus fracture upper end of left tibia
S82.169-	Torus fracture upper end of unspecified tibia
S82.811-	Torus fracture upper end of right fibula
S82.812-	Torus fracture upper end of left fibula
S82.819-	Torus fracture upper end of unspecified fibula
Note: There are no combined codes for fracture of the upper end of the fibula with tibia.	

Fracture of Shaft of Tibia/Fibula

ICD-10-CM Code/Documentation	
Unspecified Fracture	
S82.201-	Unspecified fracture of shaft of right tibia
S82.202-	Unspecified fracture of shaft of left tibia
S82.209-	Unspecified fracture of shaft of unspecified tibia
S82.401-	Unspecified fracture shaft of right fibula
S82.402-	Unspecified fracture shaft of left fibula
S82.409-	Unspecified fracture shaft of unspecified fibula
Transverse Fracture	
S82.221-	Displaced transverse fracture of shaft of right tibia
S82.222-	Displaced transverse fracture of shaft of left tibia
S82.223-	Displaced transverse fracture of shaft of unspecified tibia
S82.224-	Nondisplaced transverse fracture of shaft of right tibia
S82.225-	Nondisplaced transverse fracture of shaft of left tibia
S82.226-	Nondisplaced transverse fracture of shaft of unspecified tibia
S82.421-	Displaced transverse fracture of shaft of right fibula
S82.422-	Displaced transverse fracture of shaft of left fibula
S82.423-	Displaced transverse fracture of shaft of unspecified fibula
S82.424-	Nondisplaced transverse fracture of shaft of right fibula
S82.425-	Nondisplaced transverse fracture of shaft of left fibula
S82.426-	Nondisplaced transverse fracture of shaft of unspecified fibula
Oblique Fracture	
S82.231-	Displaced oblique fracture of shaft of right tibia
S82.232-	Displaced oblique fracture of shaft of left tibia
S82.233-	Displaced oblique fracture of shaft of unspecified tibia
S82.234-	Nondisplaced oblique fracture of shaft of right tibia
S82.235-	Nondisplaced oblique fracture of shaft of left tibia
S82.236-	Nondisplaced oblique fracture of shaft of unspecified tibia
S82.431-	Displaced oblique fracture of shaft of right fibula
S82.432-	Displaced oblique fracture of shaft of left fibula
S82.433-	Displaced oblique fracture of shaft of unspecified fibula
S82.434-	Nondisplaced oblique fracture of shaft of right fibula
S82.435-	Nondisplaced oblique fracture of shaft of left fibula
S82.436-	Nondisplaced oblique fracture of shaft of unspecified fibula
Spiral Fracture	
S82.241-	Displaced spiral fracture of shaft of right tibia
S82.242-	Displaced spiral fracture of shaft of left tibia
S82.243-	Displaced spiral fracture of shaft of unspecified tibia
S82.244-	Nondisplaced spiral fracture of shaft of right tibia
S82.245-	Nondisplaced spiral fracture of shaft of left tibia
S82.246-	Nondisplaced spiral fracture of shaft of unspecified tibia
S82.441-	Displaced spiral fracture of shaft of right fibula
S82.442-	Displaced spiral fracture of shaft of left fibula
S82.443-	Displaced spiral fracture of shaft of unspecified fibula
S82.444-	Nondisplaced spiral fracture of shaft of right fibula
S82.445-	Nondisplaced spiral fracture of shaft of left fibula
S82.446-	Nondisplaced spiral fracture of shaft of unspecified fibula
Comminuted Fracture	
S82.251-	Displaced comminuted fracture of shaft of right tibia
S82.252-	Displaced comminuted fracture of shaft of left tibia
S82.253-	Displaced comminuted fracture of shaft of unspecified tibia

ICD-10-CM Code/Documentation	
S82.254-	Nondisplaced comminuted fracture of shaft of right tibia
S82.255-	Nondisplaced comminuted fracture of shaft of left tibia
S82.256-	Nondisplaced comminuted fracture of shaft of unspecified tibia
S82.451-	Displaced comminuted fracture of shaft of right fibula
S82.452-	Displaced comminuted fracture of shaft of left fibula
S82.453-	Displaced comminuted fracture of shaft of unspecified fibula
S82.454-	Nondisplaced comminuted fracture of shaft of right fibula
S82.455-	Nondisplaced comminuted fracture of shaft of left fibula
S82.456-	Nondisplaced comminuted fracture of shaft of unspecified fibula
Segmental Fracture	
S82.261-	Displaced segmental fracture of shaft of right tibia
S82.262-	Displaced segmental fracture of shaft of left tibia
S82.263-	Displaced segmental fracture of shaft of unspecified tibia
S82.264-	Nondisplaced segmental fracture of shaft of right tibia
S82.265-	Nondisplaced segmental fracture of shaft of left tibia
S82.266-	Nondisplaced segmental fracture of shaft of unspecified tibia
S82.461-	Displaced segmental fracture of shaft of right fibula
S82.462-	Displaced segmental fracture of shaft of left fibula
S82.463-	Displaced segmental fracture of shaft of unspecified fibula
S82.464-	Nondisplaced segmental fracture of shaft of right fibula
S82.465-	Nondisplaced segmental fracture of shaft of left fibula
S82.466-	Nondisplaced segmental fracture of shaft of unspecified fibula
Other Fracture	
S82.291-	Other fracture of shaft of right tibia
S82.292-	Other fracture of shaft of left tibia
S82.299-	Other fracture of shaft of unspecified tibia
S82.491-	Other fracture of shaft of right fibula
S82.492-	Other fracture of shaft of left fibula
S82.499-	Other fracture of shaft of unspecified fibula
Note: There are no combined codes for fracture of shaft of fibula with tibia. Two codes, one from subcategory S82.2- Fracture of shaft of tibia, and one from subcategory S82.4- Fracture of shaft of fibula, are required to capture fractures of the fibula with the tibia.	

Documentation and Coding Example

Eight-year-old female brought to Urgent Care by her father after she attempted to do a flip on a **trampoline** at a **friend's house (single family home)**, but **flipped off the trampoline, landing primarily on her right leg on the grass**. She refuses to bear weight on her right leg. On examination, the right leg is bent at the knee and patient cries and becomes extremely agitated when any attempt is made to straighten or touch it. **Skin is intact** with mild swelling noted at the mid-shaft area with tenderness from knee to ankle. It is difficult to assess point tenderness because she reacts so dramatically to touch or manipulation. AP and lateral x-rays are obtained of the right lower extremity, including knee, ankle, and foot. The films show a **nondisplaced distal spiral fracture of the right tibial shaft with a displaced oblique fracture of the right fibular shaft**. Call placed to on-call pediatric orthopedist who orders splinting of the leg and medicating with Demerol 25 mg IM. He will alert ED at Children's Hospital to expect them. Medication administered, leg splinted. Mother has arrived. Parents sign patient out of Urgent Care and are given copy of x-rays. Parents are transporting to Children's by private car.

Diagnosis Code(s)

S82.244A	Nondisplaced spiral fracture of shaft of right tibia, initial encounter for closed fracture
S82.431A	Displaced oblique fracture of shaft of right fibula, initial encounter for closed fracture
W09.8XXA	Fall on or from other playground equipment
Y92.017	Garden or yard in single-family (private) house as the place of occurrence of the external cause
Y93.44	Activity, trampolining
Y99.8	Other external cause status

Coding Note(s)

Tibia and fibula fracture codes are able to capture the type of fracture for each bone. In this case, the patient has a nondisplaced spiral fracture of the right tibia with a displaced oblique fracture of the right fibula.

Physeal Fracture

Physeal fractures may also be referred to as Salter-Harris fractures or traumatic epiphyseal separations. These fractures occur along the epiphyseal (growth) plates in bones that have not reached their full growth and in which the plates are still open or partially open and filled with cartilaginous tissue.

Physeal fractures in children and adolescents with an open epiphyseal plate are differentiated from epiphyseal fractures or separation of the epiphysis in adults. For example, fracture of the lower epiphysis of the femur in an adult is reported with codes from subcategory S72.44, while Salter-Harris physeal fractures in children and adolescents of the same site are reported with codes from subcategory S79.1. Physeal fractures are listed in the alphabetic index under the main term 'fracture' and then by site under the term 'physeal'. Codes for physeal fractures are found in the following categories S49, S59, S79, S89 and S99. Refer to the section on fracture classifications for details on the Salter-Harris classification.

Coding and Documentation Requirements

Identify bone:

- Calcaneus
- Femur
- Fibula
- Humerus
- Metatarsal
- Phalanx (toe)
- Radius
- Tibia
- Ulna

Identify site (long bones excluding metatarsal and phalanx):

- Lower end physeal fracture
- Upper end physeal fracture

Identify Salter-Harris classification:

- Salter-Harris Type I
- Salter-Harris Type II
- Salter-Harris Type III
- Salter-Harris Type IV
- Other physeal fracture
- Unspecified physeal fracture

Identify laterality:

- Right
- Left
- Unspecified

Identify episode of care:

- Initial
- Subsequent with
  - Delayed healing
  - Malunion
  - Nonunion
  - Routine healing
- Sequela

Physeal Fracture Lower End of Humerus

ICD-10-CM Code/Documentation	
Unspecified Physeal Fracture	
S49.101-	Unspecified physeal fracture of lower end of humerus, right arm
S49.102-	Unspecified physeal fracture of lower end of humerus, left arm
S49.109-	Unspecified physeal fracture of lower end of humerus, unspecified arm
Salter-Harris Type I	
S49.111-	Salter-Harris Type I physeal fracture of lower end of humerus, right arm
S49.112-	Salter-Harris Type I physeal fracture of lower end of humerus, left arm
S49.119-	Salter-Harris Type I physeal fracture of lower end of humerus, unspecified arm
Salter-Harris Type II	
S49.121-	Salter-Harris Type II physeal fracture of lower end of humerus, right arm
S49.122-	Salter-Harris Type II physeal fracture of lower end of humerus, left arm
S49.129-	Salter-Harris Type II physeal fracture of lower end of humerus, unspecified arm
Salter-Harris Type III	
S49.131-	Salter-Harris Type III physeal fracture of lower end of humerus, right arm
S49.132-	Salter-Harris Type III physeal fracture of lower end of humerus, left arm
S49.139-	Salter-Harris Type III physeal fracture of lower end of humerus, unspecified arm
Salter-Harris type IV	
S49.141-	Salter-Harris Type IV physeal fracture of lower end of humerus, right arm
S49.142-	Salter-Harris Type IV physeal fracture of lower end of humerus, left arm
S49.149-	Salter-Harris Type IV physeal fracture of lower end of humerus, unspecified arm
Other Physeal Fracture	
S49.191-	Other physeal fracture of lower end of humerus, right arm
S49.192-	Other physeal fracture of lower end of humerus, left arm
S49.199-	Other physeal fracture of lower end of humerus, unspecified arm

Documentation and Coding Example

ED Note: Seven-year-old male presents to ED accompanied by mother. He was **skateboarding at the local park when the patient fell** onto his **left arm**. He c/o pain in the elbow that intensifies with movement. An off duty EMT examined him at the scene and recommended he be taken to the ED. On examination, this is a healthy appearing young boy who holds his left arm against his body with elbow bent. Color is pale, slightly diaphoretic. He is able to wiggle fingers, slightly move wrist and sensation is intact throughout the extremity. Capillary refill time WNL. Point tenderness is most pronounced along the lateral aspect just above the elbow. There is a small area of ecchymosis, mild swelling, and some displacement of the posterior fat pad at the distal end of the humerus. There is difficulty obtaining x-rays due to pain with manipulation of arm. IV started in right arm, blood drawn for CBC, electrolytes. O2 saturation 96% on RA. NSR on monitor. Medicated with MS 0.5 mg IVP. Films obtained of the elbow joint including views of the humerus, ulna, radius reveal a closed, **displaced lateral condylar fracture of the humerus extending through the growth plate and metaphysis**. Findings are consistent with a **Salter-Harris Type II fracture**. It is difficult to determine how stable the bone fragment is on x-ray and an US is obtained. The fragment appears to be quite unstable on US and decision is made to reduce the fracture in the OR.

Diagnosis Code(s)

S49.122A	Salter-Harris Type II physeal fracture of lower end of humerus, left arm, initial encounter for closed fracture
V00.131A	Fall from skateboard, initial encounter
Y92.830	Public park as place of occurrence of the external cause
Y93.51	Activity, roller skating (inline) and skateboarding
Y99.8	Other external cause status

Coding Note(s)

The code for the Salter-Harris fracture is specific to site (lower end of the humerus), type (Type II) and laterality (left side). This has also been documented as a closed fracture and it is the initial episode of care so 7th character 'A' is appended.

Injury to Blood Vessels

Codes are specific to site and also broad categories of injury including laceration (major or minor), other specified type of injury, and unspecified type of injury.

Coding and Documentation Requirements

Identify site and blood vessel:

- Neck
  - Carotid artery
  - External jugular vein
  - Internal jugular vein
  - Vertebral artery
  - Other specified blood vessel at neck level
  - Unspecified blood vessel at neck level
- Thorax
  - Innominate/subclavian
    - » Artery
    - » Vein
  - Intercostal blood vessels
  - Pulmonary blood vessels
  - Superior vena cava
  - Thoracic aorta
  - Other specified blood vessel of thorax
  - Unspecified blood vessel of thorax
- Abdomen/lower back/pelvis
  - Abdominal aorta
  - Celiac/mesenteric arteries/branches
    - » Celiac artery
    - » Inferior mesenteric artery
    - » Superior mesenteric artery
    - » Branches celiac/mesenteric artery including:
      - ◦ Gastric artery
      - ◦ Gastroduodenal artery
      - ◦ Hepatic artery
      - ◦ Splenic artery
  - Inferior vena cava (includes hepatic vein)
  - Portal/splenic vein/branches
    - » Portal vein
    - » Splenic vein
    - » Inferior mesenteric vein
    - » Superior mesenteric vein
  - Renal blood vessels
    - » Renal artery
    - » Right vein
  - Iliac blood vessels
    - » Iliac artery (includes hypogastric artery)
    - » Iliac vein (includes hypogastric vein)
    - » Uterine artery
    - » Uterine vein
    - » Other iliac blood vessel
    - » Unspecified iliac blood vessel
      - ◦ Other specified blood vessels at abdomen/lower back/pelvis level
      - ◦ Unspecified blood vessel at abdomen/lower back/pelvis level
- Shoulder/upper arm
  - Axillary artery
  - Brachial artery
  - Axillary/brachial vein
  - Superficial vein
  - Other specified blood vessels at shoulder/upper arm level
  - Unspecified blood vessel at shoulder/upper arm level
- Forearm
  - Radial artery at forearm level
  - Ulnar artery at forearm level
  - Vein at forearm level
  - Other blood vessels at forearm level
  - Unspecified blood vessel at forearm level
- Wrist/Hand
  - Radial artery at wrist/hand level
  - Ulnar artery at wrist/hand level
  - Palmar arch
    - » Superficial
    - » Deep
  - Thumb blood vessel
  - Finger blood vessel
    - » Index
    - » Middle
    - » Ring
    - » Little
  - Other blood vessels at wrist/hand level
  - Unspecified blood vessel at wrist/hand level
- Hip/thigh
  - Femoral artery at hip/thigh level
  - Femoral vein at hip/thigh level
  - Greater saphenous vein at hip/thigh level
  - Other specified blood vessels at hip/thigh level
  - Unspecified blood vessel at hip/thigh level
- Lower leg
  - Popliteal artery
  - Tibial artery
    - » Anterior tibial artery
    - » Posterior tibial artery
    - » Unspecified tibial artery
  - Peroneal artery
  - Saphenous vein
    - » Greater saphenous vein at hip/thigh level
    - » Lesser saphenous vein
  - Popliteal vein
  - Other specified blood vessels at lower leg level
  - Unspecified blood vessel at lower leg level

- Ankle/foot level
  - Dorsal artery
  - Plantar artery
  - Dorsal vein
  - Other blood vessels at ankle/foot level
  - Unspecified blood vessel at ankle/foot level

Identify injury type:

- Laceration
  - Minor which includes
    - » Incomplete transection
    - » Superficial laceration
    - » Laceration NOS
  - Major which includes
    - » Complete transection
    - » Traumatic rupture
- Other specified injury to blood vessel which includes
  - Traumatic fistula
  - Traumatic aneurysm
- Unspecified injury to blood vessel

Note: For lacerations, code also any open wound.

Identify laterality, as applicable:

- Right
- Left
- Unspecified

Identify episode of care:

- Initial encounter
- Subsequent encounter
- Sequela

Injury to Radial Artery

ICD-10-CM Code/Documentation	
Radial artery injury at forearm level	
S55.101-	Unspecified injury of radial artery at forearm level, right arm
S55.102-	Unspecified injury of radial artery at forearm level, left arm
S55.109-	Unspecified injury of radial artery at forearm level, unspecified arm
S55.111-	Laceration of radial artery at forearm level, right arm
S55.112-	Laceration of radial artery at forearm level, left arm
S55.119-	Laceration of radial artery at forearm level, unspecified arm
S55.191-	Other specified injury of radial artery at forearm level, right arm
S55.192-	Other specified injury of radial artery at forearm level, left arm
S55.199-	Other specified injury of radial artery at forearm level, unspecified arm
Radial artery injury at wrist and hand level	
S65.101-	Unspecified injury of radial artery at wrist and hand level of right arm
S65.102-	Unspecified injury of radial artery at wrist and hand level of left arm
S65.109-	Unspecified injury of radial artery at wrist and hand level of unspecified arm
S65.111-	Laceration of radial artery at wrist and hand level of right arm
S65.112-	Laceration of radial artery at wrist and hand level of left arm
S65.119-	Laceration of radial artery at wrist and hand level of unspecified arm
S65.191-	Other specified injury of radial artery at wrist and hand level of right arm
S65.192-	Other specified injury of radial artery at wrist and hand level of left arm
S65.199-	Other specified injury of radial artery at wrist and hand level of unspecified arm

Documentation and Coding Example

Thirty-five-year-old female presents to ED with a laceration to her right hand. Patient states she was **washing dishes** at home and failed to notice a **broken wine glass** in the water. She states blood was "spurting" from the wound so she wrapped her hand in a dishcloth and has applied direct pressure during the 15-minute ride to the hospital. Cloth is carefully removed to reveal a jagged laceration **4 cm long extending from the base of the thumb to the center of the palm. It is 1-2 cm deep**. The wound actively oozes bright red blood when pressure is removed. Negative modified Allen test suggests the palmer arch is intact. Pulse oximetry of each digit also reveals good blood flow throughout hand and fingers. She has full ROM, good capillary refill, and intact sensation to all digits. Patient denies significant health problems and believes her last tetanus shot was 6 or 7 years ago. The wound is infiltrated with Marcaine, copiously irrigated with sterile saline, and re-examined. There appears to be a **complete transection** of the **radial artery**, the ends can be approximated without excessive tension. Hand surgeon is in house and willing to perform the repair. Patient and her husband are in agreement.

Consult Note: Called to ED to treat patient with **right hand laceration complicated by transected radial artery**. With a portable operating microscope, the ends of the artery are easily identified and anastomosed using 6-0 chromic suture with pulsation noted distally following the repair. The wound is then closed in layers with a 3-0 Monocryl interrupted suture and skin closed with a half-buried mattress/subcuticular running stitch. Sterile dressing applied. Patient is instructed in wound care, signs and symptoms of infection, and will follow up in 7 days for a wound check.

Diagnosis Code(s)

S65.111A	Laceration of radial artery at wrist and hand level of right arm, initial encounter
S61.411A	Laceration without foreign body of right hand, initial encounter
W25.XXXA	Contact with sharp glass, initial encounter
Y92.000	Kitchen of unspecified non-institutional (private) residence as the place of occurrence of the external cause
Y93.G1	Activity, food preparation and clean up
Y99.8	Other external cause status

Coding Note(s)

In order to assign a code for an injury to the radial artery, the level of the injury must be specified as forearm level or wrist/hand level. To assign the most specific code for place of occurrence in a home or residence, the residence must be more specifically identified as to the type of residence: a single family, non-institutional private house, mobile home, apartment, or boarding house. When the place of occurrence of the external cause is specified only as "home" a code from subcategory Y92.00, Unspecified non-institutional (private) residence, is reported.

Internal Injury of the Thorax

Internal injuries with open wounds require a minimum of two codes—one for the internal injury and a second one describing the open wound. Open wounds of the thoracic region are specific to the front or back wall, laterality, whether or not the wound has penetrated the thoracic cavity, the type of wound (laceration, puncture, deep bite, or other wound), and episode of care. Each additional injury to internal organs, blood vessels, nerves, ribs, spine and/or spinal cord is reported separately.

Coding and Documentation Requirements

Open Wound of Thorax

Identify general region of open wound of thorax:

- Front wall of thorax
  - Right front wall
  - Left front wall
  - Unspecified side
  - Unspecified part of thorax
- Back wall of thorax
  - Right back wall
  - Left back wall
  - Unspecified side

Identify presence or absence of penetration:

- Without penetration into thoracic cavity
- With penetration into thoracic cavity

Identify type of wound:

- Laceration
  - Without foreign body
  - With foreign body
- Puncture
  - Without foreign body
  - With foreign body
- Bite
- Unspecified open wound

Identify episode of care:

- Initial encounter
- Subsequent encounter
- Sequela

Identify any associated injury and report with additional codes as needed:

- Heart
- Other intrathoracic organs
- Intrathoracic blood vessels
- Rib fracture
- Spinal cord injury
- Traumatic hemothorax
- Traumatic hemopneumothorax
- Traumatic pneumothorax

Identify any related wound infection

Injury to Heart

- Identify presence or absence of hemopericardium
  - Without hemopericardium
  - With hemopericardium
  - Unspecified

Identify type of injury:

- Contusion
- Laceration
  - Mild (without penetration of heart chamber)
  - Moderate (with penetration of a single heart chamber)
  - Major (with penetration of multiple heart chambers)
- Other specified injury
- Unspecified injury

Identify any associated injuries:

- Open wound of thorax
- Hemopneumothorax
- Hemothorax
- Pneumothorax

Identify episode of care:

- Initial encounter
- Subsequent encounter
- Sequela

Injury to Lung, Bronchus, and/or Thoracic Trachea

Identify site:

- Lung
- Bronchus
- Thoracic trachea

Identify type of injury:

- Contusion
- Laceration
- Primary blast injury
- Other specified injury
- Unspecified injury

Identify laterality:

- Unilateral
- Bilateral
- Unspecified
- Note: Not applicable to thoracic trachea

Identify episode of care:

- Initial encounter
- Subsequent encounter

- Sequela
- Note code also any associated open wound of thorax

Injury to Pleura, Esophagus, Diaphragm, and Other or Unspecified Intrathoracic Organs

Identify site:

- Pleura
- Esophagus
- Diaphragm
- Other specified intrathoracic organ which includes
  - Lymphatic thoracic duct
  - Thymus gland
- Unspecified intrathoracic organ

Identify type of injury:

- Contusion (not applicable to pleura)
- Laceration
- Other specified injury
- Unspecified injury

Identify episode of care:

- Initial encounter
- Subsequent encounter
- Sequela

Injury to Intrathoracic Blood Vessels

Identify site:

- Artery
  - Thoracic aorta
  - Innominate or subclavian artery
- Vein
  - Superior vena cava
  - Innominate or subclavian vein
- Pulmonary blood vessels
- Other blood vessels
  - Intercostal
  - Other blood vessels which include
    - » Azygos vein
    - » Mammary artery/vein
    - » Other specified blood vessel
- Unspecified blood vessel

Identify injury:

- Laceration
  - Minor – Incomplete transection
  - Major – Complete transection
- Other specified injury
- Unspecified injury

Identify laterality:

- Right
- Left
- Unspecified

Note: Not applicable to thoracic aorta or superior vena cava

Identify episode of care:

- Initial encounter
- Subsequent encounter
- Sequela
- Note: Code also any associated open wound (S21.-)

Rib Fractures

Identify number of ribs:

- One
- Multiple
- Identify status:
- Closed
- Open

Identify laterality:

- Right
- Left
- Unspecified

Identify episode of care:

- Initial encounter
- Subsequent encounter
  - Delayed healing
  - Nonunion
  - Routine healing
- Sequela

Fracture of Sternum

Identify location

- Body
- Manubrium
- Sternal manibural dissociation
- Xiphoid process

Identify status:

- Closed
- Open

Identify episode of care:

- Initial encounter
- Subsequent encounter
  - Delayed healing
  - Nonunion
  - Routine healing
- Sequela

Note: Code also any documented associated injury of intrathoracic organ.

Injury to Thoracic Spinal Cord

Identify type of injury:

- Concussion and edema

19. Injury/Poisoning of External Causes

- Complete lesion
- Incomplete lesion
  - Anterior cord syndrome
  - Brown-Séquard syndrome
  - Other incomplete lesion
- Unspecified lesion

Identify level:

- T1
- T2-T6
- T7-T10
- T11-T12
- Unspecified level

Identify episode of care:

- Initial encounter
- Subsequent encounter
- Sequela

Note: Code also any documented associated fracture of thoracic vertebrae, open wound of thorax, transient paralysis.

Open Wound of Thorax with Lung Injury

ICD-10-CM Code/Documentation	
Open Wound of Thorax	
For the open wound of the thorax, use one of the following subcategories with applicable 5th, 6th, and 7th characters to capture type of injury, laterality, and episode of care:	
S21.1-	Open wound of front wall of thorax without penetration into thoracic cavity
S21.2-	Open wound of back wall of thorax without penetration into thoracic cavity
S21.3-	Open wound of front wall of thorax with penetration into thoracic cavity
S21.4-	Open wound of back wall of thorax with penetration into thoracic cavity
S21.9-	Open wound of unspecified part of thorax
-WITH-	
Injury of Lung	
For lung injury, use one of the following codes with applicable 7th character for episode of care:	
S27.301-	Unspecified injury of lung, unilateral
S27.302-	Unspecified injury of lung, bilateral
S27.309-	Unspecified injury of lung, unspecified
S27.311-	Primary blast injury of lung, unilateral
S27.312-	Primary blast injury of lung, bilateral
S27.319-	Primary blast injury of lung, unspecified
S27.321-	Contusion of lung, unilateral
S27.322-	Contusion of lung, bilateral
S27.329-	Contusion of lung, unspecified
S27.331-	Laceration of lung, unilateral
S27.332-	Laceration of lung, bilateral
S27.339-	Laceration of lung, unspecified
S27.391-	Other injuries of lung, unilateral
S27.392-	Other injuries of lung, bilateral
S27.399-	Other injuries of lung, unspecified

Documentation and Coding Example

Adolescent Hispanic male found by law enforcement after a reported **gang related altercation**. On scene, the victim was discovered to be bleeding profusely from a wound in his upper back. From the blood trail it appears he walked or ran approximately 50 yards before collapsing on the **sidewalk**. A **pocket knife** with a 3-inch blade found at the scene is believed to be the weapon used in the attack. EMS assessment reveals a conscious but uncooperative, moderately obese, young Hispanic male. There is a sucking wound in the right posterior thorax, bubbling air and profusely bleeding. Patient is pale, diaphoretic with cyanotic mucus membranes. Large bore IV placed in left antecubital, O2 at 4 L/m via mask, chest wound covered with Vaseline gauze. Transported to ED.

ER Trauma Note: Patient brought in by EMS **with penetrating posterior thorax trauma s/p stabbing**. There is a **single 2 cm wound in the right posterior thorax** at the 4-5 intercostal space, sterile digital exploration estimates it to be 5 cm deep. Jugular veins are distended. He is semi-conscious with weak, flaccid muscle tone. There is no air movement on the right. Patient intubated by anesthesia and hand ventilated. PA and lateral chest films are obtained and reveal a **right pneumohemothorax**. Right chest tube placed in mid axillary line, 4-5 intercostal space. Repeat chest x-ray shows partial re-expansion of right lung. Patient transferred to OR for exploration of wound and repair of lung and vascular damage.

OR Note: Arterial and CVP lines placed. Patient positioned on left side. The entry wound is entered using a visually assisted thoracoscope. There is a **1 cm laceration of the right lung causing the pneumothorax** and brisk bleeding from completely **transected intercostal artery and vein which is the probable cause for the hemothorax**. The scope is removed and an open thoracotomy performed at the site of the stab wound. The lung is oversewn to repair the air leak and the intercostal vein and artery are both repaired successfully with end to end anastomosis. Most of the accumulated hemothorax evacuated with suction. Chest tube patent to water seal. Wound closed in layers and sterile dressing applied. Patient taken to ICU in critical condition.

Diagnosis Code(s)

S27.331A	Laceration of lung, unilateral, initial encounter
S21.431A	Puncture wound without foreign body of right back wall of thorax with penetration into thoracic cavity, initial encounter
S25.511A	Laceration of intercostal blood vessels, right side, initial encounter
S27.2XXA	Traumatic hemopneumothorax, initial encounter
X99.1XXA	Assault by knife, initial encounter
Y92.480	Sidewalk as the place of occurrence of the external cause

Coding Note(s)

In ICD-10-CM, traumatic transection of a blood vessel is coded as a laceration. External cause codes related to activity (Y93) and external cause status (Y99) are not applicable to this scenario.

Internal Injury of Abdomen

Injuries to the intra-abdominal organs (S36) are clearly differentiated from injuries to the urinary and pelvic organs (S37). As with internal injuries to the thorax, an additional code is required when there is an associated open wound of the abdomen, lower back, or pelvis (S31) and codes are specific as to whether the wound has or has not penetrated the peritoneum or retroperitoneum.

Coding and Documentation Requirements

Open Wound of Abdominal Wall

Identify general region of open wound of abdominal wall:

- Right upper quadrant
- Left upper quadrant
- Epigastric region
- Right lower quadrant
- Left lower quadrant
- Periumbilic region
- Unspecified quadrant

Identify presence or absence of penetration:

- Without penetration into peritoneal cavity
- With penetration into peritoneal cavity

Identify type of wound:

- Laceration
  - Without foreign body
  - With foreign body
- Puncture
  - Without foreign body
  - With foreign body
- Bite
- Unspecified open wound

Identify episode of care:

- Initial encounter
- Subsequent encounter
- Sequela

Identify any associated injury to intra-abdominal organs and report with additional codes as needed:

- Spleen
- Liver
- Gallbladder/Bile duct
- Pancreas
- Stomach
- Intestine
- Colon
- Rectum
- Peritoneum
- Other intra-abdominal organs
- Unspecified intra-abdominal organs

Injury of Spleen

Identify type of injury:

- Contusion
  - Minor (less than 2 cm)
  - Major (greater than 2 cm)
  - Unspecified
- Laceration
  - Superficial, which includes:
    - » Less than 1 cm
    - » Capsular
    - » Minor
  - Moderate (1-3 cm)
  - Major, which includes:
    - » Greater than 3 cm
    - » Avulsion of spleen
    - » Massive laceration
    - » Multiple moderate lacerations
    - » Stellate laceration
- Other injury
- Unspecified injury

Identify episode of care:

- Initial encounter
- Subsequent encounter
- Sequela

Injury of Liver

Identify injury:

- Contusion
- Laceration
  - Minor which includes
    - » Less than 1 cm deep
    - » Capsule only
    - » Without significant involvement of hepatic parenchyma
  - Moderate, which includes:
    - » Less than 10 cm long and less than 3 cm deep
    - » Parenchymal involvement but without major disruption of parenchyma
  - Major, which includes:
    - » Greater than 10 cm long and 3 cm deep
    - » Multiple moderate lacerations
    - » Stellate laceration
- Other injury
- Unspecified injury

Identify episode of care:

- Initial encounter
- Subsequent encounter
- Sequela

Injury of Gallbladder/Bile Duct

Identify site:

- Gallbladder
- Bile duct

For gallbladder, identify type of injury:

- Contusion
- Laceration
- Other injury
- Unspecified injury

Identify episode of care:

- Initial encounter
- Subsequent encounter
- Sequela

Injury of Pancreas

Identify injury:

- Contusion
- Laceration
  - Minor
  - Moderate
  - Major
  - Unspecified
- Other specified injury
- Unspecified

Identify region of pancreas:

- Head
- Body
- Tail
- Unspecified site

Identify episode of care:

- Initial encounter
- Subsequent encounter
- Sequela

Injury of Stomach

Identify injury type:

- Contusion
- Laceration
- Other specified injury
- Unspecified injury

Identify episode of care:

- Initial encounter
- Subsequent encounter
- Sequela

Injury of Small Intestine

Identify injury type:

- Contusion
- Laceration
- Primary blast injury
- Other specified injury
- Unspecified injury

Identify part of small intestine:

- Duodenum
- Other specified part of small intestine
- Unspecified part of small intestine

Identify episode of care:

- Initial encounter
- Subsequent encounter
- Sequela

Injury of Colon

Identify injury type:

- Contusion
- Laceration
- Primary blast injury
- Other specified injury
- Unspecified injury

Identify part of colon:

- Ascending [right] colon
- Descending [left] colon
- Sigmoid colon
- Transverse colon
- Other part of colon
- Unspecified part of colon

Identify episode of care:

- Initial encounter
- Subsequent encounter
- Sequela

Injury of Rectum

Identify injury type:

- Contusion
- Laceration
- Primary blast injury
- Other specified injury
- Unspecified injury

Identify episode of care:

- Initial encounter
- Subsequent encounter
- Sequela

Injury to Peritoneum/Other or Unspecified Intra-abdominal Organs

Identify site:

- Peritoneum
- Other specified intra-abdominal organs
- Unspecified intra-abdominal organs

For other or unspecified intra-abdominal organs, identify injury type:

- Contusion
- Laceration
- Other specified injury
- Unspecified injury

Identify episode of care:

- Initial encounter
- Subsequent encounter
- Sequela
- Note: for all, code also any associated open wound

Open Wound Right Upper Quadrant with Moderate Laceration of Liver

ICD-10-CM Code/Documentation	
S36.115-	Moderate laceration of liver
-AND ONE of the FOLLOWING CODES-	
S31.600-	Unspecified open wound of abdominal wall, right upper quadrant with penetration into peritoneal cavity
S31.610-	Laceration without foreign body of abdominal wall, right upper quadrant with penetration into peritoneal cavity
S31.620-	Laceration with foreign body of abdominal wall, right upper quadrant with penetration into peritoneal cavity
S31.630-	Puncture wound without foreign body of abdominal wall, right upper quadrant with penetration into peritoneal cavity
S31.640-	Puncture wound with foreign body of abdominal wall, right upper quadrant with penetration into peritoneal cavity
S31.650-	Open bite of abdominal wall, right upper quadrant with penetration into peritoneal cavity

Documentation and Coding Example

Patient is a twenty-one-year-old male who walks into ED with a **stab wound to the abdomen**. He states he was attempting to mediate a dispute between two employees at his **family's restaurant** when the stabbing occurred. On examination, this is a soft spoken, slightly built young man holding a bloody towel to the right abdomen. He is alert and oriented. HR 100, RR 16, BP 98/60. There is a **single wound measuring 2 cm in the RUQ**, it is not actively bleeding at this time. He states the weapon used was a small paring knife with a blade not more than 3 inches long. Abdominal examination is relatively benign except for the wound and mild tenderness to palpation in RUQ. Breath sounds are clear, equal bilaterally. HR regular with NSR on monitor. IV started in right forearm, blood drawn for CBC, Chemistry Panel, PT, PTT, Type and hold. Flat plate of abdomen is negative for free air. FAST shows some accumulation of fluid in the RUQ along the edge of the liver. Patient is hemodynamically stable. Decision made to take him to CT for abdominal scan to r/o or establish intraperitoneal injury. Spiral CT with contrast revealed a **Grade 2 liver injury with a 1.5 cm parenchymal laceration and a 1.5 cm thick subcapsular/parenchymal hematoma**. Patient will be admitted to ICU for observation. Wound irrigated, closed in layers around a drain. He is started on broad spectrum antibiotics. NPO. Transferred to unit in stable condition.

ICU Note: Patient stable overnight. Repeat CT shows no change in hematoma size. Minimal serosanguinous fluid returning from drain, the wound edges are slightly red but suture line is clean. Abdominal soft with bowel sounds present in all quadrants. Pain is localized at the site of the wound and has been well controlled with IV Morphine. Started clear liquid diet and advance as tolerated. Up in a chair, advance activity as tolerated. He is transferred to surgical floor for continued observation.

Floor Note Day 1: Continues to make good recovery. Pain controlled on oral Vicodin. Tolerating soft diet, ambulates to BR. IV hep locked. Continues on antibiotics. Wound healing well, drain removed. Repeat CT ordered for tomorrow. If no change in hematoma size, he will be discharged.

Floor Note Day 2: Rcpeat CT shows subcapsular/parenchymal hematoma to be resolving, size is now 1 cm thick. He is discharged home with oral Vicodin and antibiotics. He will be seen in Surgical Clinic in 5 days for wound check.

Diagnosis Code(s)

S36.115A	Moderate laceration of liver, initial encounter
S31.630A	Puncture wound without foreign body of abdominal wall, right upper quadrant with penetration into peritoneal cavity, initial encounter
X99.1XXA	Assault by knife, initial encounter
Y92.511	Restaurant or café as the place of occurrence of the external cause
Y99.0	Civilian activity done for income or pay

Coding Note(s)

The American Association for the Surgery of Trauma (AAST) liver injury scale provides 6 grades to identify the severity of the liver injury. The 6 grades are as follows:

- Grade 1 – Subcapsular hematoma less than 1 cm in maximal thickness, capsular avulsion, superficial parenchymal laceration less than 1 cm deep, and isolated periportal blood tracking
- Grade 2 – Parenchymal laceration 1-3 cm deep and parenchymal/subcapsular hematomas 1-3 cm thick
- Grade 3 – Parenchymal laceration more than 3 cm deep and parenchymal or subcapsular hematoma more than 3 cm in diameter
- Grade 4 – Parenchymal/subcapsular hematoma more than 10 cm in diameter, lobar destruction, or devascularization
- Grade 5 – Global destruction or devascularization of the liver
- Grade 6 – Hepatic avulsion

In ICD-10-CM, a Grade 2 injury corresponds to a moderate laceration of the liver. An activity code cannot be assigned because the activity of the person injured is not documented.

Open Wound of Extremities

Codes for open wounds of the extremities are found in categories S41, S51, S61, S71, S81, S91. Codes for open wounds are specific as to site and type of injury. Additional codes are required to report any associated injuries such as laceration of nerves, major blood vessels, muscles, or tendons. An additional code is also required to report any wound infection.

Coding and Documentation Requirements

Identify site of open wound:

- Upper limb
  - Shoulder
  - Upper arm
  - Elbow
  - Forearm
  - Wrist
  - Hand
  - Digit
    - » Specify digit
      - Thumb
      - Index finger
      - Middle finger
      - Ring finger
      - Little finger
      - Unspecified finger
    - » Specify nail involvement
      - With damage to nail
      - Without damage to nail
- Lower limb
  - Hip
  - Thigh
  - Knee
  - Lower leg
  - Ankle
  - Foot not including toes
  - Great toe
    - » With damage to nail
    - » Without damage to nail
  - Lesser toes
    - » With damage to nail
    - » Without damage to nail
  - Unspecified toe
    - » With damage to nail
    - » Without damage to nail

Identify type of open wound:

- Bite (not described as superficial)
- Puncture wound
  - With foreign body
  - Without foreign body
- Laceration
  - With foreign body
  - Without foreign body
- Unspecified open wound

Identify laterality:

- Right
- Left
- Unspecified

Identify episode of care:

- Initial encounter
- Subsequent encounter
- Sequela

Identify any associated wound infection.

Use additional code for any associated injuries to nerves, major blood vessels, muscles, or tendons.

Open Wound with Tendon Involvement, Forearm

ICD-10-CM Code/Documentation	
Unspecified Open Wound	
S51.801-	Unspecified open wound of right forearm
S51.802-	Unspecified open wound of left forearm
S51.809-	Unspecified open wound of unspecified forearm
Laceration	
S51.811-	Laceration without foreign body of right forearm
S51.812-	Laceration without foreign body of left forearm
S51.819-	Laceration without foreign body of unspecified forearm
S51.821-	Laceration with foreign body of right forearm
S51.822-	Laceration with foreign body of left forearm
S51.829-	Laceration with foreign body of unspecified forearm
Puncture Wound	
S51.831-	Puncture wound without foreign body of right forearm
S51.832-	Puncture wound without foreign body of left forearm
S51.839-	Puncture wound without foreign body of unspecified forearm
S51.841-	Puncture wound with foreign body of right forearm
S51.842-	Puncture wound with foreign body of left forearm
S51.849-	Puncture wound with foreign body of unspecified forearm
Open Bite	
S51.851-	Open bite of right forearm
S51.852-	Open bite of left forearm
S51.859-	Open bite of unspecified forearm

ICD-1Ø-CM Code/Documentation	
-WITH- Injury to flexor/extensor muscle, fascia, tendon and type of injury, forearm	
-FLEXOR-	
Unspecified Injury	
S56.2Ø1-	Unspecified injury of other flexor muscle, fascia and tendon at forearm level, right arm
S56.2Ø2-	Unspecified injury of other flexor muscle, fascia and tendon at forearm level, left arm
S56.2Ø9-	Unspecified injury of other flexor muscle, fascia and tendon at forearm level, unspecified arm
Strain	
S56.211-	Strain of other flexor muscle, fascia and tendon at forearm level, right arm
S56.212-	Strain of other flexor muscle, fascia and tendon at forearm level, left arm
S56.219-	Strain of other flexor muscle, fascia and tendon at forearm level, unspecified arm
Laceration	
S56.221-	Laceration of other flexor muscle, fascia and tendon at forearm level, right arm
S56.222-	Laceration of other flexor muscle, fascia and tendon at forearm level, left arm
S56.229-	Laceration of other flexor muscle, fascia and tendon at forearm level, unspecified arm
Other Injury	
S56.291-	Other injury of other flexor muscle, fascia and tendon at forearm level, right arm
S56.292-	Other injury of other flexor muscle, fascia and tendon at forearm level, left arm
S56.299-	Other injury of other flexor muscle, fascia and tendon at forearm level, unspecified arm
-EXTENSOR-	
Unspecified Injury	
S56.5Ø1-	Unspecified injury of other extensor muscle, fascia and tendon at forearm level, right arm
S56.5Ø2-	Unspecified injury of other extensor muscle, fascia and tendon at forearm level, left arm
S56.5Ø9-	Unspecified injury of other extensor muscle, fascia and tendon at forearm level, unspecified arm
Strain	
S56.511-	Strain of other extensor muscle, fascia and tendon at forearm level, right arm
S56.512-	Strain of other extensor muscle, fascia and tendon at forearm level, left arm
S56.519-	Strain of other extensor muscle, fascia and tendon at forearm level, unspecified arm
Laceration	
S56.521-	Laceration of other extensor muscle, fascia and tendon at forearm level, right arm
S56.522-	Laceration of other extensor muscle, fascia and tendon at forearm level, left arm
S56.529-	Laceration of other extensor muscle, fascia and tendon at forearm level, unspecified arm
Other Injury	
S56.591-	Other injury of other extensor muscle, fascia and tendon at forearm level, right arm
S56.592-	Other injury of other extensor muscle, fascia and tendon at forearm level, left arm
S56.599-	Other injury of other extensor muscle, fascia and tendon at forearm level, unspecified arm

Note: The codes listed in this table for injury of a tendon in the forearm include only those for other flexor and other extensor muscles. There are additional codes for injuries to flexor and extensor tendons of the thumb and fingers at the forearm level.

Documentation and Coding Example

Patient is a four-year-old Caucasian male bought to ED by his parents after being **bitten by the family dog**. There were no adult witnesses to the attack but older children admit that they placed the boy on the dog's back so he could "ride" her, the dog yelped, turned, **biting him on the right arm**. Crying, but fairly cooperative young boy is examined while being held by his father. The **right forearm has a 4 cm long jagged wound consistent with a dog bite**. ROM, sensation, and circulation intact to fingers and hand. There is some difficulty with pronation and supination of the forearm suggestive of brachioradialis muscle or tendon injury. Wound infiltrated with 2% Lidocaine with epinephrine and child fell asleep soon afterward. Wound copiously irrigated with dilute betadine and NS. The **wound extends into and partially severs the brachioradialis tendon near insertion at the distal styloid process of the radius**. Radial nerve is identified and appears to be intact. There are no large vascular structures damaged. The tendon is repaired with 3-Ø Chromic followed by a 2-layer wound closure. Sterile dressing and soft short arm splint applied. Patient woke up at the end of the procedure, remains quiet and cooperative. He denies pain at this time. Parents are given a prescription for Tylenol with codeine, instructed to keep dressing and splint dry. Patient has a follow up appointment in surgical clinic in 5 days.

Diagnosis Code(s)

S51.851A	Open bite of right forearm, initial encounter
S56.221A	Laceration of other flexor muscle, fascia and tendon at forearm level, right arm, initial encounter
W54.ØXXA	Bitten by dog, initial encounter
Y92.ØØ9	Unspecified place in unspecified non-institutional (private) residence as the place of occurrence of the external cause
Y93.89	Activity, other specified
Y99.8	Other external cause status

Coding Note(s)

The brachioradialis muscle assists in elbow flexion along with pronation and supination of the forearm. The partial severing of the brachioradialis tendon is coded as a laceration to a flexor muscle/fascia/tendon of the forearm.

Poisoning by, Adverse Effect of and Underdosing of Drugs, Medicaments, and Biological Substances

Drugs, medicinal and biological substances or combinations of these substances sometimes cause adverse reactions. An adverse effect is as an unwanted, negative, or dangerous reaction to a drug that was correctly prescribed and properly administered. Poisoning is a toxic reaction that may cause temporary or permanent damage occurring with improper use of a drug of substance, such as the wrong prescription or wrong dose given or taken in error. It may also occur with a correctly prescribed drug taken in combination with a nonprescribed drug or alcohol. Poisoning from a wrong prescription includes the prescription of two or more drugs that should not be taken together or should not be taken together in the doses prescribed. Poisoning from the wrong dose of a drug may be the result of either an intentional or unintentional overdose of the drug. Poisoning may also result from the wrong route of administration. A toxic effect is also a poisoning from a substance that is nonmedicinal in nature such as alcohol poisoning, lead poisoning, or poisoning from heavy metals.

Underdosing refers to taking less of a medication than was prescribed by the provider or less than the amount recommended by the manufacturer. Discontinuing a prescribed medication on the patient's initiative and not at the provider's instruction is also considered underdosing. Underdosing is never a principal or first-listed diagnosis. If the patient is seen for a medical condition such as an exacerbation of the condition for which the drug was prescribed, that is the first listed diagnosis. In addition, an additional code indicating the intent, such as noncompliance or a complication of medical care should be assigned.

Coding and Documentation Requirements

Identify the drug and external cause (single combined code), and use additional code(s) to specify the drug reaction

- Adverse effect – right prescription, right dose, properly administered
  - Code first the specific adverse effect
- Poisoning – wrong drug, wrong dose, wrong route of administration, wrong combination of drugs or alcohol
  - Identify external cause
    - » Accidental (unintentional)
    - » Intentional – self harm
    - » Intentional – assault
    - » Undetermined
  - Code the specific toxic reaction due to the poisoning additionally
- Toxic effect – nonmedicinal agent causing toxic reaction
  - Identify external cause
    - » Accidental (unintentional)
    - » Intentional – self harm
    - » Intentional – assault
    - » Undetermined
  - Code the specific toxic effect additionally
- Underdosing – taking less than prescribed or less than recommended in the manufacturer's instructions with resulting medical condition
  - Code first the specific medical condition resulting from the underdosing

Example 1

Adverse Effect of Ibuprofen

ICD-10-CM Code/Documentation
T39.315- Adverse effect of propionic acid derivatives

Note: For adverse effects, the first listed code should be the nature of the adverse effect such as vomiting, rash, ulcer.

Documentation and Coding Example 1

Twenty-four-year-old female is brought to ED by her boyfriend, a 3rd year medical student. Patient is training for her first marathon and has been **taking ibuprofen almost daily for the past 2 weeks**. Three days ago, she developed a low grade fever, sore throat, and cough. She thought she had a viral infection and decreased her workouts but continued taking ibuprofen. She woke today with a burning feeling in her eyes, sores in her mouth, and itchy red patches on her face and neck. Her boyfriend came home from an overnight call shift, recognized this as possible Stevens-Johnson Syndrome and brought her directly to the hospital. On examination, this is an ill-appearing, anxious young woman. Temperature 99.8, HR 98, RR 16, BP 98/60. **Conjunctiva is bright red without excessive tearing**. PERRL. TMs clear. No nasal drainage. **Numerous blister like sores are noted on lips, tongue and oral mucosa, oral pharynx is bright red**. Facial skin is pink with brighter red patches which are quite itchy and painful. There is a patchy reddish-purple rash on chest, abdomen, and back. Patient states these areas are not really bothersome. There is no lymphadenopathy appreciated. Breath sounds are clear, equal bilaterally. HR regular without murmur, gallop, or rub. Abdomen soft with active bowel sounds. Patient uses oral contraceptives continuously because of a history of migraine headaches, PMDD.

Impression: **Acute systemic allergic reaction to ibuprofen, manifesting as Stevens-Johnson Syndrome.**

Plan: Admit to burn service. Ophthalmology consult to evaluate ocular involvement. Gastroenterology consult to evaluate for GI lesions and whether she can tolerate oral food and fluids. IV started in right forearm. Blood drawn for CBC, electrolytes, coagulation studies. IV corticosteroids and Immunoglobulin therapy started.

Diagnosis Code(s)

L51.1	Stevens-Johnson syndrome
K12.32	Oral mucositis (ulcerative) due to other drugs
T39.315A	Adverse effect of propionic acid derivatives, initial encounter

Coding Note(s)

Stevens-Johnson Syndrome (SJS) is differentiated from Steven-Johnson Syndrome-Toxic Epidermal Necrolysis by the extent of skin involvement. In SJS, there is a red skin rash with blistering of the mucous membranes of the lips and oral mucosa, and there may be small areas of peeling skin. In SJS-TEN syndrome, there is extensive peeling of skin. This patient has symptoms consistent with SJS and the condition is documented as SJS. The patient has documented mucositis with blistering of the oral mucosa so additional codes are required to identify this manifestation. The patient may also have eye involvement and gastrointestinal involvement but other than red conjunctiva these have not been specifically documented or confirmed in the ED notes. The ED physician has requested consults from ophthalmology and gastroenterology and if involvement of the eyes or gastrointestinal tract is confirmed, those manifestations would also be reported. Coding guidelines direct to code first the nature of the adverse effect followed by the adverse effect.

Example 2

Underdosing of Lamictal Anti-seizure Medication

ICD-10-CM Code/Documentation	
T42.6x6A	Underdosing of other antiepileptic and sedative-hypnotic drugs, initial encounter

Documentation and Coding Example 2

ED Note: Seven-year-old Hispanic male brought to ED by EMS after suffering a **prolonged seizure** at school. According to the school health technician who accompanied him to ED, **patient has a history of simple partial seizure disorder and is prescribed Lamictal which is administered at home**. The witness describes generalized tonic-clonic movements. EMS called per school protocol, arrived within 3 minutes and found patient on the ground in an outside lunch area and noted the seizures were now more subtle with brief rhythmic myoclonic movements confined to upper extremities. EMS noted patient's eyes were open and staring, he did not respond to his name, did retract from painful physical stimuli. IV started during transport and Lorazepam 0.1mg/kg given slow IV push. Seizure activity decreased noticeably within 2 minutes of administering medication. O2 saturation 98% on O2 via mask at 2 L/m that was started during transport. HR 104, BP 88/50. Blood drawn for CBC, comprehensive metabolic panel, and stat calcium, magnesium, glucose, lactate, and Lamictal level. Mother arrived in ED accompanied by school principal who brought her from work. Mother states student had onset of seizures 6 months ago and had been seizure free since starting on Lamictal. **The family has no health insurance and the medication is expensive. Mother has been giving only one dose of medication a day instead of 2 for the past month to try and make it last longer**. Pediatric neurology in to see patient. PET scan requested. Stat labs reveal elevated glucose, lactate, and **sub-therapeutic Lamictal level**. Loading dose of Dilantin given IV. Patient is admitted to pediatric floor for observation and monitoring of medication.

Diagnosis Code(s)

G40.109	Localization-related (focal) (partial) symptomatic epilepsy and epileptic syndromes with simple partial seizures, not intractable, without status epilepticus
T42.6x6A	Underdosing of other antiepileptic and sedative-hypnotic drugs
Z91.120	Patient's intentional underdosing of medication regimen due to financial hardship

Coding Note(s)

Codes for underdosing are never the first-listed diagnosis. If the patient has a relapse or exacerbation of the medical condition for which the drug is prescribed due to underdosing of the drug, a code for underdosing is assigned. Lamictal is not listed in the Table of Drugs and Chemicals. However, we do know that it is used to treat epilepsy and so it would be classified as an anti-epileptic or anti-convulsant. The code for anti-epileptic/anti-convulsant NEC is used. The patient is described as having a prolonged seizure but the seizure is not documented as status epilepticus so the code for without status epilepticus is used. The patient's condition is also not described as intractable so the code for not intractable is used.

Sprain/Strain

A sprain is an injury to a ligament. A sprain occurs when the ligaments of a joint are stretched or torn. Sprains are graded by severity as:

- Grade I – Mild sprain, ligaments are stretched but not torn
- Grade II – Moderate sprain, ligaments are partially torn and there may be some loss of function
- Grade III – Severe sprains, ligament is completely torn/ruptured resulting in joint instability

A strain is an injury to muscles, fascia, and/or tendons typically resulting from strenuous activity. A strain may also be referred to as a pulled muscle. Like sprains, strains can range from mild to severe and the severity of the strain may range from stretching to tearing of the muscle or tendon. When muscles tear, small blood vessels may also be damaged resulting in bruising at the site of the injury.

Sprains because they involve the joint are categorized with dislocations. Strains are categorized with injuries of muscle, tendon and fascia. Codes for sprains are assigned a 3rd character of 3. Codes for strains are assigned a 3rd character of 6. Like other musculoskeletal injuries, codes for sprains and strains are specific to type of injury, site, laterality, and episode of care. For injuries to the ligaments of the forearms, wrists, and hands there is also a subcategory for traumatic rupture of the ligaments which may also be referred to as a Grade III sprain. For all other sites, traumatic rupture of the ligaments is coded as a sprain. If there is an open wound associated with the strain, sprain, or ruptured ligament, the open wound is reported with an additional code.

Coding and Documentation Requirements

Identify type of injury:

- Sprain (ligament injury)

19. Injury/Poisoning of External Causes

- Strain (muscle/tendon injury)
- Traumatic rupture ligament(s) (forearm, wrist and hand only)

Sprain (ligament injury)

Identify site of sprain:

- Shoulder girdle
  - Shoulder joint
    - » Coracohumeral (ligament)
    - » Rotator cuff capsule
    - » Superior glenoid labrum lesion
    - » Other specified site of shoulder joint
    - » Unspecified site of shoulder joint
  - Acromioclavicular joint
  - Sternoclavicular joint
  - Other specified parts of shoulder girdle
  - Unspecified parts of shoulder girdle
- Elbow
  - Radiohumeral
  - Radial collateral ligament
  - Ulnohumeral
  - Ulnar collateral ligament
  - Other specified part of elbow
  - Unspecified part of elbow
- Wrist
  - Carpal joint
  - Radiocarpal joint
  - Other specified part of wrist
  - Unspecified part of wrist
- Hand
  - Specify digit
    - » Thumb
    - » Index finger
    - » Middle finger
    - » Ring finger
    - » Little finger
    - » Unspecified finger
  - Specify area
    - » Interphalangeal joint
    - » Metacarpophalangeal joint
    - » Other specified part
    - » Unspecified part
- Hip
  - Iliofemoral ligament
  - Ischiocapsular ligament
  - Other specified part of hip
  - Unspecified part of hip
- Knee
  - Collateral ligament
    - » Medial collateral
    - » Lateral collateral
    - » Unspecified collateral ligament
  - Cruciate ligament
    - » Anterior cruciate
    - » Posterior cruciate
    - » Unspecified cruciate ligament
  - Superior tibiofibular joint/ligament
  - Other specified part of knee
  - Unspecified part of knee
- Ankle
  - Calcaneofibular ligament
  - Deltoid ligament
  - Tibiofibular ligament
  - Other specified part of ankle (includes internal collateral ligament and talofibular ligament)
  - Unspecified part of ankle
- Foot
  - Tarsal ligament
  - Tarsometatarsal ligament
  - Other specified part of foot
  - Unspecified part of foot
- Toes
  - Great toe
    - » Interphalangeal joint
    - » Metatarsophalangeal joint
    - » Unspecified part of toe
  - Lesser toes
    - » Interphalangeal joint
    - » Metatarsophalangeal joint
    - » Unspecified part of toe
  - Unspecified toe
    - » Interphalangeal joint
    - » Metatarsophalangeal joint
    - » Unspecified part of toe

Identify laterality:

- Right
- Left
- Unspecified

Identify episode of care:

- Initial encounter
- Subsequent encounter
- Sequela

Strain (muscle/tendon injury)

Identify site of strain:

- Shoulder and upper arm
  - Rotator cuff
  - Long head of biceps
  - Other parts of biceps
  - Triceps
  - Other specified sites of shoulder/upper arm
  - Unspecified site of shoulder/upper arm

- Forearm
  - Flexor muscle/fascia/tendon at forearm level
    - » Thumb
    - » Index finger
    - » Middle finger
    - » Ring finger
    - » Little finger
    - » Unspecified finger
    - » Other specified flexor muscle/fascia/tendon site
  - Extensor/abductor muscle/fascia/tendon at forearm level
    - » Thumb
    - » Index finger
    - » Middle finger
    - » Ring finger
    - » Little finger
    - » Unspecified finger
    - » Other specified extensor/abductor muscle/fascia/tendon site
  - Other muscles/fascia/tendons at forearm level
  - Unspecified muscle/fascia/tendon at forearm level
- Wrist/hand/finger
  - Flexor muscle/fascia/tendon at wrist/hand level
    - » Thumb
    - » Index finger
    - » Middle finger
    - » Ring finger
    - » Little finger
    - » Unspecified finger
    - » Other specified flexor muscle/fascia/tendon site
  - Extensor muscle/fascia/tendon at wrist/hand level
    - » Thumb
    - » Index finger
    - » Middle finger
    - » Ring finger
    - » Little finger
    - » Unspecified finger
    - » Other specified extensor/abductor muscle/fascia/tendon site
  - Intrinsic muscle/fascia/tendon at wrist/hand level
    - » Thumb
    - » Index finger
    - » Middle finger
    - » Ring finger
    - » Little finger
    - » Unspecified finger
    - » Other specified extensor/abductor muscle/fascia/tendon site
  - Other muscles/fascia/tendons at wrist/hand level
  - Unspecified muscle/fascia/tendon at wrist/hand level
-
- Hip/Thigh
  - Adductor muscle/fascia/tendon
  - Posterior muscle group
  - Quadriceps muscle/fascia/tendon
  - Other specified muscle/fascia/tendon at hip/thigh level
  - Unspecified muscle/fascia/tendon at hip/thigh level
- Knee/lower leg
  - Anterior muscle group
  - Peroneal muscle group
  - Posterior muscle group
    - » Achilles tendon
    - » Other posterior muscles/tendons
  - Other specified muscle/fascia/tendon at knee/lower leg level
  - Unspecified muscle/fascia/tendon at knee/lower leg level
- Ankle/foot/toe
    - » Long flexor muscle
    - » Long extensor muscle
    - » Intrinsic muscle
    - » Other specified muscle/fascia/tendon at ankle/foot/toe level
    - » Unspecified muscle/fascia/tendon at ankle/foot/toe level

Identify laterality:

- Right
- Left
- Unspecified

Identify episode of care:

- Initial encounter
- Subsequent encounter
- Sequela

Traumatic Ruptured Ligament

Identify general region of traumatic rupture:

- Forearm/wrist/hand/finger
- All other sites (including thumb) (see sprain)

Identify specific site in forearm/wrist/hand:

- Forearm
  - Radial collateral ligament
  - Ulnar collateral ligament
- Wrist
  - Collateral ligament
  - Radiocarpal ligament
  - Ulnocarpal ligament
  - Other specified ligament at wrist level
  - Unspecified ligament at wrist level
- Finger
  - Identify digit
    - » Index finger
    - » Middle finger

- » Ring finger
- » Little finger
- » Unspecified finger
- – Identify site
- » Collateral ligament
- » Palmar ligament
- » Volar plate
- » Other specified ligament
- » Unspecified ligament
- Identify laterality:
- Right
- Left
- Unspecified

Identify episode of care:

- Initial encounter
- Subsequent encounter
- Sequela

Example 1

Sprain of Ligament, Knee

ICD-10-CM Code/Documentation	
Unspecified collateral ligament	
S83.401-	Sprain of unspecified collateral ligament of right knee
S83.402-	Sprain of unspecified collateral ligament of left knee
S83.409-	Sprain of unspecified collateral ligament of unspecified knee
Medial collateral ligament	
S83.411-	Sprain of medial collateral ligament of right knee
S83.412-	Sprain of medial collateral ligament of left knee
S83.419-	Sprain of medial collateral ligament of unspecified knee
Lateral collateral ligament	
S83.421-	Sprain of lateral collateral ligament of right knee
S83.422-	Sprain of lateral collateral ligament of left knee
S83.429-	Sprain of lateral collateral ligament of unspecified knee
Unspecified cruciate ligament	
S83.501-	Sprain of unspecified cruciate ligament of right knee
S83.502-	Sprain of unspecified cruciate ligament of left knee
S83.509-	Sprain of unspecified cruciate ligament of unspecified knee
Anterior cruciate ligament	
S83.511-	Sprain of anterior cruciate ligament of right knee
S83.512-	Sprain of anterior cruciate ligament of left knee
S83.519-	Sprain of anterior cruciate ligament of unspecified knee
Posterior cruciate ligament	
S83.521-	Sprain of posterior cruciate ligament of right knee
S83.522-	Sprain of posterior cruciate ligament of left knee
S83.529-	Sprain of posterior cruciate ligament of unspecified knee

Documentation and Coding Example

Orthopedic Clinic Note #1: Patient is a 20-old lacrosse player from the university women's team. She presents today with pain, swelling, and limited ROM in her right knee. Patient states she played in the rain four days ago and **slipped on wet turf without falling but twisting her knee**. She recalls feeling a "popping" sensation in her knee but was able to finish the game without too much discomfort. An athletic trainer examined her when she came off the field and found no swelling or loss of mobility. Patient was advised to ice x 20 minutes TID and use ibuprofen for discomfort. Patient noted swelling and stiffness the next morning but was able to go about her normal routine using ice and ibuprofen. The swelling and pain has been worse each day despite rest, ice, ibuprofen, and use of a knee brace. The university is on spring recess so she has not played lacrosse since the day she was injured. On examination, this is a well-developed, well-nourished, athletic appearing Caucasian female. Good hip flexion, intact ROM in ankles/feet bilaterally, brisk reflexes present in knees, ankles, and feet. Mild swelling noted in **right knee** when compared with left. There is no crepitus or warmth appreciated. Swelling more pronounced in posterior right knee. Mild backward sag is noted with flexion but otherwise good stability noted.

Impression: **Partial posterior cruciate ligament tear, R/O avulsion fracture. X-ray of right knee obtained and avulsion fracture is R/O**. Patient scheduled for MRI in the morning and will return to clinic with the films. She is fitted with crutches and will continue with RICE and is prescribed Naproxen for pain.

Orthopedic Note #2: Patient returns following MRI. Pain has significantly improved with non-weight bearing and Naproxen. **MRI shows a partial tear of the posterior cruciate ligament and accumulation of fluid behind the patella**. No other structural abnormalities are noted. Treatment options are discussed with patient and her mother via phone call. Both are comfortable with a conservative plan of RICE, Naproxen, and PT when swelling has subsided. Letter dictated for lacrosse coach, explaining she will be benched for the remainder of the season. RTC in 2 weeks.

Orthopedic Clinic Note #3: Patient is seen today in follow-up for a right PCL sprain sustained when she slipped playing lacrosse. Patient is doing well. Right knee swelling resolved, weight bears without pain. She has had 4 sessions with physical therapist and is doing twice daily exercises at home to strengthen knee. Lacrosse coach and team members have been supportive. She attends practice but is not participating. She is no longer using Naproxen, ice but continues to use knee brace. Advised to continue with PT x 2 more weeks and RTC at that time.

Orthopedic Clinic Note #4: Patient is seen today 8 weeks following a right PCL sprain. Good ROM in right knee. No pain or swelling noted. She is discharged from PT and advised to continue with home exercises to maintain knee strength. She is cleared to resume lacrosse practice but states the season has ended for this year. RTC as needed.

Diagnosis Code(s)

Orthopedic Clinic Note #1 and #2:

S83.521A Sprain of posterior cruciate ligament of right knee, initial encounter

W18.49XA Other slipping, tripping, and stumbling without falling, initial encounter

Y92.328 Other athletic field as place of occurrence of the external cause

Y93.65 Activity, lacrosse and field hockey

Y99.8 Other external cause status (includes student)

Note: It is appropriate to use the 7th character 'A' for initial encounter for the first visit (Ortho Clinic Note #1) and for the second visit (Ortho Clinic Note #2) because both encounters are during the acute phase of treatment. At the second encounter, the patient returns with an MRI which allows confirmation of the diagnosis and this is also when the treatment plan is developed.

Subsequent episode of care:

S83.521D Sprain of posterior cruciate ligament of right knee, subsequent encounter

W18.49XD Other slipping, tripping, and stumbling without falling, subsequent encounter (visit #3 only)

Note: The 7th character 'D' for subsequent encounter is used for the third and fourth visits (Other Clinic Notes #3 and #4). During the last two visits, the patient is receiving follow-up care during the rehabilitation phase of the injury. Each clinic visit must stand alone when assigning the proper codes. Since there is no documentation in Clinic Note #4 as to how the injury happened, the external cause code cannot be assigned.

Coding Note(s)

The external cause code is used for the entire treatment period. The place of occurrence is used only once at the initial encounter for treatment. Place of occurrence codes are used in conjunction with activity codes, which are also reported only once at the initial encounter. If the activity is not stated, no activity code is used. An external cause status code is used to indicate the work status of the individual at the time of the external cause occurrence. External cause status code is used only once at the initial encounter. The code for the external cause is W18.49x- for other slipping, tripping and stumbling without falling rather than the unspecified code (W18.40x-) because it is stated that the slipping occurred due to wet turf.

Example 2

Strain of Right Index Finger, Interphalangeal Joint

ICD-10-CM Code/Documentation	
S66.110-	Strain of flexor muscle, fascia and tendon of right index finger at wrist and hand level
S66.310-	Strain of extensor muscle, fascia and tendon of right index finger at wrist and hand level
S66.510-	Strain of intrinsic muscle, fascia and tendon of right index finger at wrist and hand level
S66.811-	Strain of other specified muscles, fascia and tendons at wrist and hand level, right hand
S66.911-	Strain of unspecified muscle, fascia and tendon at right wrist and hand level, right hand

Documentation and Coding Example 2

Orthopedic Hand Clinic Note: 26-year-old **bicycle messenger** presents to clinic with c/o right index finger that he cannot straighten out. This is a well-developed, well-nourished Black male. He states approximately 3 weeks ago his finger was smashed between the **handlebar of his bike and a car door**. He felt pain immediately and his glove was ripped, but there was no break in the skin and no bleeding. He states the knuckle was swollen and tender for a few days and it especially hurt to straighten out the finger, but he could grip the handlebars and work so he just took OTC pain medication and did not bother to have it checked out. The deformity is beginning to interfere with other aspects of hand use so he presents today for an evaluation. On examination, the **right index finger is flexed downward almost to 90-degree angle at the middle PIP joint and the same degree backward at the distal PIP joint**. Patient cannot extend the finger but can manipulate it manually with only mild discomfort. There are no neurovascular deficits in the hand or fingers.

Impression: **Deformity due to extensor tendon tear right index finger**. X-ray obtained and an **avulsion fracture is r/o**. Patient fitted with a PIP flexion splint and referred to OT for hand therapy. He has no activity restrictions and may continue to work. RTC in 2 weeks.

Diagnosis Code(s)

S66.310A Strain of extensor muscle, fascia and tendon of right index finger at wrist and hand level, initial encounter

V13.4XXA Pedal cycle driver injured in collision with car, pick-up truck or van in traffic accident, initial encounter

Y92.410 Unspecified street and highway as the place of occurrence of the external cause

Y93.55 Activity, bike riding

Y99.0 Civilian activity done for income or pay

Coding Note(s)

The alphabetic index under tear, tendon refers the coder to strain which in turn refers the coder to injury, muscle, by site, strain. So, the correct code for a tear of the extensor tendon of the right hand, index finger is the code for strain. Even though the injury occurred three weeks prior to the encounter, this was the first encounter for evaluation and treatment of the injury.

Summary

Diagnosis coding for injuries, poisonings and other consequences of external causes requires detailed documentation to capture the most specific ICD-10-CM code. When evaluating documentation or developing tools to help providers understand these documentation requirements, begin by first identifying common injuries, poisonings, and other conditions due to external causes for your practice or facility. Then review the codes and documentation elements specific to those conditions. If there is no checklist in this book for the specific conditions seen in your setting, follow the format here to develop your own checklists that identify all the documentation elements for those conditions.

Resources

Documentation check lists are available in Appendix A for the following conditions:

- Burns and Corrosions
- Fractures
- Open Wound
- Sprain, Lower Extremity
- Sprain, Upper Extremity

Chapter 19 Quiz

1. A current torn ligament is reported as a:
   - a. Laceration
   - b. Rupture
   - c. Strain
   - d. Sprain
2. Malunion of a fracture is captured by:
   a. First assigning the injury code and then assigning a second code for malunion
   b. Assigning a Z-code for malunion
   c. Assigning the code for the fracture with the 7th character that captures subsequent encounter for fracture with malunion
   d. Assigning the code for the fracture with the 7th character 'A' for initial encounter because malunion is defined as occurring during the acute phase of the injury
3. How is an open wound of the extremity with a tendon injury coded?
   a. Using a code for the open wound and a second code for the tendon injury
   b. As a complication of the open wound using a 7th character extension
   c. Using a combination code for the open wound and the specific type of tendon injury
   d. Using only the code for the tendon injury
4. What documentation is required to capture the most specific code for an injury to the pancreas?
   a. Type of pancreatic injury, region of pancreatic injury, episode of care
   b. Type of open wound, type of pancreatic injury, region of pancreatic injury, episode of care
   c. Type of pancreatic injury, episode of care
   d. Region of pancreatic injury, episode of care
5. When are Glasgow coma scale codes used in addition to the intracranial injury code?
   a. When the duration of the loss of consciousness is not known
   b. There is loss of consciousness and documentation of all three elements that comprise the coma scale and/or the numeric Glasgow coma score
   c. Whenever documentation indicates that the patient has sustained a concussion
   d. When the documentation indicates that the patient has sustained a head injury
6. What is the correct code for acute care of a fracture of the lateral condyle of the left tibia?
   a. S82.125A Nondisplaced fracture of lateral condyle of left tibia, initial encounter for closed fracture
   b. S82.122A Displaced fracture of lateral condyle of left tibia, initial encounter for closed fracture
   c. S82.122D Displaced fracture of lateral condyle of left tibia, subsequent encounter for closed fracture with routine healing
   d. There is not enough information to assign a code as the fracture must be documented as closed or open and as displaced or nondisplaced
7. The classification system used for 2-part, 3-part, and 4-part fractures of the surgical neck of the humerus in an adult is called the ________________________ classification system.
   a. Gustilo
   b. Salter-Harris
   c. Physeal
   d. Neer
8. How are sprains and strains categorized?
   a. In the same categories and subcategories
   b. Sprains are categorized with dislocations and strains are categorized with other injuries
   c. Strains are categorized with dislocations and sprains are categorized with other injuries
   d. Sprains and strains are synonymous and both are categorized as tears
9. How is an encounter to treat a late effect of an injury reported?
   a. With a specific code for the late effect followed by the code for the condition being treated, such as a scar
   b. With the code that describes the condition being treated, such as a scar followed by a specific late effect code, such as late effect of a burn
   c. With the code for the condition being treated, such as a scar followed by the specific code for the injury with the 7th character 'S' to identify the scar or other condition as a sequela of the injury
   d. With the code for the injury with the 7th character 'S' followed by the code for the condition being treated, such as a scar
10. How is an ED visit for an injury documented as laceration with transection of the right radial artery at the mid forearm reported?
    a. S65.191A Other specified injury of radial artery at wrist and hand level of right arm, initial encounter
    b. S55.191A Other specified injury of radial artery at forearm level, right arm, initial encounter; S51.811A Laceration without foreign body of right forearm, initial encounter
    c. S55.111A Laceration of radial artery at forearm level, right arm, initial encounter
    d. S55.111A Laceration of radial artery at forearm level, right arm, initial encounter; S51.811A Laceration without foreign body of right forearm, initial encounter

See next page for answers and rationales.

Chapter 19 Answers and Rationales

1. A current torn ligament is reported as a:

   d. Sprain

   Rationale: *A current injury of a ligament documented only as a tear or torn ligament is reported as a sprain. This can be verified by referring to the Alphabetic Index. Under Tear, ligament, there is an instruction to See also Sprain, by site.*

2. Malunion of a fracture is captured by:

   c. Assigning the code for the fracture with the 7th character that captures subsequent encounter for fracture with malunion

   Rationale: *Malunion of a fracture is captured by the fracture code with the 7th character 'P' for subsequent encounter for [closed] fracture with malunion; 'Q' for subsequent encounter for open fracture type I or II with malunion; or 'R' for subsequent encounter for open fracture type IIIA, IIIB, or IIIC with malunion.*

3. How is an open wound of the extremity with a tendon injury coded?

   a. Using a code for the open wound and a second code for the tendon injury

   Rationale: *When coding an open wound of the extremity, additional codes are required to report any associated injuries such as laceration of nerves, major blood vessels, muscles, or tendons.*

4. What documentation is required to capture the most specific code for an injury to the pancreas?

   a. Type of pancreatic injury, region of pancreatic injury, episode of care

   Rationale: *Capturing the most specific code requires identification of the type of pancreatic injury (contusion; laceration – minor, moderate, major; other specified injury), region of pancreatic injury (head, body, tail), and the episode of care (initial, subsequent, sequela). Not all pancreatic injuries are the result of an open wound so that information is not required. If there is an open wound, a separate code is needed for the open wound.*

5. When are Glasgow coma scale codes used in addition to the intracranial injury code?

   b. There is loss of consciousness and documentation of all three elements that comprise the coma scale and/or the numeric Glasgow coma score

   Rationale: *Glasgow come scale codes should be used in addition to the intracranial injury code when there is loss of consciousness and documentation of all three elements that comprise the coma scale and/or the numeric Glasgow coma score. Because a head injury or a concussion do not always result in a loss of consciousness and because even when there is documentation of loss of consciousness, information related to the Glasgow coma scale is not always documented, the three elements that comprise the coma scale and/or the numeric coma score can only be reported when this information is documented.*

6. What is the correct code for acute care of a fracture of the lateral condyle of the left tibia?

   b. S82.122A Displaced fracture of lateral condyle of left tibia, initial encounter for closed fracture

   Rationale: *According to the chapter guidelines, traumatic fractures not indicated as open or closed are coded to closed and fractures not indicated as displaced or nondisplaced are coded to displaced. So, code S82.122ADisplaced fracture of lateral condyle of left tibia, initial encounter for closed fracture is reported. The 7th character 'A' is used to capture the acute phase of the care and the closed nature of the fracture.*

7. The classification system used for 2-part, 3-part, and 4-part fractures of the surgical neck of the humerus in an adult is called the ________________________ classification system.

   d. Neer

   Rationale: *Surgical neck fractures of the proximal or upper end of the humerus are further classified using the Neer system. The proximal humerus is divided into four parts—the humeral head, greater tubercle, lesser tubercle, and diaphysis or shaft. These four parts are separated by epiphyseal lines, also called growth plates when the bones are still growing during the developmental years. When the proximal humerus is fractured, it typically occurs at the surgical neck and along one or more of the three epiphyseal lines. The proximal humerus may fracture into 2, 3, or 4 parts at the surgical neck which is why surgical neck fractures are designated as 2-part, 3-part or 4-part fractures.*

8. How are sprains and strains categorized?

   b. Sprains are categorized with dislocations and strains are categorized with other injuries

   Rationale: *Strains are defined as injuries to the muscle, fascia, and tendons and are classified with other injuries to those tissues. Sprains are defined as injuries to the ligaments and are classified with dislocations.*

9. How is an encounter to treat a late effect of an injury reported?

   c. With the code for the condition being treated, such as a scar followed by the specific code for the injury with the 7th character 'S' to identify the scar or other condition as a sequela of the injury

   Rationale: *Late effects are called sequelae. Instructions related to coding sequelae are found in the guidelines. Two codes are required to report a sequela of an injury. The first listed diagnosis is the code describing the actual* *sequela condition. Codes for sequela of injuries are reported using the same code as the injury with a 7th character 'S' to identify that the encounter/treatment is for a sequela of the injury.*

10. How is an ED visit for an injury documented as laceration with transection of the right radial artery at the mid forearm reported?

    d. **S55.111A Laceration of radial artery at forearm level, right arm, initial encounter; S51.811A Laceration without foreign body of right forearm, initial encounter**

    Rationale: *Two codes are required, one for the open wound and one for the radial artery injury. In order to assign a code for an injury to the radial artery, the level of the injury must be specified as forearm level or wrist/hand level. Transection of an artery is synonymous with laceration so the code for a laceration of the radial artery should be used. In this case, the injury is documented as being in the mid forearm, so the code for laceration at forearm level is used, along with the code for laceration of the right forearm without foreign body since there is no documentation of the presence of a foreign body.*

Chapter 20
FACTORS INFLUENCING HEALTH AND CONTACT WITH HEALTH CARE SERVICES

Introduction

The codes for factors influencing health and contact with health care services, represent reasons for encounters. These codes are located in Chapter 20 and the initial alpha character is Z so they may be referred to as Z codes. While code descriptions in Chapter 20, such as Z00.110 Health examination of newborn under 8 days old, may appear to be a description of a service or procedure, codes in this chapter are not procedure codes. These codes represent the reason for the encounter, service or visit and the procedure *must* be reported with the appropriate procedure code. The best way to become familiar with the types of codes that are included in the supplementary section is to review the code blocks in ICD-10-CM. Below is a table outlining the blocks for factors influencing health and contact with health care services.

ICD-10-CM Blocks	
Z00-Z13	Persons Encountering Health Services for Examinations
Z14-Z15	Genetic Carrier and Genetic Susceptibility to Disease
Z16	Resistance to Antimicrobial Drugs
Z17	Estrogen Receptor Status
Z18	Retained Foreign Body Fragments
Z20-Z29	Persons With Potential Health Hazards Related to Communicable Diseases
Z30-Z39	Persons Encountering Health Services in Circumstances Related to Reproduction
Z40-Z53	Encounters for Other Specific Health Care
Z55-Z65	Persons Encountering Health Services in Circumstances Related to Socioeconomic and Psychosocial Circumstances
Z66	Do Not Resuscitate Status
Z67	Blood Type
Z68	Body Mass Index [BMI]
Z69-Z76	Persons Encountering Health Services in Other Circumstances
Z77-Z99	Persons With Potential Health Hazards Related to Family and Personal History and Certain Conditions Influencing Health Status

Even a cursory comparison of the blocks in ICD-10-CM, shows a significant reorganization of codes and code categories from historical code systems. Encounters for routine examinations such as general adult medical examination, newborn health examination, routine child health examination, and vision and hearing examinations are all included in the first block of codes in ICD-10-CM.

Coding Note(s)

The coding notes have been revised to illustrate ICD-10-CM codes classified as factors influencing health status and contact with health services. ICD-10-CM chapter level coding notes are discussed here.

Z codes represent reasons for encounters. A corresponding procedure code must accompany a Z-code if a procedure is performed. Categories Z00-Z99 are provided for occasions when circumstances other than a disease, injury or external cause classifiable to categories A00-Y89 are recorded as 'diagnoses' or 'problems'. This can arise in two main ways:

- When a person who may or may not be sick encounters the health services for some specific purpose, such as to receive limited care or service for a current condition, to donate an organ or tissue, to receive a prophylactic vaccination (immunization), or to discuss a problem which is in itself not a disease or injury
- When some circumstance, condition, or problem is present which influences the person's health status but is not in itself a current illness or injury

Exclusions

There are no chapter level exclusions listed in Chapter 21.

Chapter Guidelines

There are extensive chapter-specific coding guidelines in ICD-10-CM for factors influencing health status and contact with health services. An overview of the ICD-10-CM guidelines is provided here. For the complete guidelines consult the most current *ICD-10-CM Official Guidelines for Coding and Reporting* for the code set.

Chapter 21 guidelines provide additional information about the use of Z codes for specific types of encounters. Z codes may be used in any healthcare setting and most Z codes may be either a principal/first-listed or secondary code depending on the circumstances of the encounter. Certain Z codes may only be used as a first listed or principal diagnosis while others, such as Z55-Z65, may only be reported as secondary diagnoses. Z codes are not procedure codes. They indicate the reason for the encounter and a corresponding procedure code must accompany a Z-code to describe the service provided or the procedure performed.

Although code assignment is based on documentation by the patient's provider, there are a few exceptions in reporting Z codes. Codes for reporting social determinants of health found in categories Z55-Z65, Persons with potential health hazards related to socioeconomic and psychosocial circumstances, may be assigned based on medical record documentation from clinicians involved in the patient's care who are not the patient's provider since this information represents social information, and not medical diagnoses. Self-reported documentation by the patient can also be used for assigning social determinant codes, as long as the information is signed-off and incorporated into the health record by a clinician or provider.

Categories of Z codes

The guidelines identify 16 broad categories of Z codes. Each of these broad categories contains categories and subcategories of Z codes for similar types of patient visits/encounters with similar reporting rules. A description of each of the 16 categories and use of the codes in these categories is summarized here. Consult the most current *ICD-10-CM Official Guidelines for Coding and Reporting* for the complete guidelines for Chapter 21.

Contact/Exposure

There are two types of contact/exposure codes which may be reported as either a first-listed code to explain an encounter for testing, or as a secondary code to identify a potential risk. These two types of codes are found in two categories of contact/exposure Z codes. Category Z20 indicates contact with, and suspected exposure to communicable diseases. These codes are reported for patients who do not show signs or symptoms of a disease but are suspected to have been exposed to it either by a close personal contact with an infected individual or by being in or having been in the area where the disease is epidemic. Category Z77 indicates contact with or suspected exposure to substances that are known to be hazardous to health. Code Z77.22 Exposure to tobacco smoke (second hand smoke) is included in this category.

Inoculations and Vaccinations

There is a single code, Z23 Encounter for immunization, in this category of Z codes. Code Z23 is for encounters for inoculations and vaccinations and indicates that a patient is being seen to receive a prophylactic inoculation against a disease. A procedure code is required to capture the administration of the immunization of vaccination and to identify the specific immunization/vaccination provided. Code Z23 may be used as a secondary code if the inoculation is given as a routine part of preventive health care, such as a well-baby visit.

Status

Status codes indicate that a patient is either a carrier of a disease or has the sequelae or residual of a past disease or condition. Codes for the presence of prosthetic or mechanical devices resulting from past treatment are categorized as status codes. A status code is helpful because the status may affect the course of treatment and its outcome. Status codes should not be confused with history codes which indicate that a patient no longer has the condition. Status codes are not used with diagnosis codes that provide the same information as the status code. For example, code Z94.1 Heart transplant status, should not be used with a code from subcategory T86.2 Complications of heart transplant because codes in subcategory T86.2 already identify the patient as a heart transplant recipient. Status Z codes/categories include:

- Z14 Genetic carrier – Genetic carrier status indicates that a person carries a gene associated with a particular disease, but does not have the disease and is not at risk for developing the disease. Genetic carriers may pass the defective gene to offspring who may develop the disease.
- Z15 Genetic susceptibility to disease – Genetic susceptibility indicates that a person has a gene that increases the risk of that person developing the disease.
  - Category Z15 codes are not reported as a principal or first-listed diagnosis
  - If the patient has the condition to which he/she is susceptible, and that condition is the reason for the encounter, the code for the current condition is sequenced first
  - If the patient is seen for follow-up after completing treatment for the condition and the condition no longer exists, a follow-up code is sequenced first, followed by the appropriate personal history and genetic susceptibility codes
  - If the purpose of the encounter is genetic counseling associated with procreative management, code Z31.5 Encounter for procreative genetic counseling should be assigned as the first-listed diagnosis, followed by a code from category Z15. Additional codes should be assigned for any family or personal history
- Z16 Resistance to antimicrobial drugs – This code indicates that a patient has a condition that is resistant to antimicrobial drug treatment. Sequence the infection code first.
- Z17 Estrogen receptor status
- Z18 Retained foreign body fragments
- Z19 Hormone sensitivity malignancy status
- Z21 Asymptomatic HIV infection status – This code indicates that a patient has tested positive for HIV but has manifested no signs or symptoms of the disease.
- Z22 Carrier of infectious disease – Carrier status indicates that the person harbors the specific organisms of a disease without manifest symptoms and is capable of transmitting the infection.
- Z28.3 Underimmunization status
- Z33.1 Pregnant state, incidental – This code is a secondary code only for use when the pregnancy is in no way complicating the reason for the visit. Otherwise a code from the obstetric chapter is required.
- Z66 Do not resuscitate – This code may be used when it is documented by the provider that a patient is on do not resuscitate status at any time during the stay.
- Z67 Blood type
- Z68 Body mass index [BMI] – As with all other secondary diagnosis codes, BMI codes should only be assigned when the associated diagnosis (e.g., obesity, overweight) meets the definition of a reportable diagnosis. Do not assign BMI codes during pregnancy.
- Z74.01 Bed confinement status
- Z76.82 Awaiting organ transplant status
- Z78 Other specified health status – Code Z78.1 Physical restraint status may be used when it is documented by the provider that a patient has been put in restraints during the current encounter. Please note that this code should not be reported when it is documented by the provider that a patient is temporarily restrained during a procedure.
- Z79 Long-term (current) drug therapy – Codes from this category indicate a patient's continuous use of a prescribed

drug (including such things as aspirin therapy) for the long-term treatment of a condition or for prophylactic use.

- Assign a code from category Z79 if the patient is receiving a medication for an extended period as a prophylactic measure (such as for the prevention of deep vein thrombosis) or as treatment of a chronic condition (such as arthritis) or a disease requiring a lengthy course of treatment (such as cancer)
- Do not assign a code from category Z79 for medication being administered for a brief period of time to treat an acute illness or injury (such as a course of antibiotics to treat acute bronchitis)
- Do not use these codes for patients who have addictions to drugs
- Do not use these codes for use of medications for detoxification or maintenance programs to prevent withdrawal symptoms in patients with drug dependence (e.g., methadone maintenance for opiate dependence). Assign the appropriate code for the drug dependence instead

- Z88 Allergy status to drugs, medicaments and biological substances (except Z88.9)
- Z89 Acquired absence of limb
- Z90 Acquired absence of organs, not elsewhere classified
- Z91.0 Allergy status, other than to drugs and biological substances
- Z92.82 Status post administration of tPA (rtPA) in a different facility within the last 24 hours prior to admission to a current facility
  - Assign code Z92.82 Status post administration of tPA (rtPA) in a different facility within the last 24 hours prior to admission to current facility, as a secondary diagnosis when a patient is received by transfer into a facility and documentation indicates they were administered tissue plasminogen activator (tPA) within the last 24 hours prior to admission to the current facility
  - This guideline applies even if the patient is still receiving the tPA at the time they are received into the current facility
  - The appropriate code for the condition for which the tPA was administered (such as cerebrovascular disease or myocardial infarction) should be assigned first
  - Code Z92.82 is only applicable to the receiving facility record and not to the transferring facility record
- Z93 Artificial opening status
- Z94 Transplanted organ and tissue status
- Z95 Presence of cardiac and vascular implants and grafts
- Z96 Presence of other functional implants
- Z97 Presence of other devices
- Z98 Other postprocedural states
  - Assign code Z98.85 Transplanted organ removal status, to indicate that a transplanted organ has been previously removed. This code should not be assigned for the encounter in which the transplanted organ is removed. The complication necessitating removal of the transplant organ should be assigned for that encounter
  - See section I.C.19 for information on the coding of organ transplant complications
- Z99 Dependence on enabling machines and devices, not elsewhere classified. For encounters for weaning from a mechanical ventilator, assign a code from subcategory J96.1, Chronic respiratory failure, followed by code Z99.11, Dependence on respirator [ventilator] status.

Note: Categories Z89-Z90 and Z93-Z99 are for use only if there are no complications or malfunctions of the organ or tissue replaced, the amputation site or the equipment on which the patient is dependent.

History (of)

There are two types of history Z codes, personal and family which are defined as follows:

- Personal history codes – Explain a patient's past medical condition that no longer exists and is not receiving any treatment, but that has the potential for recurrence, and therefore may require continued monitoring
  - May be used in conjunction with follow-up codes to explain the need for a test or procedure
- Family history codes – For use when a patient has a family member who has had a particular disease that causes the patient to be at higher risk of also contracting the disease
  - May be used in conjunction with screening codes to explain the need for a test or procedure
- History codes are also acceptable on any medical record regardless of the reason for the encounter. A history of an illness, even if no longer present, is important information that may alter the type of treatment ordered

History Z codes/categories include:

- Z80 Family history of primary malignant neoplasm
- Z81 Family history of mental and behavioral disorders
- Z82 Family history of certain disabilities and chronic diseases (leading to disablement)
- Z83 Family history of other specific disorders
- Z84 Family history of other conditions
- Z85 Personal history of malignant neoplasm
- Z86 Personal history of certain other diseases
- Z87 Personal history of other diseases and conditions
- Z91.4- Personal history of psychological trauma, not elsewhere classified
- Z91.5 Personal history of self-harm
- Z91.81 History of falling
- Z91.82 Personal history of military deployment
- Z92 Personal history of medical treatment (except Z92.0 Personal history of contraception and Z92.82 Status post administration of tPA (rtPA) in a different facility within the last 24 hours prior to admission to a current facility.

Screening

Screening is testing for disease or disease precursors in seemingly well individuals so that early detection and treatment can be provided for those who test positive for the disease (e.g. screening mammogram).

- Use of screening versus signs and symptoms codes – The testing of a person to rule out or confirm a suspected diagnosis because the patient has some sign or symptom is a diagnostic examination, not a screening in these cases, and a sign or symptom code is used to explain the reason for the visit.
- First listed diagnosis versus additional code
  - A screening code may be the first-listed diagnosis if the reason for the visit is specifically the screening exam
  - A screening code may be used as an additional code if the screening is done during an office visit for other health problems
- A screening code is not necessary if the screening is inherent to a routine examination, such as a pap smear done during a routine pelvic examination
- Should a condition be discovered during the screening then the code for the condition may be assigned as an additional diagnosis
- The Z-code indicates a screening exam is planned. A procedure code is required to confirm that the screening was performed

Screening Z codes/categories include:

- Z11 Encounter for screening for infectious and parasitic diseases
- Z12 Encounter for screening for malignant neoplasms
- Z13 Encounter for screening for other diseases and disorders (except Z13.9 Encounter for screening, unspecified)
- Z36 Encounter for antenatal screening of mother

Observation

There are three observation categories for use in very limited circumstances when a person is being observed for a suspected condition that has been ruled out.

- Do not use an observation code if an injury or illness or any signs or symptoms related to the suspected condition are present. In such cases, use the diagnosis/symptom code with the corresponding external cause code
- Use observation codes primarily as a principal diagnosis. However, an observation code may be assigned as a secondary code when the patient is observed for a condition that is ruled out and unrelated to the principal diagnosis, such as when a patient receives treatment for injuries sustained in a motor vehicle accident and is also observed for suspected COVID-19 infection that is subsequently ruled out. Also, when the principal diagnosis is required to be a code from category Z38 Liveborn infants according to place of birth and type of delivery. Then, a code from category Z05 Encounter for observation and evaluation of newborn for suspected diseases and conditions ruled out, is sequenced after the Z38 code.
  - Additional codes may be used in addition to the observation code but only if they are unrelated to the suspected condition being observed
- Codes from subcategory Z03.7 Encounter for suspected maternal and fetal conditions ruled out, may be used as either a first-listed or additional code depending on the case. Use codes from Z03.7 only when the suspected condition is ruled out during that encounter. Do not use Z03.7 codes if the suspected condition is confirmed; use the code for the confirmed condition. In addition, these codes are not for use if an illness or any signs or symptoms related to the suspected condition or problem are present. In such cases the diagnosis/symptom code is used.
  - Additional codes may be used with Z03.7 codes but only if they are unrelated to the suspected condition being evaluated.
  - Do not use codes from subcategory Z03.7 for antenatal screening of mother. For encounters for suspected fetal condition that are inconclusive following testing and evaluation, assign the appropriate code from category O35, O36, O40 or O41.

Observation Z codes/categories include:

- Z03 Encounter for medical observation for suspected diseases and conditions ruled out
- Z04 Encounter for examination and observation for other reasons (except Z04.9 Encounter for examination and observation for unspecified reason)
- Z05 Encounter for observation and evaluation of newborn for suspected diseases and conditions ruled out

Aftercare

Aftercare visit codes cover situations when the initial treatment of a disease has been performed and the patient requires continued care during the healing or recovery phase, or for the long-term consequences of the disease. Reporting rules for aftercare are as follows:

- The aftercare Z-code should not be used if treatment is directed at a current, acute disease. The diagnosis code is to be used in these cases. Exceptions to this rule include:
  - Codes for encounters for antineoplastic radiation, chemotherapy and immunotherapy (Z51.0, Z51.1-) are assigned as first-listed diagnosis if the sole reason for the encounter is antineoplastic therapy even if the patient still has the neoplastic disease. The neoplasm code is reported as a secondary diagnosis.
  - Aftercare for injuries are not reported with Z codes. Assign the acute injury code with the appropriate 7th character for subsequent care
- The aftercare codes are generally the first-listed diagnosis
- An aftercare code may be used as an additional code when some type of aftercare is provided in addition to the reason for admission and no diagnosis code is applicable. An example of this would be the closure of a colostomy during an encounter for treatment of another condition
- Aftercare codes should be used in conjunction with any other aftercare codes, other diagnoses codes, or other categories

of Z codes to provide better detail on the specifics of the aftercare encounter/visit, unless otherwise directed by the classification

- Certain aftercare Z codes require a secondary diagnosis code to describe the resolving condition or sequelae. For other aftercare codes, the condition is included in the code description and a secondary diagnosis is not required
- Additional Z code aftercare category terms include fitting and adjustment, and attention to artificial openings
- Use Status Z codes with aftercare Z codes as needed to indicate the nature of the aftercare. For example, code Z95.1 Presence of aortocoronary bypass graft, may be used with code Z48.812 Encounter for surgical aftercare following surgery on the circulatory system, to indicate the surgery for which the aftercare is being performed
- Do not use a status code when the aftercare code indicates the type of status. For example, Z43.0 Encounter for attention to tracheostomy should not be used with Z93.0 Tracheostomy status

Aftercare Z codes/categories include:

- Z42 Encounter for plastic and reconstructive surgery following medical procedure or healed injury
- Z43 Encounter for attention to artificial openings
- Z44 Encounter for fitting and adjustment of external prosthetic device
- Z45 Encounter for adjustment and management of implanted device
- Z46 Encounter for fitting and adjustment of other devices
- Z47 Orthopedic aftercare
- Z48 Encounter for other postprocedural aftercare
- Z49 Encounter for care involving renal dialysis
- Z51 Encounter for other aftercare and medical care

Follow-up

The follow-up Z codes are used to explain continuing surveillance following completed treatment of a disease, condition, or injury. They imply that the condition has been fully treated and no longer exists.

- Do not confuse follow-up codes with aftercare codes or with subsequent care for injuries (7th character for subsequent encounter that explains ongoing care of a healing condition or its sequelae)
- Follow-up Z codes (sequenced first) may be used with history Z codes (reported additionally) to provide the full picture of the healed condition and its treatment. The follow-up code is sequenced first, followed by the history code
- A follow-up code may be used to explain multiple visits
- Should the condition be found to have recurred on the follow-up visit, then the diagnosis code for the condition is reported not the follow-up Z-code

Follow-up Z code/categories include:

- Z08 Encounter for follow-up examination after completed treatment for malignant neoplasm
- Z09 Encounter for follow-up examination after completed treatment for conditions other than malignant neoplasm
- Z39 Encounter for maternal postpartum care and examination

Donor

Codes in category Z52 Donors of organs and tissues, are used for living individuals who are donating blood or other body tissue. These codes are only for individuals donating for others, not for self-donations. The only exception to this rule is blood donation. There are codes for autologous blood donation in subcategory Z52.01. Codes in category Z52 are not used to identify cadaveric donations.

Counseling

Counseling Z codes are used when a patient or family member receives assistance in the aftermath of an illness or injury or when support is required in coping with family or social problems. They are not used in conjunction with a diagnosis code when the counseling component of care is considered integral to standard treatment.

Counseling Z codes/categories include:

- Z30.0- Encounter for general counseling and advice on contraception
- Z31.5 Encounter for procreative genetic counseling
- Z31.6- Encounter for general counseling and advice on procreation
- Z32.2 Encounter for childbirth instruction
- Z32.3 Encounter for childcare instruction
- Z69 Encounter for mental health services for victim and perpetrator of abuse
- Z70 Counseling related to sexual attitude, behavior and orientation
- Z71 Persons encountering health services for other counseling and medical advice, not elsewhere classified
- Z76.81 Expectant mother prebirth pediatrician visit

Encounters for Obstetrical and Reproductive Services

Z codes in pregnancy are for use in those circumstances when none of the problems or complications included in the codes for the Obstetrics chapter exist (routine prenatal visit or postpartum care). Rules for use of these codes are:

- Codes in category Z34 Encounter for supervision of normal pregnancy are always the first-listed diagnosis and are not to be used with any other code from the OB chapter
- Codes in category Z3A Weeks of gestation may be assigned to provide additional information about the pregnancy. Category Z3A codes should not be assigned for pregnancies with abortive outcomes (O00-O08), elective termination of pregnancy (Z33.2), or postpartum conditions. The date of the admission should be used to determine weeks of gestation for inpatient admissions that encompass more than one gestational week
- Codes in category Z37 Outcome of delivery should be included on all maternal delivery records. Outcome of

delivery codes are always secondary codes and are never used on the newborn record

- Z codes for family planning or procreative management and counseling should be included on an obstetric record either during the pregnancy or the postpartum stage, if applicable

See Section I.C.15 Pregnancy, Childbirth and the Puerperium for further instructions on the use of these Z codes.

Z codes/categories for obstetrical and reproductive services include:

- Z30 Encounter for contraceptive management
- Z31 Encounter for procreative management
- Z32.2 Encounter for childbirth instruction
- Z32.3 Encounter for childcare instruction
- Z33 Pregnant state
- Z34 Encounter for supervision of normal pregnancy
- Z36 Encounter for antenatal screening of mother
- Z3A Weeks of gestation
- Z37 Outcome of delivery
- Z39 Encounter for maternal postpartum care and examination
- Z76.81 Expectant mother prebirth pediatrician visit

Newborns and Infants

See Section 1.C.16 Newborn (Perinatal) Guidelines for instructions on the use of these Z codes.

Newborns and infants Z codes/categories include:

- Z76.1 Encounter for health supervision and care of foundling
- Z00.1- Encounter for routine child health examination
- Z38 Liveborn infants according to place of birth and type of delivery

Routine and Administrative Examinations

Z codes allow for the description of encounters for routine examination, such as a general check-up, or examinations for administrative purposes, such as a pre-employment physical. The codes are not to be used if the examination is for diagnosis of a suspected condition or for treatment purposes. In such cases the diagnosis code is used. During a routine exam, should a diagnosis or condition be discovered, it should be coded as an additional code. Pre-existing and chronic conditions and history codes may also be included as additional codes as long as the examination is for administrative purposes and not focused on any particular condition.

Some of the codes for routine health examinations distinguish between "with" and "without" abnormal findings. Code assignment depends on the information that is known at the time the encounter is being coded. For example, if no abnormal findings were found during the examination, but the encounter is being coded before the test results are back, it is acceptable to assign the code for "without abnormal findings". When assigning a code for "with abnormal findings," additional codes should be assigned to identify the specific abnormal findings.

Preoperative examination and pre-procedural laboratory examination Z codes are for use only in those situations when a patient is being cleared for a procedure or surgery and no treatment is given.

Z codes/categories for routine and administrative examinations include:

- Z00 Encounter for general examination without complaint, suspected or reported diagnosis
- Z01 Encounter for other special examination without complaint, suspected or reported diagnosis
- Z02 Encounter for administrative examination (except Z02.9 Encounter for administrative examinations, unspecified)
- Z32.0- Encounter for pregnancy test

Miscellaneous Z codes

The miscellaneous Z codes capture a number of other health care encounters that do not fall into one of the other categories. Certain of these codes identify the reason for the encounter; others are for use as additional codes that provide useful information on circumstances that may affect a patient's care and treatment. Prophylactic organ removal is classified as a miscellaneous Z-code, and there are specific guidelines for prophylactic organ removal as follows:

- For encounters specifically for prophylactic removal of an organ, such as the breasts, the first-listed diagnosis should be a code from category Z40 Encounter for prophylactic surgery followed by the appropriate codes to identify the associated risk factor, such as family history or genetic susceptibility
- If the patient has a malignancy of one site and is having prophylactic removal at another site to prevent either a new primary malignancy or metastatic disease, a code for the malignancy should also be assigned in addition to a code from subcategory Z40.0 Encounter for prophylactic surgery for risk factors related to malignant neoplasms. A code from subcategory Z40.0 should not be assigned if the patient is having organ removal for treatment of malignancy such as the removal of the testes for treatment of prostate cancer.

Miscellaneous Z codes/categories are as follows:

- Z28 Immunization not carried out (except Z28.3 Underimmunization status)
- Z29 Encounter for other prophylactic measures
- Z40 Encounter for prophylactic surgery
- Z41 Encounter for procedures for purposes other than remedying health state (except Z41.9 Encounter for procedure for purposes other than remedying health state, unspecified)
- Z53 Persons encountering health services for specific procedures and treatment, not carried out
- Z55 Problems related to education and literacy
- Z56 Problems related to employment and unemployment
- Z57 Occupational exposure to risk factors
- Z58 Problems related to physical environment
- Z59 Problems related to housing and economic circumstances
- Z60 Problems related to social environment
- Z62 Problems related to upbringing

- Z63 Other problems related to primary support group, including family circumstances
- Z64 Problems related to certain psychosocial circumstances
- Z65 Problems related to other psychosocial circumstances
- Z72 Problems related to lifestyle
- Z73 Problems related to life management difficulty
- Z74 Problems related to care provider dependency (except Z74.01 Bed confinement status)
- Z75 Problems related to medical facilities and other health care
- Z76.0 Encounter for issue of repeat prescription
- Z76.3 Healthy person accompanying sick person
- Z76.4 Other boarder to healthcare facility
- Z76.5 Malingerer [conscious simulation]
- Z91.1- Patient's noncompliance with medical treatment and regimen
- Z91.83 Wandering in diseases classified elsewhere
- Z91.84- Oral health risk factors
- Z91.89 Other specified personal risk factors, not elsewhere classified

Nonspecific Z codes

Certain Z codes are so non-specific or potentially redundant with other codes in the classification that there can be little justification for their use in the inpatient setting. Their use in the outpatient setting should be limited to those instances when there is no further documentation to permit more precise coding. Otherwise, any sign or symptom or any other reason for the visit that is captured in another code should be used.

Nonspecific Z codes/categories include:

- Z02.9 Encounter for administrative examinations, unspecified
- Z04.9 Encounter for examination and observation for unspecified reason
- Z13.9 Encounter for screening, unspecified
- Z41.9 Encounter for procedure for purposes other than remedying health state, unspecified
- Z52.9 Donor of unspecified organ or tissue
- Z86.59 Personal history of other mental and behavioral disorders
- Z88.9 Allergy status to unspecified drugs, medicaments and biological substances
- Z92.0 Personal history of contraception

Z codes For Use Only as Principal/First-Listed Diagnoses

The following Z codes/categories may only be reported as the principal or first listed diagnosis, except when there are multiple encounters on the same day and the medical records for the encounters are combined:

- Z00 Encounter for general examination without complaint, suspected or reported diagnosis (except Z00.6)
- Z01 Encounter for other special examination without complaint, suspected or reported diagnosis
- Z02 Encounter for administrative examination
- Z03 Encounter for medical observation for suspected diseases and conditions ruled out
- Z04 Encounter for examination and observation for other reasons
- Z33.2 Encounter for elective termination of pregnancy
- Z31.81 Encounter for male factor infertility in female patient
- Z31.83 Encounter for assisted reproductive fertility procedure cycle
- Z31.84 Encounter for fertility preservation procedure
- Z34 Encounter for supervision of normal pregnancy
- Z39 Encounter for maternal postpartum care and examination
- Z38 Liveborn infants according to place of birth and type of delivery
- Z40 Encounter for prophylactic surgery
- Z42 Encounter for plastic and reconstructive surgery following medical procedure or healed injury
- Z51.0 Encounter for antineoplastic radiation therapy
- Z51.1- Encounter for antineoplastic chemotherapy and immunotherapy
- Z52 Donors of organs and tissues (except Z52.9 Donor of unspecified organ or tissue)
- Z76.1 Encounter for health supervision and care of foundling
- Z76.2 Encounter for health supervision and care of other healthy infant and child
- Z99.12 Encounter for respirator [ventilator] dependence during power failure

General Documentation Requirements

The general documentation requirements for Z codes relate primarily to the need for more specific documentation related to the reason for the encounter or visit. Aftercare for conditions classified in Chapter 19 is captured with the code for the specific condition and a 7th character identifying the episode of care as a subsequent encounter. For most injuries and other conditions, the 7th character for a subsequent encounter is 'D', but for fractures, additional 7th characters for subsequent encounters apply.

The applicable 7th character extensions for subsequent encounters for most fractures are as follows:

D Subsequent encounter for fracture with routine healing

G Subsequent encounter for fracture with delayed healing

K Subsequent encounter for fracture with nonunion

P Subsequent encounter for fracture with malunion

The applicable 7th character extensions for fractures of the shafts of the long bones are as follows:

D Subsequent encounter for closed fracture with routine healing

E Subsequent encounter for open fracture type I or II with routine healing

F Subsequent encounter for open fracture type IIIA, IIIB, or IIIC with routine healing

G Subsequent encounter for closed fracture with delayed healing

H Subsequent encounter for open fracture type I or II with delayed healing

J Subsequent encounter for open fracture type IIIA, IIIB, or IIIC with delayed healing

K Subsequent encounter for closed fracture with nonunion

M Subsequent encounter for open fracture type I or II with nonunion

N Subsequent encounter for open fracture type IIIA, IIIB, or IIIC with nonunion

P Subsequent encounter for closed fracture with malunion

Q Subsequent encounter for open fracture type I or II with malunion

R Subsequent encounter for open fracture type IIIA, IIIB, or IIIC with malunion

See Chapter 19 of the book for additional information and new coding conventions related to episode of care.

Code-Specific Documentation Requirements

In this section, code, code categories, subcategories and subclassifications for some of the more frequently reported factors influencing health status and contact with health services are reviewed. The corresponding ICD-10-CM codes are listed and the new documentation requirements identified. The focus is on conditions with specific clinical documentation requirements. Although not all ICD-10-CM codes with significant documentation requirements are discussed, this section will provide a representative sample of the type of documentation needed for factors influencing health. The section is organized numerically by code category, subcategory, or subclassification depending on whether the documentation affects only a single code or an entire subcategory or category.

Aftercare Following Explantation of Joint Prosthesis

Two examples are listed in ICD-10-CM regarding when this code should be reported. Aftercare following explantation of joint prosthesis may be reported for a staged procedure or an encounter for evaluation of planned insertion of a new joint prosthesis following prior explantation of joint prosthesis. In ICD-10-CM, aftercare for explantation of a joint prosthesis is specific to site.

Coding and Documentation Requirements

Identify site of explantation of joint prosthesis:

- Hip
- Knee
- Shoulder

ICD-10-CM Code/Documentation	
Z47.31	Aftercare following explantation of shoulder joint prosthesis
Z47.32	Aftercare following explantation of hip joint prosthesis
Z47.33	Aftercare following explantation of knee joint prosthesis

Documentation and Coding Example

Patient is a sixty-four-year-old Caucasian male now **8 weeks post explantation of left knee prosthesis who is here today to have his left knee checked and to determine if a new prosthesis can be implanted**. This retired chemical engineer had a total knee arthroplasty 4 months ago and developed a staphylococcus coagulase negative wound infection postoperatively. After local surgical debridement and IV antibiotics failed to clear the infection, the prosthesis was removed and a vancomycin loaded polymethylmethacrylate cement spacer inserted into the suprapatellar pouch with extension to the gutters. Patient has had PT support 2-3 x week and serum CRP has been monitored weekly. CRP is WNL for the 2nd week in a row. The left knee has no redness or swelling, surgical incisions are clean and dry. **Infection appears to have cleared up**. Patient is anxious to have a new implant because he has a trip planned in 3 months. Arrangements will be made by the surgery scheduler after he has been cleared by his PMD. He is given orders for preoperative lab work, EKG, chest x-ray.

Diagnosis Code(s)

Z47.33 Aftercare following explantation of knee joint prosthesis

Coding Note(s)

In ICD-10-CM, the aftercare code is specific for aftercare following explantation of a knee joint prosthesis.

Aftercare for Healing Traumatic Fracture of Lower Leg

Aftercare of injuries in ICD-10-CM is captured with the 7th character D for routine care for most injuries. For fractures additional 7th characters for subsequent encounter apply depending on whether the fracture is open or closed and whether the healing is routine, delayed, with nonunion or with malunion.

The example below is for aftercare of a fracture of the tibial shaft.

Coding and Documentation Requirements

Identify fracture site as tibial shaft

Identify type of fracture:

- Comminuted
- Segmental
- Spiral
- Transverse
- Oblique
- Other specified fracture
- Unspecified

Identify laterality:

- Right
- Left
- Unspecified

Identify as open/closed:

- Closed
- Open

- Type I or Type II
- Type IIIA, IIIB, IIIC

Identify subsequent episode of care:

- Routine healing
- Delayed healing
- Malunion
- Nonunion

Aftercare Closed Transverse Fracture of Shaft of Tibia with Routine Healing

ICD-10-CM Code/Documentation	
S82.221D	Displaced transverse fracture of shaft of right tibia, subsequent encounter for closed fracture with routine healing
S82.222D	Displaced transverse fracture of shaft of left tibia, subsequent encounter for closed fracture with routine healing
S82.223D	Displaced transverse fracture of shaft of unspecified tibia, subsequent encounter for closed fracture with routine healing
S82.224D	Nondisplaced transverse fracture of shaft of right tibia, subsequent encounter for closed fracture with routine healing
S82.225D	Nondisplaced transverse fracture of shaft of left tibia, subsequent encounter for closed fracture with routine healing
S82.226D	Nondisplaced transverse fracture of shaft of unspecified tibia, subsequent encounter for closed fracture with routine healing

Documentation and Coding Example

Thirty-seven-year-old Caucasian male reports to Orthopedic Clinic **for cast change, possible application of functional brace.** Patient sustained a **closed, nondisplaced transverse fracture of the right tibial shaft** in a snowmobile accident 4 weeks ago. The fracture was initially treated in the ER with application of a long posterior splint and subsequently casted in plaster 4 days later from mid-thigh to metatarsal heads, knee extended and ankle in 90-degree flexion. Radiographs in plaster 2 weeks ago showed good approximation of the fracture and some callus formation, repeat films today show the same with callus size increasing. **Cast is removed and patient is fitted with a functional brace.** He will continue to use crutches until evaluated by physical therapy. First available PT appointment is in 1 week. RTC for x-ray and recheck of brace in 2 weeks, sooner if problems arise.

Diagnosis Code(s)

S82.224D Nondisplaced transverse fracture of shaft of right tibia, subsequent encounter for closed fracture with routine healing

Coding Note(s)

In ICD-10-CM, a single code identifies the visit as being for routine aftercare (subsequent encounter) and identifies the condition for which the aftercare is provided as a closed, nondisplaced, transverse tibial shaft fracture.

Infection with Drug-Resistant Microorganisms

There are a growing number of pathogenic microorganisms that are resistant to some or all of the drugs previously used to treat the resulting infections. In ICD-10-CM, combination codes are used for reporting MRSA infections. The codes are from infectious and parasitic diseases (sepsis) and respiratory body system (pneumonia) chapters. For a current infection due to MRSA that is not covered by a combination code, such as a wound infection, stitch abscess or urinary tract infection, the code for the condition is reported first followed by the code B95.62, Methicillin resistant S. aureus (MRSA) infection as the cause of diseases classified elsewhere to identify the drug resistant nature of the infection. Infections with other drug-resistant microorganisms are captured in Category Z16.

Coding and Documentation Requirements

Identify the drug (drug class) resistance:

- Beta lactam antibiotics
  - Extended spectrum beta lactamase (ESBL)
  - Penicillins, which includes:
    - Amoxicillin
    - Ampicillin
  - Other specified beta lactam antibiotics, which includes
    - Cephalosporins
- Other antibiotics
  - Single antibiotics
    - Quinolones/fluoroquinolones
    - Vancomycin
    - Vancomycin related antibiotics
    - Other specified single antibiotics, which includes:
      - Aminoglycosides
      - Macrolides
      - Sulfonamides
      - Tetracyclines
  - Multiple antibiotics
  - Unspecified antibiotic
- Other antimicrobial drugs
  - Antifungal
  - Antimycobacterial (includes tuberculostatics)
    - Single antimycobacterial drug
    - Multiple antimycobacterial drugs
  - Antiparasitic, which includes:
    - Quinine and related compounds
  - Antiviral drugs
  - Multiple antimicrobial drugs
  - Other specified antimicrobial drugs
  - Unspecified antimicrobial drugs

Note: For MRSA infections, see the appropriate body system chapter.

ICD-10-CM Code/Documentation	
Z16.10	Resistance to unspecified beta lactam antibiotics
Z16.11	Resistance to penicillins
Z16.12	Extended spectrum beta lactamase (ESBL) resistance
Z16.19	Resistance to other specified beta lactam antibiotics
Z16.20	Resistance to unspecified antibiotic
Z16.21	Resistance to vancomycin
Z16.22	Resistance to vancomycin related antibiotics

ICD-10-CM Code/Documentation	
Z16.23	Resistance to quinolones and fluoroquinolones
Z16.24	Resistance to multiple antibiotics
Z16.29	Resistance to other single specified antibiotic
Z16.30	Resistance to unspecified antimicrobial drugs
Z16.31	Resistance to antiparasitic drug(s)
Z16.32	Resistance to antifungal drug(s)
Z16.33	Resistance to antiviral drugs
Z16.341	Resistance to single antimycobacterial drug
Z16.342	Resistance to multiple antimycobacterial drugs
Z16.35	Resistance to multiple antimicrobial drugs
Z16.39	Resistance to other specified antimicrobial drug

Documentation and Coding Example

Seventy-two-year-old Caucasian male is admitted to Rehabilitation Unit from Surgical Step Down Unit. Patient underwent emergency repair of a ruptured aortic aneurysm 22 days ago. His post-operative course has been complicated by ARDS, renal failure and sepsis. He has a G-Tube for supplemental nutrition. Foley catheter was discontinued one week ago. There is a Hep-Lock in his left forearm for IV antibiotics, site has no redness or swelling. T 97.6, P 100, R 16, BP 128/90, Wt. 138 lbs. On examination, this is a thin, frail, tired appearing elderly gentleman. He is oriented to person and place but becomes a little confused when asked for the date. He does know the month and year and with prompting comes up with an appropriate day of the week. PERRL, oral mucosa is pale and dry. Skin is warm and dry. Pulses are weak in both upper and lower extremities with decreased muscle tone and muscle wasting but no edema appreciated. Heart rate regular without bruit, rub or murmur. Breath sounds have fine scattered rales throughout with decreased sounds in the bases. Respirations are somewhat shallow and labored. O2 sat on 2 L O2 via NC is 96%. **There is a surgical scar down the midline of the abdomen extending from the xyphoid to just above the pubic bone. Distal and proximal ends are healing but a 2 cm open area remains just below the umbilicus.** A 4 x 4 gauze dressing has a small amount of yellow-green drainage. G-tube site is clean and the tube is patent. Abdomen firm with active bowel sounds. Male genitalia is normal. Transfer notes indicate the **abdominal wound is positive for vancomycin resistant enterococci**. He is currently receiving IV Synercid and appears to be responding well to this antibiotic. Patient will be in wound and skin isolation but can begin PT and OT. Speech will evaluate him for swallowing and order an appropriate diet.

Diagnosis Code(s)

T81.41XA Infection following procedure, superficial incisional surgical site, subsequent encounter

B95.2 Enterococcus as the cause of diseases classified elsewhere

Z16.21 Resistance to vancomycin

Coding Note(s)

The patient is being transferred to a rehabilitation unit where he will continue to receive antibiotic therapy for the postoperative infection. This is classified as aftercare. Multiple diagnosis codes are required to capture all aspects of his condition.

The aftercare is the first-listed diagnosis. Aftercare related to a post-operative wound infection is reported with a code from subcategory T81.4- in Chapter 19 Injuries, Poisonings, and Other Consequences of External Causes, so 7th character D for subsequent encounter is reported for this phase of his care. There is no mention of the incisional wound infection reaching a depth beyond the skin and subcutaneous tissues, so the postoperative wound infection is reported at the superficial incisional surgical site level. The microorganism, enterococcus, responsible for the infection is reported secondarily as is the drug resistance to vancomycin.

Pregnancy, Normal

Codes for normal pregnancy are for use when the patient is seen for normal, uncomplicated prenatal care and are always the first-listed diagnosis. Codes in category Z34 Encounter for supervision of normal pregnancy are for use in those circumstances when none of the problems or complications included in the codes for the Obstetrics chapter exist (a routine prenatal visit or postpartum care). Codes in category Z34 Encounter for supervision of normal pregnancy are always the first-listed diagnosis and are not to be used with any other code from the OB chapter.

Coding and Documentation Requirements

Identify encounter for supervision of pregnancy:

- Normal first pregnancy
- Other normal pregnancy
- Unspecified normal pregnancy

Identify trimester:

- First trimester
- Second trimester
- Third trimester
- Unspecified trimester

ICD-10-CM Code/Documentation	
Z34.00	Encounter for supervision of normal first pregnancy, unspecified trimester
Z34.01	Encounter for supervision of normal first pregnancy, first trimester
Z34.02	Encounter for supervision of normal first pregnancy, second trimester
Z34.03	Encounter for supervision of normal first pregnancy, third trimester
Z34.80	Encounter for supervision of other normal pregnancy, unspecified trimester
Z34.81	Encounter for supervision of other normal pregnancy, first trimester
Z34.82	Encounter for supervision of other normal pregnancy, second trimester
Z34.83	Encounter for supervision of other normal pregnancy, third trimester
Z34.90	Encounter for supervision of normal unspecified pregnancy, unspecified trimester
Z34.91	Encounter for supervision of normal unspecified pregnancy, first trimester
Z34.92	Encounter for supervision of normal unspecified pregnancy, second trimester
Z34.93	Encounter for supervision of normal unspecified pregnancy, third trimester

Documentation and Coding Example

Twenty-nine-year-old Black female is seen in OB Clinic for **routine monitoring of pregnancy**. Patient is a **primigravida now at 20 weeks gestation with a singleton male fetus per ultrasound**. She states she is feeling well. Nausea and tiredness have gone away. She is starting to wear maternity clothes and is enjoying the attention as she shares the news of her pregnancy with friends and family. P 84, R 14, BP 122/72, Wt. 138 lbs. Urine sample is dipstick negative for protein and glucose. On examination, the FHB is heard via Doppler, strong and regular at 136 bpm. Fundal height is consistent with dates. Patient states she feels fetal movement daily, denies abdominal pain, discomfort with intercourse, bleeding or vaginal discharge. Her appetite is improving, she is eating a variety of foods and has no unusual cravings. Questions are answered. She is counseled regarding what to expect in the next few weeks and what symptoms should be promptly reported. RTC in 3 weeks.

Diagnosis Code(s)

Z34.02 Encounter for supervision of normal first pregnancy, second trimester

Coding Note(s)

The patient is being seen for a normal uncomplicated first pregnancy and she is in her second trimester so code Z34.02 is assigned. The timeframes for the trimesters are indicated at the beginning of Chapter 15.

Routine General Medical Examination Newborn/Infant/Child/Adult

Routine encounters for medical examinations include well newborn examination, infant/child check-ups, and annual medical examinations of adults. A newborn is defined as being under 29 days old. An infant/child is defined as being over 28 days old. Since these are some of the most frequently reported codes from Chapter 21 in ICD-10-CM, they have been arranged in the first code block, Z00-Z13 Persons encountering health services for examinations. Codes for routine medical examinations are contained in the first category, Z00 Encounters for general examination without complaint, suspected or reported diagnosis. One of the key things to note is that codes for infants, children, and adults are specific as to whether or not there are any abnormal findings on the examination. For newborns, there is a coding instruction indicating that additional codes should be assigned for any abnormal findings.

Coding and Documentation Requirements

Identify routine health check:

- Adult
- Child
- Newborn
    - Under 8 days old
    - 8-28 days old

Identify presence/absence of abnormal findings:

- With abnormal findings
- Without abnormal findings

Use an additional code for any abnormal findings.

ICD-10-CM Code/Documentation	
Z00.110	Health examination for newborn under 8 days old
Z00.111	Health examination for newborn 8 to 28 days old
Z00.121	Encounter for routine child health examination with abnormal findings
Z00.129	Encounter for routine child health examination without abnormal findings
Z00.00	Encounter for general adult medical examination without abnormal findings
Z00.01	Encounter for general adult medical examination with abnormal findings

Documentation and Coding Example

Fifty-one-year-old Hispanic male presents to PCP for **routine physical**. He is feeling well and has no health concerns since his last visit 13 months ago. Patient is a high school history teacher, his wife works in an elementary school office and their daughter is now 10 years old. He is finished with classes for the summer and looking forward to a week of relaxation before he tackles some home repair projects. He admits to a pretty sedentary lifestyle and he knows he has gained weight this past year.

T 97.4, P 90, R 14, BP 144/72, Wt. 213, Ht. 71 inches. On examination, this is a well-developed, well-nourished adult male. PERRL, neck supple without lymphadenopathy. Patent nares, there is a slight deviation of the septum toward the right but it does not obstruct air flow. Mucous membranes moist and pink, there is marked atrophy of tonsil and adenoid tissue. The posterior pharynx has a cobblestone appearance suggestive of allergies but patient denies symptoms. Heart rate regular, carotid arteries are without bruit. Peripheral pulses present and WNL. Breath sounds clear and equal bilaterally. Abdomen mildly obese with active bowel sounds. Liver palpated at 2 cm below the RCM, spleen is not palpable. No evidence of hernia. Testicles smooth, penis uncircumcised, foreskin retracts easily, hygiene excellent. Rectal exam shows good sphincter tone and a small, smooth prostate. Labs were drawn prior to this appointment and results are reviewed with patient. His BGL is normal. Cholesterol and triglycerides are in the high normal range. Of concern however is **elevated protein in his urine**.

Diagnosis: **Routine health exam, with routine labs showing elevated protein in urine.**

Plan: Patient is referred to Nephrology for complete evaluation of his renal function.

Diagnosis Code(s)

Z00.01 Encounter for general adult medical examination with abnormal findings

R80.9 Proteinuria, unspecified

Coding Note(s)

The patient has an elevated level of protein in his urine which is an abnormal finding that could be indicative of kidney disease. The code for encounter for general adult health examination with abnormal findings is sequenced first since the routine examination was the reason for the visit. The abnormal laboratory finding is reported as an additional diagnosis.

Summary

Codes that report factors influencing health and contact with health services require specific documentation of the reason for the encounter. This may involve identification of additional factors that may affect future care of the patient such as an annual adult preventive medicine examination in which there are abnormal findings. It may involve specific documentation related to the type of aftercare provided, such as aftercare related to prosthetic joint explantation which requires identification of the joint, or it may require specific documentation related to other factors influencing health such as patient medical noncompliance (Z91.1-) which now allows identification of various reasons including financial hardship or age-related debility. Coders also need to be aware of the classification of aftercare codes for injuries, poisoning, and certain other consequences of external causes and coding conventions related to reporting these aftercare services. A careful review of current documentation related to encounters/visits for these factors influencing health status is required in order to ensure that any documentation deficiencies are identified and corrected.

Resources

Documentation checklists are included in Appendix A for the following factors influencing health and contact with health care services:

- Examination, administrative
- Examination, general medical/specialty
- Examination, gynecological/contraception
- Examination, obstetrics/reproductive

Chapter 20 Quiz

1. Which code for factors influencing health and contact with health services would NOT be reported as the first listed diagnosis?
   a. Z00.01 Encounter for general adult medical examination with abnormal findings
   b. Z16.11 Resistance to penicillins
   c. Z38.00 Single liveborn infant, delivered vaginally
   d. Z51.0 Encounter for antineoplastic radiation therapy
2. Status Z codes are defined as:
   a. Codes that indicate that a patient is either a carrier of a disease or has the sequelae or residual of a past disease or condition
   b. Codes that explain a patient's past medical condition that no longer exists and is not receiving any treatment, but that has the potential for recurrence, and therefore may require continued monitoring
   c. Codes that cover situations when the initial treatment of a disease has been performed and the patient requires continued care during the healing or recovery phase, or for the long-term consequences of the disease
   d. Codes that explain continuing surveillance following completed treatment of a disease, condition, or injury
3. Identify which circumstance requires the use of a screening code.
   a. Testing is performed to rule out or confirm a suspected diagnosis because the patient has some sign or symptom
   b. A screening, such as a pap smear, is performed during a routine examination
   c. Testing is performed in an apparently well (symptomless) individual for early detection of a disease
   d. An office visit for a specific health problem in which a test is performed to more specifically identify the health problem
4. What information is required to report the most specific code for supervision of a normal first pregnancy?
   a. Number of fetuses
   b. Results of routine laboratory tests
   c. The number of prenatal visits
   d. Weeks of gestation or trimester
5. Identify which statement is true related to Z codes.
   a. Z codes may be used only in the outpatient setting
   b. Certain Z codes may only be used as a first listed or principal diagnosis.
   c. Z codes describe both reason for the encounter and the procedure performed so a procedure code is not reported additionally
   d. All of the above statements are true
6. The physician has documented that the patient is being seen for an annual preventive exam. On this visit, the physician notes that the patient has an elevated blood pressure of 150/96 which has not been present on previous visits. He wants to determine if this is an isolated finding or if the patient has hypertension and requests that the patient return for blood pressure checks. Identify the correct assignment and sequencing of the diagnosis codes.
   a. Z00.00, I10
   b. R03.0, Z00.01
   c. Z00.01, R03.0
   d. I10, Z00.01
7. A code from category Z79 Long-term (current) drug therapy would be reported under which circumstance?
   a. For a patient receiving a medication for an extended period as a prophylactic measure
   b. For a patient being administered a medication for a brief period of time to treat an acute illness or injury
   c. For a patient who is addicted to a drug
   d. For a patient receiving medications for detoxification or maintenance programs to prevent withdrawal symptoms due to drug dependence
8. Identify the false statement related to code Z92.82 Status post administration of tPA (rtPA) in a different facility within the last 24 hours.
   a. Code Z92.82 is reported on the receiving hospitals medical record when a patient is received by transfer into a facility and documentation indicates they were administered tissue plasminogen activator (tPA) within the last 24 hours prior to admission to the current facility
   b. Do not report Z92.82 if the patient is still receiving the tPA at the time they are received into the current facility
   c. The appropriate code for the condition for which the tPA was administered (such as cerebrovascular disease or myocardial infarction) should be assigned first
   d. Code Z92.82 is only applicable to the receiving facility record and not to the transferring facility record
9. In what category of Z codes is code Z77.22 Exposure to tobacco smoke (second hand smoke) classified?
   a. Status
   b. History (of)
   c. Miscellaneous
   d. Contact/Exposure
10. Preoperative examination and pre-procedural laboratory examination Z codes are for use under what circumstances?
    a. When the primary care physician is working up a patient for signs and symptoms to determine if a procedure is required
    b. When a specialist is evaluating a patient for a condition that may require surgery
    c. In those situations when a patient is being cleared for a procedure or surgery and no treatment is given
    d. All of the above

See next page for answers and rationales.

Chapter 20 Answers and Rationales

1. Which code for factors influencing health and contact with health services would NOT be reported as the first listed diagnosis?

   b. Z16.11 Resistance to penicillins

   Rationale: *Codes for drug-resistance to antibiotics are listed as secondary diagnoses. The condition being treated, in this case an infection such as bacterial pneumonia or wound infection, is reported as the first-listed diagnosis.*

2. Status Z codes are defined as:

   a. Codes that indicate that a patient is either a carrier of a disease or has the sequelae or residual of a past disease or condition

   Rationale: *Status codes indicate that a patient is either a carrier of a disease or has the sequelae or residual of a past disease. The other definitions listed are for history (personal) Z codes, aftercare Z codes, and follow-up Z codes respectively.*

3. Identify which circumstance requires the use of a screening code.

   c. Testing is performed in an apparently well (symptomless) individual for early detection of a disease

   Rationale: *Screening is performed for the early detection of disease so that prompt treatment can be provided for those who test positive for the disease. Inherent screenings such as a pap smear performed during an annual examination does not require a screening code. The other two answers describe diagnostic exams and the code for the sign, symptom, or medical condition would be reported not a screening code.*

4. What information is required to report the most specific code for supervision of a normal first pregnancy?

   d. Weeks of gestation or trimester

   Rationale: *Supervision of normal pregnancy is specific to trimester so either the weeks of gestation or the trimester must be documented.*

5. Identify which statement is true related to Z codes.

   b. Certain Z codes may only be used as a first listed or principal diagnosis.

   Rationale: *While most Z codes may be used as first-listed or additional diagnosis, certain Z codes may only be used as a first-listed or principal diagnosis. Z codes may be used in any healthcare setting not just outpatient settings. Z codes describe the reason for the encounter, but they are not used for reporting the procedure which must be reported with a CPT, HCPCS or ICD-10-PCS procedure code.*

6. The physician has documented that the patient is being seen for an annual preventive exam. On this visit, the physician notes that the patient has an elevated blood pressure of 150/96 which has not been present on previous visits. He wants to determine if this is an isolated finding or if the patient has hypertension and requests that the patient return for blood pressure checks. Identify the correct assignment and sequencing of the diagnosis codes.

   c. Z00.01, R03.0

   Rationale: *The code for encounter for general adult medical examination with abnormal findings is reported as the first listed diagnosis. Since the physician has not diagnosed the patient as having hypertension, a symptom code for the elevated blood pressure is also reported to identify the abnormal finding.*

7. A code from category Z79 Long-term (current) drug therapy would be reported under which circumstance?

   a. For a patient receiving a medication for an extended period as a prophylactic measure

   Rationale: *Codes from this category indicate a patient's continuous use of a prescribed drug for the long-term treatment of a condition or for prophylactic use. Assign a code from category Z79 if the patient is receiving a medication for an extended period as a prophylactic measure (such as for the prevention of deep vein thrombosis) or as treatment of a chronic condition (such as arthritis) or a disease requiring a lengthy course treatment (such as cancer). A code from category Z79 is not assigned for medications being administered briefly to treat an acute condition, for patients who have addictions to drugs, or for patients with drug dependency receiving drugs for detox or on maintenance programs.*

8. Identify the false statement related to code Z92.82 Status post administration of tPA (rtPA) in a different facility within the last 24 hours.

   b. Do not report Z92.82 if the patient is still receiving the tPA at the time they are received into the current facility

   Rationale: *Code Z92.82 is reported even if the patient is still receiving the tPA at the time they are received by the receiving facility.*

9. In what category of Z codes is code Z77.22 Exposure to tobacco smoke (second hand smoke) classified?

   d. Contact/Exposure

   Rationale: *Category Z77 indicates contact with or suspected exposure to substances that are known to hazardous to health. Code Z77.22 Exposure to tobacco smoke (second hand smoke) is included in this category.*

10. Preoperative examination and pre-procedural laboratory examination Z codes are for use under what circumstances?

    c. In those situations when a patient is being cleared for a procedure or surgery and no treatment is given

    Rationale: *Preoperative examination and pre-procedural laboratory examination Z codes are for use only in those situations when a patient is being cleared for a procedure or surgery and no treatment is given.*

Chapter 21
EXTERNAL CAUSES OF MORBIDITY

Introduction

Codes for external causes of morbidity are found in Chapter 21. External cause codes classify environmental events and other circumstances as the cause of injury and other adverse effects. Codes in this chapter are always reported as a secondary code with the nature of the condition or injury reported as the first-listed diagnosis. External cause codes are most frequently reported with codes in Chapter 19 Injury, Poisoning and Certain Other Consequences of External Causes (SØØ-T88). There are also conditions listed in other chapters that may also be due to an external cause. For example, when a condition such as a myocardial infarction is specifically stated as due to or precipitated by strenuous activity, such as shoveling snow, then external cause codes should be reported to identify the activity, place, and external cause status.

While not all third party payers require reporting of external cause codes, they are a valuable source of information to public health departments and other state agencies regarding the causes of death, injury, poisoning, and adverse effects. In fact, more than half of all states have mandated that hospitals collect external cause data using statewide hospital discharge data systems. Another third of all states routinely collect external cause data even though it is not mandated. There are also 15 states that have mandated statewide hospital emergency department data systems requiring collection of external cause data.

External cause of injury codes provide a framework for systematically collecting patient health related information on the external cause of death, injury, poisoning, and adverse effects. These codes define the manner of the death or injury, the mechanism, the place of occurrence of the event, the activity, and the status of the person at the time death or injury occurred. The manner of death or injury refers to whether the cause was unintentional/accidental, self-inflicted, assault, or undetermined. Mechanism describes how the injury occurred, such as a motor vehicle accident, a fall, contact with a sharp object or power tool, or being caught between moving objects. Place identifies where the injury occurred, such as a personal residence, playground, street, or place of employment. Activity indicates the activity of the person at the time the injury occurred such as swimming, running, bathing, or cooking. External cause status is used to indicate the status of the person at the time death or injury occurred such as work done for pay, military activity, or volunteer activity.

The table below lists the ICD-1Ø-CM chapter blocks for external causes.

ICD-1Ø-CM Blocks	
VØØ-V99	Transport Accidents
VØØ-VØ9	Pedestrian Injured in Transport Accident
V1Ø-V19	Pedal Cycle Rider Injured in Transport Accident
V2Ø-V29	Motorcycle Rider Injured in Transport Accident
V3Ø-V39	Occupant of 3-Wheeled Vehicle Injured in Transport Accident
V4Ø-V49	Car Occupant Injured Transport Accident
V5Ø-V59	Occupant of Pick-up Truck or Van Injured in Transport Accident
V6Ø-V69	Occupant of Heavy Transport Vehicle Injured in Transport Accident
V7Ø-V79	Bus Occupant Injured in Transport Accident
V8Ø-V89	Other Land Transport Accidents
V9Ø-V94	Water Transport Accidents
V95-V97	Air and Space Transport Accidents
V98-V99	Other and Unspecified Transport Accidents
WØØ-X58	Other External Causes of Accidental Injury
WØØ-W19	Slipping, Tripping, Stumbling and Falls
W2Ø-W49	Exposure to Inanimate Mechanical Forces
W5Ø-W64	Exposure to Animate Mechanical forces
W65-W74	Accidental Non-Transport Drowning and Submersion
W85-W99	Exposure to Electric Current, Radiation, and Extreme Ambient Air Temperature and Pressure
XØØ-XØ8	Exposure to Smoke, Fire, and Flames
X1Ø-X19	Contact with Heat and Hot Substances
X3Ø-X39	Exposure to Forces of Nature
X52-X58	Accidental Exposure to Other Specified Factors
X71-X83	Intentional Self-Harm
X92-YØ8	Assault
Y21-Y33	Event of Undetermined Intent
Y35-Y38	Legal Intervention, Operations of War, Military Operations, and Terrorism
Y62-Y84	Complications of Medical and Surgical Care
Y62-Y69	Misadventures to Patients During Surgical and Medical Care
Y7Ø-Y82	Medical Devices Associated With Adverse Incidents in Diagnostic and Therapeutic Use
Y83-Y84	Surgical and Other medical Procedures as the Cause of Abnormal Reaction of the Patient, or of Later Complication, Without Mention of Misadventure at the Time of the Procedure
Y9Ø-Y99	Supplementary Factors Related to Causes of Morbidity Classified Elsewhere
Note: Block Y9Ø-Y99 includes codes for place of occurrence, activity, and external cause status	

Alphabetic Index to External Causes

There is a separate index for external causes in ICD-10-CM. It follows the Table of Drugs and Chemicals.

Chapter Guidelines

Guidelines for Chapter 21 External Causes of Morbidity are provided so that there is standardization in the assignment of these codes. The external causes of morbidity codes should never be sequenced as the first-listed or principal diagnosis.

External cause codes are always secondary codes and can be used in any healthcare setting. External cause codes provide a means of capturing data on injuries, which is used for injury research and the development of prevention strategies.

Most recent guidelines added in 2014 clarify that there is no national requirement for mandatory ICD-10-CM external cause code reporting. Unless a provider is subject to a state-based external cause code reporting mandate or these codes are required by a particular payer, reporting of ICD-10-CM codes in Chapter 20, External Causes of Morbidity, is not required. However, in the absence of a mandatory reporting requirement, providers are encouraged to voluntarily report external cause codes, as they provide valuable data for injury research and evaluation of injury prevention strategies.

General External Cause Coding Guidelines

The general external cause coding guidelines relate to all external cause codes, including those that describe the cause, the intent, the place of occurrence, the activity of the patient, and the patient's status at the time of the injury. There are more specific guidelines that relate to each particular type of external cause codes. The general guidelines are as follows:

External cause codes may be used with any code in ranges A00.0-T88.9 or Z00-Z99 when the health condition is due to an external cause. The most common health conditions related to external causes are those for injuries in categories S00-T88

- It is appropriate to assign external cause codes to infections and diseases in categories A00-R99 and Z00-Z99 that are the result of an external cause, such as a heart attack resulting from strenuous activity.
- There are multiple types of external cause codes that are used to completely identify the cause, intent, place of occurrence, activity and status for injuries. The majority of external cause codes are assigned for the entire length of treatment for the condition resulting from the external cause. Some of the external cause codes are only reported on the initial visit.
- The appropriate 7th character must be assigned to identify the encounter as the initial encounter, subsequent encounter, or sequela
- Assign as many external cause codes as needed to fully explain each cause. If only one external cause code can be recorded, assign the code most related to the principal diagnosis
- Selection of the appropriate external cause code is guided by the Alphabetic Index to External Causes and by Includes and Excludes notes in the Tabular List
- External cause codes are never the principal or first-listed diagnosis
- Certain external cause codes are combination codes that describe sequential events resulting in an injury, such as a fall from striking against an object. The injury may be due to either or both events. The code assigned should correspond to the sequence of events regardless of which event caused the most serious injury
- No external cause code is required if the external cause and intent are captured by a code from another chapter. Codes for poisoning, adverse effect, and underdosing of drugs, medicaments, and biological substances in categories T36-T50 and toxic effects of substances chiefly nonmedicinal as to source in categories T51-T65 capture both the external cause and the intent.

Place of Occurrence, Activity, and Status Codes

When applicable, place of occurrence (Y92), activity (Y93), and external cause status (Y99) codes are sequenced after the main external cause codes. Regardless of the number of external cause codes assigned to describe the cause generally, only one place of occurrence, one activity, and one external cause status code is assigned. In the rare instance that a new injury occurs during hospitalization, an additional place of occurrence code may be assigned.

Place of Occurrence Guidelines

A code from category Y92 Place of occurrence of the external cause is assigned to identify the location of the patient at the time of injury or other health condition. Place of occurrence codes are secondary codes for use after other external cause codes.

- A place of occurrence code is used only *once* at the initial encounter for treatment
- 7th characters are not used for place of occurrence codes in category Y92
- Only one code from category Y92 is recorded in the medical record unless a new injury occurs during hospitalization, then an additional place of occurrence code may be assigned
- A place of occurrence code is used in conjunction with an activity code from category Y93
- If the place of occurrence is not documented or not applicable, DO NOT assign code Y92.9 Unspecified place or not applicable

Activity Code Guidelines

A code from category Y93 Activity code is assigned to describe the activity of the patient at the time the injury or other health condition occurred.

- An activity code is used only *once* at the initial encounter for treatment
- Only one code from category Y93 is recorded in the medical record
- An activity code is used with a place of occurrence code from category Y92
- Use an activity code with external cause and intent codes if identifying the activity provides additional information about the event
- Activity codes DO NOT apply to poisonings, adverse effects, misadventures, or sequela

- If the activity is not stated, DO NOT assign code Y93.9 Unspecified activity

External Cause Status Guidelines

A code from category Y99 External cause status should be assigned whenever any other external cause code is assigned for an encounter, including an activity code, except for the events noted below. Guidelines are as follows:

- Assign a code from category Y99 to indicate the work status of the person at the time the event occurred
- The status code indicates that the event occurred during a
- Civilian work activity
- Military work activity
- Non-work activity, such as a student, volunteer, or leisure activity
- Assign a code from category Y99 when applicable with other external cause codes, such as transport accidents or falls
- External cause status codes do not apply to poisoning, adverse effects, misadventures, or late effects
- DO NOT assign a code from category Y99 if no other external cause codes (cause, activity) are applicable to the encounter
- An external cause status code is used only *once* at the initial encounter for treatment
- Only one code from category Y99 should be recorded in the medical record
- DO NOT assign code Y99.9 Unspecified external cause status if the status is not stated

Reporting Format Limits to the Number of External Cause Codes

If the reporting format limits the number of external cause codes that can be reported, external cause codes should be reported in the following order:

- First report the code for the external cause/intent most related to the principal diagnosis
- If the reporting format allows capture of additional external cause codes, next report the cause/intent, including medical misadventures of additional events
- Codes for the above described external cause(s)/intent(s) should be reported rather than the codes for place, activity, or external cause status

Multiple External Cause Coding Guidelines

Some external cause circumstances may require that more than one external cause code be reported to fully describe the external cause of an illness, injury, or poisoning. Sequencing of external cause codes are prioritized as follows:

- For two or more events causing separate injuries, the external cause codes should be assigned in the following order:
  - External cause codes for child and adult abuse take priority over all other external cause codes
  - External cause codes for terrorism events take priority over all other external cause codes except child and adult abuse
  - External cause codes for cataclysmic events take priority over all other external cause codes except child and adult abuse, and terrorism
  - External cause codes for transport accidents take priority over all other external cause codes except child and adult abuse, terrorism, and cataclysmic events
- Activity and external cause status codes are assigned following all causal (intent) external cause codes
- The first-listed external cause code should correspond to the cause of the most serious diagnosis due to an assault, accident, or self-harm following the order of hierarchy listed above

Child and Adult Abuse Guidelines

Adult and child abuse and neglect are classified as assault. Assault codes may be used to indicate the external cause of an injury resulting from the confirmed abuse. For confirmed cases of abuse, neglect, and maltreatment, when the perpetrator is known, a code from Y07 Perpetrator of maltreatment and neglect should accompany any other assault codes.

Unknown or Undetermined Intent Guidelines

The following guidelines apply to assignment of codes for unknown or undetermined intent:

- If the intent (accident, self-harm, assault) of the cause of an injury or other condition is unknown or unspecified, code the intent as accidental
- All transport accident categories assume accidental intent
- A code for undetermined intent is assigned only when the documentation in the medical record specified that the intent cannot be determined

Sequelae (Late Effects) of External Cause Guidelines

Sequelae are reported using the code for the external cause with the 7th character extension 'S' for sequela:

- Use for any condition described as a late effect or sequela resulting from a previous injury
- A sequela external cause code should never be used with a related current nature of injury code
- Use a sequela external cause code for subsequent visits when a late effect of the initial injury is being treated
- Do not use a late effect external cause code for subsequent visits for follow-up care (e.g., to assess healing or to receive rehabilitative therapy) of the injury or poisoning when no late effect of the injury has been documented

Terrorism Guidelines

External cause codes for terrorism are used to identify injuries resulting from the unlawful use of force or violence against persons or property to intimidate or coerce a government, the civilian population, or any segment thereof, in furtherance of a political or social objective. Terrorism external cause codes are assigned when the cause of an injury is identified by the Federal Government (FBI) as terrorism and should be assigned as follows:

- The first listed external cause code should be a code from category Y38 Terrorism
- Use an additional code from category Y92 to identify the place of occurrence
- More than one code from category Y38 may be assigned if the injury is the result of more than one mechanism of terrorism

When the cause of injury is the result of suspected terrorism:

- DO NOT assign a code from category Y38
- Suspected terrorism is classified as assault

For conditions occurring subsequent to the terrorist event:

- Assign code Y38.9 Terrorism, secondary effects
- DO NOT assign code Y38.9 for conditions that are due to the initial terrorist act
- Code Y38.9 may be assigned with another code from category Y38 when there is an injury due to the initial terrorist event and an injury that is a subsequent result of the terrorist event

General Documentation Requirements

Increased granularity in ICD-10-CM codes requires specific documentation of cause, intent, place of occurrence, and activity at the time of the injury or other health condition. With the ICD-10-CM code set, separate external cause codes are not required for poisoning, adverse effects, or underdosing of drugs and other substances (T36-T50), or for toxic effect of nonmedicinal substances (T51-T65), since the external cause is now captured in a combination code from Chapter 19. External cause codes do require a 7th character to identify the episode of care. The 7th characters used in Chapter 20 are the same as those used in Chapter 19 and the characters have the same definitions. The characters and definitions are as follows:

A Initial encounter. This is the period when the patient is receiving active treatment for the injury, poisoning, or other consequences of an external cause. An 'A' may be assigned on more than one claim.

D Subsequent encounter. This is an encounter after the active phase of treatment when the patient is receiving routine care for the injury or poisoning during the period of healing or recovery.

S Sequela. The 7th character extension 'S' is assigned for complications or conditions that arise as a direct result of an injury.

Classification of Codes

Reviewing the code blocks provides a good overview of how the general classifications of external causes are arranged. More detailed information on classification of codes is provided in the code specific examples that follow.

Combination Codes

As was discussed in Chapter 19 Injury, Poisoning, and Other Consequences of External Causes, there are combination codes for two blocks of codes including: T36-T50 Poisoning by, adverse effect of and underdosing of drugs, medicaments, and biological substances; and T51-T65 Toxic effects of substances chiefly nonmedicinal as to source. These combination codes identify both the substance and the intent which includes accidental (unintentional), intentional self-harm, assault, and undetermined for poisoning and toxic effects of nonmedicinal substances. This means that there are no external cause codes for these conditions in the external cause chapter.

Code-Specific Documentation Requirements

Many examples of external cause coding were provided in Chapter 19 covering injury and poisoning. Some of the same scenarios are used in this chapter but the focus of the discussion here is on the documentation elements required to capture the most specific external cause codes. In this section, ranges of codes used to describe the same type of accidents are first discussed and then a specific example is provided of the documentation elements for a specific accident category or subcategory in that range of codes.

Accidental Falls

The external cause code categories that capture falls are found in block W00-W19 Slipping, tripping, stumbling, and falls. Category W09 Fall on and from playground equipment has three specific codes—for slide (W09.0-), swing (W09.1-), and jungle gym (W09.2-) with a fourth code for other playground equipment (W09.8-). Another example of code specificity is found in category W13 Fall from, out of or through building or structure. Codes in category W13 are specific to balcony (W13.0), bridge (W13.1-), roof (W13.2-), through floor (W13.3-), and from, out of, or through window (W13.4-). There are additional codes for fall from, out of or through other building or structure (W13.8-) and fall from, out of or through building, not otherwise specified (W13.9-).

Codes for falls also capture external causes of accidental injury due to jumping or diving into water in addition to falling into water. Codes in categories W00-W19 are specific to accidental fall injuries. Falls involving an assault are found in categories Y01-Y02. Falls involving assault are specific to pushing from high place (Y01) and pushing in front of moving object (Y02).

Other Fall from One Level to Another

An example of the coding and documentation requirements for other fall from one level to another along with some of the ICD-10-CM external cause codes is provided below.

Coding and Documentation Requirements

Identify other fall from one level to another:

- Fall down embankment
- Fall from/out of grocery cart
- Fall from tree
- Other fall from one level to another, which includes
  - Fall from cherry picker
  - Fall from lifting device
  - Fall from mobile elevated work platform
  - Fall from sky lift

Identify episode of care:

- Initial
- Subsequent
- Sequela

ICD-10-CM Code/Documentation	
W14.-	Fall from tree
W17.81-	Fall down embankment (hill)
W17.82-	Fall from (out of) grocery cart
W17.89-	Other fall from one level to another
Note: A 7th digit is required to identify the episode of care.	

Documentation and Coding Example

Thirty-nine-year-old male presents to ED with c/o moderate to severe pain in his back after **falling** approximately 15 feet from a boulder while **rock climbing**. Accident occurred approximately 2 hours ago. Patient is a well-developed, well-nourished male who looks younger than his stated age. He is muscular and very tan. He states he is a professional guide leading hiking tours and rock climbing expeditions. The accident today occurred in his **leisure time** on a familiar rock face and was witnessed by friends. As he descended from the top of the rock, his equipment malfunctioned and he dropped rapidly landing with a hard jolt upright on both legs. He felt an immediate sharp pain in the mid back which is relieved somewhat by lying flat. He denies pain in his hips, knees, or ankles and was able to hike approximately 0.5 miles to a vehicle. On examination: Temperature 99 degrees, HR 72, RR 12, BP 114/60. Skin warm, slightly diaphoretic, outdoor temperature is in upper 80s. O2 saturation on RA 96%. PERRL, oriented x 3. No cervical spine tenderness and cranial nerves are grossly intact. Motor and sensory function is intact to upper extremities. Breath sounds clear and equal bilaterally, HR regular, no murmur or muffling of heart sounds appreciated. No visual deformities to spine but there is exquisite tenderness with muscle guarding at level of T10 to L4. There is no sign of crepitus. He has limited ROM when attempting flexion, extension, and rotation of spine due to pain. There are no neurological deficits in lower extremities. IV started in left forearm, D5 LR infusing. Medicated for pain with MS 2 mg IV push with good relief. AP and lateral spine x-rays reveal a possible **wedge compression fracture at T12. CT confirms wedge compression fracture involving the anterior column at T12**. Orthopedic consult obtained. Patient fitted with TLSO brace and discharged home with oral narcotic pain medication and instructions to schedule a follow-up in orthopedic clinic in 1 week.

Diagnosis Code(s)

S22.080A Wedge compression fracture of T11-T12 vertebra, initial encounter for closed fracture

W17.89XA Other fall from one level to another, initial encounter

Y93.31 Activity, mountain climbing, rock climbing, and wall climbing

Y92.838 Other recreation area as the place of occurrence of the external cause

Y99.8 Other external cause status

Coding Note(s)

There is no specific code for a fall from a boulder so code W17.89xA is assigned to identify the fall from one level to another and the episode of care as the initial encounter. The code for the place of occurrence is more specific, identifying the place as "other recreation area." Y99.8 Other external cause status, which includes leisure activity, is used instead of Y99.0 Civilian activity done for income or pay, because the injury occurred during a leisure activity.

Assault Injuries

Injuries caused by an assault are classified in block X92-Y09. The Includes note under assault lists homicide. There are separate codes for various types of firearms including: handgun, rifle, shotgun, and larger firearm. Examples of codes classified in this code block also include assaults by drowning or submersion; explosive material; smoke, fire, and flames; steam, hot vapors, and hot objects; sharp or blunt objects; pushing from a high place; pushing or placing victim in front of a moving object; motor vehicle; and bodily force. Also included in this code block are codes that identify the perpetrator of an assault classified as maltreatment or neglect (Y07). Codes in category Y07 are to be used only in cases of confirmed abuse which is coded to category T74 Adult and child abuse, neglect, and other maltreatment, confirmed.

The example used in the scenario below is an assault by a sharp object. The coding and documentation requirements and code comparisons for this type of scenario are listed below.

Coding and Documentation Requirements

Identify the sharp object:

- Knife
- Glass
- Sword/dagger
- Other sharp object
- Unspecified sharp object

Identify the episode of care:

- Initial encounter
- Subsequent encounter
- Sequela

Assault with Sharp Object

ICD-10-CM Code/Documentation	
X99.0-	Assault by sharp glass
X99.1-	Assault by knife
X99.2-	Assault by sword or dagger
X99.8-	Assault by other sharp object
X99.9-	Assault by unspecified sharp object

Documentation and Coding Example

Patient is a 21-year-old male who walks into ED with a **stab wound to the abdomen**. He states he was at work attempting to mediate a dispute between two employees at his **family's restaurant** when the stabbing occurred. On examination, this is a soft spoken, slightly built young man holding a bloody towel to the right abdomen. He is alert and oriented. HR 100, RR 16, BP 98/60. There is a **single wound measuring 2 cm in the RUQ**, which is not actively bleeding at this time. He states the weapon used was a small paring knife with a blade not more than 3 inches long. Abdominal examination is relatively benign except for the wound and mild tenderness to palpation in RUQ. Breath sounds are clear, equal bilaterally. HR regular with NSR on monitor. IV started in right forearm, blood drawn for CBC, Chemistry Panel, PT, PTT, Type and hold. Flat plate of abdomen is negative for free air. FAST shows some accumulation of fluid in the RUQ along the edge of the liver. Patient is hemodynamically stable. Decision made to take him to CT for abdominal scan to r/o or establish intra-peritoneal injury. Spiral CT with contrast revealed a **Grade 2 liver injury with a 1.5 cm parenchymal laceration and a 1.5 cm thick subcapsular/parenchymal hematoma**. Patient will be admitted to ICU for observation. Wound irrigated, closed in layers around a drain. He is started on broad spectrum antibiotics. NPO. Transferred to unit in stable condition.

ICU Note: Patient stable overnight. Repeat CT shows no change in hematoma size. Minimal serosanguinous fluid returning from drain, the wound edges are slightly red but suture line is clean. Abdomen soft with bowel sounds present in all quadrants. Pain is localized at the site of the wound and has been well controlled with IV Morphine. Started clear liquid diet and advance as tolerated. Up in a chair, advance activity as tolerated. He is transferred to surgical floor for continued observation.

Floor Note Day 1: Continues to make good recovery. Pain controlled on oral Vicodin. Tolerating soft diet, ambulates to BR. IV heplocked. Continues on antibiotics. Wound healing well, drain removed. Repeat CT ordered for tomorrow. If no change in hematoma size, he will be discharged.

Floor Note Day 2: Repeat CT shows subcapsular/parenchymal hematoma to be resolving, size is now 1 cm thick. He is discharged home with oral Vicodin and antibiotics. He will be seen in Surgical Clinic in 5 days for wound check.

Diagnosis Code(s)

S36.115A	Moderate laceration of liver, initial encounter
S31.630A	Puncture wound without foreign body of abdominal wall, right upper quadrant with penetration into peritoneal cavity, initial encounter
X99.1XXA	Assault by knife, initial encounter
Y92.511	Restaurant or café as the place of occurrence of the external cause
Y99.0	Civilian activity done for income or pay

Coding Note(s)

The code for the cause and intent is specific to an assault with a knife. The place of occurrence is specific to a restaurant or café. The patient was at work, so the external cause status is a civilian activity done for income or pay.

Natural and Environmental Accidents

Some of the external causes listed as exposure to forces of nature are listed in Chapter 19 Injury, Poisoning, and Certain Other Consequences of External Causes. External cause codes in this chapter are combination codes that identify the injury or health condition and the external cause. Codes that are listed in Chapter 19 include:

- Bites and stings by venomous animals and insects, and poisoning by toxic plants in category T63 Toxic effect of contact with venous animals and plants
- Abandonment or neglect of helpless individuals in category T74 Adult and child abuse, neglect, and other maltreatment
- Effects of lightning and motion sickness in category T75 Other and unspecified effects of other external causes

Codes for external causes of injury caused by nonvenomous animals due to mechanical forces such as bites, scratches, or being struck or gored by the animal are listed in categories W53-W64. All of the external causes related to forces of nature are listed in categories X30-X39. External causes of injury and health conditions classified in this code block include: excessive natural heat and cold; sunlight; earthquakes, avalanches, and volcanoes; landslides and other earth movements; cataclysmic storms such as hurricanes, tornadoes, blizzards, and dust storms; tidal waves and floods; and exposure to other forces of nature.

Coding and Documentation Requirements

Identify the animal:

- Alligator
- Amphibians
  - Frogs
  - Toads
  - Other nonvenomous amphibians
- Arthropod/insect
- Birds
  - Chicken
  - Duck
  - Goose
  - Psittacines
    - Macaw
    - Parrot
    - Other psittacines
  - Turkey
  - Other birds
- Crocodile
- Mammal (other than marine mammal)
  - Cat
  - Dog
  - Hoof stock
    - Cow
    - Horse
    - Other hoof stock
  - Pig
  - Raccoon

  - Rodent
    - Mouse
    - Rat
    - Squirrel
    - Other rodent
  - Other nonvenomous mammal
- Marine animal
  - Marine mammal
    - Dolphin
    - Orca
    - Sea lion
    - Other marine mammal
  - Fish
    - Shark
    - Other fish
  - Other nonvenomous marine animal
- Reptiles
  - Lizards
  - Snakes
  - Turtles
  - Other nonvenomous reptile
- Other/unspecified nonvenomous animal

Identify type of contact with nonvenomous animal:

- Bite
- Crushed by
- Pecked
- Scratch
- Struck by
- Other type of contact causing injury or a health condition, which includes contact with
  - Feces
  - Saliva
  - Urine

Identify episode of care:

- Initial encounter
- Subsequent encounter
- Sequela

External Cause – Contact with Dog

ICD-10-CM Code/Documentation	
W54.0-	Bitten by dog
W54.1-	Struck by dog
W54.8-	Other contact with dog
Note: A 7th digit is required to identify the episode of care.	

Documentation and Coding Example

Patient is a 4-year-old Caucasian male bought to ED by his parents after being **bitten by the family dog**. There were no adult witnesses to the attack, but older children admit that they placed the boy on the dog's back so he could "ride" her. The dog yelped and turned, **biting him on the right arm**. Crying but fairly cooperative, young boy is examined while being held by his father. The **right forearm has a 4 cm long jagged wound consistent with a dog bite**. ROM, sensation, and circulation intact to fingers and hand. There is some difficulty with pronation and supination of the forearm suggestive of brachioradialis muscle or tendon injury. Wound infiltrated with 2% Lidocaine with epinephrine and child fell asleep soon afterward. Wound copiously irrigated with dilute betadine and NS. The **wound extends into and partially severs the brachioradialis tendon near insertion at the distal styloid process of the radius**. Radial nerve is identified and appears to be intact. There are no large vascular structures damaged. The tendon is repaired with 3-0 Chromic followed by a 2-layer wound closure. Sterile dressing and soft short arm splint applied. Patient woke up at the end of the procedure, remains quiet and cooperative. He denies pain at this time. Parents are given a prescription for Tylenol with codeine, instructed to keep dressing and splint dry. Patient has a follow up appointment in surgical clinic in 5 days.

Diagnosis Code(s)

S51.851A	Open bite of right forearm, initial encounter
S56.221A	Laceration of other flexor muscle, fascia, and tendon at forearm level, right arm, initial encounter
W54.0XXA	Bitten by dog, initial encounter
Y92.009	Unspecified place in unspecified non-institutional (private) residence as the place of occurrence of the external cause
Y93.89	Activity, other specified
Y99.8	Other external cause status

Coding Note(s)

There is a specific code for a dog bite as the cause of the wound, which is identified additionally as the initial encounter. Although the place of occurrence was at home, a noninstitutional private residence, there is not enough information to assign a specific code because the documentation does not state whether the injury occurred in a single-family residence, an apartment, or other type of private residence, nor is the room or area of the residence where the injury occurred identified. An activity is provided but there is not a specific code for that activity. Since the patient is a child and was playing, the code for other external cause status is reported.

Transport Accidents

External cause codes for transport accidents are found in categories V00-V99 and the definition of a transport accident is any accident involving a device designed primarily for, or being used at the time primarily for, conveying persons or goods from one place to another. In order to assign codes accurately for transport accidents, definitions related to transport accidents, which are found under the code block (V00-V99), must be applied in order to select the appropriate code.

In ICD-10-CM, code block V00-V99 for transport accidents is structured into 12 groups as follows:

- V00-V09 Pedestrian Injured in Transport Accident
- V10-V19 Pedal Cycle Rider Injured in Transport Accident
- V20-V29 Motorcycle Rider Injured in Transport Accident
- V30-V39 Occupant of Three-Wheeled Vehicle Injured in Transport Accident
- V40-V49 Car Occupant Injured Transport Accident
- V50-V59 Occupant of Pick-up Truck or Van Injured in Transport Accident
- V60-V69 Occupant of Heavy Transport Vehicle Injured in Transport Accident
- V70-V79 Bus Occupant Injured in Transport Accident
- V80-V89 Other Land Transport Accidents
- V90-V94 Water Transport Accidents
- V95-V97 Air and Space Transport Accidents
- V98-V99 Other and Unspecified Transport Accidents

The first nine groups (V00-V89), excluding category V00 for pedestrian conveyance accidents, relate to land-transport accidents and reflect the victim's mode of transport. The groups are then subdivided into categories to identify the victim's counterpart or the type of event. The type of vehicle of which the injured person is an occupant is identified in the first two characters of the code since this is seen as the most important factor to identify for prevention purposes. To be classified as a transport accident, the vehicle involved must be moving or running or in use for transport purposes at the time of the accident.

In the section below, the documentation elements for a motor vehicle/pedestrian accident are described.

Coding and Documentation Requirements

Identify the mode of transport of the accident victim as a pedestrian in the motor vehicle/pedestrian accident and further specify the mode of pedestrian conveyance:

- On foot
- On roller skates
- On standing micromobility conveyance
- On skateboard
- With other conveyance

Identify the victim's (patient's) counterpart in the motor vehicle/pedestrian accident:

- 2 or 3-wheeled vehicle
- Car, pick-up truck, or van
- Heavy transport vehicle or bus
- Railway train or vehicle

Identify type of accident:

- Non-traffic
- Traffic
- Unspecified

Identify episode of care:

- Initial
- Subsequent
- Sequela

Use additional codes to identify place of occurrence, activity, and external cause status as appropriate.

Pedestrian/Motor Vehicle Accident

Note: a 7th character to identify the episode of care is required

ICD-10-CM Code/Documentation	
Two- or Three-Wheeled Motor Vehicle	
V02.00-	Pedestrian on foot injured in collision with two- or three-wheeled motor vehicle in nontraffic accident
V02.01-	Pedestrian on roller-skates injured in collision with two- or three-wheeled motor vehicle in nontraffic accident
V02.031-	Pedestrian on standing electric scooter injured in collision with two- or three-wheeled motor vehicle in nontraffic accident
V02.038-	Pedestrian on other standing micro-mobility pedestrian conveyance injured in collision with two- or three-wheeled motor vehicle in nontraffic accident
V02.02-	Pedestrian on skateboard injured in collision with two- or three-wheeled motor vehicle in nontraffic accident
V02.09-	Pedestrian with other conveyance injured in collision with two- or three-wheeled motor vehicle in nontraffic accident
V02.10-	Pedestrian on foot injured in collision with two- or three-wheeled motor vehicle in traffic accident
V02.11-	Pedestrian on roller skates injured in collision with two- or three-wheeled motor vehicle in traffic accident
V02.12-	Pedestrian on skateboard injured in collision with two- or three-wheeled motor vehicle in traffic accident
V02.131-	Pedestrian on standing electric scooter injured in collision with two- or three-wheeled motor vehicle in traffic accident
V02.138-	Pedestrian on other standing micro-mobility pedestrian conveyance injured in collisionwith two- or three-wheeled motor vehicle in traffic accident
V02.19-	Pedestrian with other conveyance injured in collision with two- or three-wheeled motor vehicle in traffic accident
V02.90-	Pedestrian on foot injured in collision with two- or three-wheeled motor vehicle, unspecified whether traffic or nontraffic accident
V02.91-	Pedestrian on roller skates injured in collision with two- or three-wheeled motor vehicle, unspecified whether traffic or nontraffic accident
V02.92-	Pedestrian on skateboard injured in collision with two- or three-wheeled motor vehicle, unspecified whether traffic or nontraffic accident
V02.931-	Pedestrian on standing electric scooter injured in collision with two- or three wheeled motor vehicle, unspecified whether traffic or nontraffic accident
V02.938-	Pedestrian on other standing micro-mobility pedestrian conveyance injured in collision with two- or three wheeled motor vehicle, unspecified whether traffic or nontraffic accident
V02.99-	Pedestrian with other conveyance injured in collision with two- or three-wheeled motor vehicle, unspecified whether traffic or nontraffic accident

Other and Unspecified Vehicles	
V09.00-	Pedestrian injured in nontraffic accident involving unspecified motor vehicles
V09.01-	Pedestrian injured in nontraffic accident involving military vehicle
V09.09-	Pedestrian injured in nontraffic accident involving other motor vehicles
V09.20-	Pedestrian injured in traffic accident involving unspecified motor vehicles
V09.21-	Pedestrian injured in traffic accident involving military vehicles
V09.29-	Pedestrian injured in traffic accident involving other motor vehicles

Documentation and Coding Example

ED Note: Patient is a fifty-three-year-old female involved in a **pedestrian vs. van accident**. Patient was crossing the street in a marked crosswalk when she was struck by a van making a left turn. The van struck the patient on her **right side** with the impact propelling her into the air, landing approximately 10 feet away on the pavement. She is complaining of pain in her right hip. On examination, this is a well-developed, well-nourished female who is alert and oriented x 3. HR 94, RR 16, BP 150/86. O2 saturation 97 % on oxygen at 2 L/m via NC. PERRL. Breath sounds clear, equal bilaterally, HR regular without murmur or muffling. No abdominal or flank tenderness, bladder is not palpated. There is bruising over the right hip area with visual limb length inequality. Bedside US reveals no free fluid in peritoneum. Foley catheter placed with some difficulty due to hip pain and deformity. Urine returned is dark yellow, dipstick negative for blood. Blood drawn for CBC, electrolytes, PT, PTT, Type and hold. EKG obtained. AP and oblique views of pelvis reveal a transverse-posterior wall fracture of the right acetabulum. CT scan of pelvis and abdomen R/O intra-abdominal organ injury and enhanced 3D reconstruction shows a **nondisplaced transverse acetabular fracture with an associated moderately displaced posterior wall fracture on the right**. Care of patient is assumed by orthopedic team as patient awaits transfer to OR.

Diagnosis Code(s)

S32.461A Displaced associated transverse-posterior fracture of right acetabulum, initial encounter for closed fracture

V03.10XA Pedestrian on foot injured in collision with car, pick-up truck or van in traffic accident, initial encounter

Y92.410 Unspecified street and highway as the place of occurrence of the external cause

Coding Note(s)

The external cause code provides more information about the type of accident and the injured person. The code captures information about the pedestrian by identifying that the pedestrian was on foot and not using a pedestrian conveyance. It also identifies the type of vehicle specifically and identifies the encounter as the initial encounter. A second external cause code is assigned to identify the place of occurrence as an unspecified street/highway. Neither the activity nor the patient's work status is documented, so no codes are assigned from categories V93 or V99.

Place of Occurrence

Place of occurrence codes are found in category Y92. For a non-institutional residence there are subcategories for single family home, mobile home, apartment (includes condominium), boarding house, other non-institutional residence, and unspecified non-institutional residence. Specific codes within these subcategories identify the specific room or areas of the house or premises where the injury or health condition occurred, such as the kitchen, dining room, bathroom, bedroom, driveway, garage, swimming pool, garden/yard, other specified place, or unspecified place. The greater specificity extends to all places of occurrence including institutional residences, schools, sports and athletic areas, streets and highways, trade and service areas, industrial and construction areas, farms, and other places.

Coding and documentation requirements are provided below for a home or noninstitutional residence as the place of occurrence.

Coding and Documentation Requirements

Identify non-institutional (private) residence:

- Apartment
- Boarding house
- Mobile home
- Single family house
- Other specified non-institutional residence
- Unspecified non-institutional residence

Identify room or area of premises where accident occurred:

- Room
  - Bathroom
  - Bedroom
  - Dining room
  - Kitchen
- Other specific area
  - Driveway
  - Garage
  - Garden/yard
  - Swimming pool
- Other specified place of residence or premises
- Unspecified place

Single-Family Noninstitutional House as Place of Occurrence

ICD-10-CM Code/Documentation	
Y92.010	Kitchen of single-family (private) house as the place of occurrence of the external cause
Y92.011	Dining room of single-family (private) house as the place of occurrence of the external cause
Y92.012	Bathroom of single-family (private) house as the place of occurrence of the external cause
Y92.013	Bedroom of single-family (private) house as the place of occurrence of the external cause

Y92.014	Private driveway to single-family (private) house as the place of occurrence of the external cause
Y92.015	Private garage of single-family (private) house as the place of occurrence of the external cause
Y92.016	Swimming pool in single-family (private) house or garden as the place of occurrence of the external cause
Y92.017	Garden or yard in single-family (private) house as the place of occurrence of the external cause
Y92.018	Other place in single-family (private) house as the place of occurrence of the external cause
Y92.019	Unspecified place in single-family (private) house as the place of occurrence of the external cause

Documentation and Coding Example

Twenty-three-year-old Black male **employed as a gardener** on a private estate presents to Urgent Care Clinic with a right shoulder injury sustained about 6 hours ago. He reports that he **fell approximately 5 feet off a ladder while trimming hedges**, landing on his outstretched right arm and hand. He describes a "popping" feeling in the shoulder followed by numbness in the arm and hand. He was able to move the extremity after a few minutes and the numbness subsided in approximately one hour, but the shoulder has continued to feel loose all day. PMH includes asthma for which he takes Singulair, Advair daily and Albuterol when needed; and TB treated with INH seven years ago. On examination, this is a soft spoken, slightly built, thin young man. Temperature 97.4, HR 62, RR 14, BP 116/70. Alert and oriented x 3, PERRL, patient denies striking head, neck, or back in the fall. Heart rate regular without murmur, breath sounds have a few expiratory wheezes but otherwise clear and equal bilaterally. Left upper extremity is normal in appearance. Right clavicle has slight prominence but otherwise normal contour, there is no shoulder sag. Moderate point tenderness is localized over the AC joint which can be easily manipulated out of position. There are no obvious neurovascular deficits. X-rays obtained including AP and lateral views of shoulder, lateral projection of scapula and weight bearing view (AP projection w/15 lb. weight). No fractures visible and no obvious dislocation of clavicle or humerus.

Impression: **Subluxation of right acromioclavicular joint**.

Treatment: Patient is fitted with a sling which can be worn for comfort. He is instructed to ice shoulder x 20 minutes, 3-4 x day and may continue with exercise/activity as tolerated. He is prescribed Ibuprofen 600 mg TID for pain. He will F/U with PMD in one week with possible referral to orthopedist and/or physical therapy for strengthening exercises if the right shoulder joint continues to feel loose.

Diagnosis Code(s)

S43.111A	Subluxation of right acromioclavicular joint, initial encounter
W11.XXXA	Fall on and from ladder, initial encounter
Y92.017	Garden or yard in single-family (private) house as the place of occurrence of the external cause
Y93.H2	Activity, gardening and landscaping
Y99.0	Civilian activity done for income or pay

Coding Note(s)

ICD-10-CM codes are assigned for the external cause, place of occurrence, activity, and external cause status. The external cause is a fall from a ladder. The place of occurrence is the garden/yard of a single family private residence. The activity the patient was performing at the time of the fall is gardening and landscaping and this activity was being done for pay, so the external cause status is the code for civilian activity done for income or pay.

Summary

Even though external cause codes are not required on all claims or by all payers, they do provide valuable information related to the cause, intent, place, activity, and work status of the patient at the time of the injury. Codes for cause, intent, and place are specific in ICD-10-CM which requiring precise documentation by the physician. It is particularly important to document sufficient detail about the external cause of injury when it results in an emergency department visit or an inpatient stay because the majority of states either mandate or routinely collect external cause data for these two places of service.

Chapter 21 Quiz

1. What external cause is not reported with a cause code from Chapter 21 External Causes of Morbidity, in ICD-10-CM?
   a. Accidental fall
   b. Accidental drowning
   c. Unintentional poisoning
   d. Assault by a handgun
2. If the documentation does not identify the activity of the patient that resulted in the injury and it is not possible to query the provider, what is reported in ICD-10-CM?
   a. No activity code is reported
   b. Code Y93.9 Activity unspecified is reported
   c. Code Y93.89 Activity other specified is reported
   d. Code Y99.9 Unspecified external cause status is assigned
3. Intentional poisoning with barbiturates reported with code T42.3X2 requires an additional code from block X71-X83 to indicate self-harm.
   a. True
   b. False
4. When the intent of an injury or another condition resulting from an external cause is not documented or not known, how should the intent be reported?
   a. No intent code is assigned
   b. It is reported with a code for undetermined intent
   c. It depends on the other circumstances related to the injury or other condition
   d. It is reported as accidental intent
5. Code block V00-V99 is structured into 12 groups. How are land transport accident codes categorized?
   a. The type of accident is categorized, such as a two-car collision, roll-over, or other type of accident.
   b. Categories identify the mode of transportation of the victim and the victim's counterpart (vehicle) or the type of event.
   c. Categories first designate the accident as a traffic or nontraffic transport accident and then designate the victim.
   d. Categories first identify the type of vehicle or vehicles involved in the accident such as auto-pedestrian, car-bus, or single car accident.
6. Identify the true statement about place of occurrence codes.
   a. A place of occurrence code is required for all injuries and other health conditions resulting from an external cause.
   b. A place of occurrence code requires a 7th character extension to identify the episode of care.
   c. A place of occurrence code is reported only once at the initial encounter for treatment.
   d. A place of occurrence code is a supplemental code and is not reported unless requested by the payer.
7. The external cause code for a dog bite is found in what block of codes?
   a. Exposure to forces of nature (X30-X39)
   b. Exposure to inanimate mechanical forces (W20-W49)
   c. S and T codes that describe open wounds (S00-T88)
   d. Exposure to animate mechanical forces (W50-W64)
8. External cause codes for land transport accidents V00-V09 capture what information related to pedestrians?
   a. Whether the pedestrian is on foot or using a pedestrian conveyance
   b. The place of occurrence
   c. The external cause status
   d. All of the above
9. What type of falls are classified in categories W00-W19 Slipping, tripping, stumbling, and falls?
   a. Accidental falls
   b. Falls involving assault
   c. Intentionally jumping from a high place
   d. Falls resulting from being pushed from a high place
10. Identify the false statement regarding external cause codes.
    a. External cause codes are never the principal or first listed diagnosis
    b. Only one external cause code may be reported for a specific injury or episode of care
    c. External cause codes may be used with any code in ranges A00.0-T88.9 or Z00-Z99 when the health condition is due to an external cause
    d. External cause codes are assigned for the entire length of treatment for the condition resulting from the external cause

See next page for answers and rationales.

Chapter 21 Answers and Rationales

1. What external cause is not reported with a code from Chapter 20 External Causes of Morbidity, in ICD-10-CM?

    c. **Unintentional poisoning**

    Rationale: *Both the cause and intent of an unintentional poisoning are now captured with a combination code from Chapter 19 Injury, Poisoning, and Certain Other Consequences of External Causes, so no accidental poisoning codes are reported from Chapter 20.*

2. If the documentation does not identify the activity of the patient that resulted in the injury and it is not possible to query the provider, what is reported in ICD-10-CM?

    a. **No activity code is reported**

    Rationale: *Coding guideline I.C.20.c states "DO NOT assign code Y93.9 Unspecified activity, if the activity is not stated." This means that if the activity is not documented and the physician cannot be queried, no activity code is reported.*

3. Intentional poisoning with barbiturates reported with code T42.3X2 requires an additional code from block X71-X83 to indicate self-harm, True or false?

    b. **False**

    Rationale: *Poisoning codes have a 5th or 6th character that already identifies intent. Coding guideline I.C.20 states that no external cause code from chapter 20 is needed if the external cause and intent are included in a code from another chapter.*

4. When the intent of an injury or another condition resulting from an external cause is not documented or not known, how should the intent be reported?

    d. **It is reported as accidental intent**

    Rationale: *Coding guideline I.C.20.i states "If the intent (accident, self-harm, assault) of the cause of an injury or other condition is unknown or unspecified, code the intent as accidental intent." The code for undetermined intent is only assigned when documentation in the medical record states that the intent cannot be determined.*

5. Code block V00-V99 is structured into 12 groups. How are land transport accident codes categorized?

    b. **Categories identify the mode of transportation of the victim and the victim's counterpart (vehicle) or the type of event.**

    Rationale: *According to the note under the code block Transport Accidents V00-V99, land accident categories identify the victim's mode of transport first and then identify the victim's counterpart or the type of event. This can be verified by reviewing the code categories for land transport accidents. For example, if the injured person is a bicyclist (pedal cycle rider) who was hit by a car, a code from category V13 Pedal cycle rider injured in collision with car, pick-up truck or van is reported. This category identifies the victim as the pedal cycle rider and the victim's counterpart as a car, pick-up truck, or van.*

6. Identify the true statement about place of occurrence codes.

    c. **A place of occurrence code is reported only once at the initial encounter for treatment.**

    Rationale: *Place of occurrence codes are reported only once at the initial encounter for treatment. Place of occurrence codes are not required for all injuries or other health care conditions resulting from an external cause. For example, place of occurrence codes are not required for poisoning, adverse effects, and underdosing of drugs. Place of occurrence codes do not require a 7th character for episode of care. Place of occurrence codes may be required by the state for certain care settings (emergency department and inpatient) even if the payer does not require reporting of external cause codes.*

7. The external cause code for a dog bite is found in what block of codes?

    d. **Exposure to animate mechanical forces (W50-W64)**

    Rationale: *The external cause dog bite is classified as exposure to animate mechanical forces (W50-W64). The injury would be reported with a code from categories S00-T88, but codes for bites in the injury chapter do not identify the external cause.*

8. External cause codes for land transport accidents V00-V09 capture what information related to pedestrians?

    a. **Whether the pedestrian is on foot or using a pedestrian conveyance**

    Rationale: *ICD-10-CM external cause codes for land transport accidents involving pedestrians capture information on whether the pedestrian is on foot, on roller-skates, on a skateboard, or using another type of pedestrian conveyances well as the type of vehicle is captured. The external cause codes for the transport do not capture the place of occurrence or the external cause status to capture that information, additional codes are required from category Y92 and Y99.*

9. What type of falls are classified in categories W00-W19 Slipping, tripping, stumbling, and falls?

    a. **Accidental falls**

    Rationale: *Codes in categories W00-W19 are specific to accidental injuries. Falls involving an assault are found in categories Y01-Y02. Falls involving assault are specific to pushing from a high place (Y01) and pushing in front of a moving object (Y02). Falls involving self-harm are found in categories (X80-X81).*

10. Identify the false statement regarding external cause codes.

    b. **Only one external cause code may be reported for a specific injury or episode of care**

    Rationale: *Coding guideline I.C.20.a.4 state "Assign as many external cause codes as necessary to fully explain each cause. If only one external cause code can be recorded, assign the code most related to the principal diagnosis."*

Chapter 22
CODES FOR SPECIAL PURPOSES (UØØ-U85)

This chapter is for the provisional assignment of new diseases of uncertain etiology or emergency use. Specifically, codes U00-U49 are to be used by WHO for the provisional assignment of new diseases of uncertain etiology or emergency use. Included in Chapter 22 are two codes:

- U07.0 Vaping-related disorder
- U07.1 COVID-19

UØ7.Ø Vaping-Related Disorder

The purpose of U07.0 is for coding encounters related to E-cigarette, or vaping, product use.

Code U07.0 Vaping-related disorder, has been implemented in response to the recent occurrences of vaping-related disorders. The incorporation of this diagnosis code is consistent with certain provisions of the Health Insurance Portability and Accountability Act of 1996 (HIPAA) for diagnosis coding, including the *Official ICD-10-CM Guidelines for Coding and Reporting,* as maintained and distributed by the U.S. Department of Health and Human Services.

The code is consistent with the emergency code established by the World Health Organization (WHO). The code resulted from a meeting of the WHO Framework Convention on Tobacco Control and the WHO Family of International Classifications (WHOFIC) Network Classification and Statistics Advisory Committee (CSAC).

Clinical Explanation

According to the U.S. Centers for Disease Control and Prevention (CDC), using an electronic cigarette (e-cigarette) is commonly called vaping. E-cigarette or vaping product use associated lung injury (EVALI) is the name given by the CDC to the dangerous lung disease linked to vaping. Symptoms include cough, shortness of breath, acute respiratory distress, chest pain, fever, stomach pain, diarrhea, nausea, vomiting, and weight loss. Damaging lung effects can be so severe as to stop the lungs from functioning.

E-cigarettes, also known as vape pens, mods, tanks, e-hookahs, and electronic nicotine delivery systems (ENDS) work by heating a liquid in a pod or cartridge into an aerosol that the user then inhales. Vaping liquids are composed of base ingredients, such as glycerol (vegetable glycerin) and propylene glycol that create the vapor when heated, combined with other additives like nicotine, artificial flavorings, THC (tetrahydrocannabinol) or CBD (cannabinoid) oil, and vitamin E acetate. THC is the psychoactive mind-altering compound of marijuana that produces the "high".

Although no single ingredient alone has been identified to cause EVALI, and it is unclear how the condition develops, it is known that harmful acetals form as chemical byproducts when other additives or flavorings are mixed in with the base ingredients and heated into a vapor. THC diluted with vitamin E acetate is linked to hospitalized cases of the initial outbreak in 2019. It is thought that vitamin E acetate, or other harmful chemical byproduct produced by the heated liquid, disrupts the lung's surfactant lining or otherwise interferes with the lung's ability to expand. Treatment includes the use of a ventilator or supplemental oxygen depending on illness severity, corticosteroids to reduce inflammation, and antibiotics or antivirals until test results for EVALI are finalized.

The U.S. Food and Drug Administration (FDA) and the U.S. Centers for Disease Control and Prevention (CDC) continue to investigate the incidents of severe respiratory illness associated with the use of vaping products.

Coding Guidance for Assigning UØ7.Ø

For patients documented with electronic cigarette (e-cigarette), or vaping product use associated lung injury (EVALI), or acute lung injury but without further documentation identifying a specific condition (pneumonitis, bronchitis), assign only code U07.0.

Per tabular instructions, when assigning U07.0, use additional code(s) to identify manifestations, such as:

- abdominal pain (R10.84)
- acute respiratory distress syndrome (J80)
- diarrhea (R19.7)
- drug-induced interstitial lung disorder (J70.4)
- lipoid pneumonia (J69.1)
- weight loss (R63.4)

Lung-Related Complications

For patients presenting with conditions related to vaping, assign code U07.0 as the principal diagnosis. Assign additional codes for other specified respiratory manifestations, such as:

- J68.0 Bronchitis and pneumonitis due to chemicals, gases, fumes and vapors
- J69.1 Pneumonitis due to inhalation of oils and essences
- J80 Acute respiratory distress syndrome
- J82.8- Pulmonary eosinophilia, not elsewhere classified
- J84.114 Acute interstitial pneumonitis
- J96.0- Acute respiratory failure

Associated respiratory signs and symptoms due to vaping, such as cough, shortness of breath, etc., are not coded separately, when a definitive diagnosis has been established. However, it would be appropriate to code separately any gastrointestinal symptoms, such as diarrhea and abdominal pain.

Poisoning and Toxicity

Acute nicotine exposure can be toxic. Children and adults have been poisoned by swallowing, breathing, or absorbing e-cigarette liquid through their skin or eyes. For these patients assign code:

- T65.291-, Toxic effect of other nicotine and tobacco, accidental (unintentional); includes Toxic effect of other tobacco and nicotine NOS.

For a patient with acute tetrahydrocannabinol (THC) toxicity, assign code:

- T40.7X1- Poisoning by cannabis (derivatives), accidental (unintentional).

Substance Use, Abuse and Dependence

For patients with documented substance use/abuse/dependence, additional codes identifying the substance(s) used should be assigned.

When the provider documentation refers to use, abuse and dependence of the same substance (e.g. nicotine, cannabis, etc.), only one code should be assigned to identify the pattern of use based on the following hierarchy:

- If both use and abuse are documented, assign only the code for abuse
- If both abuse and dependence are documented, assign only the code for dependence
- If use, abuse and dependence are all documented, assign only the code for dependence
- If both use and dependence are documented, assign only the code for dependence.

Assign as many codes, as appropriate. Examples:

- Cannabis related disorders: F12.---
- Nicotine related disorders: F17.----

For vaping of nicotine with dependence, assign code F17.29-, Nicotine dependence, other tobacco products. Electronic nicotine delivery systems (ENDS) are non-combustible tobacco products.

This coding guidance is effective Oct. 1, 2020. The guidelines for proper assignment of U07.0 can be found in the official coding guidelines for Chapter 10.

U07.1 COVID-19

The purpose of U07.1 is for coding encounters related to infections due to SARS-CoV-2.

Code U07.1, COVID-19, has been implemented in response to the recent pandemic. A national emergency has been declared in the United States concerning the COVID-19 Outbreak. Given these developments, and the critical need to report COVID-19 in claims and surveillance data, the Centers for Disease Control (CDC), under the National Emergencies Act Section 201 and 301, announced a change in the effective date of new diagnosis code U07.1, COVID-19, as April 1, 2020. This off-cycle update was unprecedented and is an exception to the code set updating process established under HIPAA. Code U07.1 was also included in the FY2021 code update, effective Oct. 1, 2020. The guidelines for proper assignment of U07.1 can be found in Chapter 1 of the official coding guidelines.

Clinical Explanation

COVID-19, also known as the 2019 novel coronavirus, is a newly discovered strain of coronavirus emerging in December of 2019 causing respiratory illness with flu-like symptoms that range from mild to severe illness and death. The official name of this new virus is "SARS-CoV-2", and the disease it causes is named "coronavirus disease 2019", which is abbreviated COVID-19. This virus is genetically related to the virus causing the SARS outbreak of 2003, but causes a different illness. Many infected with COVID-19 will experience mild to moderate respiratory illness and recover without special treatment. Severe cases require hospitalization and ventilator assistance. Most patients recover with supportive care. Symptoms may appear 2-14 days after exposure and include cough, fever, shortness of breath, or difficulty breathing in serious cases. Older persons and those with an existing medical condition such as heart or lung disease, cancer, or diabetes are at greater risk for developing more serious illness. Emergency warning signs for COVID-19 infection that require immediate medical attention include trouble breathing; continual pain or pressure in the chest; a newly altered mental state such as confusion or the inability to be aroused; and a bluish tint to the lips or face.

The virus is spread primarily through contact with an infected person by saliva droplets or nasal discharge whenever the person coughs or sneezes. COVID-19 is also spread by touching contaminated surfaces such as doorknobs, and then touching the eyes, nose, or mouth. There are currently no specific vaccines or treatment for COVID-19 although many are under investigation and clinical trial. Infection is slowed by following the official guidelines for protective measures and practicing good respiratory hygiene.

Coding Guidance for Assigning U07.1

Code only a confirmed diagnosis of the 2019 novel coronavirus disease (COVID-19) as documented by the provider or documentation of a positive COVID-19 test result. For a confirmed diagnosis, assign code U07.1, COVID-19. This is an exception to the hospital inpatient guideline Section II, H. In this context, "confirmation" does not require documentation of a positive test result for COVID-19; the provider's documentation that the individual has COVID-19 is sufficient.

If the provider documents "suspected," "possible," "probable," or "inconclusive" COVID-19, do not assign code U07.1. Instead, code the signs and symptoms reported.

Sequencing of Codes

When COVID-19 meets the definition of principal diagnosis, code U07.1 COVID-19, should be sequenced first, followed by the appropriate codes for associated manifestations, except when another guideline requires that certain codes be sequenced first. *(See Section I.C.1.d. Sepsis, and Septic Shock for a COVID-19 infection that progresses to sepsis. See Section I.C.19.g.3.a. Transplant complications other than kidney for a COVID-19 infection in a lung transplant patient.)*

During pregnancy, childbirth, or the puerperium, when COVID-19 is the reason for the admission or encounter, assign code O98.5- Other viral diseases complicating pregnancy, childbirth and the puerperium, as the principal diagnosis, and code U07.1 COVID-19 and the appropriate code(s) for any associated manifestation(s) as additional diagnoses. Codes from Chapter 15 always take sequencing priority. *(See Section I.C.15.s. for COVID-19 infection in pregnancy, childbirth, and the puerperium.)*

For a newborn that tests positive for COVID-19, assign code U07.1 COVID-19, and the appropriate codes for any associated manifestation(s) in neonates/newborns in the absence of documentation indicating a specific type of transmission. For a newborn that tests positive for COVID-19 and the provider documents the condition was contracted in utero or during the birth process, assign codes P35.8 Other congenital viral diseases, and U07.1 COVID-19. When coding the birth episode in a newborn record, the appropriate code from category Z38 Liveborn infants according to place of birth and type of delivery, should be assigned as the principal diagnosis. *(See Section I.C.16.h. for COVID-19 infection in newborn.)*

Acute Respiratory Illnesses Due to COVID-19

When the reason for the encounter/admission is a respiratory manifestation of COVID-19, assign U07.1 as the principal/first-listed diagnosis and assign code(s) for the respiratory manifestation(s) as additional diagnoses.

The following conditions are examples of common respiratory manifestations of COVID-19:

- **Pneumonia:** Assign codes U07.1 (COVID-19) and J12.89 (Other viral pneumonia).
- **Acute bronchitis:** Assign codes U07.1 and J20.8 (Acute bronchitis due to other specified organisms). Note: Bronchitis not otherwise specified (NOS) due to COVID-19 should be coded using code U07.1 and J40 (Bronchitis, not specified as acute or chronic).
- **Lower respiratory infection:** If the COVID-19 is documented as being associated with a lower respiratory infection, not otherwise specified (NOS), or an acute respiratory infection, NOS, assign codes U07.1 and J22 (Unspecified acute lower respiratory infection). If the COVID-19 is documented as being associated with a respiratory infection, NOS, assign codes U07.1 and J98.8 (Other specified respiratory disorders).
- **Acute respiratory distress syndrome:** Assign codes U07.1 and J80 (Acute respiratory distress syndrome).
- **Acute respiratory failure:** Assign codes U07.1 and J96.0- (Acute respiratory failure).

Note: When the reason for the encounter/admission is a non-respiratory manifestation (e.g., viral enteritis) of COVID-19, assign code U07.1 COVID-19, as the principal diagnosis and assign the appropriate code(s) for the manifestation(s) as additional diagnoses.

Additional COVID-19 Guidance

- **Exposure:** For asymptomatic individuals with actual or suspected exposure to COVID-19, assign code Z20.828 Contact with and (suspected) exposure to other viral communicable diseases. For symptomatic individuals with actual or suspected exposure to COVID-19 and the infection has been ruled out, or test results are inconclusive or unknown, assign code Z20.828.
- **Screening:** During the COVID-19 pandemic, a screening code is generally not appropriate. For encounters for COVID-19 testing, including preoperative testing, code as exposure to COVID-19.
- **Signs and symptoms without definitive diagnosis of COVID-19:** For patients who have any symptoms that are associated with COVID-19, but a definitive diagnosis has not be confirmed, assign the appropriate codes for each of the symptoms such as R05 (Cough), R06.02 (Shortness or breath) or R50.9 (Fever, unspecified). If a patient with signs/symptoms associated with COVID-19 also has an actual or suspected contact with or exposure to COVID-19, assign Z20.828.
- **Asymptomatic individuals who test positive for COVID-19:** For patients who are asymptomatic and test positive for COVID-19, assign U07.1.
- **Personal history of COVID-19:** For patients with a history of COVID-19, assign code Z86.19 Personal history of other infectious and parasitic diseases.
- **Follow-up visits after COVID-19 infection has resolved:** For individuals who previously had COVID-19 and are being seen for follow-up evaluation, and COVID-19 test results are negative, assign codes Z09 Encounter for follow-up examination after completed treatment for conditions other than malignant neoplasm, and Z86.19 Personal history of other infectious and parasitic diseases.

Appendix A

DOCUMENTATION CODING CHECKLISTS

Introduction

Appendix A provides checklists for common diagnoses and other conditions which are designed to be used for review of current records to help identify any documentation deficiencies. The checklists begin with the applicable ICD-10-CM categories, subcategories, and/or codes being covered. ICD-10-CM definitions and other information pertinent to coding the condition are then provided. This is followed by a checklist that identifies each element needed for assignment of the most specific code. If one or more of the required elements are not documented, this information should be shared with the physician and a corrective action plan initiated to ensure that the necessary information is captured in the future.

Similar documentation and coding checklists for conditions not addressed in this book can be created using the checklists provided as a template. There are a few different formats and styles of checklists so users can determine which style works best for their practice and then create additional checklists using that format and style.

Angina Pectoris

ICD-10-CM Categories/Subcategories

Angina is classified based on whether it occurs alone or with documented atherosclerosis as follows:

I20	Angina pectoris
I25.11	Atherosclerotic heart disease with angina
I25.7	Atherosclerosis of coronary artery bypass graft(s) and coronary artery of transplanted heart with angina pectoris
I23.7	Postinfarction angina

ICD-10-CM Definitions

Angina – Pain or discomfort, pressure or squeezing, usually centered in the chest, or other atypical symptoms that result from diseased coronary arteries with restricted blood flow to the heart muscle. Also called angina pectoris. Angina is classified in ICD-10-CM by the types described below.

Angina equivalent – Instead of decreased blood flow to the heart causing classic angina symptoms such as chest pain or discomfort, pressure or squeezing, atypical symptoms occur, such as indigestion, shortness of breath, weakness, or malaise. These symptoms are the patient's angina equivalent, that is the symptoms that the patient gets instead of classic angina symptoms. Use the ICD-10-CM code for other forms of angina pectoris (I20.8).

Angina of effort – Angina that occurs as a result of exertion. Use the ICD-10-CM code for other forms of angina pectoris (I20.8).

Coronary slow flow syndrome – Angina that occurs in the absence of angiographic evidence indicating atherosclerotic disease or narrowing of the coronary arteries. The cause is believed to be due to disease or narrowing in the microvasculature of the heart. Use the code for other forms of angina pectoris (I20.8).

Prinzmetal angina – Rare type of angina caused by spasm of the coronary arteries that temporarily restricts blood flow to the heart muscle. Pain usually occurs at rest, is often severe, and is typically relieved by angina medication. Also called angiospastic angina, spasm-induced angina, and variant angina. Use the ICD-10-CM code for angina with documented spasm (I20.1).

Stable angina – The most common form of angina. Typically occurs with exertion and subsides with rest. The type and severity of pain is usually predictable; pain is of short duration, usually 5 minutes or less and responds to angina medication. Use the ICD-10-CM code for unspecified angina (I20.8).

Unstable angina – A medical emergency that may signal an impending myocardial infarction, characterized by chest pain or discomfort that is unexpected in that it may occur at rest, increase in severity, last longer than is typical (30 minutes or more), and may not respond to angina medications. Also called accelerated angina, crescendo angina, de novo effort angina, intermediate coronary syndrome, preinfarction syndrome, or worsening effort angina. Use the ICD-10-CM code for unstable angina (I20.0).

Appendix A: Coding Checklists

Checklist

1. Identify angina pectoris as with/without atherosclerotic disease:
   - ☐ With coronary atherosclerosis – See Coronary Atherosclerosis Check List
   - ☐ Without coronary atherosclerosis
2. For angina without a diagnosis of coronary atherosclerosis, identify type of angina pectoris:
   - ☐ Unstable angina, which includes:
     - ☐ Accelerated angina
     - ☐ Crescendo angina
     - ☐ De novo effort angina
     - ☐ Intermediate coronary syndrome
     - ☐ Preinfarction syndrome
     - ☐ Worsening effort angina
   - ☐ Angina with documented spasm, which includes:
     - ☐ Angiospastic angina
     - ☐ Prinzmetal angina
     - ☐ Spasm-induced angina
     - ☐ Variant angina
   - ☐ Other forms of angina pectoris, which include:
     - ☐ Angina equivalent
     - ☐ Angina of effort
     - ☐ Coronary slow flow syndrome
     - ☐ Stenocardia
     - ☐ Stable angina
   - ☐ Unspecified angina pectoris, which includes:
     - ☐ Angina NOS
     - ☐ Anginal syndrome
     - ☐ Cardiac angina
     - ☐ Ischemic chest pain
   - ☐ Postinfarction angina

Asthma

ICD-10-CM Categories

In ICD-10-CM, asthma is classified by cause, such as exercise induced; by symptoms, such as cough variant; and by severity in the following categories:

J44 Other chronic obstructive pulmonary disease – Note: use a code from category J44 in conjunction with a code from category J45 for the following documented conditions:

- asthma and chronic obstructive pulmonary disease
- chronic asthmatic bronchitis
- chronic obstructive asthma

J45 Asthma

ICD-10-CM Definitions

Definitions of asthma severity:

Mild intermittent asthma – Asthma symptoms that come and go. Daytime symptoms occur 2 days or less per week, nighttime symptoms 2 days per month or less, use of rescue inhaler 2 times or less per week. Asthma does not interfere with daily activities, and FEV1 (forced expiratory volume in 1 second) is normal.

Mild persistent asthma – Asthma symptoms that occur almost weekly, but can be controlled with a single medication. Daytime symptoms occur more than 2 days per week but not daily, nighttime symptoms 3-4 nights per month, rescue inhaler more than 2 days per week but not daily. There is minor interference with daily activities, and FEV1 > 80% of predicted or normal most of the time.

Moderate persistent asthma – Asthma symptoms that occur almost daily, but can be controlled with two medications. Daily daytime asthma symptoms, nighttime symptoms more than 1 night per week but not every night, rescue inhaler use daily. Asthma moderately interferes with daily activities, and FEV1 > 60% but < 80% of predicted.

Severe persistent asthma – Daily asthma symptoms despite the use of more than two medications. Symptoms throughout the day, nightly asthma, use of rescue inhaler multiple times per day, extreme interference with daily activities, and FEV1 < 60% of predicted.

Definitions of other types of asthma:

Cough variant asthma – Asthma in which a cough is the only symptom

Exercise induced bronchospasm – Asthma that occurs during or after exercise

Asthma complications:

Acute exacerbation – Episode of progressively worsening shortness of breath, coughing, wheezing, and chest tightness or any combination of these; also called an asthma attack.

Status asthmaticus – Acute, severe, life-threatening asthma attack that does not respond to inhaled bronchodilators and is accompanied by symptoms of potential respiratory failure.

Checklist

1. Identify severity/type of asthma:
   - ☐ Mild
     - ☐ Intermittent
     - ☐ Persistent
   - ☐ Moderate persistent
   - ☐ Severe persistent
   - ☐ Other specified type
     - ☐ Cough variant asthma
     - ☐ Exercise induced bronchospasm
     - ☐ Other asthma
   - ☐ Unspecified asthma
2. Identify complications:
   - ☐ With acute exacerbation
   - ☐ With status asthmaticus
   - ☐ Uncomplicated

Note: Complications do not apply to other specified types of asthma (cough variant, exercise induced bronchospasm, other specified type)

3 For chronic obstructive asthma, assign a code from category J44 Other chronic obstructive pulmonary disease and a code from category J45 Asthma

4. Use additional code to identify:
   - ☐ Exposure to environmental tobacco smoke (Z77.22)
   - ☐ Exposure to tobacco smoke in the perinatal period (P96.81)
   - ☐ History of tobacco dependence (Z87.891)
   - ☐ Occupational exposure to environmental tobacco smoke (Z57.31)
   - ☐ Tobacco dependence (F17.-)
   - ☐ Tobacco use (Z72.0)

Bronchitis/Bronchiolitis, Acute Infection

ICD-10-CM Categories

Acute bronchitis and bronchiolitis are classified in the following categories:

J20	Acute bronchitis
J21	Acute bronchiolitis

ICD-10-CM Definitions

Bronchiolitis, acute infection – Inflammation and swelling of the mucous membranes lining the bronchioles, the smallest airways in the lungs, most often caused by a viral infection/illness. Primarily affects infants and children under the age of 2 years. Symptoms can include productive cough, wheezing, tachypnea (fast breathing), nasal flaring, and intercostal retractions.

Bronchitis, acute infection – Inflammation of the mucous membranes lining the bronchi caused by a viral or bacterial infection/illness with symptoms that include cough with production of mucus. Bronchi are the large to medium-size airways that branch from the trachea carrying air to distal portions of the lungs.

Checklist

1. Identify site of infection:
   - ☐ Bronchitis (bronchi)
   - ☐ Bronchiolitis (bronchioles)
2. For bronchitis, identify organism:
   - ☐ Coxsackievirus
   - ☐ Echovirus
   - ☐ Haemophilus influenzae
   - ☐ Mycoplasma pneumoniae
   - ☐ Parainfluenza virus
   - ☐ Respiratory syncytial virus (RSV)
   - ☐ Rhinovirus
   - ☐ Streptococcus
   - ☐ Other specified organism – Specify ________
   - ☐ Unspecified
3. For bronchiolitis, identify organism:
   - ☐ Human metapneumovirus
   - ☐ Respiratory syncytial virus (RSV)
   - ☐ Other specified organism – Specify ________
   - ☐ Unspecified

Burns, Corrosions, and Frostbite

ICD-10-CM Categories

Burns and corrosions are classified in the following ICD-10-CM categories:

T20	Burn and corrosion of head, face and neck
T21	Burn and corrosion of trunk
T22	Burn and corrosion of shoulder and upper limb, except wrist and hand
T23	Burn and corrosion of wrist and hand
T24	Burn and corrosion of lower limb, except ankle and foot
T25	Burn and corrosion of ankle and foot
T26	Burn and corrosion confined to eye and adnexa
T27	Burn and corrosion of respiratory tract
T28	Burn and corrosion of internal organ
T30	Burn and corrosion, body region unspecified
T31	Burns classified according to extent of body surface involved
T33	Superficial frostbite

ICD-10-CM Definitions

Burn – A thermal injury due to a heat source such as fire, a hot appliance, friction, hot objects, hot air, hot water, electricity, lightning, and radiation. Burns due to exposure to the sun are not considered burns in ICD-10-CM.

Corrosion – A thermal injury due to chemicals.

Episode of Care – There are three (3) possible 7th character values for burns and corrosions. The 7th character defines the stage of treatment and residual effects related to the initial injury.

A **Initial encounter.** The period when the patient is receiving active treatment for the injury, poisoning, or other consequences of an external cause. An 'A' may be assigned on more than one claim.

D **Subsequent encounter.** Encounter after the active phase of treatment and when the patient is receiving routine care for the injury during the period of healing or recovery.

S **Sequela.** Encounter for complications or conditions that arise as a direct result of an injury.

Extent of body surface – The amount of body surface burned is governed by the rule of nines. These percentages may be modified for infants and children or adults with large buttocks, thighs, and abdomens when those regions are burned.

Head and neck – 9%

Each arm – 9%

Each leg – 18%

Anterior trunk – 18%

Posterior trunk – 18%

Genitalia – 1%

Levels of Burns:

First Degree – Affects only the epidermis causing pain, redness, and swelling.

Second Degree – Affects both the dermis and epidermis causing pain, redness, white or blotchy skin, and swelling. Blistering may occur and pain can be intense. Scarring can develop.

Third Degree – Affects the fat or subcutaneous layer of the skin. The skin will appear white or charred black or may look leathery. Third degree burns can destroy nerves resulting in numbness.

Note: Burns noted as non-healing are coded as acute burns and necrosis of burned skin should be coded as a non-healing burn.

Checklist

1. Identify the type of thermal injury:
   - ☐ Burn
   - ☐ Corrosion
   - ☐ Frostbite (Proceed to #9)
2. Identify the body region:
   - ☐ Eye
   - ☐ Internal organs
   - ☐ Skin (external body surface)
   - ☐ Multiple areas
   - ☐ Unspecified body region

Note: Codes from category T30 Burn and corrosion, body region unspecified, is extremely vague and should rarely be used.

3. Identify the body area
   - ☐ Eye and adnexa
     - ☐ Eyelid and periocular area
     - ☐ Cornea and conjunctival sac
     - ☐ With resulting rupture and destruction of eyeball
     - ☐ Unspecified site – review medical record/query physician
   - ☐ External body surface
     - ☐ Head, face and neck
       - ☐ Scalp
       - ☐ Forehead and cheek
       - ☐ Ear
       - ☐ Nose
       - ☐ Lips
       - ☐ Chin
       - ☐ Neck
       - ☐ Multiple sites of head, face, and neck
       - ☐ Unspecified site – review medical record/query physician
       - ☐ Trunk
         - ☐ Chest wall
         - ☐ Abdominal wall

- ☐ Upper back
- ☐ Lower back
- ☐ Buttocks
- ☐ Genital region
  - ☐ Female
  - ☐ Male
- ☐ Other site
- ☐ Unspecified site – review medical record/query physician

☐ Shoulder and upper limb (excluding wrist and hand)
- ☐ Scapula
- ☐ Shoulder
- ☐ Axilla
- ☐ Upper arm
- ☐ Elbow
- ☐ Forearm
- ☐ Multiple sites shoulder and upper limb (excluding wrist and hand)
- ☐ Unspecified site – review medical record/query physician

☐ Wrist and hand
- ☐ Wrist
- ☐ Hand
  - ☐ Back of hand
  - ☐ Palm
  - ☐ Finger
    - ☐ Multiple fingers not including thumb
    - ☐ Multiple fingers including thumb
    - ☐ Single except thumb
    - ☐ Thumb
    - ☐ Unspecified site hand – review medical record/query physician
  - ☐ Multiple sites of wrist and hand

☐ Lower limb except ankle and foot
- ☐ Thigh
- ☐ Knee
- ☐ Lower leg
- ☐ Multiple sites of lower limb
- ☐ Unspecified site lower limb – review medical record/query physician

☐ Ankle and foot
- ☐ Ankle
- ☐ Foot
- ☐ Toe(s)
- ☐ Multiple sites of ankle and foot
- ☐ Unspecified site ankle or foot – review medical record/query physician

☐ Internal Organs
- ☐ Ear drum
- ☐ Esophagus
- ☐ Genitourinary organs, internal
- ☐ Mouth and pharynx
- ☐ Other parts of alimentary tract
- ☐ Respiratory tract
  - ☐ Larynx and trachea
  - ☐ Larynx and trachea with lung
  - ☐ Other parts of respiratory tract (thoracic cavity)
  - ☐ Unspecified site respiratory tract- review medical record/query physician
- ☐ Other internal organ
- ☐ Unspecified internal organ

4. Identify degree of burn:
   - ☐ First degree
   - ☐ Second degree
   - ☐ Third degree
   - ☐ Unspecified degree – review medical record/query physician
5. Identify laterality:
   - ☐ Left
   - ☐ Right
   - ☐ Unspecified – review medical record/query physician

Note: Laterality only applies to burns and corrosions involving the extremities, ears, and eyes.

6. Identify episode of care/stage of healing/complication
   - ☐ A Initial encounter
   - ☐ D Subsequent encounter
   - ☐ S Sequela
7. Identify extent of body surface involved and percent of third degree burns, if over 10% of body surface:
   - ☐ Less than 10% of body surface
   - ☐ 10-19% of body surface
     - ☐ 0% to 9% of third degree burns
     - ☐ 10-19% of third degree burns
   - ☐ 20-29% of body surface
     - ☐ 0% to 9% of third degree burns
     - ☐ 10-19% of third degree burns
     - ☐ 20-29% of third degree burns
   - ☐ 30-39% of body surface
     - ☐ 0% to 9% of third degree burns
     - ☐ 10-19% of third degree burns
     - ☐ 20-29% of third degree burns
     - ☐ 30-39% of third degree burns
   - ☐ 40-49% of body surface
     - ☐ 0% to 9% of third degree burns
     - ☐ 10-19% of third degree burns
     - ☐ 20-29% of third degree burns
     - ☐ 30-39% of third degree burns
     - ☐ 40-49% of third degree burns
   - ☐ 50-59% of body surface
     - ☐ 0% to 9% of third degree burns
     - ☐ 10-19% of third degree burns
     - ☐ 20-29% of third degree burns
     - ☐ 30-39% of third degree burns
     - ☐ 40-49% of third degree burns
     - ☐ 50-59% of third degree burns
   - ☐ 60-69% of body surface
     - ☐ 0% to 9% of third degree burns

- ☐ 10-19% of third degree burns
- ☐ 20-29% of third degree burns
- ☐ 30-39% of third degree burns
- ☐ 40-49% of third degree burns
- ☐ 50-59% of third degree burns
- ☐ 60-69% of third degree burns

☐ 70-79% of body surface
- ☐ 0% to 9% of third degree burns
- ☐ 10-19% of third degree burns
- ☐ 20-29% of third degree burns
- ☐ 30-39% of third degree burns
- ☐ 40-49% of third degree burns
- ☐ 50-59% of third degree burns
- ☐ 60-69% of third degree burns
- ☐ 70-79% of third degree burns

☐ 80-89% of body surface
- ☐ 0% to 9% of third degree burns
- ☐ 10-19% of third degree burns
- ☐ 20-29% of third degree burns
- ☐ 30-39% of third degree burns
- ☐ 40-49% of third degree burns
- ☐ 50-59% of third degree burns
- ☐ 60-69% of third degree burns
- ☐ 70-79% of third degree burns

☐ 80-89% of third degree burns 90% or more of body surface
- ☐ 0% to 9% of third degree burns
- ☐ 10-19% of third degree burns
- ☐ 20-29% of third degree burns
- ☐ 30-39% of third degree burns
- ☐ 40-49% of third degree burns
- ☐ 50-59% of third degree burns
- ☐ 60-69% of third degree burns
- ☐ 70-79% third degree burns
- ☐ 80-89% third degree burns
- ☐ 90% or more third degree burns

Note: Extent of body surface is to be coded as a supplementary code for burns of an external body surface when the site is specified. It should only be used as the primary code when the site of the burn is unspecified.

8. Identify the external cause source/chemical agent, intent and place:
   - ☐ If burn, identify the source and intent X00-X19, X75-X77, X96-X98
   - ☐ If corrosion, code first the chemical agent and intent (T51-T65)
   - ☐ Place Y92
9. For frostbite, identify extent of tissue involvement:
   - ☐ Superficial
   - ☐ With tissue necrosis
10. For frostbite, identify body area:
    - ☐ Head
      - ☐ Ear
      - ☐ Nose
      - ☐ Other part of head
    - ☐ Neck
    - ☐ Thorax
    - ☐ Abdominal wall, lower back and pelvis
    - ☐ Arm
    - ☐ Wrist, hand, and fingers
      - ☐ Wrist
      - ☐ Hand
      - ☐ Finger(s)
    - ☐ Hip and thigh
    - ☐ Knee and lower leg
    - ☐ Ankle, foot, and toes
      - ☐ Ankle
      - ☐ Foot
      - ☐ Toe(s)
    - ☐ Other sites
    - ☐ Unspecified site
11. Identify laterality (excluding nose, neck, thorax, abdominal wall, lower back and pelvis):
    - ☐ Left
    - ☐ Right
    - ☐ Unspecified – review medical record/query physician
12. For sequencing of multiple burns and/or burns with related conditions:
    - Multiple external burns only. When more than one external burn is present, the first listed diagnosis code is the code that reflects the highest degree burn
    - Internal and external burns. The circumstances of the admission or encounter govern the selection of the principle or first-listed diagnosis
    - Burn injuries and other related conditions such as smoke inhalation or respiratory failure. The circumstances of the admission or encounter govern the selection of the principal or first-listed diagnosis.
    - Assign separate codes for each burn site
    - Classify burns of the same local site (three-digit category level) but of different degrees to the subcategory identifying the highest degree recorded in the diagnosis.

Cataract

ICD-10-CM Categories/Codes

Cataracts are classified in Chapter 7 Diseases of the Eye and Adnexa based on whether they are age related or due to other underlying conditions. There is also a code for congenital cataract classified in Chapter 17 Congenital Malformations, Deformations, and Chromosomal Abnormalities. The codes are as follows:

For Diabetic Cataracts, see:

E08.36	Diabetes mellitus due to underlying condition with diabetic cataract
E09.36	Drug or chemical induced diabetes mellitus with diabetic cataract
E10.36	Type I diabetes mellitus with diabetic cataract
E11.36	Type II diabetes mellitus with diabetic cataract
E13.36	Other specified diabetes mellitus with diabetic cataract
H25	Age-related cataract
H26	Other cataract
H28	Cataract in diseases classified elsewhere
Q12.0	Congenital cataract

ICD-10-CM Definitions

Cataract – Opacity or clouding of the lens of the eye that can cause blurring, haziness of vision, and blindness.

Age-related cataract – Cataract that occurs as a result of aging. Also called a senile cataract.

Congenital cataract – Cataract that is present at birth.

Incipient – Initial stage, beginning to happen or develop

Presenile cataract – Cataract that is not a result of aging, trauma, drug toxicity, or another condition or disease process. In the Alphabetic Index, a See note for Cataract, presenile is provided when the terms Cataract, infantile or Cataract, juvenile are referenced. Cataract, presenile lists codes in subcategory H26.0 Infantile and juvenile cataract.

Checklist

1. Identify cataract as age-related, congenital, or other type:
   - ☐ Age-related – Proceed to #2
   - ☐ Congenital – Use code Q12.0
   - ☐ Other type – Proceed to #3
   - ☐ In diseases classified elsewhere – Proceed to #4
2. Age-Related Cataract
   a. Identify type:
      - ☐ Combined forms
      - ☐ Incipient
        - ☐ Anterior subcapsular polar
        - ☐ Cortical
        - ☐ Posterior subcapsular polar
        - ☐ Other incipient type
      - ☐ Morgagnian type
      - ☐ Nuclear
      - ☐ Other specified type
      - ☐ Unspecified age-related cataract

   b. Specify laterality:
      - ☐ Right
      - ☐ Left
      - ☐ Bilateral
      - ☐ Unspecified eye
3. Cataract – Other Type

   Excludes age-related types and congenital cataract.

   a. Identify type:
      - ☐ Infantile and juvenile
        - ☐ Combined forms
        - ☐ Cortical/lamellar/zonular
        - ☐ Nuclear
        - ☐ Subcapsular polar
          - ☐ Anterior
          - ☐ Posterior
        - ☐ Other specified infantile/juvenile
        - ☐ Unspecified
      - ☐ Traumatic – Use additional code from Chapter 20 to identify external cause
        - ☐ Localized
        - ☐ Partially resolved
        - ☐ Total
        - ☐ Unspecified traumatic cataract
      - ☐ Complicated
        - ☐ Glaucomatous – Specify and code first glaucoma type (see category H40-H42) ______________
        - ☐ Secondary to ocular disorder – Specify associated ocular disorder ______________
        - ☐ With neovascularization – Specify associated condition ______________
        - ☐ Unspecified complication
      - ☐ Toxic – Use additional code for adverse effect T36-T50
      - ☐ Secondary
        - ☐ Soemmering's ring
        - ☐ Other specified type secondary cataract
        - ☐ Unspecified secondary cataract
      - ☐ Other specified type
      - ☐ Unspecified cataract

   b. Specify laterality:
      - ☐ Right
      - ☐ Left
      - ☐ Bilateral
      - ☐ Unspecified eye
4. Cataract in Diseases Classified Elsewhere
   a. Code first underlying disease
      - ☐ Hypoparathyroidism E20.-
      - ☐ Myxedema E03.-
      - ☐ Myotonia G71.1-

Cholecystitis, Cholelithiasis, Choledocholithiasis and Cholangitis

ICD-10-CM Categories/Codes

K80	Cholelithiasis
K81	Cholecystitis
K82.A1	Gangrene of gallbladder in cholecystitis
K82.A2	Perforation of gallbladder in cholecystitis
K83.0	Cholangitis

ICD-10-CM Definitions

Cholangitis – Inflammation of the bile ducts most often caused by the presence of stones or calculi in the bile ducts.

Cholecystitis – Inflammation of the gallbladder most often caused by the presence of calculi or sludge that blocks the flow of bile. Cholecystitis may be acute or chronic and chronic cases may be complicated by an acute inflammation.

Choledocholithiasis – Calculi in the bile ducts that may also cause inflammation of the bile ducts, referred to as cholangitis. A complication of calculi in the bile ducts is obstruction of the flow of bile.

Cholelithiasis – The presence of stones or calculi in the gallbladder. Cholelithiasis may occur alone or with cholecystitis. A complication of calculi in the gallbladder is obstruction of the flow of bile.

Checklist

1. Cholecystitis
   - ☐ With cholelithiasis or choledocholithiasis – Proceed to 3
   - ☐ Without cholelithiasis or choledocholithiasis
     - ☐ Acute (K81.0)
     - ☐ Acute with chronic (K81.2)
     - ☐ Chronic (K81.1)
     - ☐ Unspecified (K81.9) – review medical record/query physician
   - ☐ Gallbladder gangrene (K82.A1)
   - ☐ Gallbladder perforation (K82.A2)
2. Cholangitis
   - ☐ With choledocholithiasis – Proceed to 3
   - ☐ Without choledocholithiasis (K83.0)
3. Cholelithiasis – Identify site of calculus:
   - ☐ Bile duct only – Proceed to 5
   - ☐ Gallbladder only – Proceed to 4
   - ☐ Gallbladder and bile duct – Proceed to 6
   - ☐ Other
     - ☐ With obstruction (K80.81)
     - ☐ Without obstruction (K80.80)
4. Calculus of gallbladder only
   - ☐ With cholecystitis
     - ☐ Acute
       - ☐ With obstruction (K80.01)
       - ☐ Without obstruction (K80.00)
     - ☐ Acute and chronic
       - ☐ With obstruction (K80.13)
       - ☐ Without obstruction (K80.12)
     - ☐ Chronic
       - ☐ With obstruction (K80.11)
       - ☐ Without obstruction (K80.10)
     - ☐ Other
       - ☐ With obstruction (K80.19)
       - ☐ Without obstruction (K80.18)
   - ☐ Without cholecystitis
     - ☐ With obstruction (K80.21)
     - ☐ Without obstruction (K80.20)
5. Calculus of bile duct only
   - ☐ With cholangitis
     - ☐ Acute
       - ☐ With obstruction (K80.33)
       - ☐ Without obstruction (K80.32)
     - ☐ Acute and chronic
       - ☐ With obstruction (K80.37)
       - ☐ Without obstruction (K80.36)
     - ☐ Chronic
       - ☐ With obstruction (K80.35)
       - ☐ Without obstruction (K80.34)
     - ☐ Unspecified
       - ☐ With obstruction (K80.31) – review medical record/query physician
       - ☐ Without obstruction (K80.30) – review medical record/query physician
   - ☐ With cholecystitis (includes cholangitis if present)
     - ☐ Acute
       - ☐ With obstruction (K80.43)
       - ☐ Without obstruction (K80.42)
     - ☐ Acute and chronic
       - ☐ With obstruction (K80.47)
       - ☐ Without obstruction (K80.46)
     - ☐ Chronic
       - ☐ With obstruction (K80.45)
       - ☐ Without obstruction (K80.44)
     - ☐ Unspecified
       - ☐ With obstruction (K80.41) – review medical record/query physician
       - ☐ Without obstruction (K80.40) – review medical record/query physician
   - ☐ Without cholangitis or cholecystitis
     - ☐ With obstruction (K80.51)
     - ☐ Without obstruction (K80.50)
6. For calculus of gallbladder and bile duct, identify:
   - ☐ With cholecystitis
     - ☐ Acute
       - ☐ With obstruction (K80.63)
       - ☐ Without obstruction (K80.62)
     - ☐ Acute and chronic
       - ☐ With obstruction (K80.67)
       - ☐ Without obstruction (K80.66)
     - ☐ Chronic
       - ☐ With obstruction (K80.65)
       - ☐ Without obstruction (K80.64)
     - ☐ Unspecified

- ☐ With obstruction (K80.61) – review medical record/query physician
- ☐ Without obstruction (K80.60) – review medical record/query physician

☐ Without cholecystitis

- ☐ With obstruction (K80.71)
- ☐ Without obstruction (K80.70)

Conjunctivitis

ICD-10-CM Categories/Subcategories

B30	Viral conjunctivitis
H10.0	Mucopurulent conjunctivitis
H10.1	Acute atopic conjunctivitis
H10.2	Other acute conjunctivitis
H10.3	Unspecified acute conjunctivitis
H10.4	Chronic conjunctivitis
H10.5	Blepharoconjunctivitis
H10.8	Other conjunctivitis
H10.9	Unspecified conjunctivitis

Refer to ICD-10-CM Alphabetic Index for newborn conjunctivitis, conjunctivitis due to other specific organisms, and other less common types of conjunctivitis.

ICD-10-CM Definitions

Conjunctivitis – Inflammation of the conjunctiva, the clear membrane lining the inner surface of the eyelid and outer surface of the eye. Inflammation may be caused by bacteria, viruses, allergens, or chemicals. Symptoms include redness, swelling, drainage, and discomfort, but visual acuity and pupil response should be normal.

Checklist

1. Identify type of conjunctivitis:
   - ☐ Acute conjunctivitis
     - ☐ Atopic
     - ☐ Pseudomembranous
     - ☐ Serous
     - ☐ Toxic (chemical) – Code first chemical and intent (T51-T65)
     - ☐ Unspecified acute conjunctivitis
   - ☐ Blepharoconjunctivitis
     - ☐ Angular
     - ☐ Contact
     - ☐ Ligneous
     - ☐ Unspecified blepharoconjunctivitis
   - ☐ Chronic conjunctivitis
     - ☐ Follicular
     - ☐ Giant papillary
     - ☐ Simple
     - ☐ Vernal
     - ☐ Other chronic allergic
     - ☐ Unspecified chronic conjunctivitis
   - ☐ Mucopurulent conjunctivitis
     - ☐ Acute follicular
     - ☐ Other mucopurulent type
   - ☐ Pingueculitis
   - ☐ Viral
     - ☐ Acute epidemic hemorrhagic (enteroviral)
     - ☐ Due to adenovirus
       - ☐ Conjunctivitis
       - ☐ Keratoconjunctivitis
     - ☐ Pharyngoconjunctivitis
     - ☐ Other viral conjunctivitis – Specify ______________
     - ☐ Unspecified viral conjunctivitis
   - ☐ Other conjunctivitis – Specify ______________
   - ☐ Unspecified
2. Specify laterality (excluding viral conjunctivitis):
   - ☐ Right
   - ☐ Left
   - ☐ Bilateral
   - ☐ Unspecified eye

Coronary Atherosclerosis With/Without Angina

ICD-10-CM Subcategories

Atherosclerotic heart disease is classified as with or without angina pectoris in the following subcategories:

I25.1 Atherosclerotic heart disease of native coronary artery

I25.7 Atherosclerosis of coronary artery bypass graft(s) and coronary artery of transplanted heart with angina pectoris

I25.81 Atherosclerosis of other coronary vessels without angina pectoris

ICD-10-CM Definitions

A combination code is used to identify coronary atherosclerosis as with or without angina in ICD-10-CM. Use codes from subcategories I25.1, I25.7, and I25.8 to capture both the coronary atherosclerosis, the presence/absence of angina, and when angina is present, the type of angina. For angina without documented coronary atherosclerosis, see category I20.

Angina – Pain or discomfort, pressure or squeezing, usually centered in the chest, or other atypical symptoms that result from diseased coronary arteries with restriction of blood flow to the heart muscle. Also called angina pectoris. Angina is classified in ICD-10-CM by the type of angina, which includes: unstable, angina with documented spasm, other forms of angina, and unspecified angina. For detailed definitions of each type, see the Angina check list.

Coronary Atherosclerosis – Condition affecting arterial blood vessels in the heart and characterized by inflammation and accumulation of macrophage white blood cells and low-density lipoproteins along the arterial walls leading to narrowing of the vessels and decreased blood flow to the heart muscle. Synonymous terms include:

- Atherosclerotic cardiovascular disease
- Atherosclerotic heart disease
- Coronary (artery) atheroma
- Coronary (artery) disease
- Coronary (artery) sclerosis
- Chronic ischemic heart disease

Checklist

1. Identify site of coronary atherosclerosis:
   - ☐ Native coronary artery
   - ☐ Graft
     - ☐ Autologous artery bypass graft
     - ☐ Autologous vein bypass graft
     - ☐ Nonautologous biological bypass graft
     - ☐ Other specified type of bypass graft
     - ☐ Unspecified type of bypass graft
   - ☐ Transplanted heart
     - ☐ Native coronary artery of transplanted heart
     - ☐ Bypass graft (artery/vein) of transplanted heart
2. Identify presence/absence and type of angina pectoris:
   - ☐ With angina pectoris
     - ☐ Unstable
     - ☐ With documented spasm
     - ☐ With other documented form of angina pectoris
     - ☐ Unspecified angina pectoris
   - ☐ Without angina pectoris
3. Identify and assign additional code for any:
   - ☐ Chronic total occlusion of coronary artery (I25.82)
   - ☐ Coronary atherosclerosis due to
     - ☐ Calcified coronary lesion (I25.84)
     - ☐ Lipid rich plaque (I25.83)
4. Use additional code to identify exposure to tobacco smoke or history of, current use of, or dependence on tobacco:
   - ☐ Exposure to environmental tobacco smoke (Z77.22)
   - ☐ History of tobacco use (Z87.891)
   - ☐ Occupational exposure to environmental tobacco smoke (Z57.31)
   - ☐ Tobacco dependence (F17.-)
   - ☐ Tobacco use (Z72.0)

Dermatitis, Contact

ICD-10-CM Categories

Contact dermatitis is classified in the following categories:

L23	Allergic contact dermatitis
L24	Irritant contact dermatitis
L25	Unspecified contact dermatitis

ICD-10-CM Definitions

In ICD-10-CM, the terms dermatitis and eczema are used synonymously and interchangeably in the classification.

Contact dermatitis (eczema) – Inflammation of the skin resulting from direct contact with a substance which causes the inflammatory skin reaction. Skin inflammation may be due to an allergy to the substance or due to irritants in the substance.

Allergic contact dermatitis (eczema) – Inflammation of the skin resulting from an allergy to a substance that has come in direct contact with the skin.

Irritant contact dermatitis (eczema) – Inflammation of the skin resulting from irritation by a chemical or other substance that has come in direct contact with the skin.

Checklist

1. Identify type of contact dermatitis:
   - ☐ Allergic – Proceed to #2
   - ☐ Irritant – Proceed to #3
   - ☐ Unspecified – Proceed to #4
2. Allergic Contact Dermatitis
   a. Specify cause:
      - ☐ Animal (cat) (dog) dander
      - ☐ Adhesives
      - ☐ Cosmetics
      - ☐ Drugs in contact with skin – Specify drug ___________
      - ☐ Dyes
      - ☐ Food in contact with skin
      - ☐ Metals
      - ☐ Plants (except food)
      - ☐ Other chemical products
      - ☐ Other specified agents – Specify agent ___________
      - ☐ Unspecified cause
3. Irritant Contact Dermatitis
   a. Specify cause:
      - ☐ Cosmetics
      - ☐ Detergents
      - ☐ Drugs in contact with skin – Specify drug ___________
      - ☐ Food in contact with skin
      - ☐ Metals
      - ☐ Plants (except food)
      - ☐ Oils and greases
      - ☐ Solvents
      - ☐ Other chemical products
      - ☐ Other specified agents – Specify agent ___________
      - ☐ Unspecified cause
4. Unspecified Contact Dermatitis
   a. Specify cause:
      - ☐ Cosmetics
      - ☐ Drugs in contact with skin – Specify drug ___________
      - ☐ Dyes
      - ☐ Food in contact with skin
      - ☐ Other chemical products
      - ☐ Plants (except food)
      - ☐ Other specified agents – Specify agent ___________
      - ☐ Unspecified cause

For contact dermatitis caused by drugs, use additional code for adverse effect, if applicable, to identify drug (T36-T50 with fifth character 5)

Diabetes Mellitus

ICD-10-CM Categories

E08	Diabetes mellitus due to underlying condition
E09	Drug or chemical induced diabetes mellitus
E10	Type 1 diabetes mellitus
E11	Type 2 diabetes mellitus
E13	Other specified diabetes mellitus

ICD-10-CM Definitions

Codes for diabetes mellitus are combination codes that reflect the type of diabetes, the body system affected, and any specific complications/manifestations affecting that body system.

Other specified diabetes (E13) includes secondary diabetes specified as:

- Due to genetic defects of beta-cell function
- Due to genetic defects in insulin action
- Postpancreatectomy
- Postprocedural
- Secondary diabetes not elsewhere classified

Checklist

1. Identify the type of diabetes mellitus:
   - ☐ Type 1
   - ☐ Type 2 (includes unspecified)
   - ☐ Secondary diabetes
     - ☐ Drug or chemical induced
     - ☐ Due to underlying condition
     - ☐ Other specified diabetes mellitus
2. Identify the body system affected and any manifestations/complications:
   - ☐ No complications
   - ☐ Arthropathy
     - ☐ Neuropathic
     - ☐ Other arthropathy
   - ☐ Circulatory complications
     - ☐ Peripheral angiopathy
       - ☐ With gangrene
       - ☐ Without gangrene
     - ☐ Other circulatory complication
   - ☐ Hyperglycemia
   - ☐ Hyperosmolarity (except type 1)
     - ☐ With coma
     - ☐ Without coma
   - ☐ Hypoglycemia
     - ☐ With coma
     - ☐ Without coma
   - ☐ Ketoacidosis
     - ☐ With coma
     - ☐ Without coma
   - ☐ Kidney complications
     - ☐ Nephropathy
     - ☐ Chronic kidney disease – Use additional code (N18.1-N18.6) for stage of CKD
     - ☐ Other diabetic kidney complication
   - ☐ Neurological complications
     - ☐ Amyotrophy
     - ☐ Autonomic (poly)neuropathy
     - ☐ Mononeuropathy
     - ☐ Polyneuropathy
     - ☐ Other diabetic neurological complication
     - ☐ Unspecified diabetic neuropathy
   - ☐ Ophthalmic complications
     - ☐ Diabetic retinopathy
       - ☐ Mild nonproliferative
         - ☐ With macular edema
         - ☐ Without macular edema
       - ☐ Moderate nonproliferative
         - ☐ With macular edema
         - ☐ Without macular edema
       - ☐ Severe nonproliferative
         - ☐ With macular edema
         - ☐ Without macular edema
       - ☐ Proliferative
         - ☐ With traction retinal detachment involving the macula
         - ☐ With traction retinal detachment not involving the macula
         - ☐ With combined traction retinal detachment and rhegmatogenous retinal detachment
         - ☐ With macular edema
         - ☐ Without macular edema
       - ☐ Unspecified
         - ☐ With macular edema
         - ☐ Without macular edema
       - ☐ Identify laterality (*except with diabetic cataract, unspecified diabetic retinopathy, and other diabetic ophthalmic complication*)
         - ☐ Right eye
         - ☐ Left eye
         - ☐ Bilateral
         - ☐ Unspecified eye
     - ☐ Diabetic cataract
     - ☐ Diabetic macular edema, resolved following treatment
     - ☐ Other diabetic ophthalmic complication
   - ☐ Oral complications
     - ☐ Periodontal disease
     - ☐ Other oral complications
   - ☐ Skin complications
     - ☐ Dermatitis
     - ☐ Foot ulcer, chronic, non-pressure – Use additional code (L97.4-, L97.5-) to identify site and severity of ulcer

- ☐ Other chronic, non-pressure skin ulcer – Use additional code (L97.1-, L97.2-, L97.3-, L97.8-, L98.41-, L98.49-) to identify site and severity of ulcer
- ☐ Other skin complication

☐ Other specified complication – Use additional code to identify complication

☐ Unspecified complication

For Type II (E11) and secondary diabetes types (E08, E09, E13), use additional code to identify any long-term insulin use (Z79.4).

For diabetes due to underlying disease (E08), code first the underlying condition.

For diabetes due to drugs or chemicals (E09):

- Code first poisoning due to drug or toxin (T36-T65 with 5th or 6th character 1-4 or 6) – OR-
- Use additional code for adverse effect, if applicable, to identify drug (T36-T50 with 5th or 6th character 5)

For other specified diabetes mellitus (E13) documented as due to pancreatectomy:

- Assign first code E89.1 Postprocedural hypoinsulinemia
- Assign the applicable codes from category E13
- Assign a code from Z90.41- Acquired absence of pancreas
- Use additional code (Z79.4, Z79.84) to identify type of control

Examination, Administrative

ICD-10-CM Categories

Codes for encounters for examination are found in categories Z00-Z13.

Administrative examinations are listed in category Z02 Encounter for administrative examination.

ICD-10-CM Definitions

Administrative examination – Examinations that are performed for specific administrative purposes such as pre-employment, school, sports, and insurance.

Checklist

Identify reason for administrative examination:

- ☐ Admission to
  - ☐ Educational institution
  - ☐ Residential institution
- ☐ Adoption services
- ☐ Alcohol/drug test
- ☐ Armed forces recruitment
- ☐ Certificate for
  - ☐ Disability
  - ☐ Other medical certificate
- ☐ Driver's license
- ☐ Insurance
- ☐ Paternity testing
- ☐ Pre-employment
- ☐ Sports participation
- ☐ Other administrative purposes
- ☐ Unspecified administrative purposes

Examination, General Medical

ICD-10-CM Categories

Codes for encounters for examination are found in categories Z00-Z13. Categories for encounter for general examinations and special examinations include:

Z00	Encounter for general examination without complaint, suspected or reported diagnosis
Z01	Encounter for other special examination without complaint, suspected or reported diagnosis

While gynecological examinations are reported with codes in category Z01, examinations related to pregnancy and reproduction are not – see categories Z30-Z36 and Z39.

ICD-10-CM Definitions

General examination – Codes for encounters for general examinations are reported for patients who are seen without a medical complaint or a suspected or reported diagnosis, such as an annual examination for an adult or a well-child examination. Codes for adults and infants/children are specific as to whether the examination was with or without abnormal findings. Codes identifying any abnormal findings are reported additionally.

Special examination – Special examinations include: eyes/vision, ears/hearing, dental exam/cleaning, blood pressure, gynecological, preprocedural, allergy testing, blood typing, and antibody response.

Checklist

1. Identify purpose of examination:
   - ☐ General examination – Proceed to #2
   - ☐ Special examination – Proceed to #3
2. For general examination identify:
   - ☐ Adult
     - ☐ With abnormal findings
     - ☐ Without abnormal findings
   - ☐ Child (Over 28 days old)
     - ☐ Adolescent development state
     - ☐ Period of delayed growth
       - ☐ With abnormal findings
       - ☐ Without abnormal findings
     - ☐ Period of rapid growth
     - ☐ Routine
       - ☐ With abnormal findings
       - ☐ Without abnormal findings
   - ☐ Newborn (Under 29 days old)
     - ☐ Under 8 days old
     - ☐ 8-28 days old
   - ☐ Other reason
     - ☐ Normal comparison and control in clinical research program
     - ☐ Other general examination
     - ☐ Potential organ/tissue donor
3. For special examination, identify type/reason:
   - ☐ Allergy testing
   - ☐ Antibody response examination
   - ☐ Blood pressure
     - ☐ With abnormal findings
     - ☐ Without abnormal findings
   - ☐ Blood typing
   - ☐ Dental exam and cleaning
     - ☐ With abnormal findings
     - ☐ Without abnormal findings
   - ☐ Ears/Hearing
     - ☐ Hearing conservation treatment
     - ☐ Evaluation
       - ☐ With abnormal findings
         - ☐ Following failed hearing screening
         - ☐ With other abnormal findings
       - ☐ Without abnormal findings
   - ☐ Eyes/Vision
     - ☐ With abnormal findings
     - ☐ Without abnormal findings
   - ☐ Gynecological
     - ☐ Cervical smear to confirm findings of normal smear following initial abnormal smear
     - ☐ Examination (routine)
       - ☐ With abnormal findings
       - ☐ Without abnormal findings
   - ☐ Preprocedural
     - ☐ Cardiovascular examination
     - ☐ Laboratory examination
     - ☐ Other preprocedural examination
     - ☐ Respiratory examination
   - ☐ Other specified special examination

Use additional code(s) to identify any abnormal findings.

Examination, Gynecological/Contraception

ICD-10-CM Categories/Subcategories

Z01.4	Encounter for gynecological examination
Z08	Encounter for gynecological exam status post hysterectomy for malignant condition
Z12.4	Encounter for screening for malignant neoplasm of cervix
Z30	Encounter for contraceptive management

ICD-10-CM Definitions

Contraceptive Management – General counseling and advice on contraception; prescribing and surveillance of contraceptive pills, injectable contraceptives, and emergency contraception; insertion, removal, and replacement of intrauterine device; and other contraceptive advice and services such as natural family planning and sterilization.

Gynecological Examination – An annual or periodic pelvic examination that may or may not include a cervical pap smear.

Screening for malignant neoplasm of cervix – A screening pap smear of the cervix to evaluate and detect any cytological abnormalities that might be indicative of malignant neoplasm.

Checklist

1. Identify purpose of examination:
   - ☐ Gynecological – Proceed to #2
   - ☐ Cervical pap smear only (not performed as part of general gynecological examination) – Use code Z12.4
   - ☐ Contraceptive management – Proceed to #3
2. Gynecological Examination
   a. Identify reason for visit:
      - ☐ Cervical smear to confirm findings of recent normal smear following initial abnormal smear
      - ☐ Gynecological exam status post hysterectomy for malignancy
      - ☐ Routine gynecological examination with or without cervical smear
        - ☐ With abnormal findings
        - ☐ Without abnormal findings

   b. Use additional code(s) to identify any abnormal findings

   c. Use additional code to identify:
      - ☐ Screening for human papillomavirus, if applicable, (Z11.51)
      - ☐ Screening vaginal pap smear, if applicable (Z12.72)
      - ☐ Acquired absence of uterus, if applicable (Z90.71-)
3. Contraceptive Management
   a. Identify type of encounter for contraceptive management:
      - ☐ Contraceptive pills
        - ☐ Initial prescription
        - ☐ Surveillance
      - ☐ Emergency contraception
      - ☐ General counseling and advice on contraception
      - ☐ Implantable subdermal contraceptive
        - ☐ Initial prescription
        - ☐ Surveillance
      - ☐ Injectable contraceptive
        - ☐ Initial prescription
        - ☐ Surveillance
      - ☐ Intrauterine contraceptive device
        - ☐ Initial prescription
        - ☐ Insertion (without removal of previously placed IUD)
        - ☐ Routine checking of device
        - ☐ Removal
        - ☐ Removal with reinsertion (replacement)
      - ☐ Natural family planning instruction to avoid pregnancy
      - ☐ Other contraception (barrier/diaphragm)
        - ☐ Initial prescription
        - ☐ Surveillance
      - ☐ Transdermal patch hormonal contraceptive
        - ☐ Initial prescription
        - ☐ Surveillance
      - ☐ Sterilization
      - ☐ Other contraceptive management
      - ☐ Vaginal ring hormonal contraceptive
        - ☐ Initial prescription
        - ☐ Surveillance
      - ☐ Unspecified contraceptive management

Examination, Obstetric/Reproductive

ICD-10-CM Categories

Z31	Encounter for procreative management
Z32	Encounter for pregnancy test and childbirth and childcare instruction
Z33	Pregnant state
Z34	Encounter for supervision of normal pregnancy
Z36	Encounter for antenatal screening of mother
Z39	Encounter for maternal postpartum care and examination

Note: For contraceptive management, see Examination, Gynecological/Contraceptive checklist.

ICD-10-CM Definitions

Pregnancy Z-codes – Z-codes for pregnancy are used when none of the problems or complications included in the Obstetrics chapter exist. Z-codes are used to report antenatal screening, procreative management, routine prenatal visits, and postpartum care.

Checklist

Identify purpose of visit:

- ☐ Assisted reproductive fertility procedure cycle (Z31.83)
- ☐ Antenatal screening of mother (Z36)
- ☐ Procreative management
  - ☐ Fertility
    - ☐ Male factor infertility in female patient (Z31.81)
    - ☐ Preservation
      - ☐ Counseling (Z31.62)
      - ☐ Procedure (Z31.84)
    - ☐ Testing (Z31.41)
  - ☐ Genetic counseling (Z31.5)
  - ☐ Genetic testing, female/mother
    - ☐ Disease carrier status (Z31.430)
    - ☐ Other genetic testing (Z31.438)
  - ☐ Genetic testing, male/father
    - ☐ Disease carrier status (Z31.440)
    - ☐ Recurrent pregnancy loss in partner (Z34.441)
    - ☐ Other genetic testing (Z31.448)
  - ☐ General procreative counseling/advice, other (Z31.69)
  - ☐ Gestation carrier counseling/management (Z31.7)
  - ☐ Investigation and testing, other procreative (Z31.49)
  - ☐ Natural family planning (Z31.61)
  - ☐ Sterilization reversal
    - ☐ Reversal services (Z31.0)
    - ☐ Aftercare (Z31.42)
  - ☐ Rh incompatibility status (Z31.82)
  - ☐ Other procreative management services (Z31.89)
- ☐ Pregnancy – other services
  - ☐ Childbirth instruction (Z32.2)
  - ☐ Childcare instruction (Z32.3)
  - ☐ Elective termination (Z33.2)
  - ☐ State
    - ☐ Gestational carrier (Z33.3)
    - ☐ Incidental (Z33.1)
  - ☐ Test
    - ☐ Positive (Z32.01)
    - ☐ Negative (Z32.02)
    - ☐ Result unknown (Z32.00)
- ☐ Supervision of normal pregnancy
  - ☐ First pregnancy
    - ☐ First trimester (Z34.01)
    - ☐ Second trimester (Z34.02)
    - ☐ Third trimester (Z34.03)
    - ☐ Unspecified trimester (Z34.00)
  - ☐ Other normal pregnancy
    - ☐ First trimester (Z34.81)
    - ☐ Second trimester (Z34.82)
    - ☐ Third trimester (Z34.83)
    - ☐ Unspecified trimester (Z34.80)
  - ☐ Unspecified normal pregnancy
    - ☐ First trimester (Z34.91)
    - ☐ Second trimester (Z34.92)
    - ☐ Third trimester (Z34.93)
    - ☐ Unspecified trimester (Z34.90)
- ☐ Postpartum care/examination
  - ☐ Immediately after delivery (Z39.0)
  - ☐ Lactation supervision (Z39.1)
  - ☐ Routine follow-up examination (Z39.2)

Feeding Problems, Newborn

ICD-10-CM Categories

P92 Feeding problems of newborn

ICD-10-CM Definitions

Codes in category P92 are used for feeding problems in a newborn which is defined as 28 days old or younger. For feeding problems in a child over 28 days old, see R63.3.

Failure to thrive in a newborn is reported with code P92.6. For failure to thrive in a child over 28 days old, see R62.51.

Vomiting of a newborn is reported with codes in subcategory P92.0. For vomiting of a child over 28 days old, see subcategory R11.1-

Checklist

Specify condition:

- ☐ Difficulty feeding at breast
- ☐ Failure to thrive
- ☐ Overfeeding
- ☐ Regurgitation/rumination
- ☐ Slow feeding
- ☐ Underfeeding
- ☐ Vomiting
    - ☐ Bilious
    - ☐ Other vomiting
- ☐ Other feeding problem – Specify ________________
- ☐ Unspecified feeding problem

Fractures

ICD-10-CM Categories

Fractures are classified according to whether the fracture is a result of trauma or due to overuse or an underlying disease process (nontraumatic).

Nontraumatic fractures are classified in the following ICD-10-CM categories:

M48.4	Fatigue fracture of vertebra
M48.5	Collapsed vertebra, not elsewhere classified
M80	Osteoporosis with current pathological fracture
M84.3	Stress fracture
M84.4	Pathological fracture, not elsewhere classified
M84.5	Pathological fracture in neoplastic disease
M84.6	Pathological fracture in other disease
M84.75	Atypical femoral fracture

Traumatic fractures are classified in the following ICD-10-CM categories:

S02	Fracture of skull and facial bones
S12	Fracture of cervical vertebra and other parts of neck
S22	Fracture of ribs, sternum and thoracic spine
S32	Fracture of lumbar spine and pelvis
S42	Fracture of shoulder and upper arm
S49.0	Physeal fracture of upper end of humerus
S49.1	Physeal fracture of lower end of humerus
S52	Fracture of forearm
S59.0	Physeal fracture of lower end of ulna
S59.1	Physeal fracture of upper end of radius
S59.2	Physeal fracture of lower end of radius
S62	Fracture at wrist and hand level
S72	Fracture of femur
S79.0	Fracture of upper end of femur
S79.1	Fracture of lower end of femur
S82	Fracture of lower leg, including ankle
S89.0	Physeal fracture of upper end of tibia
S89.1	Physeal fracture of lower end of tibia
S89.2	Physeal fracture of upper end of fibula
S89.3	Physeal fracture of lower end of fibula
S92	Fracture of foot and toe, except ankle
S99.0	Physeal fracture of calcaneus
S99.1	Physeal fracture of metatarsal
S99.2	Physeal fracture of phalanx of toe

ICD-10-CM Definitions

Closed – A fracture that does not have contact with the outside environment.

Comminuted – A fracture that has more than two pieces.

Displaced – Bone breaks in two or more parts that are not in normal alignment.

Episode of Care – There are sixteen (16) possible 7th character values to select from for fractures depending upon the fracture category. The 7th character defines the stage of treatment, fracture condition for traumatic fractures (open vs. closed), status of healing and residual effects related to the initial fracture.

A. Initial encounter. The period when the patient is receiving active treatment for the injury, poisoning, or other consequences of an external cause. An 'A' may be assigned on more than one claim.

B. Initial encounter for open fracture or (Gustilo) type I or II.

C. Initial encounter for open fracture (Gustilo) type IIIA, IIIB or IIIC.

D. Subsequent encounter for (closed) fracture with routine healing. Encounter after the active phase of treatment and when the patient is receiving routine care for the fracture during the period of healing or recovery.

E. Subsequent encounter for open fracture (Gustilo) type I or II. Encounter after the active phase of treatment and when the patient is receiving routine care for the fracture during the period of healing or recovery.

F. Subsequent encounter for open fracture (Gustilo) type IIIA, IIIB, IIIC with routine healing. Encounter after the active phase of treatment when the patient is receiving routine care for the fracture during the period of healing or recovery.

G. Subsequent encounter for (closed) fracture with delayed healing.

H. Subsequent encounter for open fracture (Gustilo) type I or II with delayed healing.

J. Subsequent encounter for open fracture (Gustilo) type IIIA, IIIB, IIIC with delayed healing.

K. Subsequent encounter for (closed) fracture with nonunion.

M. Subsequent encounter for open fracture (Gustilo) type I or II with nonunion.

N. Subsequent encounter for open fracture (Gustilo) type IIIA, IIIB, IIIC with nonunion.

P. Subsequent encounter for (closed) fracture with malunion.

Q. Subsequent encounter for open fracture (Gustilo) type I or II with malunion.

R. Subsequent encounter for open fracture (Gustilo) type IIIA, IIIB, IIIC with malunion.

S. Sequela. Encounter for complications or conditions that arise as a direct result of a fracture.

Fracture – A disruption or break of the continuity of a bone, epiphyseal plate or cartilaginous surface.

Greenstick – Incomplete fracture in children where one side of the bone breaks, the other side bends. Tends to occur in the shaft of a long bone.

Oblique – A diagonal fracture of a long bone.

Open fracture – An open wound at the site of the fracture resulting in communication with the outside environment. The open may be produced by the bone or the opening can produce the fracture.

Gustilo classification – Classification of open fractures of the forearm (S52), femur (S72) and lower leg (S82) based upon the size of the open wound and the amount of soft tissue injury.

Osteochondral – A break of tear of the articular cartilage along with a fracture of the bone.

Pathologic – Fracture that involves an underlying disease process. It may involve an injury but of the type that would not typically result in a fracture.

Physeal – Fracture in growing children that involves the growth plate.

Spiral – Twisting fracture usually of a long bone resulting in a spiral-shaped fracture line.

Stress – Fracture due to repetitive activity or overexertion without trauma.

Torus – Incomplete fracture of a long bone in children where one side buckles and the other side bulges. Occurs towards the ends of the shaft of the bone.

Transverse – A fracture line that goes across the shaft of a long bone.

Checklist

1. Identify whether the fracture is due to trauma or non-traumatic:
   - ☐ Nontraumatic fracture
     - ☐ Atypical femoral fracture
     - ☐ Pathological fracture
       - ☐ Due to osteoporosis
         - ☐ Age-related
         - ☐ Other
       - ☐ Due to neoplastic disease
         - ☐ Define neoplasm
       - ☐ Due to other disease
         - ☐ Define underlying disease
       - ☐ Not otherwise specified
     - ☐ Stress fracture
   - ☐ Traumatic fracture
2. If non-traumatic, identify nature and anatomic site of fracture:
   - ☐ Due to osteoporosis
     - ☐ Shoulder
     - ☐ Humerus
     - ☐ Forearm
     - ☐ Hand
     - ☐ Femur
     - ☐ Lower leg
     - ☐ Ankle and foot
     - ☐ Vertebra
   - ☐ Pathological, other disease process
     - ☐ Shoulder
     - ☐ Humerus
     - ☐ Radius
     - ☐ Ulna
     - ☐ Hand
     - ☐ Finger(s)
     - ☐ Pelvis
     - ☐ Femur
     - ☐ Hip, unspecified
     - ☐ Tibia
     - ☐ Fibula
     - ☐ Ankle
     - ☐ Foot
     - ☐ Toe(s)
     - ☐ Other site (includes vertebra)
   - ☐ Stress
     - ☐ Shoulder
     - ☐ Humerus
     - ☐ Radius
     - ☐ Ulna
     - ☐ Hand
     - ☐ Finger(s)
     - ☐ Pelvis
     - ☐ Femur
     - ☐ Hip, unspecified
     - ☐ Tibia
     - ☐ Fibula
     - ☐ Ankle
     - ☐ Foot
     - ☐ Toe(s)
     - ☐ Vertebra
       - a. Identify type:
         - ☐ Collapsed/Compression/Wedging
         - ☐ Fatigue
       - b. Identify spinal region:
         - ☐ Occipito-atlanto-axial region
         - ☐ Cervical region
         - ☐ Cervicothoracic region
         - ☐ Thoracic region
         - ☐ Thoracolumbar region
         - ☐ Lumbar region
         - ☐ Lumbosacral region
         - ☐ Sacral/sacrococcygeal region
     - ☐ Other site

- ☐ Rib (s)
  - ☐ One
  - ☐ Multiple
  - ☐ Flail chest
- ☐ Sternum
  - ☐ Body
  - ☐ Manubrium
  - ☐ Manubrium dissociation
  - ☐ Xiphoid process

4. For atypical femoral fractures and traumatic fractures, identify fracture configuration/type, where appropriate:
   - ☐ Atypical femoral fracture
     - ☐ Complete oblique
     - ☐ Complete transverse
     - ☐ Incomplete
   - ☐ Vertebral fractures
     - ☐ C1
       - ☐ Stable burst
       - ☐ Unstable burst
     - ☐ Thoracic and Lumbar
       - ☐ Wedge
       - ☐ Stable burst
       - ☐ Unstable burst
       - ☐ Other
     - ☐ Humerus
       - ☐ Surgical neck
         - ☐ 2-part
         - ☐ 3-part
         - ☐ 4-part
       - ☐ Upper or lower end
         - ☐ Physeal
           - ☐ Salter-Harris Type I
           - ☐ Salter-Harris Type II
           - ☐ Salter-Harris Type III
           - ☐ Salter-Harris Type IV
           - ☐ Other
           - ☐ Unspecified – review medical record/query physician
         - ☐ Torus
       - ☐ Shaft
         - ☐ Comminuted
         - ☐ Greenstick
         - ☐ Oblique
         - ☐ Segmental
         - ☐ Spiral
         - ☐ Transverse
         - ☐ Other
         - ☐ Unspecified – review medical record/query physician
       - ☐ Supracondylar without intercondylar fracture
         - ☐ Comminuted
         - ☐ Simple
     - ☐ Ulna
       - ☐ Olecranon process
         - ☐ with intercondylar extension
         - ☐ without intercondylar extension
       - ☐ Upper or lower end
         - ☐ Physeal
           - ☐ Salter-Harris Type I
           - ☐ Salter-Harris Type II
           - ☐ Salter-Harris Type III
           - ☐ Salter-Harris Type IV
           - ☐ Other
           - ☐ Unspecified – review medical record/query physician
         - ☐ Torus
       - ☐ Shaft
         - ☐ Bent bone
         - ☐ Comminuted
         - ☐ Greenstick
         - ☐ Monteggia
         - ☐ Oblique
         - ☐ Segmental
         - ☐ Spiral
         - ☐ Transverse
         - ☐ Other
         - ☐ Unspecified – review medical record/query physician
     - ☐ Radius
       - ☐ Upper or lower end
         - ☐ Physeal
           - ☐ Salter-Harris Type I
           - ☐ Salter-Harris Type II
           - ☐ Salter-Harris Type III
           - ☐ Salter-Harris Type IV
           - ☐ Other
           - ☐ Unspecified – review medical record/query physician
         - ☐ Torus
       - ☐ Shaft
         - ☐ Bent bone
         - ☐ Comminuted
         - ☐ Galeazzi's
         - ☐ Greenstick
         - ☐ Oblique
         - ☐ Segmental
         - ☐ Spiral
         - ☐ Transverse
         - ☐ Other
         - ☐ Unspecified – review medical record/query physician
       - ☐ Lower end
         - ☐ Extraarticular
           - ☐ Colles'
           - ☐ Smith's
           - ☐ Other

        - ☐ Intraarticular
            - ☐ Barton's
            - ☐ Other
        - ☐ Torus
- ☐ Pelvis
    - ☐ Ilium
        - ☐ Avulsion
        - ☐ Other
    - ☐ Ischium
        - ☐ Avulsion
        - ☐ Other
    - ☐ Multiple fractures of pelvis
        - ☐ with stable disruption of pelvic ring
        - ☐ with unstable disruption of pelvic ring
        - ☐ without disruption of pelvic ring
- ☐ Femur
    - ☐ Physeal upper end
        - ☐ Salter-Harris Type I
        - ☐ Other
        - ☐ Unspecified
    - ☐ Shaft
        - ☐ Comminuted
        - ☐ Oblique
        - ☐ Segmental
        - ☐ Spiral
        - ☐ Transverse
        - ☐ Other
        - ☐ Unspecified – review medical record/query physician
    - ☐ Lower end
        - ☐ Physeal
            - ☐ Salter-Harris Type I
            - ☐ Salter-Harris Type II
            - ☐ Salter-Harris Type III
            - ☐ Salter-Harris Type IV
            - ☐ Other
            - ☐ Unspecified – review medical record/query physician
        - ☐ Torus
    - ☐ Other
- ☐ Patella
    - ☐ Comminuted
    - ☐ Longitudinal
    - ☐ Osteochondral
    - ☐ Transverse
    - ☐ Other
    - ☐ Unspecified – review medical record/query physician
- ☐ Tibia
    - ☐ Upper or lower end
        - ☐ Physeal
            - ☐ Salter-Harris Type I
            - ☐ Salter-Harris Type II
            - ☐ Salter-Harris Type III
            - ☐ Salter-Harris Type IV
            - ☐ Other
            - ☐ Unspecified – review medical record/query physician
        - ☐ Torus
        - ☐ Other
    - ☐ Shaft
        - ☐ Comminuted
        - ☐ Oblique
        - ☐ Segmental
        - ☐ Spiral
        - ☐ Transverse
        - ☐ Other
        - ☐ Unspecified – review medical record/query physician
- ☐ Fibula
    - ☐ Upper or lower end
        - ☐ Physeal
            - ☐ Salter-Harris Type I
            - ☐ Salter-Harris Type II
            - ☐ Other
            - ☐ Unspecified – review medical record/query physician
        - ☐ Torus
        - ☐ Other
    - ☐ Shaft
        - ☐ Comminuted
        - ☐ Oblique
        - ☐ Segmental
        - ☐ Spiral
        - ☐ Transverse
        - ☐ Other
        - ☐ Unspecified – review medical record/query physician
- ☐ Talus
    - ☐ Avulsion
- ☐ Calcaneus
    - ☐ Avulsion
    - ☐ Physeal
        - ☐ Salter-Harris Type I
        - ☐ Salter-Harris Type II
        - ☐ Salter-Harris Type III
        - ☐ Salter-Harris Type IV
        - ☐ Other
        - ☐ Unspecified – review medical record/query physician
- ☐ Metatarsal
    - ☐ Physeal
        - ☐ Salter-Harris Type I
        - ☐ Salter-Harris Type II
        - ☐ Salter-Harris Type III
        - ☐ Salter-Harris Type IV

- ☐ Other
- ☐ Unspecified – review medical record/query physician

- ☐ Phalanx
  - ☐ Physeal
    - ☐ Salter-Harris Type I
    - ☐ Salter-Harris Type II
    - ☐ Salter-Harris Type III
    - ☐ Salter-Harris Type IV
    - ☐ Other
    - ☐ Unspecified – review medical record/query physician

5. For traumatic fractures excluding torus and greenstick, identify displacement unless inherent to fracture configuration:
   - ☐ Displaced
   - ☐ Nondisplaced

Note: Fractures not documented as displaced or nondisplaced, default to displaced.

6. Identify laterality, excluding vertebral fractures:
   - ☐ Left
   - ☐ Right
   - ☐ Unspecified – review medical record/query physician
7. For traumatic fractures, identify status:
   - ☐ Closed
   - ☐ Open
     - ☐ If S52, S72, S82
       - ☐ Gustilo Type I
       - ☐ Gustilo Type II
       - ☐ Gustilo Type IIIA
       - ☐ Gustilo Type IIIB

Note: Fractures not identified as open or closed, default to closed.

8. Identify episode of care/stage of healing/complication:
   - ☐ Pathologic fracture
     - ☐ A Initial encounter
     - ☐ D Subsequent encounter with routine healing
     - ☐ G Subsequent encounter with delayed healing
     - ☐ K Subsequent encounter with nonunion
     - ☐ P Subsequent encounter with malunion
     - ☐ S Sequela
   - ☐ Stress fracture (excluding vertebra)
     - ☐ A Initial encounter
     - ☐ D Subsequent encounter with routine healing
     - ☐ G Subsequent encounter with delayed healing
     - ☐ K Subsequent encounter with nonunion
     - ☐ P Subsequent encounter with malunion
     - ☐ S Sequela
   - ☐ Stress fracture vertebra (fatigue, collapsed vertebra)
     - ☐ A Initial encounter
     - ☐ D Subsequent encounter with routine healing
     - ☐ G Subsequent encounter with delayed healing
     - ☐ S Sequela
   - ☐ Traumatic fracture vertebra
     - ☐ A Initial encounter for closed fracture
     - ☐ B Initial encounter for open fracture
     - ☐ D Subsequent encounter with routine healing
     - ☐ G Subsequent encounter with delayed healing
     - ☐ K Subsequent encounter with nonunion
     - ☐ S Sequela
   - ☐ Traumatic (excluding torus and greenstick and S52, S62, S72, S82)
     - ☐ A Initial encounter for closed fracture
     - ☐ B Initial encounter for open fracture
     - ☐ D Subsequent encounter with routine healing
     - ☐ G Subsequent encounter with delayed healing
     - ☐ K Subsequent encounter with nonunion
     - ☐ P Subsequent encounter with malunion
     - ☐ S Sequela
   - ☐ Traumatic torus and greenstick
     - ☐ A Initial encounter
     - ☐ D Subsequent encounter with routine healing
     - ☐ G Subsequent encounter with delayed healing
     - ☐ K Subsequent encounter with nonunion
     - ☐ P Subsequent encounter with malunion
     - ☐ S Sequela
   - ☐ Traumatic (S52 forearm, S72 femur, S82 lower leg)
     - ☐ A Initial encounter for closed fracture
     - ☐ B Initial encounter for Gustilo type I or II
     - ☐ C Initial encounter for Gustilo type III A or IIIB
     - ☐ D Subsequent encounter closed fracture with routine healing
     - ☐ E Subsequent encounter Gustilo type I or II with routine healing
     - ☐ F Subsequent encounter Gustilo type IIIA or IIIB with routine healing
     - ☐ G Subsequent encounter closed fracture with delayed healing
     - ☐ H Subsequent encounter Gustilo type I or II with delayed healing
     - ☐ J Subsequent encounter Gustilo type IIIA or IIIB with delayed healing
     - ☐ K Subsequent encounter closed fracture with nonunion
     - ☐ M Subsequent encounter Gustilo type I or II with nonunion
     - ☐ N Subsequent encounter Gustilo type IIIA or IIIB with nonunion
     - ☐ P Subsequent encounter closed fracture with malunion
     - ☐ Subsequent encounter Gustilo type I or II with malunion
     - ☐ R Subsequent encounter Gustilo type IIIA or IIIB with malunion
     - ☐ S Sequela

9. Identify any associated injuries:
   - ☐ Fracture of skull and facial bones any associated intracranial injuries S06.-
   - ☐ Fracture of cervical vertebra any associated spinal cord injury S14.0, S14.1-
   - ☐ Fracture of thoracic vertebra any associated spinal cord injury S24.0, S24.1-
   - ☐ Fracture of lumbar vertebra any associated spinal cord/nerve injury S34.0-, S34.1-
   - ☐ Fracture of rib(s) and sternum any associated injury intrathoracic organ S27.-
10. Identify the external cause, intent, activity, place, and status where applicable

Gestational Diabetes/Abnormal Glucose Tolerance

ICD-10-CM Code Subcategories

O24.4	Gestational diabetes mellitus
O99.81	Abnormal glucose complicating pregnancy, childbirth and the puerperium

ICD-10-CM Definitions

Abnormal glucose – An abnormal glucose tolerance test without specific documentation of gestational diabetes mellitus.

Gestational diabetes mellitus – Glucose intolerance during pregnancy with specific documentation of gestational diabetes mellitus.

ICD-10-CM Guidelines

Gestational diabetes can occur during the second and third trimesters in women without a pre-pregnancy diagnosis of diabetes mellitus. Gestational diabetes may cause complications similar to those in patients with pre-existing diabetes mellitus. Coding guidelines for reporting gestational diabetes are as follows:

- Assign a code from subcategory O24.4 Gestational diabetes mellitus
- Do not assign any other codes in category O24 Diabetes mellitus in pregnancy, childbirth and the puerperium, in conjunction with codes in subcategory O24.4
- The provider must document whether the gestational diabetes is being controlled by diet, insulin, or oral hypoglycemic drugs
- If documentation indicates the gestational diabetes is being controlled with both diet and insulin, report only the code for insulin-controlled
- Do not assign code Z79.4, Long-term use of insulin, with codes in subcategory O24.4.
- Do not assign a code in subcategory O24.4 for documentation of an abnormal glucose tolerance test in pregnancy without specific documentation by the provider that the patient has gestational diabetes. Use a code from subcategory O99.81 Abnormal glucose complicating pregnancy, childbirth, and the puerperium

Checklist

1. Identify condition:
   - ☐ Abnormal glucose
   - ☐ Gestational diabetes
2. Identify maternal episode of care:
   - ☐ Pregnancy
   - ☐ Childbirth
   - ☐ Puerperium
3. For gestational diabetes, specify method of control:
   - ☐ Controlled by oral hypoglycemics
   - ☐ Diet controlled
   - ☐ Insulin controlled
   - ☐ Unspecified control

Glaucoma

ICD-10-CM Categories/Subcategories

H40	Glaucoma
H42	Glaucoma in diseases classified elsewhere
Q15.0	Congenital glaucoma

ICD-10-CM Definitions

Glaucoma – Group of eye disorders characterized by elevated intraocular pressure that can cause optic nerve damage.

Checklist

1. Identify type:
   - ☐ Glaucoma in diseases classified elsewhere – Specify underlying condition ________________
   - ☐ Glaucoma suspect
     - ☐ Anatomical narrow angle (primary angle closure suspect)
     - ☐ Open angle with borderline findings
       - ☐ High risk
       - ☐ Low risk
     - ☐ Ocular hypertension
     - ☐ Preglaucoma
     - ☐ Primary angle closure without glaucoma damage
     - ☐ Steroid responder
   - ☐ Open-angle glaucoma
     - ☐ Capsular glaucoma with pseudoexfoliation of lens
     - ☐ Low-tension glaucoma
     - ☐ Pigmentary glaucoma
     - ☐ Primary open-angle glaucoma
     - ☐ Residual stage of open-angle glaucoma
     - ☐ Unspecified open angle glaucoma
   - ☐ Primary angle-closure glaucoma
     - ☐ Acute angle-closure glaucoma (attack) (crisis)
     - ☐ Chronic angle-closure glaucoma
     - ☐ Intermittent angle-closure glaucoma
     - ☐ Residual stage of angle-closure glaucoma
     - ☐ Unspecified primary angle-closure glaucoma
   - ☐ Secondary glaucoma (due to)
     - ☐ Drugs – Specify drug ____________________
     - ☐ Eye inflammation – Specify underlying condition ________________
     - ☐ Eye trauma – Specify underlying condition ________________
     - ☐ Other eye disorders – Specify underlying condition ________________\
   - ☐ Other specified type of glaucoma
     - ☐ Aqueous misdirection (malignant glaucoma)
     - ☐ Glaucoma with increased episcleral venous pressure
     - ☐ Hypersecretion glaucoma
     - ☐ Other specified type – Specify ________________
   - ☐ Unspecified type
2. Specify laterality:
   - ☐ Right eye
   - ☐ Left eye
   - ☐ Bilateral
   - ☐ Unspecified eye
3. Specify stage using the appropriate 7th character:
   - ☐ 0 – Stage unspecified
   - ☐ 1 – Mild stage
   - ☐ 2 – Moderate stage
   - ☐ 3 – Severe stage
   - ☐ 4 – Indeterminate stage

Note: Stage is not required for conditions listed under the following:

- Angle-closure glaucoma
  - Acute
  - Intermittent
  - Residual stage
- Glaucoma suspect
- Open-angle
  - Residual stage
- Other specified type of glaucoma
  - Aqueous misdirection
  - Hypersecretion
  - With increased episcleral venous pressure
  - Other specified glaucoma
- Unspecified glaucoma

4. Use additional code for adverse effect, if applicable, to identify the drug (T36-T50 with 5th or 6th character 5) for glaucoma secondary to drugs
5. Code also the underlying condition for:
   - Glaucoma secondary to eye trauma
   - Glaucoma secondary to eye inflammation
   - Glaucoma secondary to other eye disorders
6. For glaucoma in diseases classified elsewhere, code underlying condition first

Gout

ICD-10-CM Categories

Gout is classified in two categories in Chapter 13 as a disease of the musculoskeletal system and connective tissue:

M1A	Chronic gout
M10	Gout

ICD-10-CM Definitions

Chronic gout – Long term gout that develops in cases where uric acid levels remain consistently high over a number of years, resulting in more frequent attacks and pain that may remain constant.

Gout – A complex type of arthritis characterized by the accumulation of uric acid crystals within the joints, causing severe pain, redness, swelling, and stiffness, particularly in the big toe. The needle-like crystal deposits in a joint cause sudden attacks or flares of severe pain and inflammation that intensify before subsiding.

Uric acid – A chemical compound of ions and salts formed by the metabolic breakdown of purines, found in foods such as meats and shellfish, and in cells of the body.

Checklist

1. Identify type of gout:
   - ☐ Acute (attack) (flare)
   - ☐ Chronic
   - ☐ Unspecified
2. Identify cause:
   - ☐ Drug-induced
     - ☐ Use additional code to identify drug and adverse effect, if applicable
   - ☐ Due to renal impairment
     - ☐ Code first causative renal disease
   - ☐ Idiopathic (primary)
   - ☐ Lead-induced
     - ☐ Code first toxic effects of lead and lead compounds
   - ☐ Secondary
     - ☐ Code first associated condition
   - ☐ Unspecified
3. Identify site:
   - ☐ Lower extremity
     - ☐ Ankle/foot
     - ☐ Hip
     - ☐ Knee
   - ☐ Upper extremity
     - ☐ Elbow
     - ☐ Hand
     - ☐ Shoulder
     - ☐ Wrist
   - ☐ Vertebrae
   - ☐ Multiple sites
   - ☐ Unspecified site
4. Identify laterality for extremities:
   - ☐ Left
   - ☐ Right
   - ☐ Unspecified
5. For chronic gout, identify presence/absence of tophi:
   - ☐ With tophi
   - ☐ Without tophi
6. For all types of gout, identify any accompanying conditions with the underlying gout:
   - ☐ Autonomic neuropathy
   - ☐ Cardiomyopathy
   - ☐ Disorders of external ear, iris, or ciliary body
   - ☐ Glomerular disorders
   - ☐ Urinary calculus

Headache Syndromes

ICD-10-CM Subcategories

G44.0	Cluster headaches and other trigeminal autonomic cephalgias (TAC)
G44.1	Vascular headache, not elsewhere classified
G44.2	Tension-type headache
G44.3	Post-traumatic headache
G44.4	Drug-induced headache, not elsewhere classified
G44.5	Complicated headache syndromes
G44.8	Other specified headache syndromes
R51.0	Headache with orthostatic component, not elsewhere classified
R51.9	Headache NOS

ICD-10-CM Definitions

Headache NOS – Headache not further documented as a migraine or other specific headache syndrome is reported with the sign/symptom code R51.9 in Chapter 18 of ICD-10-CM.

Intractable headache – A headache that is not responding to treatment. Synonymous terms include: pharmacoresistant (pharmacologically resistant) headache, treatment resistant headache, refractory headache, and poorly controlled headache.

Not intractable headache – Headache that is responding to treatment.

Tension headache – Tension headache is synonymous with tension-type headache in ICD-10-CM. Use codes in subcategory G44.2 for headache documented as tension headache.

Checklist

1. Identify the specific type of headache or syndrome:
   - ☐ Cluster headaches and trigeminal autonomic cephalgias
     - ☐ Cluster headache
       - ☐ Chronic
       - ☐ Episodic
       - ☐ Unspecified
     - ☐ Paroxysmal hemicranias
       - ☐ Chronic
       - ☐ Episodic
     - ☐ Short lasting unilateral neuralgiform headache with conjunctival injection and tearing (SUNCT)
     - ☐ Other trigeminal autonomic cephalgias (TAC)
   - ☐ Vascular headache, not elsewhere classified
   - ☐ Tension-type headache
     - ☐ Chronic
     - ☐ Episodic
     - ☐ Unspecified
   - ☐ Post-traumatic headache
     - ☐ Acute
     - ☐ Chronic
     - ☐ Unspecified
   - ☐ Drug-induced headache, not elsewhere classified – Use additional code for adverse effect, if applicable, to identify drug (T36-T50 with 5th or 6th character 5)
   - ☐ Complicated headache syndromes
     - ☐ Hemicrania continua
     - ☐ New daily persistent headache (NDPH)
     - ☐ Primary thunderclap headache
     - ☐ Other complicated headache syndrome
   - ☐ Other specified headache syndromes
     - ☐ Hypnic headache
     - ☐ Headache associated with sexual activity
     - ☐ Primary cough headache
     - ☐ Primary exertional headache
     - ☐ Primary stabbing headache
     - ☐ Other specified type headache syndrome – Specify ____________
2. Identify response to treatment for the following types: cluster, paroxysmal hemicranias, SUNCT, other TAC, tension-type, post-traumatic, and drug-induced
   - ☐ Intractable
   - ☐ Not intractable

Appendix A: Coding Checklists

Hearing Loss

ICD-10-CM Categories/Subcategories

H83.3	Noise effects on inner ear
H90	Conductive and sensorineural hearing loss
H91	Other and unspecified hearing loss

ICD-10-CM Definitions

Conductive hearing loss – Conductive hearing loss (CHL) is a mechanical problem involving the outer ear, tympanic membrane (ear drum), or bones (ossicles) in the middle ear.

Mixed hearing loss – Mixed hearing loss is conductive hearing loss (CHL) in combination with sensorineural hearing loss (SNHL). Damage or a disorder is present in the outer and/or middle ear along with damage or a disorder to the inner ear (cochlea) and/or Cranial Nerve VIII (vestibulocochlear nerve).

Noise effects on inner ear – Noise as the cause of hearing loss or noise causing other acoustic trauma to the ear.

Sensorineural hearing loss – Sensorineural hearing loss (SNHL) can occur when problems arise with Cranial Nerve VIII (vestibulocochlear nerve), the inner ear, or central processing centers of the brain. SNHL may be mild, moderate, or severe, or result in total deafness.

Checklist

1. Identify type of hearing loss:
   - ☐ Conductive and sensorineural
     - ☐ Conductive hearing loss (deafness)
     - ☐ Mixed conductive and sensorineural hearing loss
     - ☐ Sensorineural hearing loss
   - ☐ Other and unspecified hearing loss
     - ☐ Noise effects on inner ear
     - ☐ Ototoxic hearing loss – Specify drug (see #4)
     - ☐ Presbycusis
     - ☐ Sudden idiopathic
     - ☐ Other specified
   - ☐ Unspecified
2. For conductive, sensorineural, and mixed types, specify laterality:
   - ☐ Bilateral
   - ☐ Unilateral, left ear, with unrestricted hearing on the contralateral side
   - ☐ Unilateral, right ear, with unrestricted hearing on the contralateral side
   - ☐ Unspecified
3. For other and unspecified types, specify laterality:
   - ☐ Bilateral
   - ☐ Left ear
   - ☐ Right ear
   - ☐ Unspecified ear
4. For ototoxic hearing loss, specify as poisoning or adverse effect
   - ☐ For poisoning, code the poisoning first (T36-T65 with 5th or 6th character 1-4 or 6)
   - ☐ For adverse effect, use an additional code to identify the drug (T36-T50 with 5th or 6th character 5)

Influenza

ICD-10-CM Categories

Influenza is classified in the following categories:

J09	Influenza due to certain identified influenza viruses
J10	Influenza due to other identified influenza virus
J11	Influenza due to unidentified influenza virus

ICD-10-CM Definitions

Novel influenza A virus – Includes the following types of influenza:

- Avian
- Bird
- A/H5N1
- Other influenza of animal origin (not bird, not swine)
- Swine

Influenza due to other identified influenza virus – Any specified type of influenza not of animal origin and not listed as one of the included types under novel influenza A virus.

Influenza due to unspecified influenza virus – Influenza not specified as to type.

Checklist

1. Identify type of influenza virus:
   - ☐ Novel influenza A – Proceed to #2
   - ☐ Other identified influenza virus – Proceed to #3
   - ☐ Unidentified type of influenza virus – Proceed to #4
2. Novel influenza A – Identify complications/manifestations:
   - ☐ Gastrointestinal manifestations (J09.X3)
   - ☐ Pneumonia (J09.X1)
   - ☐ Use additional code to identify any associated:
     - ☐ Lung abscess
     - ☐ Infectious organism for pneumonia or other specified type of pneumonia
   - ☐ Other respiratory manifestations (J09.X2)
   - ☐ Use additional code to identify any associated:
     - ☐ Pleural effusion
     - ☐ Sinusitis
   - ☐ Other specified manifestations (J09.X9)
   - ☐ Use additional codes to identify manifestations:
     - ☐ Encephalopathy
     - ☐ Myocarditis
     - ☐ Otitis media
     - ☐ Other specified
3. Other identified influenza virus – Identify complications/manifestations:
   - ☐ Encephalopathy (J10.81)
   - ☐ Gastrointestinal manifestations (J10.2)
   - ☐ Myocarditis (J10.82)
   - ☐ Otitis media (J10.83) – Use additional code to identify ruptured tympanic membrane
   - ☐ Pneumonia
     - ☐ With same influenza virus pneumonia (J10.01)
     - ☐ With other specified pneumonia (J10.08) – Code also other specified type
     - ☐ Unspecified type (J10.00)

     Note: Use additional code to identify any associated lung abscess
   - ☐ Other respiratory manifestations (J10.1)
   - ☐ Use additional code to identify any associated:
     - ☐ Pleural effusion
     - ☐ Sinusitis
   - ☐ Other manifestations(J10.89) – Use additional code to identify manifestation
4. Unidentified influenza virus – Identify complications/manifestations:
   - ☐ Encephalopathy (J11.81)
   - ☐ Gastrointestinal manifestations (J11.2)
   - ☐ Myocarditis (J11.82)
   - ☐ Otitis media (J11.83) – Use additional code to identify ruptured tympanic membrane
   - ☐ Pneumonia
     - ☐ Specified type (J11.08) – Code also other specified type of pneumonia
     - ☐ Unspecified type (J11.00)

   Note: Use additional code to identify any associated lung abscess
   - ☐ Other respiratory manifestations (J11.1)
   - ☐ Use additional code to identify any associated:
     - ☐ Pleural effusion
     - ☐ Sinusitis
   - ☐ Other specified manifestations – Specify

     ____

Jaundice, Neonatal

ICD-10-CM Categories

P55	Hemolytic disease of newborn
P56	Hydrops fetalis due to hemolytic disease
P57	Kernicterus
P58	Neonatal jaundice due to other excessive hemolysis
P59	Neonatal jaundice from other and unspecified causes

ICD-10-CM Definitions

Excessive hemolysis of newborn – Excessive breakdown of red blood cells in a newborn that is not caused by hemolytic disease.

Hemolytic disease of the newborn (HDN) – Also called erythroblastosis fetalis, isoimmunization, or blood group incompatibility. HDN occurs when fetal red blood cells (RBCs) that have an antigen that the mother lacks, cross the placenta into the maternal circulation and stimulate antibody production in the mother. The maternal antibodies cross back over to the fetal circulation where they attack the fetal red blood cells causing red blood cell destruction in the fetus. A symptom of hemolytic disease of the newborn is jaundice.

Hydrops fetalis– Abnormal accumulation of fluid in two or more fetal compartments, such as edema, ascites, pleural effusion, and pericardial effusion. When caused by the destruction of large numbers of red blood cells, it can lead to severe or total body swelling that disrupts organ function.

Kernicterus – Brain damage occurring in the newborn with severe jaundice due to such high amounts of bilirubin in the blood that it moves out of blood serum and into brain tissue.

Checklist

1. Specify cause of neonatal jaundice:
   - ☐ Jaundice due to hemolytic disease
     - ☐ ABO isoimmunization of newborn
     - ☐ Rh isoimmunization of newborn
     - ☐ With hydrops fetalis
       - ☐ Due to isoimmunization
       - ☐ Due to other hemolytic disease – Specify ________
       - ☐ Due to unspecified hemolytic disease
     - ☐ With kernicterus
       - ☐ Due to isoimmunization
       - ☐ Other specified
       - ☐ Unspecified
     - ☐ Other hemolytic diseases of newborn – Specify ________________
     - ☐ Unspecified hemolytic disease
   - ☐ Jaundice due to other excessive hemolysis
     - ☐ Due to bleeding
     - ☐ Due to bruising
     - ☐ Due to drugs/toxins
       - ☐ Transmitted from mother – Specify drug ________________
       - ☐ Given to newborn – Specify drug ____________________
     - ☐ Due to infection
     - ☐ Due to polycythemia
     - ☐ Due to swallowed maternal blood
     - ☐ Other specified excessive hemolysis – Specify ________________
     - ☐ Unspecified excessive hemolysis
   - ☐ Jaundice from other/unspecified causes
     - ☐ Breast milk inhibitor
     - ☐ Hepatocellular damage
       - ☐ Inspissated bile syndrome
       - ☐ Other specified hepatocellular damage – Specify ______________
       - ☐ Unspecified hepatocellular damage
     - ☐ Prematurity (associated with preterm delivery)
     - ☐ Other specified cause – Specify________________
     - ☐ Unspecified neonatal jaundice

Lymphoma – Follicular

ICD-10-CM Category

C82 Follicular lymphoma

ICD-10-CM Definitions

Follicular lymphoma – Lymphoma is a cancer of the lymph system. Follicular lymphoma is an indolent (slow growing), non-Hodgkin lymphoma (NHL) that arises from B-lymphocytes, which means that it is a B-cell lymphoma.

Follicular lymphoma is subdivided into several different types with some types being further differentiated by grade. The grading system used in ICD-10-CM was developed by the Revised European-American Classification of Lymphoid Neoplasms (REAL) which has also been adopted by the World Health Organization (WHO). The REAL/WHO classification grades follicular lymphoma based on the number of centroblasts per high-power field (hpf). The grades are as follows:

- Grade I (1) 0-5 centroblasts per hpf with a predominance of small centrocytes
- Grade II (2) 6-15 centroblasts per hpf with centrocytes present
- Grade III (3) >15 centroblasts per hpf with a decreased number or no centrocytes present
  - Grade IIIa (3A) >15 centroblasts per hpf with centrocytes still present
  - Grade IIIb (3B) >15 centroblasts per hpf presenting as solid sheets with no centrocytes present

The REAL/WHO classification also recognizes 2 variants of follicular lymphoma—cutaneous follicle center lymphoma and diffuse follicle center lymphoma, which have specific ICD-10-CM codes.

Checklist

1. Review notes and/or pathology report and identify the non-Hodgkin follicular lymphoma:
   - ☐ Follicular lymphoma
     - ☐ Grade I
     - ☐ Grade II
     - ☐ Grade IIIa
     - ☐ Grade IIIb
     - ☐ Grade III, unspecified – review medical record/query physician
   - ☐ Diffuse follicle center lymphoma
   - ☐ Cutaneous follicle center lymphoma
   - ☐ Other types of follicular lymphoma
   - ☐ Unspecified follicular lymphoma – review medical record/query physician
2. Identify site or sites:
   - ☐ Lymph nodes
     - ☐ Head/face/neck
     - ☐ Intrathoracic
     - ☐ Intra-abdominal
     - ☐ Axilla and upper limb
     - ☐ Inguinal region and lower limb
     - ☐ Intrapelvic
     - ☐ Multiple lymph node sites
   - ☐ Spleen
   - ☐ Extranodal/solid organ sites
   - ☐ Unspecified site – review medical record/query physician

Melanoma/Melanoma In Situ

ICD-10-CM Categories

C43	Malignant melanoma of skin
D03	Melanoma in situ

ICD-10-CM Definitions

Melanoma in situ – Malignant neoplasm of the melanin (brown pigment producing) cells that is documented as in situ, which includes melanoma that is described as:

- Stage 0
- TIS (tumor in situ)
- Epidermal layer only

Melanoma – Malignant neoplasm of the melanin (brown pigment producing) cells that is described as having invaded the dermis or as one of the following stages:

- Stage I – localized
  - Stage IA – less than 1.0 mm thick, no ulceration, no lymph node involvement, no distant metastases
  - Stage 1B – less than 1.0 mm thick with ulceration or less than 2.0 mm thick without ulceration, no lymph node involvement, no distant metastases
- Stage II – localized
  - Stage IIA – 1.01-2.00 mm thick with ulceration, no lymph node involvement, no distant metastases
  - Stage IIB – 2.01-4.00 mm thick without ulceration, no lymph node involvement, no distant metastases
  - Stage IIC – greater than 4.00 mm thick with ulceration, no lymph node involvement, no distant metastases
- Stage III – tumor spread to regional lymph nodes or development of in transit metastases or satellites without spread to distant sites. Three substages IIIA, IIIB, IIIC.
- Stage IV – tumor spread beyond regional lymph nodes with metastases to distant sites

Checklist

1. Review physician notes and/or pathology report and identify as:
   - ☐ Melanoma In Situ (see category D03)
   - ☐ Malignant melanoma (see category C43)

2. Identify site:
   - ☐ Head and Neck
     - ☐ Lip
     - ☐ Eyelid/canthus
       - ☐ Right
         - ☐ Lower
         - ☐ Upper
       - ☐ Left
         - ☐ Lower
         - ☐ Upper
       - ☐ Unspecified side – review medical record/query physician
     - ☐ Ear/external auricular canal
       - ☐ Right
       - ☐ Left
       - ☐ Unspecified side – review medical record/query physician
     - ☐ Nose (C43.31)
     - ☐ Other parts of face (includes nose for melanoma in situ)
     - ☐ Unspecified part of face – review medical record/query physician
     - ☐ Scalp/neck
   - ☐ Trunk
     - ☐ Anal skin
     - ☐ Skin of breast
     - ☐ Other parts of trunk
   - ☐ Extremities
     - ☐ Upper limb, including shoulder
       - ☐ Right
       - ☐ Left
       - ☐ Unspecified side – review medical record/query physician
     - ☐ Lower limb, including hip
       - ☐ Right
       - ☐ Left
       - ☐ Unspecified side – review medical record/query physician
   - ☐ Other sites (D03.8)
   - ☐ Overlapping sites of skin (C43.8)
   - ☐ Unspecified site – review medical record/query physician

   Note: Overlapping sites of skin applies only to malignant melanoma.

   Other sites apply only to melanoma in situ.

   Reference the Alphabetic Index carefully as there are other identified body sites listed under Melanoma (malignant), skin, but they are not coded to C43. These include male and female external genital organs.

Migraine

ICD-10-CM Subcategories

G43.0	Migraine without aura
G43.1	Migraine with aura
G43.4	Hemiplegic migraine
G43.5	Persistent migraine aura without cerebral infarction
G43.6	Persistent migraine aura with cerebral infarction
G43.7	Chronic migraine without aura
G43.A	Cyclical vomiting
G43.B	Ophthalmoplegic migraine
G43.C	Periodic headache syndromes in child or adult
G43.D	Abdominal migraine
G43.8	Other migraine
G43.9	Migraine, unspecified

ICD-10-CM Definitions

Migraine – Common neurological disorder that often manifests as a headache. Usually unilateral and pulsating in nature, the headache results from abnormal brain activity along nerve pathways and brain chemical (neurotransmitter) changes. These affect blood flow in the brain and surrounding tissue and may trigger an "aura" or warning sign (visual, sensory, language, motor) before the onset of pain. Migraine headache is frequently accompanied by autonomic nervous system symptoms (nausea, vomiting, sensitivity to light and/or sound).

Intractable headache – A headache that is not responding to treatment. Synonymous terms include: pharmacoresistant (pharmacologically resistant) headache, treatment resistant headache, refractory headache, and poorly controlled headache.

Not intractable headache – Headache that is responding to treatment.

Status migrainosus – Migraine that has lasted more than 72 hours.

Checklist

1. Identify migraine type:
   - ☐ Abdominal
   - ☐ Chronic without aura
   - ☐ Cyclical vomiting
   - ☐ Hemiplegic
   - ☐ Menstrual – Code also associated premenstrual tension syndrome (N94.3)
   - ☐ Ophthalmoplegic
   - ☐ Periodic headache syndromes in child or adult
   - ☐ Persistent aura
     - ☐ With cerebral infarction – Code also type of cerebral infarction (I63.-)
     - ☐ Without cerebral infarction
   - ☐ With aura – Code also any associated seizure (G40.-, R56.9)
   - ☐ Without aura
   - ☐ Other specified migraine
   - ☐ Unspecified migraine
2. Identify presence/absence of intractability:
   - ☐ Intractable
   - ☐ Not intractable
3. Identify presence/absence of status migrainosus (not required for migraines documented as abdominal, cyclical vomiting, ophthalmoplegic, or periodic headache syndromes in child/adult):
   - ☐ With status migrainosus
   - ☐ Without (mention of) status migrainosus
4. Use additional code for adverse effect, if applicable, to identify drug (T36-T50 with 5th or 6th character 5)

Mood Disorders

ICD-10-CM Categories/Subcategories

Codes for mood [affective] disorders are found in block F30-F39, with mood disorders due to known physiological condition reported in subcategory F06.3. Codes for substance-induced mood disorders are spread throughout block F10-F19 Mental and behavioral disorders due to psychoactive substance use.

F06.3	Mood disorder due to known physiological condition
F30	Manic episode
F31	Bipolar disorder
F32	Major depressive disorder, single episode
F33	Major depressive disorder, recurrent
F34	Persistent mood [affective] disorders
F39	Unspecified mood [affective] disorder

ICD-10-CM Definitions

Bipolar disorder – Also known as manic depressive disorder; a brain disorder causing mental illness marked by unusual, clear shifts in mood, energy, and activity levels that leave the person experiencing intense emotion, extreme changes in sleep and activity, and unusual behaviors that can interfere with normal day-to-day activity.

Cyclothymic disorder – Mood disorder marked by numerous periods of both hypomanic and depressive symptoms that do not meet requirements of a manic episode or a depressive episode, lasting 2 years in an adult and 1 year in adolescents.

Dysthymic disorder – A persistent, continuous, long-term form of depression that is usually mild or moderate as opposed to severe, lasting at least 2 years, and significantly interfering with relationships, work, or daily activity.

Mood disorders – A group of psychiatric diseases made up mainly of bipolar disorder and depression. Symptoms are mild to severe and characterized by significant disturbances in a person's persistent emotional state; the two primary types of moods are depression and mania.

Checklist

1. Identify causative type of mood disorder:
   - ☐ Due to known physiological condition – Proceed to #2
   - ☐ Due to substance use/abuse – Proceed to #3
   - ☐ Not due to any known physiological condition – Proceed to #4
2. Mood disorder due to known physiological condition
   a. Identify accompanying diagnostic features:
      - ☐ Depressive features
      - ☐ Major depressive-like episode
      - ☐ Manic features
      - ☐ Mixed features
      - ☐ Unspecified
3. Mood disorder due to substance use/abuse
   a. Identify substance and use status:
      - ☐ Alcohol
        - ☐ Abuse (mild use disorder)
        - ☐ Dependence (moderate/severe use disorder)
        - ☐ Use, unspecified
      - ☐ Cocaine
        - ☐ Abuse (mild use disorder)
        - ☐ Dependence (moderate/severe use disorder)
        - ☐ Use, unspecified
      - ☐ Hallucinogen
        - ☐ Abuse (mild use disorder)
        - ☐ Dependence (moderate/severe use disorder)
        - ☐ Use, unspecified
      - ☐ Inhalant
        - ☐ Abuse (mild use disorder)
        - ☐ Dependence (moderate/severe use disorder)
        - ☐ Use, unspecified
      - ☐ Opioid
        - ☐ Abuse (mild use disorder)
        - ☐ Dependence (moderate use disorder)
        - ☐ Use, unspecified
      - ☐ Other psychoactive substance
        - ☐ Abuse (mild use disorder)
        - ☐ Dependence (moderate/severe use disorder)
        - ☐ Use, unspecified
      - ☐ Other stimulant
        - ☐ Abuse (mild use disorder)
        - ☐ Dependence (moderate/severe use disorder)
        - ☐ Use, unspecified
      - ☐ Sedative/Hypnotic/Anxiolytic
        - ☐ Abuse (mild use disorder)
        - ☐ Dependence (moderate/severe use disorder)
        - ☐ Use, unspecified
4. Mood disorder not due to any known physiological condition
   a. Identify specific mood disorder:
      - ☐ Bipolar disorder
        - ☐ Current episode
          - ☐ Depressed
            - ☐ Mild
            - ☐ Mild or moderate severity, unspecified
            - ☐ Moderate
            - ☐ Severe
              - ☐ With psychotic features
              - ☐ Without psychotic features
          - ☐ Hypomanic
          - ☐ Manic, without psychotic features
            - ☐ Mild
            - ☐ Moderate
            - ☐ Severe
            - ☐ Unspecified
          - ☐ Manic, with psychotic features (severe)

- ☐ Mixed
  - ☐ Mild
  - ☐ Moderate
  - ☐ Severe
    - ☐ With psychotic features
    - ☐ Without psychotic features
  - ☐ Unspecified
- ☐ In remission
  - ☐ Full (most recent episode):
    - ☐ Depressed
    - ☐ Hypomanic
    - ☐ Manic
    - ☐ Mixed
  - ☐ Partial
    - ☐ Depressed
    - ☐ Hypomanic
    - ☐ Manic
    - ☐ Mixed
  - ☐ Unspecified
- ☐ Other bipolar disorder
  - ☐ Bipolar II
  - ☐ Recurrent manic episodes
- ☐ Unspecified bipolar disorder

☐ Major depressive disorder
- ☐ Recurrent
  - ☐ In full remission
  - ☐ In partial remission
  - ☐ In unspecified remission
  - ☐ Mild
  - ☐ Moderate
  - ☐ Other
  - ☐ Severe
    - ☐ With psychotic features
    - ☐ Without psychotic features
  - ☐ Unspecified
- ☐ Single episode
  - ☐ In full remission
  - ☐ In partial remission
  - ☐ Mild
  - ☐ Moderate
  - ☐ Severe
    - ☐ With psychotic features
    - ☐ Without psychotic features
  - ☐ Unspecified

☐ Manic episode
- ☐ In full remission
- ☐ In partial remission
- ☐ Other/Hypomania
- ☐ Unspecified
- ☐ With psychotic symptoms (severe)
- ☐ Without psychotic symptoms
  - ☐ Mild
  - ☐ Moderate
  - ☐ Severe
  - ☐ Unspecified

☐ Persistent mood disorder
- ☐ Cyclothymic
- ☐ Disruptive mood dysregulation disorder
- ☐ Dysthymic
- ☐ Other specified
- ☐ Unspecified

☐ Other depressive episodes
- ☐ Atypical/Post-schizophrenic/Other specified
- ☐ Premenstrual dysphoric disorder

☐ Unspecified mood disorder

Myocardial Infarction

ICD-10-CM Categories

Acute myocardial infarction is classified in the following ICD-10-CM categories:

I21	ST elevation (STEMI) and non-ST elevation (NSTEMI) myocardial infarction
I22	Subsequent ST elevation (STEMI) and non-ST elevation (NSTEMI) myocardial infarction

ICD-10-CM Definitions

Myocardial infarction – An interruption of blood flow to an area of the heart muscle leading to cell damage or death. Myocardial infarctions are classified as either STEMI or NSTEMI. STEMI stands for ST segment elevation myocardial infarction and is the more severe type. STEMI occurs when a coronary artery is totally occluded and virtually all the heart muscle dependent on blood supplied by the affected artery begins to die. NSTEMI is the milder form of myocardial infarction and stands for non-ST segment elevation myocardial infarction. In NSTEMI, the coronary artery is only partially occluded, and only the inner portion of the heart muscle supplied by the affected artery dies. NSTEMI is also referred to as a subendocardial infarction.

Initial acute myocardial infarction (AMI) – Assign a code from category I21 ST elevation (STEMI) and non-ST elevation (NSTEMI) myocardial infarction.

Subsequent AMI – Assign a code from category I22 Subsequent ST elevation (STEMI) and non-ST elevation (NSTEMI) myocardial infarction for a new AMI occurring during the 4-week healing phase of a previous AMI. A code from category I21 is also assigned for the initial AMI.

Treatment/healing phase for a new AMI – For ICD-10-CM coding purposes, the initial treatment and healing phase of a new AMI is 4 weeks (28 days). During the first 4 weeks, a code from category I21 or codes from categories I21 and I22 are assigned for an admission or encounter for the care of the AMI. After the 4- week healing period has passed, the appropriate aftercare code is assigned for any care related to the myocardial infarction.

Old/healed myocardial infarction (MI) – Documentation of history of MI, old MI, or healed MI is reported with code I25.2 Old myocardial infarction.

Checklist

1. Identify episode of care:
   - ☐ Initial (care for an initial AMI)
   - ☐ Subsequent (care for a subsequent new AMI within the 4- week time frame of a previous AMI)
2. Identify type of myocardial infarction:
   - ☐ ST elevation myocardial infarction (STEMI)
   - ☐ Other
     - ☐ Type 2
     - ☐ Other Types 3-5
   - ☐ Non-ST elevation myocardial infarction (NSTEMI)
   - ☐ Unspecified acute myocardial infarction
3. For initial episode of care of STEMI identify site:
   - ☐ Anterior wall
     - ☐ Left main coronary artery
     - ☐ Left anterior descending artery
     - ☐ Other coronary artery of anterior wall
   - ☐ Inferior wall
     - ☐ Right coronary artery
     - ☐ Other coronary artery of inferior wall
   - ☐ Other specified sites
     - ☐ Left circumflex coronary artery
     - ☐ Other specified site
   - ☐ Unspecified site
4. For Type 2 myocardial infarction, identify the underlying cause, if applicable:
   - ☐ Anemia (D50.0-D64.9)
   - ☐ Chronic obstructive pulmonary disease (J44-)
   - ☐ Paroxysmal tachycardia (I47.0-I47.9)
   - ☐ Shock (R57.0-R57.9)
5. For Types 3-5 myocardial infarction, identify relationship to cardiac surgery and any complications, if known and applicable:
   - ☐ Postprocedural during cardiac surgery
   - ☐ Postprocedural following cardiac surgery
   - ☐ Complications
     - ☐ (Acute) Stent occlusion (T82.897-)
     - ☐ (Acute) Stent stenosis (T82.857-)
     - ☐ (Acute) Stent thrombosis (T82.867-)
     - ☐ Cardiac arrest due to underlying cardiac condition (I46.2)
     - ☐ Complication of percutaneous coronary intervention (PCI) (I97.89)
     - ☐ Occlusion of coronary artery bypass graft (T82.218-)
6. For subsequent episode of care STEMI identify site:
   - ☐ Anterior wall
   - ☐ Inferior wall
   - ☐ Other sites
   - ☐ Unspecified site

Note: For NSTEMI no site-specific information is required. Select code based on episode of care only.

7. Identify any current complications of STEMI or NSTEMI (within initial 28-day period) and report additionally:
   - ☐ Atrial septal defect (I23.1)
   - ☐ Hemopericardium (I23.0)
   - ☐ Rupture of cardiac wall (I23.3)
   - ☐ Rupture of chordae tendineae (I23.4)
   - ☐ Rupture of papillary muscle (I23.5)
   - ☐ Ventricular septal defect (I23.2)
   - ☐ Thrombosis of atrium, auricular appendage, ventricle (I23.6)
   - ☐ Postinfarction angina (I23.7)
   - ☐ Other specified type of current complication of AMI (I23.8)
8. Use additional code, if applicable, to identify any exposure to tobacco smoke, history of tobacco use, current tobacco use, or tobacco dependence:
   - ☐ Exposure to environmental tobacco smoke (Z77.22)
   - ☐ History of tobacco dependence (Z87.891)
   - ☐ Occupational exposure to environmental tobacco smoke (Z57.31)
   - ☐ Tobacco dependence (F17.-)
   - ☐ Tobacco use (Z72.0)
9. Use additional code to identify presence of hypertension (I10-I15)
10. For transfer patient, use additional code, if applicable, to identify status post administration of tPA (rtPA) in a different facility within the last 24 hours prior to admission to current facility (Z92.82)

Obstetrics – Multiple Gestation

ICD-10-CM Category

O30	Multiple gestation
O31.1	Continuing pregnancy after spontaneous abortion of one fetus or more
O31.2	Continuing pregnancy after intrauterine death of one fetus or more
O31.3	Continuing pregnancy after elective fetal reduction of one fetus or more

ICD-10-CM Additional Multiple Gestation Coding Information

Some complications of pregnancy and childbirth occur more frequently in multiple gestation pregnancies than in single gestation pregnancies and these complications may affect one or more of the fetuses. To address this, 14 code categories and subcategories in ICD-10-CM require identification of the fetus affected by the complication using a 7th character. The categories requiring identification of the fetus include:

O31	Complications specific to multiple gestation
O32	Maternal care for malpresentation of fetus
O33.3	Maternal care for disproportion due to outlet contraction of pelvis
O33.4	Maternal care for disproportion of mixed maternal and fetal origin
O33.5	Maternal care for disproportion due to unusually large fetus
O33.6	Maternal care for disproportion due to hydrocephalic fetus
O35	Maternal care for known or suspected fetal abnormality and damage
O36	Maternal care for other fetal problems
O40	Polyhydramnios
O41	Other disorders of amniotic fluid and membranes
O60.1	Preterm labor with preterm delivery
O60.2	Term delivery with preterm labor
O64	Obstructed labor due to malposition and malpresentation of fetus
O69	Labor and delivery complicated by umbilical cord complications

7th Characters Identifying Fetus

The 7th character identifies the fetus to which the complication code applies and are as follows:

- 0 – Unspecified fetus/not applicable
- 1 – Fetus 1
- 2 – Fetus 2
- 3 – Fetus 3
- 4 – Fetus 4
- 5 – Fetus 5
- 9 – Other fetus

Single Gestation/Unspecified Fetus

For single gestation or when the documentation is insufficient to identify the fetus, the 7th character '0' for not applicable/unspecified is assigned.

Multiple Gestation

For multiple gestations, each fetus should be identified with a number as Fetus 1, Fetus 2, Fetus 3, etc. The fetus or fetuses affected by the condition should be documented using the number assigned to the fetus. The complication code is then assigned for each fetus affected by the complication.

Checklist

1. Identify multiple gestation and number of placenta/amniotic sacs
   - ☐ Twin pregnancy
     - ☐ Conjoined twin pregnancy
     - ☐ One placenta/one amniotic sac (monochorionic/monoamniotic)
     - ☐ One placenta/two amniotic sacs (monochorionic/diamniotic)
     - ☐ Two placentae/two amniotic sacs (dichorionic/diamniotic)
     - ☐ Unable to determine number of placenta/amniotic sacs
     - ☐ Unspecified number of placenta/amniotic sacs
   - ☐ Triplet pregnancy
     - ☐ Two or more monochorionic fetuses
     - ☐ Two or more monoamniotic fetuses
     - ☐ Trichorionic/triamniotic
     - ☐ Unable to determine number of placenta/amniotic sacs
     - ☐ Unspecified number of placenta/amniotic sacs
   - ☐ Quadruplet pregnancy
     - ☐ Two or more monochorionic fetuses
     - ☐ Two or more monoamniotic fetuses
     - ☐ Quadrachorionic/quadra-amniotic
     - ☐ Unable to determine number of placenta/amniotic sacs
     - ☐ Unspecified number of placenta/amniotic sacs
   - ☐ Other specified multiple gestation
     - ☐ Two or more monochorionic fetuses
     - ☐ Two or more monoamniotic fetuses
     - ☐ Number of chorions and amnions equal to the number of fetuses
     - ☐ Unable to determine number of placenta/amniotic sacs
     - ☐ Unspecified number of placenta/amniotic sacs
   - ☐ Unspecified multiple gestation
2. Identify trimester
   - ☐ First (less than 14 weeks 0 days)
   - ☐ Second (14 weeks 0 days to less than 28 weeks 0 days)
   - ☐ Third (28 weeks 0 days until delivery)
   - ☐ Unspecified
3. Assign additional code for continuing pregnancy following fetal loss or elective fetal reduction of one or more fetuses

4. Specify as continuing pregnancy after
   - ☐ Spontaneous abortion of one or more fetuses
   - ☐ Intrauterine death of one or more fetuses
   - ☐ Elective fetal reduction of one or more fetuses
5. Identify trimester as
   - ☐ First (less than 14 weeks 0 days)
   - ☐ Second (14 weeks 0 days to less than 28 weeks 0 days)
   - ☐ Third (28 weeks 0 days until delivery)
   - ☐ Unspecified
6. Identify fetus affected by complication (fetal loss/reduction) as:
   - ☐ Fetus 1
   - ☐ Fetus 2
   - ☐ Fetus 3
   - ☐ Fetus 4
   - ☐ Fetus 5
   - ☐ Other fetus
   - ☐ Unspecified fetus/not applicable

Open Wound

ICD-10-CM Categories

Open wound codes are used for wounds caused by trauma. Do not assign a code for "open wound" unless the etiology of the wound is related to trauma. Open wounds are classified in the following ICD-10-CM categories:

S01	Open wound of head
S11	Open wound of neck
S21	Open wound of thorax
S31	Open wound of abdomen, lower back, pelvis, and external genitalia
S41	Open wound of shoulder and upper arm
S51	Open wound of elbow and forearm
S61	Open wound of wrist, hand, and fingers
S71	Open wound of hip and thigh
S81	Open wound of knee and lower leg
S91	Open wound of ankle, foot, and toes

ICD-10-CM Definitions

Episode of Care – There are three (3) possible 7th character values to select from for open wounds. The 7th character defines the stage of treatment and residual effects related to the initial injury.

> **A Initial encounter.** The period when the patient is receiving active treatment for the injury, poisoning, or other consequences of an external cause. An 'A' may be assigned on more than one claim.
>
> **D Subsequent encounter.** Encounter after the active phase of treatment and when the patient is receiving routine care for the injury during the period of healing or recovery.
>
> **S Sequela.** Encounter for complications or conditions that arise as a direct result of an injury.

Laceration – A tear, cut or gash caused by a sharp object producing edges that may be jagged or straight.

Puncture wound – A wound caused by an object that pierces the skin or an organ, creating a small hole.

Checklist

1. Identify the type of open wound:
   - ☐ Bite
   - ☐ Laceration
     - ☐ With foreign body
     - ☐ Without foreign body
   - ☐ Puncture wound
     - ☐ With foreign body
     - ☐ Without foreign body
   - ☐ Unspecified open wound – review medical record/query physician
2. Identify the body area:
   - ☐ Head
     - ☐ Scalp
     - ☐ Eyelid and periocular area
     - ☐ Ear
     - ☐ Nose
     - ☐ Cheek and temporomandibular area
     - ☐ Lip and oral cavity
     - ☐ Other parts of head
     - ☐ Unspecified part of head – review medical record/query physician
   - ☐ Neck
     - ☐ Larynx
     - ☐ Trachea
     - ☐ Vocal cord
     - ☐ Thyroid gland
     - ☐ Pharynx and cervical esophagus
     - ☐ Other specified parts of neck
     - ☐ Unspecified part of neck – review medical record/query physician
   - ☐ Thorax
     - ☐ Front wall of thorax
       - ☐ With penetration into thoracic cavity
       - ☐ Without penetration into thoracic cavity
     - ☐ Back wall of thorax
       - ☐ With penetration into thoracic cavity
       - ☐ Without penetration into thoracic cavity
     - ☐ Unspecified part of thorax – review medical record/query physician
   - ☐ Abdomen, lower back, pelvis, and external genitalia
     - ☐ Abdominal wall
       - ☐ Upper quadrant
         - ☐ With penetration into peritoneal cavity
         - ☐ Without penetration into peritoneal cavity
       - ☐ Epigastric region
         - ☐ With penetration into peritoneal cavity
         - ☐ Without penetration into peritoneal cavity
       - ☐ Lower quadrant
         - ☐ With penetration into peritoneal cavity
         - ☐ Without penetration into peritoneal cavity
     - ☐ Penis
     - ☐ Scrotum and testis
     - ☐ Vagina and vulva
     - ☐ Unspecified external genital organs – review medical record/query physician
     - ☐ Lower back and pelvis
       - ☐ With penetration into retroperitoneum
       - ☐ Without penetration into retroperitoneum
     - ☐ Buttock
     - ☐ Anus
   - ☐ Shoulder and upper arm
     - ☐ Shoulder

- ☐ Upper arm
- ☐ Elbow and forearm
  - ☐ Elbow
  - ☐ Forearm
- ☐ Wrist, hand, and fingers
  - ☐ Wrist
  - ☐ Hand
  - ☐ Thumb
    - ☐ With damage to nail
    - ☐ Without damage to nail
  - ☐ Other finger
    - ☐ Index finger
      - ☐ With damage to nail
      - ☐ Without damage to nail
    - ☐ Middle finger
      - ☐ With damage to nail
      - ☐ Without damage to nail
    - ☐ Ring finger
      - ☐ With damage to nail
      - ☐ Without damage to nail
    - ☐ Little finger
      - ☐ With damage to nail
      - ☐ Without damage to nail
- ☐ Hip and thigh
  - ☐ Hip
  - ☐ Thigh
- ☐ Knee and lower leg
  - ☐ Knee
  - ☐ Lower leg
- ☐ Ankle, foot, and toes
  - ☐ Ankle
  - ☐ Foot
  - ☐ Toe
    - ☐ Great toe
      - ☐ With damage to nail
      - ☐ Without damage to nail
    - ☐ Lesser toe
      - ☐ With damage to nail
      - ☐ Without damage to nail

3. Identify laterality:
   - ☐ Left
   - ☐ Right
   - ☐ Unspecified – review medical record/query physician

Note: Not all codes require laterality. Laterality is pertinent whenever there are two sides for the same structure, such as but not limited to eyelids, cheeks, extremities, buttocks, upper and lower abdominal quadrants, breasts, and chest wall.

4. Identify episode of care/stage of healing/complication:
   - ☐ A Initial encounter
   - ☐ D Subsequent encounter
   - ☐ S Sequela
5. Code also any associated wound infection
6. Identify any associated injury and report with additional codes
   - ☐ Open wound of head
     - ☐ Cranial nerve injury (S04)
     - ☐ Intracranial injury (S06)
     - ☐ Muscle and tendon of head (S09.1-)
   - ☐ Open wound of neck
     - ☐ Associated spinal cord injury (S14.0–S14.1-)
     - ☐ Blood vessel injury (S15)
     - ☐ Dislocation and subluxation (S13)
   - ☐ Open wound of thorax
     - ☐ Blood vessel injury (S25)
     - ☐ Dislocation and subluxation (S23)
     - ☐ Injury of heart (S26)
     - ☐ Injury of intrathoracic organs (S27)
     - ☐ Injury of muscle and tendon of thorax (S29)
     - ☐ Rib fracture (S22.3-, S22.4-)
     - ☐ Spinal cord injury (S24.0, S24.1-)
     - ☐ Traumatic hemopneumothorax (S27.32)
     - ☐ Traumatic hemothorax (S27.1)
     - ☐ Traumatic pneumothorax (S27.0)
   - ☐ Open wound of abdomen, lower back, pelvis, and external genitalia
     - ☐ Associated spinal cord injury (S24.0, S24.1-, S34.0-, S34.1-)
     - ☐ Blood vessel injury (S35)
     - ☐ Dislocation and subluxation of lumbar vertebra (S33)
     - ☐ Injury of intra-abdominal organ (S36)
     - ☐ Injury of muscle, fascia, and tendon of abdomen, lower back and pelvis (S39)
     - ☐ Injury of urinary and pelvic organs (S37)
   - ☐ Open wound of shoulder and upper arm
     - ☐ Blood vessel injury (S45)
     - ☐ Dislocation and subluxation (S43)
     - ☐ Muscle, fascia, and tendon injury (S46)
     - ☐ Nerve injury (S44)
   - ☐ Open wound of elbow and forearm
     - ☐ Blood vessel injury (S55)
     - ☐ Dislocation and subluxation (S53)
     - ☐ Muscle, fascia, and tendon injury (S56)
     - ☐ Nerve injury (S54)
   - ☐ Open wound of wrist, hand, and fingers
     - ☐ Blood vessel injury (S65)
     - ☐ Dislocation and subluxation (S63)
     - ☐ Muscle, fascia, and tendon injury (S66)
     - ☐ Nerve injury (S64)
   - ☐ Open wound of hip and thigh
     - ☐ Blood vessel injury (S75)
     - ☐ Dislocation and subluxation (S73)
     - ☐ Muscle, fascia, and tendon injury (S76)
     - ☐ Nerve injury (S74)
   - ☐ Open wound of knee and lower leg
     - ☐ Blood vessel injury (S85)

        - ☐ Dislocation and subluxation (S83)
        - ☐ Muscle, fascia, and tendon injury (S86)
        - ☐ Nerve injury (S84)
    - ☐ Open wound of foot, ankle, and toes
        - ☐ Blood vessel injury (S95)
        - ☐ Dislocation and subluxation (S93)
        - ☐ Muscle, fascia, and tendon injury (S96)
        - ☐ Nerve injury (S94)

7. Identify the external cause, intent, activity, place and status where applicable.

Osteomyelitis

ICD-10-CM Categories

Osteomyelitis is classified in the following ICD-10-CM categories:

A02.24	Salmonella osteomyelitis
A54.43	Gonococcal osteomyelitis
B67.2	Echinococcus granulosus infection of bone
H05.02	Osteomyelitis of orbit
H05.3	Periostitis of orbit
H70.2	Petrositis
M46.2	Osteomyelitis of vertebra
M86	Osteomyelitis

ICD-10-CM Definitions

Acute osteomyelitis – The sudden onset of pyogenic inflammation in bone developing within 2 weeks of an initial injury, disease, or other infection; most commonly occurring in children.

Brodie's abscess – A form of subacute osteomyelitis creating an intraosseous abscess.

Chronic osteomyelitis – Long term pyogenic inflammation in bone that develops a few months after an initial injury, disease, or other infection; uncommon in children.

Hematogenous osteomyelitis – Osteomyelitis caused by bacterial seeding from the blood. Acute hematogenous osteomyelitis may have a slow clinical development with insidious onset; it occurs more often in children than adults and tends to affect the metaphysis in children in the acute phase. Hematogenous osteomyelitis has a high incidence of occurrence in the vertebra, but can also occur in the pelvis and clavicle.

Multifocal osteomyelitis – A rare, chronic, and recurrent non-pyogenic autoinflammatory form of osteomyelitis that primarily affects children and results in multiple lesions in the bone in multiple sites. The lesions can occur in any bone, are lytic and destructive in the early phase of the disease and sclerotic and reactive in the late phase. There may be skin, eye, and/or bowel manifestations. Also called chronic recurrent multifocal osteomyelitis (CRMO) and SAPHO syndrome (synovitis, acne, pustulosis, hyperostosis, osteitis).

Osteomyelitis – Inflammation of bone due to a pyogenic organism, most commonly bacterial in origin. May occur as a result of an injury to bone and the surrounding soft tissue, following surgery, or resulting from infection elsewhere in the body. Osteomyelitis may be localized or may involve the periosteum, cortex, marrow, and cancellous tissue of the bone. The tibia, femur, humerus, maxilla, mandible and vertebra are the most common bones affected.

Periostitis – Inflammation of the outer covering of bone known as the periosteum. The acute form is due to infection and results in severe pain, fever, malaise, and pus within the periosteum. Congenital forms are generally caused by syphilis.

Petrositis – Also known as petrous apicitis and Gradenigo's syndrome or Gradenigo-Lannois syndrome, petrositis is an infection of the temporal bone usually resulting from suppurative mastoiditis and otitis media. The most common causative organisms are *Streptococcus pneumoniae*, *Haemophilus influenzae*, *Staphylococcus aureus* or *Pseudomonas* and occasionally tuberculosis.

Subacute osteomyelitis – Pyogenic inflammation in bone that develops within one to several months after an initial injury, disease, or other infection.

Checklist

1. Identify the type of osteomyelitis:
   - ☐ Acute
     - ☐ Hematogenous
     - ☐ Other
   - ☐ Chronic
     - ☐ Hematogenous
     - ☐ Multifocal
     - ☐ Other
     - ☐ With draining sinus
   - ☐ Organism specific (no additional criteria needed)
     - ☐ Gonococcal osteomyelitis
     - ☐ Echinococcus granulosus infection of bone
     - ☐ Salmonella osteomyelitis
   - ☐ Petrositis (go to 3)
     - ☐ Acute
     - ☐ Chronic
   - ☐ Subacute
   - ☐ Other (includes Brodie's abscess)
   - ☐ Unspecified (includes periostitis without osteomyelitis)

Note: Osteomyelitis of the vertebral column and orbit is not subclassified as acute, subacute, or chronic.

2. Identify the body area:
   a. For osteomyelitis of vertebral column:
      - ☐ Occipito-atlantal-axial region
      - ☐ Cervical region
      - ☐ Cervicothoracic region
      - ☐ Thoracic region
      - ☐ Thoracolumbar region
      - ☐ Lumbar region
      - ☐ Lumbosacral region
      - ☐ Sacrococcygeal region
      - ☐ Multiple sites in spine
      - ☐ Unspecified site, vertebra – review medical record/ query physician

   b. For acute, chronic, or subacute osteomyelitis:
      - ☐ Humerus
      - ☐ Radius and ulna
      - ☐ Hand
      - ☐ Femur
      - ☐ Tibia and fibula

- ☐ Ankle and foot
- ☐ Other sites
- ☐ Unspecified site – review medical record/query physician

c. If other osteomyelitis:

- ☐ Shoulder
- ☐ Upper arm
- ☐ Forearm
- ☐ Hand
- ☐ Thigh
- ☐ Lower leg
- ☐ Ankle and foot
- ☐ Multiple sites
- ☐ Other site
- ☐ Unspecified sites – review medical record/query physician

3. Identify laterality (excluding osteomyelitis of vertebra, multiple, other, and unspecified site):
   - ☐ Bilateral (petrositis only)
   - ☐ Left
   - ☐ Right
   - ☐ Unspecified – review medical record/query physician
4. Code also infectious agent, if known (B95-B97)
5. Code also major osseous defect, if applicable

Otitis Media

ICD-10-CM Categories/Codes

H65	Nonsuppurative otitis media
H66	Suppurative and unspecified otitis media
H67	Otitis media in diseases classified elsewhere

ICD-10-CM Definitions

Do not report otitis media in influenza, measles, scarlet fever, or tuberculosis with codes listed in the categories above. Codes for otitis media in influenza, measles, scarlet fever, and tuberculosis are as follows:

A18.6	Tuberculosis of (inner) (middle) ear
A38.0	Scarlet fever with otitis media
B05.3	Measles complicated by otitis media
J09.X9	Influenza due to identified novel influenza A virus with other manifestations (use additional code to identify manifestation)
J10.83	Influenza due to other identified influenza virus with otitis media
J11.83	Influenza due to unidentified influenza virus with otitis media

Checklist

1. Identify as nonsuppurative, suppurative/unspecified, in diseases classified elsewhere:
   - ☐ In diseases classified elsewhere – Proceed to #2
   - ☐ Nonsuppurative otitis media – Proceed to #3
   - ☐ Suppurative/unspecified otitis media – Proceed to #4
2. Otitis Media In Diseases Classified Elsewhere
   a. Specify otitis media due to/with:
      - ☐ Influenza due to identified novel influenza A virus with other manifestations (J09.X9) – Use additional code to identify manifestation ____________
      - ☐ Influenza due to other identified influenza virus with otitis media (J10.83)
      - ☐ Influenza due to unidentified influenza virus with otitis media (J11.83)
      - ☐ Measles complicated by otitis media (B05.3)
      - ☐ Scarlet fever with otitis media (A38.0)
      - ☐ Tuberculosis of (inner) (middle) ear (A18.6)
      - ☐ Other diseases classified elsewhere – Code first underlying disease (such as viral disease B00-B34) ____________

   b. Specify laterality:
      - ☐ Bilateral
      - ☐ Left
      - ☐ Right
      - ☐ Unspecified ear

   c. Assign additional code for any associated perforated tympanic membrane (H72.-)
3. Nonsuppurative Otitis Media
   a. Identify status:
      - ☐ Acute (and subacute) – Proceed to #3b, #3d
      - ☐ Chronic – Proceed to #3c, #3d
      - ☐ Unspecified – Proceed to #3d

   b. For acute/subacute nonsuppurative otitis media:
      - ☐ Specify type
        - ☐ Allergic otitis media
        - ☐ Serous otitis media
        - ☐ Other acute (includes mucoid, sanguineous, seromucinous, other/unspecified, acute nonsuppurative)
      - ☐ Specify not recurrent/recurrent
        - ☐ Not specified as recurrent
        - ☐ Recurrent

   c. For chronic nonsuppurative otitis media:
      - ☐ Specify type
        - ☐ Allergic otitis media
        - ☐ Mucoid otitis media
        - ☐ Serous otitis media
        - ☐ Other chronic (includes exudative, seromucinous, with effusion, other/unspecified, chronic nonsuppurative)

   d. For nonsuppurative otitis media:
      - ☐ Specify laterality
        - ☐ Bilateral
        - ☐ Left
        - ☐ Right
        - ☐ Unspecified ear
      - ☐ Assign additional code for any associated perforated tympanic membrane (H72.-)
      - ☐ Assign additional code for any causative infectious agent (B95-B97)
4. Suppurative/Unspecified Otitis Media
   a. Identify status:
      - ☐ Acute (and subacute) suppurative – Proceed to #4b, #4d
      - ☐ Chronic suppurative – Proceed to #4c, #4d
      - ☐ Unspecified
        - ☐ Suppurative otitis media (not specified as acute or chronic) – Proceed to #4d
        - ☐ Not specified as nonsuppurative or suppurative – Assign code

   b. For acute/subacute suppurative otitis media:
      - ☐ Specify any spontaneous ear drum rupture
        - ☐ With spontaneous rupture of ear drum
        - ☐ Without spontaneous rupture of ear drum
      - ☐ Specify not recurrent/recurrent
        - ☐ Not specified as recurrent
        - ☐ Recurrent

c. For chronic suppurative otitis media:
   - ☐ Specify type
     - ☐ Atticoantral
     - ☐ Tubotympanic
   - ☐ Other chronic suppurative otitis media

d. For suppurative otitis media:
   - ☐ Specify laterality
     - ☐ Bilateral
     - ☐ Left
     - ☐ Right
     - ☐ Unspecified ear

Note: Assign addition code for any associated perforated tympanic membrane (H72.-) – Excludes codes in subcategories H66.0 and H66.01

5. For all types of otitis media, identify any exposure to tobacco smoke, history of tobacco use, current use/dependence on tobacco
   - ☐ Exposure to environmental tobacco smoke (Z77.22)
   - ☐ Exposure to tobacco smoke in the perinatal period (P96.81)
   - ☐ History of tobacco dependence (Z87.891)
   - ☐ Occupational exposure to environmental tobacco smoke (Z57.31)
   - ☐ Tobacco dependence (F17.-)
   - ☐ Tobacco use (Z72.0)

Pharyngitis/Tonsillitis, Acute

ICD-10-CM Categories

J02	Acute pharyngitis
J03	Acute tonsillitis

ICD-10-CM Definitions

Acute Pharyngitis – Acute inflammation of the throat including the mucous membrane and underlying part of the pharynx. Additional terms used to describe acute pharyngitis include: gangrenous pharyngitis, infective pharyngitis, sore throat, suppurative pharyngitis, ulcerative pharyngitis.

Acute Tonsillitis – Acute inflammation of the palatine tonsils. Tonsillitis may be a single acute inflammation or may occur repeatedly in which case it is classified as acute recurrent. Additional terms used to describe acute tonsillitis include: follicular tonsillitis, gangrenous tonsillitis, infective tonsillitis, ulcerative tonsillitis.

Streptococcal Pharyngitis – Acute inflammation of the throat including the mucous membrane and underlying part of the pharynx due to Group A, beta-hemolytic streptococcus (GABHS) infection. Additional terms used to describe streptococcal pharyngitis include: septic pharyngitis, streptococcal sore throat.

Streptococcal Tonsillitis – Acute inflammation of the palatine tonsils due to Group A, beta-hemolytic streptococcus (GABHS) infection. Streptococcal tonsillitis may be a single acute infection or may occur repeatedly in which case it is classified as acute recurrent.

Checklist

1. Identify as acute pharyngitis/tonsillitis
   - ☐ Acute Pharyngitis
   - ☐ Acute Tonsillitis
2. Identify organism
   - ☐ Streptococcus
   - ☐ Assign additional code to identify organism (B95-B97) ____________________
   - ☐ Unspecified organism
3. For acute tonsillitis, identify as:
   - ☐ Acute (single episode)
   - ☐ Acute recurrent (multiple repeat episodes)

Pneumonia

ICD-10-CM Categories/Subcategories

Codes for pneumonia are located across multiple categories, found mainly in Chapter 10 Diseases of the Respiratory System with some codes listed in Chapter 1 Certain Infectious and Parasitic Diseases. Congenital pneumonia is coded in Chapter 17 Congenital Malformations, Deformations, and Chromosomal Abnormalities.

Coding pneumonia may require more than one code to capture the type of pneumonia, infecting organism, associated or underlying conditions, and any related abscess. Follow all coding instructions carefully for sequencing and assigning pneumonia codes for the specific type of organism, and all other related conditions or factors.

The main categories and some specific codes for pneumonia are listed below, although the list is not all inclusive of codes that report pneumonia or conditions occurring with pneumonia:

A15.0	Tuberculous pneumonia
B01.2	Varicella pneumonia
J12	Viral pneumonia, not elsewhere classified
J13	Pneumonia due to Streptococcus pneumoniae
J14	Pneumonia due to Haemophilus influenzae
J15	Bacterial pneumonia, not elsewhere classified
J16	Pneumonia due to infectious organisms, not elsewhere classified
J17	Pneumonia in diseases classified elsewhere
J18	Pneumonia, unspecific organism
J69	Pneumonitis due to solids and liquids
J84.11	Idiopathic interstitial pneumonia
J95.851	Ventilator associated pneumonia
P23	Congenital pneumonia
P24.01	Meconium aspiration pneumonia

ICD-10-CM Definitions

Pneumonia – An inflammation or infection of the lung(s) caused by microorganisms such as bacteria, viruses, or fungi; aspiration of foreign material; or inhalation of chemicals or hazardous materials, causing an accumulation of fluid, inflammatory cells, and fibrin that impairs the exchange of oxygen and carbon dioxide in the alveoli.

Checklist

1. Identify the type of pneumonia:
   - ☐ Aspiration/Inhalation – Proceed to #2
   - ☐ Bacterial – Proceed to #3
   - ☐ Congenital – Proceed to #4
   - ☐ Fungal – Proceed to #5
   - ☐ Interstitial – Proceed to #6
   - ☐ Other specified types – Proceed to #7
   - ☐ Viral – Proceed to #8
2. Aspiration/Inhalation pneumonia
   a. Identify causative aspirate:
      - ☐ Anesthesia
        - ☐ During labor and delivery (O74.0)
        - ☐ During pregnancy (O29.01-)
        - ☐ During puerperium (O89.01)
        - ☐ Postprocedural, chemical (J95.4)
      - ☐ Fumes, Vapors, Gases (J68.0)
      - ☐ Solids and liquids
        - ☐ Blood (J69.8)
        - ☐ Detergent (J69.8)
        - ☐ Food (J69.0)
        - ☐ Gastric Secretions (J69.0)
        - ☐ Oils and Essences (J69.1)
        - ☐ Other Solids and Liquids (J69.8)
        - ☐ Vomit (J69.0)
      - ☐ Unspecified (J69.0)
3. Bacterial pneumonia
   a. Identify causative bacteria:
      - ☐ Actinomyces (A42.0)
      - ☐ Bacillus anthracis (A22.1)
      - ☐ Bacteroides (J15.8)
      - ☐ Bordetella
        - ☐ Other (A37.81)
        - ☐ Parapertussis (A37.11)
        - ☐ Pertussis (A37.01)
      - ☐ Burkholderia pseudomallei (A24.1)
      - ☐ Butyrivibrio fibriosolvens (J15.8)
      - ☐ Chlamydia (J16.0)
        - ☐ Psittaci (A70)
      - ☐ Clostridium (J15.8)
      - ☐ Eaton's agent (J15.7)
      - ☐ Enterobacter (J15.6)
      - ☐ Escherichia coli (J15.5)
      - ☐ Friedlander's bacillus (J15.0)
      - ☐ Fusobacterium nucleatum (J15.8)
      - ☐ Gram-negative, other (J15.6)
      - ☐ Gram-positive (J15.9)
      - ☐ Haemophilus influenzae (J14)
      - ☐ Klebsiella pneumoniae (J15.0)
      - ☐ Melioidosis (A24.1)
      - ☐ Mycoplasma pneumoniae (J15.7)
      - ☐ Neisseria gonorrhoeae (A54.84)
      - ☐ Nocardia asteroides (A43.0)
      - ☐ Other specified (J15.8)
      - ☐ Proteus (J15.6)
      - ☐ Pseudomonas (J15.1)
      - ☐ Salmonella (A02.22)
        - ☐ typhi (A01.03)
      - ☐ Serratia marcescens (J15.6)
      - ☐ Staphylococcus

- ☐ Aureus, Methicillin resistant (J15.212)
- ☐ Aureus, Methicillin susceptible (J15.211)
- ☐ Other (J15.29)
- ☐ Unspecified staphylococcus (J15.20)

☐ Streptococcus
- ☐ Group B (J15.3)
- ☐ Other (J15.4)
- ☐ S. pneumoniae (J13)

☐ Tuberculosis (A15.0)

☐ Unspecified bacteria (J15.9)

4. Congenital pneumonia
   a. Identify causative source:
   - ☐ Aspiration
     - ☐ Amniotic fluid and mucus (P24.11)
     - ☐ Blood (P24.21)
     - ☐ Meconium (P24.01)
     - ☐ Milk and regurgitated food (P24.31)
     - ☐ Other/Unspecified (P24.81)
   - ☐ Infectious Agent
     - ☐ Chlamydia (P23.1)
     - ☐ Escherichia coli (P23.4)
     - ☐ Francisella tularensis (A21.2)
     - ☐ Haemophilus influenzae (P23.6)
     - ☐ Klebsiella pneumoniae (P23.6)
     - ☐ Mycoplasma (P23.6)
     - ☐ Other bacterial agent (P23.6)
     - ☐ Other organisms (P23.8)
     - ☐ Pseudomonas (P23.5)
     - ☐ Rubella (P35.0)
     - ☐ Staphylococcus (P23.2)
     - ☐ Streptococcus
       - ☐ Group B (P23.3)
       - ☐ Other (P23.6)
     - ☐ Syphilitic, early (A50.04)
     - ☐ Viral agent (P23.0)
     - ☐ Unspecified (P23.9)
5. Fungal pneumonia
   a. Identify causative type:
   - ☐ Aspergillosis
     - ☐ Invasive (B44.0)
     - ☐ Other (B44.1)
   - ☐ Blastomycosis
     - ☐ Acute (B40.0)
     - ☐ Chronic (B40.1)
     - ☐ Unspecified (B40.2)
   - ☐ Candidiasis (B37.1)
   - ☐ Coccidioidomycosis
     - ☐ Acute (B38.0)
     - ☐ Chronic (B38.1)
     - ☐ Unspecified (B38.2)
   - ☐ Cryptococcosis (B45.0)
   - ☐ Histoplasmosis
     - ☐ Acute (B39.0)
     - ☐ Chronic (B39.1)
     - ☐ Unspecified (B39.2)
   - ☐ Paracoccidioidomycosis (B41.0)
   - ☐ Pneumocystosis (B59)
   - ☐ Sporotrichosis (B42.0)
6. Interstitial pneumonia
   a. Identify type:
   - ☐ Idiopathic
     - ☐ Acute (J84.114)
     - ☐ Cryptogenic organizing (J84.116)
     - ☐ Desquamative (J84.117)
     - ☐ Fibrosing (J84.112)
     - ☐ Hamman-Rich (J84.114)
     - ☐ Nonspecific (J84.113)
     - ☐ Not otherwise specified (J84.111)
     - ☐ Respiratory bronchiolitis (J84.115)
   - ☐ In diseases classified elsewhere (J84.178)
   - ☐ Lymphoid (J84.2)
7. Other specified types
   a. Identify type, other causative agent, or site:
   - ☐ Allergic (J82.89)
   - ☐ Ascariasis (B77.81)
   - ☐ Bronchopneumonia (J18.0)
   - ☐ Due to other specified infectious organism (J16.8)
   - ☐ Eosinophilic (J82.81, J82.82)
   - ☐ Hypostatic (J18.2)
   - ☐ In diseases classified elsewhere (J17)
   - ☐ Lobar (J18.1)
   - ☐ Other (J18.8)
   - ☐ Passive (J18.2)
   - ☐ Toxoplasma gondii (B58.3)
   - ☐ Ventilator associated (J95.851)
8. Viral pneumonia
   a. Identify causative virus:
   - ☐ Adenoviral (J12.0)
   - ☐ COVID-19 (U07.1 and J12.89)
   - ☐ Human metapneumovirus (J12.3)
   - ☐ Other virus (J12.89)
   - ☐ Parainfluenza (J12.2)
   - ☐ Postmeasles (B05.2)
   - ☐ Respiratory syncytial virus (J12.1)
   - ☐ Rubella (B06.81)
   - ☐ SARS-associated coronavirus (J12.81)
   - ☐ Varicella (B01.2)
   - ☐ Unspecified (J12.9)
9. Unspecified pneumonia (J18.9)

Rheumatoid Arthritis

ICD-10-CM Categories

Rheumatoid arthritis may be classified as a combination code according to the type of rheumatoid arthritis, the joint, and organ system involved. Conditions related to rheumatoid arthritis are also included in this category.

Rheumatoid arthritis is classified in the following ICD-10-CM categories/subcategories:

M05	Rheumatoid arthritis with rheumatoid factor
M06	Other rheumatoid arthritis
M08.0	Unspecified juvenile rheumatoid arthritis
M08.1	Juvenile ankylosing spondylitis
M08.2	Juvenile rheumatoid arthritis with systemic onset
M08.3	Juvenile rheumatoid polyarthritis (seronegative)
M08.4	Pauciarticular juvenile rheumatoid arthritis
M45.0	Ankylosing spondylitis

ICD-10-CM Definitions

Ankylosing spondylitis – Also known as Marie-Strumpell disease, rheumatoid spondylitis, and Bechterew's syndrome, ankylosing spondylitis is a chronic, progressive, autoimmune arthropathy that affects the spine and sacroiliac joints, eventually leading to spinal fusion and rigidity. Almost all of the autoimmune spondylarthropathies share a common genetic marker, HLA-B27, although the cause is still unknown. The disease appears in some predisposed people after exposure to bowel or urinary tract infections. The most common patient is a young male, aged 15-30. It affects men about three times more than women. Swelling occurs in the intervertebral discs and in the joints between the spine and pelvis. Patients have persistent buttock and low back pain and stiffness alleviated with exercise. Over time, the vertebrae may become fused together, progressing up the spine and affecting other organs.

Felty's Syndrome – An atypical form of rheumatoid arthritis that presents with fever, an enlarged spleen, recurring infections, and a decreased white blood count.

Juvenile rheumatoid arthritis with systemic onset – Systemic onset juvenile rheumatoid arthritis (JRA), also known as Still's Disease in children, is an autoimmune inflammatory disease that develops in children up to the age of 16. It is the most uncommon form of JRA. It begins with periods of recurrent high fever spikes up to 103 degrees accompanied by a rash that lasts for at least two weeks. Other symptoms can include enlarged lymph nodes, enlarged liver or spleen, or inflammation of the lining of the heart or lungs (pericarditis or pleuritis). Joint swelling and joint damage may not appear for months or years after the fevers begin. In addition to the joints, other connective tissue organs such as the liver and spleen may also be affected.

Pauciarticular juvenile rheumatoid arthritis – Pauciarticular JRA, also known as oligoarticular JRA, is an autoimmune inflammatory disease that develops in children any time up to 16 years of age that presents with an initial onset affecting 5 or fewer joints. The larger joints, such as the knees, ankles, and elbows are the most commonly affected. Pauciarticular JRA is the most common form of JRA occurring more commonly in girls. Children, particularly boys, who develop the disease after the age of 7 tend to have other joints, including the spine, become affected and will frequently continue with the disease into adulthood. Children who develop the disease at a younger age tend to go into remission and become asymptomatic.

Rheumatoid arthritis – Rheumatoid arthritis (RA) is an autoimmune, systemic, inflammatory disease that normally occurs between the ages of 30 and 50. RA affects the synovial lining of joints resulting in swelling, pain, warmth, and stiffness around the joint, followed by thickening of the synovial lining; bone and cartilage destruction leading to pain; joint deformity and instability; and loss of function. RA commonly begins in the small joints of the hands and wrists and is often symmetrical, affecting the same joints on both sides. RA is accompanied by other physical symptoms including morning pain and stiffness or pain with prolonged sitting; flu-like low grade fever and muscle ache; disease flare-ups followed by remission; and sometimes rheumatoid nodules under the skin, particularly over the elbows. Some people also have an increase in rheumatoid factor antibody that helps direct the production of normal antibodies.

Rheumatoid factor – Rheumatoid factor is an antibody (protein) in the blood that binds with other antibodies and is not present in normal individuals. A value of 14IU/ml or greater is considered positive.

Rheumatoid nodule – Benign lumps or masses that develop under the skin of some patients with rheumatoid arthritis. These masses are firm and generally located near a joint, most commonly occurring on the fingers, elbows, forearm, knees, and backs of the heels.

Still's disease (adult-onset) – Adult-onset Still's disease is a rare inflammatory disease that develops in adults over the age of 45 and affects multiple joints and organ systems. There is no known cause of Still's disease. Common symptoms include fever, joint pain, sore throat, muscle pain, and a rash. This disease may be an isolated episode or reoccur. The knees and wrists are the most common joints destroyed by the disease.

Checklist

1. Identify the type of arthritis:
   - ☐ Ankylosing spondylitis
     - ☐ Ankylosing spondylitis
     - ☐ Juvenile ankylosing spondylitis
   - ☐ Juvenile rheumatoid arthritis
     - ☐ Juvenile rheumatoid arthritis with systemic onset
     - ☐ Juvenile rheumatoid polyarthritis
     - ☐ Pauciarticular juvenile rheumatoid arthritis
     - ☐ With or without rheumatoid factor/unspecified
   - ☐ Rheumatoid arthritis
     - ☐ With rheumatoid factor (seropositive)
       - ☐ Felty's syndrome
       - ☐ Rheumatoid arthritis
       - ☐ Other

- ☐ Other rheumatoid arthritis
  - ☐ Adult-onset Still's disease
  - ☐ Rheumatoid bursitis
  - ☐ Rheumatoid nodule
  - ☐ Other specified
  - ☐ Without rheumatoid factor (seronegative)

Note: For Adult-onset Still's disease and juvenile rheumatoid polyarthritis there is no further classification for the code. For Still's disease in children, see juvenile rheumatoid arthritis with systemic onset.

2. For other than ankylosing spondylitis, identify joint:
   - ☐ Shoulder
   - ☐ Elbow
   - ☐ Wrist
   - ☐ Hand
   - ☐ Hip
   - ☐ Knee
   - ☐ Ankle and foot
   - ☐ Vertebrae (excluding Felty's syndrome)
   - ☐ Multiple sites (excluding Felty's syndrome and pauciarticular JRA)
   - ☐ Other specific site
   - ☐ Unspecified site– review medical record/query physician
3. For ankylosing spondylitis (M45), identify vertebral level/region:
   - ☐ Occipito-atlanto-axial spine
   - ☐ Cervical region
   - ☐ Cervicothoracic region
   - ☐ Thoracic region
   - ☐ Thoracolumbar region
   - ☐ Lumbar region
   - ☐ Lumbosacral region
   - ☐ Sacral and sacrococcygeal region
   - ☐ Multiple sites in spine
   - ☐ Unspecified sites in spine– review medical record/query physician

   Note: Juvenile ankylosing spondylitis (M08.1) is not defined by vertebral level/region.
4. For rheumatoid arthritis with rheumatoid factor (excluding other), identify organ system involvement:
   - ☐ Rheumatoid heart disease
   - ☐ Rheumatoid myopathy
   - ☐ Rheumatoid lung disease
   - ☐ Rheumatoid polyneuropathy
   - ☐ Rheumatoid vasculitis
   - ☐ Other organs and systems
   - ☐ Without organ or system involvement
5. Identify laterality excluding vertebrae, multiple sites, and ankylosing spondylitis:
   - ☐ Left
   - ☐ Right
   - ☐ Unspecified – review medical record/query physician

Seizures

ICD-10-CM Categories/Subcategories

Codes for seizures are located across multiple categories in different chapters. Epileptic seizures are the only group classified to Chapter 6 Diseases of the Nervous System. Other types of nonepileptic seizures such as new onset, febrile, or hysterical seizure are classified to other chapters.

F44.5	Conversion disorder with seizures or convulsions
G40	Epilepsy and recurrent seizures
P90	Convulsions of newborn
R56	Convulsions, not elsewhere classified

ICD-10-CM Definitions

Absence seizure – A type of seizure common in children that appears as brief, sudden lapses in attention or vacant staring spells during which the child is unresponsive; often accompanied by other signs such as lip smacking, chewing motions, eyelid fluttering, and small finger or hand movements; formerly called petit mal seizure.

Epilepsy – Disorder of the central nervous system characterized by long-term predisposition to recurring episodes of sudden onset seizures, muscle contractions, sensory disturbance, and loss of consciousness caused by excessive neuronal activity in the brain and resulting in cognitive, psychological, and neurobiological consequences.

Generalized tonic clonic seizure – A type of seizure involving the entire body that usually begins on both sides of the brain and manifests with loss of consciousness, muscle stiffness, and convulsive, jerking movements; also called grand mal seizure.

Juvenile myoclonic epilepsy – A form of generalized epilepsy manifesting in mid or late childhood typically emerging first as absence seizures, then the presence of myoclonic jerks upon awakening from sleep in another 1-9 years as its hallmark feature, followed by generalized tonic clonic seizures some months later in nearly all cases.

Lennox-Gastaut syndrome – Severe form of epilepsy characterized by multiple different seizure types that are hard to control that may be absence, tonic (muscle stiffening), atonic (muscle drop), myoclonic, tonic clonic (grand mal); usually beginning before age 4 and associated with impaired intellectual functioning, developmental delay, and behavioral disturbances.

Localization-related epilepsy – Focal epilepsy generating seizures from one localized area of the brain where excessive or abnormal electrical discharges begin; synonymous with partial epilepsy.

Myoclonic jerks – Irregular, shock-like movements in the arms or legs that occur upon awakening, usually seen affecting both arms but sometimes restricted to the fingers, and may occur unilaterally, typically occurring in clusters and often a warning sign before generalized tonic clonic seizure.

Seizure – A transient occurrence of abnormal or uncontrolled electrical discharges in the brain resulting in an event of physical convulsions, thought and sensory disturbances, other minor physical signs, and possible loss of consciousness.

Checklist

1. Identify type of seizure(s):
   - ☐ Epileptic – Proceed to #2
   - ☐ Other (nonepileptic) type – Proceed to #3
2. Epilepsy and recurrent seizures
   a. Identify type of epilepsy or epileptic syndrome:
      - ☐ Absence epileptic syndrome (G40.A-)
      - ☐ Dravet syndrome (G40.83-)
      - ☐ Epileptic spasms (G40.82-)
      - ☐ Generalized
        - ☐ Idiopathic (G40.3-)
        - ☐ Other (G40.4-)
      - ☐ Juvenile myoclonic epilepsy (G40.B-)
      - ☐ Lennox-Gastaut syndrome (G40.81-)
      - ☐ Localization-related (focal) (partial)
        - ☐ Idiopathic (G40.0-)
        - ☐ Symptomatic
          - ☐ With complex partial seizures (G40.2-)
          - ☐ With simple partial seizures (G40.1-)
      - ☐ Other epilepsy (G40.80-)
      - ☐ Other seizures (G40.89)
      - ☐ Related to external causes (G40.5-)
      - ☐ Unspecified epilepsy (G40.9-)

   b. Determine intractability status:
      - ☐ Intractable
      - ☐ Not intractable

   Note: Intractable status does not apply to other seizures or to epileptic seizures related to external causes, while not intractable does not apply to Dravet syndrome.

   c. Determine status epilepticus:
      - ☐ With status epilepticus
      - ☐ Without status epilepticus

   Note: Status epilepticus does not apply to other seizures.
3. Other (nonepileptic) type seizures
   a. Identify type of other nonepileptic seizure:
      - ☐ Febrile
        - ☐ Complex (R56.01)
        - ☐ Simple (R56.00)
      - ☐ Hysterical (F44.5)
      - ☐ Newborn (P90)
      - ☐ Post-traumatic (R56.1)
      - ☐ Unspecified (R56.9)

Sepsis, Severe Sepsis, Septic Shock

ICD-10-CM Categories/Subcategories

Codes for sepsis, severe sepsis, septic shock, and SIRS often require multiple codes to capture the organism, the severity of the sepsis, and additional information related to complications of care. The most frequently reported codes related to sepsis and related conditions are listed. Consult the ICD-10-CM code book and follow all coding instructions carefully for sequencing and assigning all the sepsis codes required, such as those identifying the specific type or organism, as well as other factors related to the sepsis diagnosis.

A40	Streptococcal sepsis
A41	Other sepsis
O85	Puerperal sepsis
P36	Bacterial sepsis of newborn
R65	Symptoms and signs specifically associated with inflammation and infection (includes codes for SIRS and severe sepsis)

ICD-10-CM Definitions

Episode of Care – Designates the episode of care as initial (A), subsequent (D) or a sequela (S) for injuries, poisonings, and certain other conditions; and, in some instances, provides additional information about the injury.

Sepsis – Systemic infection. Immune response to an infection caused by infectious micro-organisms in the bloodstream. May also be referred to as systemic inflammatory response syndrome (SIRS) due to infectious process.

Septic shock – Circulatory failure associated with severe sepsis

Severe sepsis – Systemic infection with associated acute organ dysfunction or failure

Checklist

1. Sepsis due to or following procedure (postprocedural following immunization, infusion, transfusion, therapeutic injection)
   - ☐ Yes – Follow instructions in 4, 7, and 8
   - ☐ No – Go to 2
2. Sepsis complicating pregnancy, labor, puerperium (postpartum) period
   - ☐ Yes – Follow instructions in 5, 8
   - ☐ No – Go to 3
3. Sepsis during the neonatal period
   - ☐ Yes – Follow instructions in 6, 8
   - ☐ No – Follow instructions in 7, 8
4. Identify the sepsis as (code first):
   - ☐ Postprocedural sepsis
     - ☐ Initial Encounter (T81.44XA)
     - ☐ Subsequent Encounter (T81.44XD)
     - ☐ Sequela (T81.44XS) OR
     - ☐ Obstetrical (O86.04)

     For postprocedural sepsis, assign first the infection site, if known (T81.40-T81.43 or O86.00-O86.03)
   - ☐ Infection following immunization
     - ☐ Initial Encounter (T88.0XXA)
     - ☐ Subsequent Encounter (T88.0XXD)
     - ☐ Sequela (T88.0XXS)

     Assign additional code to identify the specific sepsis infection.
   - ☐ Sepsis following infusion, transfusion, therapeutic injection

     Select appropriate code from T80.2- and add required seventh digit. Assign additional code to identify the specific sepsis infection.
     - ☐ Initial Encounter
     - ☐ Subsequent Encounter
     - ☐ Sequela
5. Sepsis during or following pregnancy, labor, puerperal (postpartum).

   a. *Identify sepsis as (code first):*
   - ☐ Puerperal (postpartum) sepsis (O85)
   - ☐ Sepsis during labor (O75.3)
   - ☐ Sepsis following abortion
     - ☐ Incomplete spontaneous (O03.37)
     - ☐ Complete spontaneous or unspecified (O03.87)
     - ☐ Induced termination (O04.87)
   - ☐ Failed attempted termination (O07.37)
   - ☐ Sepsis following ectopic or molar pregnancy (O08.82)

   b. *Identify (code also) infectious organism in diseases classified elsewhere from the following categories B95, B96, B97 (consult ICD-10-CM book for specific codes)*
6. Sepsis during the neonatal period (sepsis of newborn). Identify as due to:
   - ☐ Anaerobes (P36.5)
   - ☐ Escherichia coli (P36.4)
   - ☐ Other bacteria (P36.8 and additional code from category B96)
   - ☐ Staphylococcus
     - ☐ Aureus (P36.2)
     - ☐ Unspecified (P36.30)
     - ☐ Other specified (P36.39)
   - ☐ Streptococcus
     - ☐ Group B (P36.0)
     - ☐ Unspecified (P36.10)
     - ☐ Other specified (P36.19)
   - ☐ Unspecified (P36.9)

7. Identify the infectious organism:
   - ☐ Bacterial
     - ☐ Anaerobes (A41.4)
     - ☐ Gonococcal (A54.86)
     - ☐ Haemophilus influenzae (A41.3)
     - ☐ Listerial (A32.7)
     - ☐ Meningococcal/Meningococcemia
       - ☐ Acute (A39.2)
       - ☐ Chronic (A39.3)
       - ☐ Unspecified (query provider or A39.4)
     - ☐ Other gram negative organisms
       - ☐ Unspecified (A41.50)
       - ☐ E. coli (A41.51)
       - ☐ Pseudomonas (A41.52)
       - ☐ Serratia (A41.53)
       - ☐ Other gram-negative sepsis (A41.59)
     - ☐ Other specified type
       - ☐ Enterococcus (A41.81)
       - ☐ Other (A41.89)
     - ☐ Staphylococcal
       - ☐ Methicillin susceptible S. aureus (MSSA) (A41.01)
       - ☐ Methicillin resistant S. aureus (MRSA) (A41.02)
       - ☐ Other specified (A41.1)
       - ☐ Unspecified (A41.2)
     - ☐ Streptococcal
       - ☐ Group A (A40.0)
       - ☐ Group B (A40.1)
       - ☐ S. pneumoniae (A40.3)
       - ☐ Other specified (A40.8)
       - ☐ Unspecified (A40.9)
       - ☐ Unspecified bacteria (A41.9)
   - ☐ Other types
     - ☐ Candidal (B37.7)
     - ☐ Herpesviral (B00.7)
     - ☐ Salmonella (A02.1)
     - ☐ Other specified types – Consult ICD-10-CM book
8. With documented severe sepsis/associated organ dysfunction/septic shock
   - ☐ Yes
     - ☐ Without septic shock (R65.20)
     - ☐ With septic shock (R65.21)

     For postprocedural septic shock, assign code T81.12 with the appropriate seventh digit. Do not assign code R65.21.
     - ☐ Code any documented acute organ dysfunction
   - ☐ No – no additional code required

Appendix A: Coding Checklists

Skin Ulcer, Chronic, Non-Pressure

ICD-10-CM Category/Subcategory

Codes for non-pressure chronic ulcers of the skin are found in the following categories/subcategories:

L97 Non-pressure chronic ulcer lower limb, not elsewhere classified

L98.4 Non-pressure chronic ulcer of skin, not elsewhere classified

ICD-10-CM Definitions

Non-pressure chronic skin ulcer – Breakdown in the skin not caused by pressure and usually due to an underlying condition. The non-pressure chronic skin ulcer may involve only the skin, extend into the subcutaneous tissue and fat layer, or even deeper into the muscle and bone. Other terms for non-pressure chronic skin ulcers include:

- Atrophic ulcer of skin
- Chronic ulcer of skin
- Neurogenic ulcer of skin
- Non-healing ulcer of skin
- Non-infected sinus of skin
- Perforating ulcer of skin
- Trophic ulcer of skin
- Tropical ulcer of skin

Checklist

1. Identify site of non-pressure chronic skin ulcer:
   - ☐ Back
   - ☐ Buttocks
   - ☐ Lower leg
     - ☐ Ankle
     - ☐ Calf
     - ☐ Foot
       - ☐ Heel and midfoot
       - ☐ Other part of foot
     - ☐ Other part of lower leg
     - ☐ Unspecified part of lower leg
   - ☐ Thigh
   - ☐ Other/unspecified site
2. Specify laterality:
   - ☐ Right
   - ☐ Left
   - ☐ Unspecified

Note: Laterality does not apply to subcategory L98.4.

3. Specify ulcer severity:
   - ☐ Limited to breakdown of skin
   - ☐ With fat layer exposed
   - ☐ With muscle involvement
     - ☐ with necrosis
     - ☐ without necrosis
     - ☐ Other specified severity
   - ☐ With bone involvement
     - ☐ with necrosis
     - ☐ without necrosis
   - ☐ Other specified severity
   - ☐ Unspecified severity
4. For ulcer of lower limb, identify and code first any documented underlying condition:
   - ☐ Atherosclerosis of the lower extremities with ulceration (I70.23-, I70.24-, I70.33-, I70.34-, I70.43-, I70.44-, I70.53-, I70.54-, I70.63-, I70.64-, I70.73-, I70.74-)
   - ☐ Chronic venous hypertension with ulcer (I87.31-, I87.33-)
   - ☐ Diabetic ulcers (E08.621, E08.622, E09.621, E09.622, E10.621, E10.622, E11.621, E11.622, E13.621, E13.622)
   - ☐ Post-phlebitic syndrome with ulcer (I87.01-, I87.03-)
   - ☐ Post-thrombotic syndrome with ulcer (I87.01-, I87.03-)
   - ☐ Varicose ulcer (I83.0-, I83.2-)
5. Identify and code first any associated gangrene (I96)

Skin Ulcer, Pressure

ICD-10-CM Category

Pressure ulcers of the skin are classified in category:

L89 Pressure Ulcer

ICD-10-CM Definitions

Pressure ulcer – Skin ulceration caused by prolonged pressure occurring most often over bony prominences of the body. The ulcer is caused by ischemia of the underlying structures of the skin, fat, and muscles as a result of the sustained and constant pressure. Pressure ulcer severity is classified as Stage 1-4, unstageable, and unspecified. Other terms used to describe a pressure ulcer include:

- Bed sore
- Decubitus ulcer
- Plaster ulcer
- Pressure area
- Pressure sore

Stage 1 pressure ulcer – Pre-ulcer skin changes limited to persistent focal edema.

Stage 2 pressure ulcer – Pressure ulcer with abrasion, blister, partial thickness skin loss involving epidermis and/or dermis.

Stage 3 pressure ulcer – Pressure ulcer with full thickness skin loss involving damage or necrosis of subcutaneous tissue.

Stage 4 pressure ulcer – Pressure ulcer with necrosis of soft tissues through to underlying muscle, tendon, or bone.

Unstageable pressure ulcer – Pressure ulcers whose stage cannot be clinically determined. Unstageable pressure ulcers may be covered by slough or eschar or may have been treated with a skin or muscle graft. If the slough or eschar is removed, a stage 3 or 4 pressure ulcer will usually be revealed.

Unspecified pressure ulcer stage – The stage of the pressure ulcer has not been documented.

Checklist

1. Identify site of pressure ulcer:
   - ☐ Ankle
   - ☐ Back (except contiguous site back, buttock, hip)
     - ☐ Lower (except sacral region)
     - ☐ Sacral region (includes coccyx)
     - ☐ Upper
     - ☐ Unspecified part
   - ☐ Buttock (except contiguous site back, buttock, hip)
   - ☐ Contiguous site of back, buttock, hip
   - ☐ Elbow
   - ☐ Head (includes face)
   - ☐ Heel
   - ☐ Hip (except contiguous site back, buttock, hip)
   - ☐ Other specified site
   - ☐ Unspecified site
2. Specify laterality:
   - ☐ Right
   - ☐ Left
   - ☐ Unspecified

Note: Laterality does not apply to sacral region; contiguous site of back, buttock, and hip; or other unspecified site.

3. Specify pressure ulcer stage:
   - ☐ Pressure ulcer stage 1
   - ☐ Pressure ulcer stage 2
   - ☐ Pressure ulcer stage 3
   - ☐ Pressure ulcer stage 4
   - ☐ Unstageable (based on the clinical documentation)
   - ☐ Unspecified stage
4. Code first any associated gangrene (I96)

Sprain, Lower Extremity

ICD-10-CM Code Categories

S73	Dislocation and sprain of joint and ligaments of hip
S83	Dislocation and sprain of joints and ligaments of knee
S93	Dislocation and sprain of joints and ligaments at ankle, foot and toe level

ICD-10-CM Definitions

Sprain – A sprain is an injury to a ligament. A sprain occurs when the ligaments of a joint are stretched or torn. Sprains are graded by severity:

- Grade I – Mild sprain, ligaments are stretched but not torn
- Grade II – Moderate sprain, ligaments are partially torn and there may be some loss of function
- Grade III – Severe sprains, ligament is completely torn/ruptured

Episode of Care – There are three (3) 7th character values to select from for sprains:

A **Initial encounter.** The period when the patient is receiving active treatment for the injury, poisoning, or other consequences of an external cause. An 'A' may be assigned on more than one claim.

D **Subsequent encounter.** Encounter after the active phase of treatment and when the patient is receiving routine care for the injury or poisoning during the period of healing or recovery.

S **Sequela.** Encounter for complications or conditions that arise as a direct result of an injury.

Note: For strain of muscle, fascia, or tendon, see Strain in ICD-10-CM code book.

Checklist

1. Identify site of sprain:
   - ☐ Hip
     - ☐ Iliofemoral ligament
     - ☐ Ischiocapsular ligament
     - ☐ Other specified part of hip
     - ☐ Unspecified sprain of hip– review medical record/query physician
   - ☐ Knee
     - ☐ Collateral ligament
       - ☐ Medial collateral
       - ☐ Lateral collateral
       - ☐ Unspecified collateral ligament– review medical record/query physician
     - ☐ Cruciate ligament
       - ☐ Anterior cruciate
       - ☐ Posterior cruciate
       - ☐ Unspecified cruciate ligament – review medical record/query physician
     - ☐ Superior tibiofibular joint/ligament
     - ☐ Other specified part of knee
     - ☐ Unspecified part of knee – review medical record/query physician
   - ☐ Ankle
     - ☐ Calcaneofibular ligament
     - ☐ Deltoid ligament
     - ☐ Tibiofibular ligament
     - ☐ Other specified ligament of ankle (includes internal collateral ligament and talofibular ligament)
     - ☐ Unspecified ligament of ankle – review medical record/query physician
   - ☐ Foot
     - ☐ Tarsal ligament
     - ☐ Tarsometatarsal ligament
     - ☐ Other sprain of foot
     - ☐ Unspecified sprain of foot – review medical record/query physician
   - ☐ Toes
     - ☐ Great toe
       - ☐ Interphalangeal joint
       - ☐ Metatarsophalangeal joint
       - ☐ Unspecified sprain of great toe – review medical record/query physician
     - ☐ Lesser toes
       - ☐ Interphalangeal joint
       - ☐ Metatarsophalangeal joint
       - ☐ Unspecified sprain of lesser toe – review medical record/query physician
     - ☐ Unspecified toe
       - ☐ Interphalangeal joint
       - ☐ Metatarsophalangeal joint
       - ☐ Unspecified sprain of toe – review medical record/query physician
2. Identify laterality
   - ☐ Right
   - ☐ Left
   - ☐ Unspecified– review medical record/query physician
3. Identify episode of care:
   - ☐ Initial encounter
   - ☐ Subsequent encounter
   - ☐ Sequela

Sprain, Upper Extremity

ICD-10-CM Code Categories

S43	Dislocation and sprain of joints and ligaments of shoulder girdle
S53	Dislocation and sprain of joints and ligaments of elbow
S63	Dislocation and sprain of joints and ligaments at wrist and hand level

ICD-10-CM Definitions

Sprain – A sprain is an injury to a ligament. A sprain occurs when the ligaments of a joint are stretched or torn. Sprains are graded by severity:

- Grade I – Mild sprain, ligaments are stretched but not torn
- Grade II – Moderate sprain, ligaments are partially torn and there may be some loss of function
- Grade III – Severe sprains, ligament is completely torn/ruptured

Episode of Care – There are three (3) 7th character values to select from for sprains:

A **Initial encounter.** The period when the patient is receiving active treatment for the injury, poisoning, or other consequences of an external cause. An 'A' may be assigned on more than one claim.

D **Subsequent encounter.** Encounter after the active phase of treatment and when the patient is receiving routine care for the injury or poisoning during the period of healing or recovery.

S **Sequela.** Encounter for complications or conditions that arise as a direct result of an injury.

Note: Traumatic rupture of the ligaments of the forearm, wrist, and hand are not coded as sprains. See Traumatic rupture of ligaments in ICD-10-CM code book. For strain of muscle, fascia, or tendon, see Strain in ICD-10-CM code book.

Checklist

1. Identify site of sprain:
   - ☐ Shoulder girdle
     - ☐ Shoulder joint
       - ☐ Coracohumeral (ligament)
       - ☐ Rotator cuff capsule
       - ☐ Superior glenoid labrum lesion
       - ☐ Other sprain of shoulder joint
       - ☐ Unspecified sprain of shoulder joint– review medical record/query physician
     - ☐ Acromioclavicular joint
     - ☐ Sternoclavicular joint
     - ☐ Other specified parts of shoulder girdle
     - ☐ Unspecified parts of shoulder girdle– review medical record/query physician
   - ☐ Elbow
     - ☐ Radiohumeral (joint)
     - ☐ Radial collateral ligament
     - ☐ Ulnohumeral (joint)
     - ☐ Ulnar collateral ligament
     - ☐ Other sprain of elbow
     - ☐ Unspecified sprain of elbow– review medical record/query physician
   - ☐ Wrist
     - ☐ Carpal joint
     - ☐ Radiocarpal joint
     - ☐ Other specified sprain of wrist
     - ☐ Unspecified sprain of wrist– review medical record/query physician
   - ☐ Thumb/fingers
     - ☐ Thumb
       - ☐ Interphalangeal joint
       - ☐ Metacarpophalangeal joint
       - ☐ Other sprain of thumb
       - ☐ Unspecified sprain of thumb– review medical record/query physician
     - ☐ Index finger
       - ☐ Interphalangeal joint
       - ☐ Metacarpophalangeal joint
       - ☐ Other sprain of index finger
       - ☐ Unspecified sprain of index finger– review medical record/query physician
     - ☐ Middle finger
       - ☐ Interphalangeal joint
       - ☐ Metacarpophalangeal joint
       - ☐ Other sprain of middle finger
       - ☐ Unspecified sprain of middle finger– review medical record/query physician
     - ☐ Ring finger
       - ☐ Interphalangeal joint
       - ☐ Metacarpophalangeal joint
       - ☐ Other sprain of ring finger
       - ☐ Unspecified sprain of ring finger– review medical record/query physician
     - ☐ Little finger
       - ☐ Interphalangeal joint
       - ☐ Metacarpophalangeal joint
       - ☐ Other sprain of little finger
       - ☐ Unspecified sprain of little finger– review medical record/query physician
     - ☐ Unspecified finger
       - ☐ Interphalangeal joint
       - ☐ Metacarpophalangeal joint
       - ☐ Other sprain of unspecified finger
       - ☐ Unspecified sprain of unspecified finger– review medical record/query physician
2. Identify laterality
   - ☐ Right
   - ☐ Left
   - ☐ Unspecified– review medical record/query physician
3. Identify episode of care:
   - ☐ Initial encounter
   - ☐ Subsequent encounter
   - ☐ Sequela

Substance Use, Abuse, Dependence

ICD-10-CM Code Categories

F10	Alcohol related disorders
F11	Opioid related disorders
F12	Cannabis related disorders
F13	Sedative, hypnotic, or anxiolytic related disorders
F14	Cocaine related disorders
F15	Other stimulant related disorders
F16	Hallucinogen related disorders
F17	Nicotine dependence
F18	Inhalant related disorders
F19	Other psychoactive substance related disorders

ICD-10-CM Guidelines

The codes for psychoactive substance use (F10.9-, F11.9-, F12.9-, F13.9-, F14.9-, F15.9-, F16.9-, F18.9-, F19.9-) should only be assigned based on provider documentation and when they meet the definition of a reportable diagnosis.

The codes for psychoactive substance use are only used when the psychoactive substance use is associated with a mental or behavioral disorder in the documentation by the provider.

ICD-10-CM classifies "history of alcohol or drug abuse" as "in remission" which is identified with a 5th or 6th character.

In categories for **Mental and behavioral disorders due to psychoactive substance use**, selection of codes for "in remission" (F10-F19 with -.21) requires the provider's documentation of "in remission".

When the provider documents use, abuse, and dependence of the same substance, assign only one code to identify the pattern of use as follows:

- Assign only the code for abuse if both use and abuse are documented
- Assign only the code for dependence when the documentation specifies both abuse and dependence; or both use and dependence; or when use, abuse, and dependence are all documented

Appendix A: Coding Checklists

Checklist

1. Is the psychoactive substance use associated with a mental or behavioral disorder in the provider documentation?
   - ☐ Yes – assign the appropriate code(s) for psychoactive substance use (F10.9-, F11.9-, F12.9-, F13.9-, F14.9-, F15.9-, F16.9-, F18.9-, F19.9-)
   - ☐ No – do not assign codes from this section unless clarification is documented
2. Is the provider's clinical judgment of the patient's current condition as "in remission" clearly documented?
   - ☐ Yes – assign the appropriate 5th or 6th character for "in remission"
   - ☐ No – do not assign the 5th or 6th character indicating "in remission" without documentation by the provider
3. Are both use and abuse documented by the provider?
   - ☐ Yes – Assign only the code for abuse – for alcohol use/abuse/dependence, go to #7, #8 and #9; for other psychoactive substance disorders go to #8 and #9
   - ☐ No – see #4
4. Are both use and dependence documented?
   - ☐ Yes – assign only the code for dependence – for alcohol use/abuse/dependence, go to #7, #8 and #9; for other psychoactive substance disorders go to #8 and #9
   - ☐ No – see #5
5. Are both abuse and dependence documented?
   - ☐ Yes – assign only the code for dependence – for alcohol use/abuse/dependence, go to #7, #8 and #9; for other psychoactive substance disorders go to #8 and #9
   - ☐ No – see #6
6. Are use, abuse, and dependence all documented?
   - ☐ Yes – assign only the code for dependence – for alcohol use/abuse/dependence, go to #7, #8 and #9; for other psychoactive substance disorders go to #8 and #9
   - ☐ No – for alcohol use/abuse/dependence, go to #7, #8 and #9; for other psychoactive substance disorders go to #8 and #9
7. In cases with alcohol intoxication, does the documentation specify the blood alcohol level?
   - ☐ Yes – assign an additional code to indicate the patient's blood alcohol level from category Y90 (Evidence of alcohol involvement determined by blood alcohol level)
   - ☐ No – if the record indicates blood alcohol levels were obtained but does not specify the level, assign code Y90.9 (Presence of alcohol in blood, level not specified) and query the physician for clarification as necessary
8. Is the presence of intoxication or intoxication delirium indicated in the provider documentation?
   - ☐ Yes – assign the specific code to indicate the associated intoxication or intoxication delirium
   - ☐ No – proceed to #9
9. If the condition is documented as with withdrawal, are the withdrawal symptoms described in the provider documentation?
   - ☐ Yes – assign the specific code describing the associated withdrawal symptoms
   - ☐ No – assign the unspecified code and query the physician for clarification as necessary

Undescended/Retractile Testes

ICD-10-CM Categories/Codes

Q53	Undescended and ectopic testicle
Q55.22	Retractile testis

ICD-10-CM Definitions

Abdominal testis – An undescended testis that does not descend into the scrotum before birth, remaining instead in the retroperitoneum or abdomen which is where the testes originate during fetal development.

Cryptorchidism (undescended testis) – Congenital anomaly in which one or both testes do not descend into the normal position in the scrotum before birth.

Ectopic testis – Variant of undescended testis in which the testis lies outside the usual pathway of descent.

Perineal ectopic testis – An ectopic testis that has descended into an abnormal position between the penoscrotal raphe and the genitofemoral fold.

Retractile testis – The tendency of a descended testis to ascend to the upper part of the scrotum or into the inguinal canal.

Checklist

1. Identify condition:
   - ☐ Abdominal testis
     - ☐ inguinal
     - ☐ intraabdominal
   - ☐ Ectopic perineal testis
   - ☐ Ectopic testis
   - ☐ High scrotal
   - ☐ Retractile testis
   - ☐ Unspecified undescended testicle
2. Specify laterality:
   - ☐ Bilateral
   - ☐ Unilateral
   - ☐ Unspecified

Note: Laterality is not required for retractile testis.

Varicose Veins, Lower Extremities

ICD-10-CM Category

Varicose veins of the lower extremities are classified in category:

I83 Varicose veins of lower extremities

ICD-10-CM Definitions

Varicose vein – Enlarged, tortuous (twisted) veins that may be complicated by pain, inflammation, ulcer, swelling, edema, or other complications.

Non-pressure chronic skin ulcer – Breakdown in the skin not caused by pressure and usually due to an underlying condition. The non-pressure chronic skin ulcer may involve only the skin, extend into the subcutaneous tissue and fat layer, or even deeper into the muscle and bone. For more information see checklist for Skin Ulcer, Chronic, Non-Pressure.

Checklist

1. Identify any lower extremity varicose vein complication:
   - ☐ Asymptomatic
   - ☐ Complicated by
     - ☐ Inflammation
     - ☐ Pain
     - ☐ Ulcer
     - ☐ Ulcer and inflammation
     - ☐ Other complication. Specify ______________
2. Specify laterality:
   - ☐ Right
   - ☐ Left
   - ☐ Unspecified
3. For varicose vein of the lower extremity with ulcer or ulcer and inflammation:
   a. Identify site of ulcer:
      - ☐ Ankle
      - ☐ Calf
      - ☐ Foot
        - ☐ Heel
        - ☐ Midfoot
        - ☐ Other part of foot
      - ☐ Thigh
      - ☐ Other part of leg
      - ☐ Unspecified site of leg

   b. Use additional code (L97.-) to identify severity of ulcer:
      - ☐ Limited to breakdown of skin
      - ☐ Fat layer exposed
      - ☐ Muscle involvement
        - ☐ with necrosis
        - ☐ without necrosis
      - ☐ Bone involvement
        - ☐ with necrosis
        - ☐ without necrosis
      - ☐ Unspecified severity

Appendix B
CLINICAL DOCUMENTATION IMPROVEMENT (CDI) CHECKLISTS

Introduction

Appendix B provides bulleted lists that can be used for clinical documentation improvement. These are different from the Documentation and Coding Checklists in that they are designed to be used by clinical documentation improvement (CDI) specialists and would be used primarily in the inpatient setting for chart review to help identify missed diagnoses or under-documented conditions.

Physicians often don't realize that coding specialists need a specifically documented diagnosis to assign a code especially if the physician believes that the documentation clearly identifies the reason for the admission and any concurrent conditions or complications affecting the patient's medical care. For example, if the discharge diagnosis is pneumonia and laboratory results of sputum cultures and the medications administered clearly indicate a specific bacterial infection as the cause of the pneumonia, the coding specialist cannot assign a code for bacterial pneumonia without this being specifically documented by the physician. Physicians may not recognize that coders cannot interpret information in the medical record. Codes must be assigned based solely on the physician's documentation. However, coding specialists and CDI specialists can review the documentation for specific clinical indicators to determine whether a condition may be present and then they can query the physician regarding the condition to determine if the condition does in fact exist. CDI specialists work with physicians and coders to ensure that the documentation supports the assignment of a more specific code.

Appendix B provides clinical documentation improvement bulleted lists for three conditions that are often lacking sufficient documentation in the inpatient setting. The information in these lists identifies common indicators of the condition so that the physician can be queried to determine if the condition should be included as a diagnosis or a more specific diagnosis in the medical record.

CDI Checklist – Chronic Obstructive Pulmonary Disease (COPD)

Definitions

- COPD may also be referred to as: Chronic Obstructive Lung Disease (COLD), Chronic Obstructive Airway Disease (COAD), Chronic Airflow Limitation (CAL) or Chronic Obstructive Respiratory Disease (CORD). An individual may have chronic bronchitis, a long-term cough with mucus production or emphysema, destruction of lung tissue that occurs over time. Most people diagnosed with COPD will have a combination of both
- Forced expiratory volume in one second (FEV1)–The amount of air forcibly exhaled in the first second of a forced exhalation
- Forced volume vital capacity (FVC)-The amount of air forcibly exhaled after taking in the deepest breath possible

Types

- Chronic bronchitis–Defined symptomatically as a cough with sputum production, on a majority of days, three months of the year, for 2 consecutive years. Clinically there are also:
  - Increased number (hyperplasia) and increased size (hypertrophy) of goblet cells and mucus glands in the airway
  - Scarring of airway walls from infiltration of inflammatory cells
  - Squamous metaplasia, an abnormal change in the tissue lining of the airway causing fibrosis, thickening, and narrowing of the airway and limiting airflow
- Emphysema–Damage to the lung with inflammation of the air sacs (alveoli) and increase in the size of air space distal to the terminal bronchioles. The increased size of the air sacs:
  - Reduces the surface area for gas exchange (oxygen and carbon dioxide)
  - Inhibits the elasticity and support of the interstitial tissue
  - Four types identified:
    - » Centriacinar/centrilobular: Disease is located in the proximal and central acini (air space close to bronchioles).
    - » Panacinar/panlobular: Disease is found in air spaces from bronchioles to alveoli. This type is most often associated with alpha-1-antitrypsin deficiency
    - » Distal/paraseptal: The proximal acinus is normal and disease affects the distal area
    - » Irregular: Scattered areas of the acini are affected. This type is most often associated with fibrosis

Stages

Stages are categorized by airflow limitation which is a measurement of forced expiratory volume in one second (FEV1)/forced volume vital capacity (FVC) < 0.70

- Stage I – Mild COPD
  - Mild airflow limitations
  - FEV1/FVC < 0.70; FEV1 ≥ 80% of predicted
  - Other possible symptoms
    - » Chronic cough
    - » Sputum production
- Stage II – Moderate COPD
  - Worsening airflow limitations
  - FEV1/FVC < 0.70; FEV1 = 50-79% of predicted
  - Shortness of breath (SOB), especially on exertion
  - Other possible symptoms
    - » Chronic cough
    - » Sputum production
- Stage III – Severe COPD
  - Worsening airflow limitations
  - FEV1/FVC < 0.70; FEV1 = 30-49% of predicted
  - Shortness of breath (SOB)
  - Reduced exercise capacity
  - Fatigue
  - Exacerbations that affect quality of life
  - Other possible symptoms
    - » Chronic cough
    - » Sputum production
- Stage IV – Very severe COPD
  - Severe airflow limitations
  - FEV1/FVC < 0.70
    - » FEV1 < 30% predicted

    OR
    - » FEV1 < 50% with presence of chronic respiratory failure defined as PaO2 < 8.0 kPa (60 mm/Hg) with or without PaCO2 > 6.7 kPa (50 mm/Hg) while breathing air at sea levels
  - Shortness of breath (SOB)
  - Reduced exercise capacity
  - Fatigue
  - Quality of life significantly impaired
  - Exacerbations life-threatening and requiring admission to intensive care unit of acute care facility
  - Other possible symptoms
    - » Right heart failure (cor pulmonale)
    - » Elevated jugular venous pressure
    - » Pitting edema of lower extremities (ankles)
    - » Chronic cough
    - » Sputum production

Signs/Symptoms

- Chronic cough, dry or mucus producing
- Fatigue
- Frequent respiratory infections
- Shortness of breath (SOB, dyspnea), often worse with exercise/activity
- Wheezing

Risk factors

- Smoking
- Non-smokers with congenital absence of the protein, Alpha-1 antitrypsin
- Exposure to certain (workplace) chemicals (cadmium, isocyanates)
- Coal and gold mining, working in cotton textile plants, welding
- Exposure to second hand smoke and air pollution
- Exposure to cooking fires with poor ventilation
- Gastroesophageal reflux disease (GERD)

Diagnostic Indicators

- Positive history for risk factors
- Chronic cough with sputum production
- Dyspnea
- Rhonchi, wheezing, rales present with auscultation of breath sounds
- Use of accessory muscles (neck, abdomen) to help with breathing
- Change in chest shape/circumference (Barrel chest)
- Abnormal pulmonary function test that is not fully reversible and usually progressive

Treatment

- Stop smoking, reduce exposure to pollutants/chemicals
- Medications
  - Bronchodilators-reduce airway constriction
    - » Albuterol (ProAir)
    - » Ipratropium (Atrovent)
    - » Tiotropium (Spiriva)
    - » Salmeterol (Serevent)
    - » Formoterol (Foradil)
  - Inhaled corticosteroids-decrease inflammation
    - » Flunisolide (Aerobid)
    - » Budesonide (Pulmicort)
    - » Fluticasone (Flovent)
    - » Beclomethasone (Qvar)
    - » Mometasone (Asmanex)
    - » Ciclesonide (Alvesco)
  - Oral anti-inflammatory-site specific to lungs
    - » Montelukast (Singulair)
    - » Roflimulast
- Pulmonary Rehabilitation–Learning to breath in ways that allow for exercise/physical activity and maintenance of muscle strength
- Surgery to remove damaged section of lung may allow other areas to work more effectively
- Lung transplant

Treatment-Severe COPD-In addition to above:

- Systemic corticosteroids (oral and/or intravenous)
- Antibiotics if infection is present
- Inhaled bronchodilators and/or corticosteroids delivered via nebulizer
- Supplemental oxygen
- Assisted breathing: Mask, BiPAP, endotracheal tube with mechanical ventilation

Complications

- Irregular heart rate (cardiac arrhythmias)
- Need for supplemental oxygen and/or mechanical ventilation
- Pulmonary hypertension–Elevated blood pressure in the arteries/blood vessels in the right side of the heart
- Cor pulmonale – Right side heart enlargement with subsequent pumping failure usually caused by pulmonary hypertension
- Pneumonia
- Pneumothorax
- Weight Loss/Malnutrition
- Osteoporosis due to decreased exercise/activity and corticosteroid use

CDI Checklist – Pneumonia

Definition

Pneumonia is a respiratory condition, usually due to an infection, which causes inflammation in the lungs and an accumulation of fluid, inflammatory cells and fibrin ultimately impairing oxygen/carbon dioxide exchange in the alveoli (air sacs).

Types

- Aspiration–Occurs when foreign material is inhaled causing inflammation of the airway (bronchial tubes) and lungs. Other names include: Anaerobic pneumonia, Aspiration pneumonitis (Mendelson's syndrome), Necrotizing pneumonia
  - Aspiration of vomit/gastric acid most often leads to a chemical pneumonitis
  - Aspiration of oral/pharyngeal fluid most often results in bacterial pneumonia (anaerobic)
  - Aspiration of oil (vegetable, cooking) causes an exogenous lipoid pneumonia
- Bacterial–This includes both gram negative and gram positive organisms
  - Streptococcus pneumoniae (Pneumococcus), is most common type
  - Staphylococcus aureus
  - Haemophilus influenzae
  - Enterococcus bacteriaceae
  - Pseudomonas aeruginosa
  - Bacteria-like organisms:
    - » Mycoplasma pneumoniae
    - » Chlamydophila pneumoniae
    - » Legionella pneumophila
    - » Pneumocystis jiroveci
- Community acquired–An infection that develops from commonplace germs encountered during an individual's normal routine. The most common causative organisms of community acquired pneumonia are:
  - Streptococcus pneumoniae (Pneumococcus)
  - Staphylococcus aureus
  - Haemophilus influenzae
  - Enterococcus bacteriaceae
  - Adenovirus
- Fungal–Certain areas of the United States have specific fungi that cause pneumonia in both healthy and immune compromised individuals. The three most commonly found are:
  - Coccidioidomycosis (Coccidioides immitis), found in the Southwestern US and may be referred to as "San Joaquin fever" or "Valley Fever".
  - Histoplasmosis (Histoplasma capsulatum), most prevalent in the Midwest
  - Blastomycosis (Blastomyces dermatitidis), found in the Southeast.
- Hospital acquired pneumonia (HAP)–Hospitalization, including residing in a long term care facility and/or receiving dialysis or infusion therapy in an outpatient center/clinic, places individuals at increased risk for developing pneumonia. The most common causative bacteria are:
  - Pseudomonas aeruginosa
  - Methicillin-resistant Staphylococcus aureus (MRSA).
- Pneumonia caused by opportunistic organisms–Opportunistic organisms most often cause illness in a host with congenital or acquired immune deficits or defenses, such as:
  - Fungi
    - » Candida species
    - » Aspergillus species
    - » Mucor species
    - » Cryptococcus neoformans
  - Bacteria-like organisms
    - » Pneumocystis jiroveci
    - » Mycobacterium avium.
- Ventilator-associated pneumonia (VAP)–VAP is a subtype of HAP and occurs in patients who have endotracheal tubes or a tracheostomy and receive respiratory support via mechanical ventilation
  - Baseline respiratory cultures should be obtained at the initiation of ventilator support
  - Signs/symptoms of pneumonia with subsequent cultures that contain bacteria different from baseline are determined to be VAP
  - Common causative bacteria include:
    - » Pseudomonas aeruginosa
    - » Klebsiella pneumoniae
    - » Serratia marcescens
    - » Enterobacter
    - » Citrobacter
    - » Acinetobacter
    - » Stenotrophomonas maltophilia
    - » Burkholderia cepacia
    - » Methicillin-resistant Staphylococcus aureus (MRSA)
- Viral–Many viral infections can lead to pneumonia including:
  - Influenza virus ("Flu") which affects all population groups
  - Respiratory Syncytial Virus (RSV) is most common in infants (especially infants born prematurely) and adults with impaired immunity
  - Coronaviruses, which cause Severe Acute Respiratory Syndrome, or SARS-associated coronavirus pneumonia and the newly emerged COVID-19 respiratory disease
  - Human Parainfluenza virus found most often in children, elderly and persons with impaired immunity
  - Adenoviruses which are most common in children
  - Herpes Virus
  - Avian influenza
  - Cytomegalovirus (CMV)
- Workplace acquired–Certain work environments may predispose an individual to pneumonia, such as:

- Manufacturing plant accidents may cause workers to inhale chemicals or other hazardous materials that lead to inflammation and fluid accumulation in the lungs
- Farming or slaughterhouses may expose workers to:
  - » Anthrax
  - » Brucella
  - » Coxiella burnetii
- Exposure to birds or bird droppings can cause Psittacosis pneumonia from Chlamydia psittaci
- Exposure to rodent droppings may cause Hantavirus infection of the lungs

Types Classified by Site

- Lobar pneumonia
  - Acute onset
  - Inflammation and consolidation affecting a large and continuous area of one or more lobes of the lung
  - Causative organisms include:
    - » Streptococcus pneumoniae (Pneumococcus)
    - » Haemophilus influenzae
    - » Moraxella catarrhalis
    - » Mycobacterium tuberculosis
- Bronchial pneumonia (Bronchopneumonia)
  - Inflammation of the walls of the bronchioles (air tubes) in multiple areas of one or both lungs
  - Most often found in infants, children, elderly and persons with impaired immunity
  - Rarely caused by the bacteria, Streptococcus pneumoniae (Pneumococcus)
- Acute interstitial pneumonia
  - Fine, lace-like, vascular tissue found throughout the lungs as a support system for the alveoli (air sacs)
  - Normally not visualized on X-ray or CT scans
  - Bacteria, virus and fungi can cause pneumonia in this tissue
  - Causative organism is most often the bacteria-like, Mycoplasma pneumoniae

Classification of Types in Children

- Non-severe
  - Symptoms may include cough, difficulty breathing, increased respiratory rate (RR)
    - » <2 months=RR >60/minute
    - » 2 – 12 months=RR >50/minute
    - » 12 months-5 years=RR >40/minute
  - One or more of the following on auscultation:
    - » Crackles (rales)
    - » Areas of decreased breath sounds
    - » Areas of bronchial breathing
  - Infection can be treated with antibiotics as an outpatient
- Severe
  - Include signs and symptoms of non-severe plus one or more of the following:
    - » Crackles (rales)
    - » Retractions
    - » Nasal flaring
    - » Grunting
  - On auscultation includes findings from non-severe and may also have:
    - » Abnormal vocal resonance
    - » Pleural rub
  - Admit to hospital for antibiotics and supportive therapy.
- Very severe
  - Includes signs and symptoms of non-severe and severe plus one or more of the following:
    - » Central cyanosis
    - » Dehydration
    - » Lethargy
    - » Seizures
  - Admit to hospital for antibiotics and supportive care including:
    - » Oxygen therapy
    - » Intravenous fluids
    - » Intubation and mechanical ventilation

Signs/Symptoms

- Cough, dry or productive (mucus producing) – Mucus is often thick and colored (brown, yellow, green and/or blood tinged)
- Chills – feeling suddenly cold, shivering and/or shaking
- Fever – Body temperature > 100.4° F (38° C)
- Difficulty breathing/shortness of breath (dyspnea)
- Sweating (diaphoresis), including night sweats
- Sharp/stabbing pain in chest especially with inspiration or cough
- Cyanosis (blue color to skin, nail beds, mucous membranes)
- Fatigue – Extreme tiredness
- Headache
- Vomiting, decreased appetite, weight loss
- Confusion, decreased level of consciousness
- Decreased blood pressure (↓BP)
- Increased heart rate (↑HR), respiratory rate (↑RR)
- In infants: grunting, retractions, poor perfusion

General Risk Factors

- Recent surgery or trauma (injury)
- General anesthesia
- Serious chronic or acute illness/disease, such as diabetes mellitus, renal failure, cirrhosis of the liver, heart failure/ cardiac disease, cancer
- Chronic or acute respiratory conditions, such as asthma, chronic obstructive pulmonary disease (COPD), bronchiectasis, cystic fibrosis
- Impaired immunity from HIV/AIDS, chemotherapy
- Cigarette, cigar or pipe smoking/smoke inhalation
- Residing in a hospital, long term care facility, shelter, receiving dialysis or infusions at an outpatient treatment center.

- Impaired swallowing due to conditions such as stroke, dementia, Parkinson's disease, degenerative muscular or neurological diseases (muscular dystrophy, multiple sclerosis, myasthenia gravis)
- Esophageal strictures or reflux
- Impaired mobility such as cerebral palsy, spinal cord injuries
- Altered level of consciousness caused by drugs/alcohol, neurological diseases, brain injury/tumor, seizure disorder
- Recent upper respiratory infections such as influenza, laryngitis, common cold

Risk Factors For Increased Morbidity/Mortality

- Age > 65 or <5 years
- Severely underweight or obese
- Malnourished/poor nutritional status
- Concurrent chronic or acute disease or condition

Other Factors That Predispose To Certain Types of Pneumonia

- Admitted from SNF
  - Aspiration pneumonia
  - Bacterial pneumonia
  - Hospital acquired pneumonia (HAP)
  - Opportunistic
- History of cerebral vascular accident (CVA) w/dysphagia
  - Aspiration pneumonia
  - Opportunistic
- Alzheimer's or other type of dementia
  - Aspiration pneumonia
  - Opportunistic

Diagnostic Tests/Procedures

- Chest X-ray or CT scan
- Arterial blood gases
- CBC w/differential
- Culture and gram stain of sputum
- Blood cultures
- Culture of pleural fluid
- Swallowing studies
- Bronchoscopy

Complications

- Acute respiratory distress syndrome (ARDS)
- Pleural effusion (fluid/inflammation in the lining around the lung)
- Lung abscess
- Respiratory failure (requiring intubation and ventilator assistance)
- Sepsis or severe sepsis with septic shock or organ failure
- Myelodysplastic syndromes
- Fungal infection (specific) complications
  - Mediastinal fibrosis
  - Broncholithiasis (histoplasmosis)
  - Dissemination to other organs, blood vessel invasion causing:
    - » Emboli and infarction
    - » Fistula formation
    - » Sepsis syndrome

Treatment

Common Antibiotics, Antiviral, Antifungal Medications

- Aspiration Pneumonia
  - Antibiotics may be prescribed following aspiration because of the increased risk that bacteria may proliferate in the area of inflammation. See list under Bacterial pneumonia
- Bacterial Pneumonia
  - Often treated with a combination of antibiotics until the causative organism has been identified by culture and the specific antibiotic(s) have been identified by sensitivity testing
  - Macrolides
    - » Azithromycin (Zithromax)
    - » Clarithromycin (Biaxin)
    - » Erythromycin
  - Tetracyclines
    - » doxycycline
  - Fluoroquinolones
    - » Gemifloxacin (Factive)
    - » Levofloxacin (Levaquin)
    - » Moxifloxaccin (Avelox)
  - Cephalosporins
    - » Cefaclor
    - » Cefadroxil
    - » Cefprozil
    - » Cefuroxime (Ceftin)
    - » Cephalexin (Keflex)
  - Penicillins
    - » Amoxicillin
    - » Amoxicillin with clavulanate (Augmentin)
    - » Ampicillin
    - » Piperacillin
    - » Ticarcillin with clavulanate (Timentin)
  - Vancomycin (Vancocin)
- Fungal Pneumonia
  - Amphotericin B-Fundamental drug for severe/life threatening infections. Effective against:
    - » Aspergillus
    - » Cryptococcosis
    - » Systemic candidiasis
    - » Histoplasmosis
    - » Blastomycosis
    - » Coccioidomycosis
    - » Zygomycosis.
  - Triazoles
    - » Itraconazole, effective against:
      - o Aspergillus

Appendix B: CDI Checklists

      - Mucosal candidal infections
      - Histoplasmosis
      - Blastomycosis
      - Coccidioidomycosis
    - Fluconazole, effective against:
      - Candida albicans (mucosal and invasive)
      - Cryptococcosis
      - Coccidioidomycosis
    - Voriconazole
      - Invasive aspergillosis
      - Other molds
    - Posaconazole
      - Oral candidiasis
      - Aspergillus
      - Coccidioidomycosis.
  - Echinocandin
    - Caspofungin
      - Candida species
      - Aspergillus species
    - Micafungin
      - Candida species
      - Aspirgillus species
    - Anidulafungin
      - Candida
      - Aspergillus species.
- Viral Pneumonia–Antiviral drugs may lessen the severity and shorten the length of time an individual has symptoms. Although antibiotics are not effective in killing viruses, some physicians will prescribe them because of the high incidence of secondary bacterial infection.
  - Antiviral medications include:
    - Amantadine (Symadine)
    - Rimantadine (Flumadine)
    - Oseltamivir (Tamiflu)
    - Zanamivir (Relenza).
  - For varicella pneumonia:
    - Acyclovir (Zovirax).
  - For Respiratory Syncytial Virus (RSV):
    - Ribavirin (Rebetol)

Other Treatment

- Breathing treatments
  - Usually administered by a Respiratory Therapist and may include:
    - Medication to thin/loosen mucus so it can be removed by suction (if intubated) or coughed up by the patient
    - A patient who has underlying respiratory disease such as COPD or asthma, and is experiencing airway constriction may further benefit from inhaled bronchodilator medication such as albuterol
    - Percussion (gentle tapping on chest over lungs to loosen mucus) and postural drainage (positioning to help drain mucus/fluids into bronchial tubes to be suctioned out or coughed up)
- Humidifier or vaporizer
  - Warm or cold moisture added to the air to help thin and loosen mucus
- Supplemental oxygen delivered by nasal cannula/prongs or a mask
- Ventilator support for patients with:
  - Respiratory failure
  - ARDS

CDI Checklist – Sepsis, Severe Sepsis, Septic Shock, and SIRS

Definitions

The definitions of sepsis, severe sepsis, septic shock and systemic inflammatory response syndrome have changed in ICD-10-CM. The signs/symptoms below reflect the conditions as they are defined for ICD-10-CM coding purposes. Physicians may not use the same terms in their documentation. For example, physicians may use the term SIRS or sepsis interchangeably to describe sepsis due to an infection. However, for coding purposes when SIRS is due to an infection, the code for sepsis is reported even if the physician used SIRS to describe the disease process.

Sepsis Signs and Symptoms

A documented infection (by culture, stain or polymerase chain reaction) with two or more of the following signs/symptoms may be indicative of sepsis:

- Temperature
  - Elevated – 100.4°F/38°C

  OR
  - Decreased – 96.8°F/36°C
- Tachycardia/elevated heart rate (HR)
  - > 90 BPM
- Respiratory rate (RR) or $PaCO_2$
  - RR > 20 breaths per minute

  OR
  - PaCO < 32 mm Hg (4.3 kPa)
- White Blood Cell (WBC) Count
  - >12,000 (mm3)

  OR
  - <4,000 (mm3)

  OR
  - 10% bands (immature WBCs)
    - » White blood cells in (normally) sterile fluid (i.e., urine, cerebral spinal fluid)
    - » Evidence of free air in abdomen (perforated viscus) by x-ray or CT scan
    - » Focal opacification consistent with pneumonia on chest x-ray

Additional signs/symptoms of sepsis:

- Peripheral vasodilation
- Change in mental status, such as lack of attention, confusion/disorientation, agitation
- Hemorrhagic skin rash (petechiae, purpura)
- Hypotension, dizziness
- Decreased platelet counts

Signs/symptoms of severe sepsis:

- Reduced urine output (oliguria) or no urine output (anuria)
- Reduced oxygen levels in the blood (hypoxemia)
- Increased lactic acid levels (>4 mmol/L) in blood (lactic acidosis)
- Altered mental status (cerebral function)
- Acute organ dysfunction, such as
  - Acute kidney failure (oligoria, anuria, serum electrolyte imbalance, volume overload)
  - Acute respiratory failure-Acute lung injury (ALI) PaO2/FiO2 <300 OR acute respiratory distress syndrome (ARDS) PaO2/FiO2 <200
  - Critical illness myopathy/polymyopathy (widespread muscle weakness and neurological dysfunction that can delay recovery and cause prolonged ventilator dependence)
  - Disseminated intravascular coagulopathy (DIC) (elevated fibrin degradation products from clot disintegration
  - Encephalopathy (agitation, confusion or coma due to ischemia, hemorrhage, microthrombi, microabscesses, multifocal necrotizing leukoencephalopathy)
  - Hepatic failure (disruption in the function of protein synthesis leading to bleeding disorders from low levels of clotting factors and a disruption of bilirubin metabolism with a subsequent elevation of indirect bilirubin levels)
  - Acute cardiac failure (systolic or diastolic heart failure due to cytokines and decreased myocyte function or cellular damage manifested as a troponin leak)

Signs/symptoms of septic shock

- Same symptoms as severe sepsis

  AND
- Systolic blood pressure < 90 mm/HG (hypotension) that
  - Does not return to normal with intravenous hydration (>6 L or 40mg/kg crystalloid fluid)
  - Requires the use of medication to maintain blood pressure (vasopressors/inotropes)

SIRS Signs and Symptoms

A documented injury or trauma with the following signs/symptoms may be indicative of systemic inflammatory response (SIRS):

- Temperature
  - Elevated – 100.4°F/38°C

  OR
  - Decreased – 96.8°F/36°C
- Tachycardia/elevated heart rate (HR)
  - > 90 BPM
- Respiratory rate (RR) or PaCO
  - RR > 20 breaths per minute

  OR
  - PaCO < 32 mm Hg (4.3 kPa)
- Elevated WBC (leukocytosis) or severely decreased WBC levels (leukopenia)

A diagnosis of SIRS with acute organ failure requires documentation of one or more of the following:

- Acute kidney failure (oligoria, anuria, electrolyte abnormalities, volume overload)
- Acute respiratory failure-Acute lung injury (ALI) PaO2/FiO2 <300 OR acute respiratory distress syndrome (ARDS) PaO2/ FiO2 <200
- Critical illness myopathy/polymyopathy (widespread muscle weakness and neurological dysfunction that can delay recovery and cause prolonged ventilator dependence.
- Disseminated intravascular coagulopathy (DIC) elevated fibrin degradation products from clot disintegration
- Encephalopathy (agitation, confusion or coma due to ischemia, hemorrhage, microthrombi, microabscesses, multifocal necrotizing leukoencephalopathy
- Hepatic failure (disruption in the function of protein synthesis leading to bleeding disorders from low levels of clotting factors and a disruption of bilirubin metabolism with a subsequent elevation of indirect bilirubin levels)
- Other acute organ failure-acute cardiac failure (systolic or diastolic heart failure due to cytokines and decreased myocyte function or cellular damage manifested as a troponin leak)

Diagnostic Tests

The following tests are commonly performed to establish or rule-out a diagnosis of sepsis:

- White Blood Cell (WBC) count w/differential
- Gram stain
- Urinalysis for bacteria/infectious agents (sterile catheterization or bladder tap)
- Urine for gram stain and culture
- Blood cultures
- Platelet count, bleeding time, fibrin degradation studies
- Lumbar puncture (spinal tap) for examination of cerebral spinal fluid
- Catheter tip culture for suspected central line sepsis
- Arterial blood gases to monitor metabolic or respiratory acidosis/alkalosis
- Chest x-ray to evaluate for pneumonia
- Abdominal x-ray or CT to evaluate for perforated viscus (free air in abdomen)
- Ultrasound exam may be performed for suspected biliary sepsis.

Therapeutic Measures

To treat sepsis the following measures are often employed:

- Intravenous antibiotics (empiric monotherapy or combination of antimicrobial agents are given until culture and sensitivity have been reported, then the most therapeutic drug(s) are continued for a minimum of 2 weeks)
- Intravenous fluids – well defined (500 mL) and rapidly infused colloid and crystalloid fluid boluses
- Transfusion of platelets or red blood cells if coagulopathy is present.
- Supplemental oxygen with continuous monitoring by pulse oximetry.
- Intubation and Mechanical ventilation – necessary due to increased work of breathing and as airway protection due to encephalopathy or decreased level of consciousness
- Central venous catheter for central venous pressure (CVP) monitoring (normal range 8-12 mmHg)
- Vasopressors (norepinephrine or phenylephrine) to maintain mean arterial pressure (MAP) > or = to 65
- Inotropes (Dobutamine) if vasopressors do not stabilize MAP
- Dialysis if urine output is >0.5 ml/kg/hr and there is evidence of kidney damage in blood chemistries (elevated BUN, creatine, potassium) or fluid overload from fluid bolus
- Surgical treatment of the underlying infection, such as incision and drainage

Appendix C
GLOSSARY

Abnormal gait – Deviation in normal walking usually caused by a disruption or disintegration of strength, sensation or coordination in the central nervous system and/or the musculoskeletal system.

Abnormal involuntary movements – Abnormal involuntary movements (AIM) may also be referred to as dyskinesias. These movements can include athetosis (sinuous, writhing movements of hands/fingers), choreas (continuous jerking movements of head/face/body), dystonia (sustained muscle contraction), hemiballism (sudden flinging/throwing motion of an extremity), myoclonus (rapid, repetitive muscle jerks), torticollis (neck spasm), tardive dyskinesia (neuroleptic orofacial movements), tics and tremors.

Abruptio placentae – Obstetrical complication in which the placenta separates from the wall of the uterus prior to delivery of the fetus.

Abscess – Collection of pus (white blood cells) that accumulates within tissue. It is an inflammatory response precipitated by an infectious process or foreign body (splinter, thorn, nail).

Acne – Skin condition that occurs when hair follicles become clogged with oil and dead skin cells. Non-inflammatory acne lesions are called comedones and may appear black or white. Inflammatory acne lesions include papules (small red bumps), pustules or pimples (small, red, pus filled bumps), nodules (large solid lumps) and cysts (large, painful, pus filled lumps).

Adherent prepuce – Foreskin of the penis extends past the head of the penis (glans) and cannot be retracted back to expose the glans.

Akathisia (acathisia) – Syndrome characterized by a feeling of inner restlessness with symptoms that may range from a sense of disquiet or anxiety to severe discomfort especially in the knees and legs that may make it impossible to sit still or be motionless.

Allergic contact dermatitis – Inflammation of the skin characterized by redness, swelling and itching; and may include blisters/lesions with fluid drainage/oozing caused by sensitization to an allergen that has come into contact with the skin.

Alzheimer's Disease – Type of dementia affecting memory, thoughts, and behavior that worsens over time. In early onset Alzheimer's, symptoms occur before age 60. In late onset Alzheimer's, symptoms occur after age 60.

Amaurosis fugax – Transient loss of vision in one eye.

Amenorrhea – Absence of menstruation in a woman of reproductive age.

Anal fissure – Linear break or tear in the skin surrounding the anal opening.

Anal/Rectal abscess – Inflammation and infection with collection of pus (white blood cells) near the anal opening or inside the anus or rectum.

Anal/Rectal fistula – Abnormal connection or passage between the anal canal or rectum and the skin surrounding the anal opening.

Anal/Rectal prolapse – Section of the rectal wall sags down from the normal anatomical position and may protrude through the anal opening.

Anal/Rectal stenosis – Unusual narrowing or tightness of the anal sphincter and/or rectum, making it difficult to have a bowel movement (pass feces, defecate).

Anemia – Reduced number of red blood cells (RBCs) and/or a low concentration of hemoglobin, a protein found on RBCs.

Anencephaly – Congenital neural tube defect in which the telencephalon (large section of brain containing the cerebral hemispheres) fails to form. The skull and scalp may also fail to form leaving the brain exposed.

Angina Pectoris – Chest pain caused by decreased blood flow to the heart muscle, usually from a spasm or occlusion in the coronary arteries.

Ankyloglossia – Congenital short, thick or tight lingual frenulum (membrane that connects underside of tongue to floor of mouth) which inhibits range of motion in the tip of the tongue. The condition may also be referred to as "tongue tie".

Anorexia nervosa – Complex eating disorder characterized by food restrictions that can lead to malnutrition and/or starvation

Aortic valve – Heart valve located between the left ventricle of the heart and the aorta that is formed by 3 leaflets.

Appendicitis – Inflammation of the (vermiform, cecal) appendix, a finger shaped, blind pouch that extends from the intestine in the area of the cecum (junction of the large and small intestine).

Arhinencephaly – Congenital defect of the face and brain, more frequently called holoprosencephaly (HPE) resulting from early embryonic failure of the forebrain to divide into two hemispheres.

Asthma – Chronic inflammatory condition that causes narrowing of the bronchi (large upper airways connecting the trachea to the lungs), characterized by swelling, increased mucus production, and muscle tightness.

Atopic dermatitis – Chronic, inflammatory, non-contagious skin disorder characterized by pruritus (itching) that precedes redness or rash.

Azoospermia – Absent or non-measurable level of sperm present in semen (ejaculate).

Balanoposthitis – Inflammation of the glans penis (head of the penis) and the prepuce (foreskin) in an uncircumcised male.

Barrett's esophagus – Changes in the lining of the esophagus (tube that connects the throat to the stomach) that occurs as a complication of gastroesophageal reflux disease (GERD).

Barton's fracture – Intra-articular fracture of the distal radius with dislocation/displacement of the radio-carpal joint.

Bennet's fracture – Fracture of the thumb involving the intra-articular joint at the base of the first metacarpal bone and extending into the carpometacarpal joint often with subluxation/dislocation of that joint.

Bent bone – Type of greenstick fracture that occurs in soft bone tissue of infants/young children.

Biliary atresia (stenosis) (stricture), congenital – A condition that is present at birth and characterized by a blockage of the ducts that carry bile from the liver to the gallbladder.

Biliary stenosis – Narrowing of the bile ducts which impedes the flow of bile.

Binge eating disorder (BED) – Complex eating disorder characterized by recurrent episodes of overeating not followed by purging, exercise or fasting. Individuals who engage in this behavior are usually overweight or obese and experience guilt, shame and distress which perpetuates the cycle.

Body Mass Index (BMI) – A measurement of height and weight that is used to assess the total proportion of fat in the body. BMI is not however a direct measure of body fat.

Bronchiectasis – Localized, irreversible dilation of the bronchi (large airways) due to destruction of muscle and elastic tissue in the airway lining. The condition may be congenital (present at birth) or acquired later in life.

Bronchiolitis – Inflammation and swelling of the mucous membranes lining the bronchioles, the smallest airways in the lungs.

Bronchitis – Inflammation of the mucous membranes lining the bronchi, the large to medium-size airways that branch from the trachea carrying air to distal portions of the lungs.

Bulimia nervosa – Complex eating disorder characterized by frequent, recurrent episodes of overeating (binging) followed by (singly or in combination) forced vomiting, ingestion of laxatives and/or diuretics (purging), fasting or exercise. Individuals with this binge/purge disorder are more likely to have a normal (healthy) body weight or be slightly overweight.

Carbuncle – Infection of several furuncles that come together in the same area, characterized by a red, swollen lump filled with fluid, pus, and dead tissue, that may appear white or yellow at the center.

Cardiac arrest – Failure of the heart muscle to contract effectively which impedes the normal circulation of blood and prevents oxygen delivery to the body.

Cellulitis – Inflammation of the connective (soft) tissue often extending into the deep dermal and subcutaneous layers of the skin.

Cerebral cysts, congenital – Also called porencephaly, this is a rare condition present at birth and characterized by the formation of cavities in the cerebral cortex of the brain.

Cerebral Palsy – Group of disorders that affect the brain and central nervous system with impairment to sight, hearing, movement and/or cognition caused by an injury to the brain occurring in utero, during delivery, or in the first 2 years of life when the brain is still growing.

Chemotherapy – Treatment with one or more cytotoxic or antineoplastic drugs that act upon cancerous or malignant cells that divide more rapidly than normal cells to kill or destroy the cancerous or malignant cells.

Cholangitis – Inflammation and/or infection of the cystic (bile) duct.

Cholecystitis – Inflammation and/or infection of the gallbladder.

Choledochal cyst – Congenital cystic dilatation of the bile ducts.

Cholelithiasis – Presence of stones or calculi in the gallbladder or cystic (bile) duct.

Chorea – Abnormal, involuntary, hyperkinetic muscle movement disorder characterized by irregular, repetitive, dance-like rhythmic muscle movements which seem to flow from one muscle or group of muscles to another. The movements may also include twisting or writhing into odd postures that make walking difficult.

Chorioamnionitis – Inflammation of the chorion (maternal side) and/or amnion (fetal side) of the fetal membrane, usually caused by a bacterial infection.

Choroid – Layer of tissue comprised of blood vessels and connective tissue located between the sclera and retina in the eye.

Choroidal degeneration – Group of eye disorders characterized by loss of cellular or tissue function and subsequent structural changes in the choroid layer of the eye.

Cleft lip – Congenital anomaly of the upper lip characterized by indentation or gap in the upper lip (partial or incomplete cleft lip) that may continue into the nose (complete cleft lip) resulting from failure of the maxillary and/or medial nasal processes to fuse during fetal development. Also called cheiloschisis, the defect may be unilateral (one sided) or bilateral (two sided).

Cleft palate – Congenital anomaly of the palate characterized by a gap in the bony hard palate or roof of mouth and/or muscular soft palate/uvula (area behind the hard palate). Also called palatoschisis, it results from failure of the lateral palatine process, nasal septum and/or the median palatine process to fuse during fetal development. A complete cleft involves both the hard and soft palates (and may include a gap in the maxilla). An incomplete cleft involves either the hard or soft palate but does not extend through both.

Colles' fracture – Fracture that occurs just above the radio-carpal junction, usually presenting as a transverse break of the distal radius with displacement posteriorly (dorsally) of the hand/wrist.

Coma – Coma is a prolonged period (>6 hours) of unresponsiveness. It is characterized by the inability to arouse or failure to respond normally to noxious stimuli (pain), light and sound.

Conductive hearing loss – Hearing loss caused by a mechanical problem involving the outer ear, tympanic membrane (ear drum), or bones (ossicles) in the middle ear.

Conjoined twins – Identical twins with a shared (fused) area of the body, most commonly the head, chest or pelvis. This rare type of twin develops from a single fertilized egg cell with a common chorion, placenta and amniotic sac.

Conjunctivitis – Inflammation of the conjunctiva which is the inner surface of the eyelid and outer surface of the eye.

Contracture muscle/tendon sheath – Shortening of the muscle and/or tendon sheath which prevents normal movement and flexibility.

Coronary atherosclerosis – Condition affecting arterial blood vessels in the heart and characterized by inflammation and accumulation of macrophage white blood cells and low-density lipoproteins along the arterial walls leading to narrowing of the vessels and decreased blood flow to the heart muscle.

Craniorachischisis – Severe neural tube defect present at birth characterized by a total or partial fissure involving the skull and spinal column. The condition is very rare and includes both anencephaly and spina bifida (myelomeningocele).

Cushing syndrome – Endocrine disorder that occurs when the body is exposed to high levels of the hormone cortisol either from an exogenous source, such as corticosteroid drugs or from an endogenous source such as overproduction of cortisol in the adrenal glands.

Cystic liver disease, congenital – Liver disease that is present at birth and is characterized by formation of thin walled sacs in the liver, usually in clusters, that contain fluid, gas, or a semi-solid material.

Cystitis – Inflammation of the urinary bladder.

Down's syndrome (Trisomy 21) – Genetic disorder caused by the presence of 3 copies (trisomy) of chromosome number 21. There are three recognized variations of Trisomy 21, nonmosaicism, mosaicism and Robertsonian translocation. Nonmosaicism is the most common and occurs when either the male sperm or female egg has an extra copy of chromosome 21. Mosaicism is uncommon and results from a nondisjunction event that occurs on chromosome 21 during early cell division in a normal (46 chromosome) fertilized egg causing some cells to have 47 chromosomes. Robertsonian translocation (Familial Down Syndrome) is also uncommon and occurs when the long arm of chromosome 21 attaches to another chromosome (usually chromosome 14). The parent is phenotypically normal but a gamete can be formed that has an extra 21st chromosome.

Drug resistant microorganisms – Pathogenic microorganisms that have developed strains that are resistant to some or all of the drugs previously used to treat the resulting infections.

Dysmenorrhea – Dysmenorrhea is pain associated with the menstrual cycle. Primary dysmenorrhea has no underlying disease or condition. Secondary dysmenorrhea has an underlying cause such as endometriosis, ovarian cysts, pelvic inflammatory disease, intrauterine devices, premenstrual syndrome, premenstrual dysphoric disorder, uterine leiomyoma or fibroid tumors.

Dyspareunia – Recurrent or persistent pain associated with sexual intercourse.

Eclampsia – A life threatening obstetrical condition with onset anytime between the 20th week of pregnancy and up to 6 weeks postpartum characterized by hypertension, proteinuria (protein present in urine), and tonic-clonic (motor) seizures. hypertension may be pre-existing or pregnancy-induced.

Edema – Swelling caused by fluid accumulation in the interstitial tissue.

Ehlers-Danlos syndromes (Cutis hyperelastica) – Rare group of genetically inherited connective tissue disorders caused by defects in collagen synthesis, which can manifest in the musculoskeletal system with joint hyper-flexibility or instability and pain, in the skin with hyper-elasticity or fragility, and in the cardiovascular system with fragile blood vessels and valvular heart defects.

Emphysema – Chronic type of obstructive pulmonary disease characterized by the slow destruction of elastic tissue forming the alveoli (air sacs) in the lungs. This leads to an increase in alveoli size and subsequent wall collapse with expiration, trapping air (carbon dioxide) and limiting oxygen availability.

Encephalocele – Rare congenital defect of the neural tube, the channel that forms the brain and spinal cord during fetal development. The condition is characterized by a sac-like protrusion of the meningeal membrane containing cerebral spinal fluid (meningocele) or cerebral spinal fluid (CSF) and brain tissue (encephalomeningocele).

Endometriosis – Presence of cells that are normally found in the uterus outside the uterine cavity, most often in the peritoneum. Endometrial cells react to hormone stimulation during the menstrual cycle causing them to thicken and bleed. This can lead to irritation, development of scar tissue and adhesions, pain, and often problems with fertility.

Epilepsy – Epilepsy is a brain disorder characterized by seizures which are episodic changes in attention or behavior. Seizures occur when an area of the brain becomes over excited and creates abnormal signals. Seizures can manifest as simple staring (absence) or involve whole body shaking (motor, tonic-clonic).

Erectile dysfunction (impotence) – Inability to form or maintain an erection firm enough for sexual intercourse.

Esophageal stenosis, congenital – Narrowing of the esophagus which is present at birth. This narrowing restricts the passage of food/fluid/saliva from the mouth to the stomach.

Esophageal varices – Dilated, submucosal veins in the esophagus.

Esophageal web (ring) – Thin membrane of (normal) mucosal or submucosal tissue that protrudes and obstructs the esophagus. The condition can be congenital (present at birth) or acquired later in life.

Essential hypertension – Abnormally elevated blood pressure levels that have no underlying cause; also called primary or idiopathic hypertension.

Failure to thrive – A condition in which an individual fails to meet expected growth standards due to an inability to consume, retain or utilize nutrients needed to gain weight and grow. It is most common in infants and young children but can occur at any age. Identifying the underlying problem is usually necessary before the condition can be treated effectively.

Fasciculation – Local, involuntary muscle twitch often visible under the skin or detected by electromyography (EMG).

Foodborne infection – Illness that results from food contaminated with microorganisms such as bacteria, and the microorganism continue to grow in the gastrointestinal tract causing the illness.

Foodborne intoxication – Illness that results from consumption of toxins produced in food contaminated by some types by bacteria, such as Staphylococcus aureus and Clostridium botulinum. It is the toxins, not the bacteria, that causes the illness.

Frostbite – Localized damage to skin and soft tissue due to loss of blood circulation from exposure to extremely low temperatures. It usually occurs in distal body parts (fingers, toes, nose).

Functional quadriplegia (quadriparesis) – Partial or complete inability to move due to disability or fragility without physical injury or damage to the central nervous system (brain, spinal cord).

Furuncle – Infection of a hair follicle that extends into the sebaceous gland (pilosebaceous unit), characterized by a red, swollen bump filled with fluid, pus (neutrophils), dead tissue, that may appear white or yellow at the center.

Galeazzi's fracture – Fracture occurring at the junction of the distal and middle third of the radial shaft with subluxation/dislocation of the distal radio-ulnar joint.

Gastric varices – Dilated, submucosal veins in the stomach that are prone to bleeding.

Gastroesophageal reflux disease (GERD) – Chronic digestive disorder that occurs when the muscular valve between the esophagus and stomach fails to function properly allowing gastric acid to flow backward (reflux) from the stomach into the esophagus. The mucosal tissue lining the esophagus becomes irritated causing symptoms such as frequent heartburn, difficulty swallowing, chronic cough and laryngitis.

Gastroschisis – Rare defect in the anterior wall of the abdomen, occurring more often on the right side of the umbilicus in which the abdominal muscles and peritoneum fail to develop normally, exposing abdominal organs to amniotic fluid. The bowel (intestine) can shorten, twist and swell leading to problems with feeding, digestion and absorption of nutrients.

Gestational diabetes – A type of diabetes characterized by glucose intolerance that develops during pregnancy. Hormones produced by the placenta block insulin receptors in the mother causing maternal blood glucose levels to rise. Maternal blood glucose levels usually return to normal post-delivery.

Gestational hypertension – Pregnancy-induced hypertension, characterized by arterial blood pressure >140/90 mmHg, without proteinuria (protein present in urine) in a pregnant woman without previously documented hypertension.

Glaucoma – Group of eye disorders characterized by elevated intraocular pressure that can cause optic nerve damage.

Glomerulonephritis – Disorder of the renal system characterized by inflammation of the glomeruli or small blood vessels in the kidneys.

Glycoprotein metabolism – Glycoprotein metabolic disorders are rare inherited genetic diseases characterized by a failure to synthesize or degrade glycoprotein molecules causing them to accumulate in body organs and tissue.

Glycosaminoglycan metabolism – Metabolic disorder, such as Hurler's, Hurler-Scheie, Morquio, and Sanfilippo, that is usually an inherited genetic disease that causes a failure in the breakdown of long chain sugar molecules which then accumulate and damage body organs.

Gout – An arthritis-like condition caused by an accumulation of uric acid in the blood which leads to inflammation of the joints. Acute gout typically affects one joint. Chronic gout is characterized by repeated episodes of pain and inflammation in one or more joints.

Greenstick fracture – Fracture occurring in soft bone tissue which bends and only partially breaks. It is most common in infants and young children.

HELLP Syndrome – HELLP syndrome is a serious, often life-threatening condition that can progress from pre-eclampsia/eclampsia and includes hemolytic anemia, elevated liver enzymes and decreased platelet count.

Hematosalpinx – Accumulation of blood in the fallopian tube leading to blockage and dilation of the tube.

Hemiparesis (acquired) – Weakness (of muscles/motor function) that affects one side of the body.

Hemiplegia (acquired) – Paralysis (loss of motor function) that affects one side of the body.

Hemolytic anemia – Abnormal breakdown of red blood cells causing a reduced number of red blood cells (RBCs) and/or a low concentration of hemoglobin, the iron-containing protein found on RBCs.

Haemophilus influenzae – Haemophilus influenzae is a bacterium with six encapsulated strains (a-f) and some untypable, unencapsulated strains. H. influenzae is an opportunistic pathogen known to cause pneumonia, meningitis, epiglottitis and other infection/illness, most often in children.

Hepatic cirrhosis – Liver cirrhosis arises from liver fibrosis and is characterized by pseudo-lobule formation with changes to the liver's fundamental structure and subsequent framework collapse.

Hepatic fibrosis – Histological change in liver cells caused by liver inflammation. This change is characterized by an increase in collagen fiber deposits in the extra-cellular spaces of the liver causing a decrease in blood perfusion and hardening of the liver cells.

Hepatitis, chronic, non-viral – Liver inflammation lasting longer than 6 months and characterized by hepatocellular necrosis with infiltration of inflammatory cells.

Hiatal hernia, congenital – Rare condition present at birth, characterized by the protrusion of all or part of the stomach though the diaphragm (sheet of muscle that separates the chest and abdominal cavities) into the esophagus.

Hirschsprung's disease (congenital aganglionic megacolon) – Congenital absence of certain ganglion cells in one or more sections of the gastrointestinal (GI) tract, which causes decreased peristalsis (contraction of intestinal muscles), constipation, and possible bowel obstruction.

Holoprosencephaly (HPE) – Congenital defect of the face and brain, also called arhinencephaly caused by an early embryonic failure of the forebrain to divide into two hemispheres. Three forms of HPE have been identified. Alobar HPE is the most severe and is characterized by almost complete failure of forebrain separation, the nose is missing and the eyes merged into a single median structure. Semilobar HPE has some forebrain separation and facial anomalies may or may not be present. Lobar HPE may have a considerable amount of forebrain separation, rare facial anomalies and brain function can be nearly normal.

Hydrocele (testis) – Accumulation of serous fluid in the scrotum, usually in a remnant piece of peritoneum called the tunica vaginalis that wraps around the testicle.

Hydrocephalus, congenital – Abnormal accumulation of cerebral spinal fluid (CSF) in the ventricles of the brain that is present at birth, usually due to obstruction to the outflow of CSF from the ventricles or subarachnoid space. Congenital hydrocephalus may cause increased intracranial pressure and an enlarged head.

Hydronephrosis – Dilation/distention of the kidney resulting from urine overfill usually caused by an obstruction in the ureter, bladder or urethra.

Hydrops fetalis – Accumulation of excess fluid in two or more fetal compartments, usually arising from an initial overproduction of interstitial fluid, followed by inadequate lymphatic drainage. These compartments can include subcutaneous tissue/scalp, pleural space (pleural effusion), pericardium (pericardial effusion) and the abdomen (ascites).

Hydrosalpinx – Accumulation of serous fluid in the fallopian tube leading to blockage and dilation of the tube. The condition may be unilateral or bilateral and is often associated with infertility.

Hyperesthesia, skin – Sensory dysfunction in any area of the skin, characterized by increased sensation to a normally non-noxious stimulus or sensation without any stimuli input.

Hypertrophic pyloric stenosis, congenital – A condition present at birth, characterized by thickening of the muscles that form the pylorus (valve between the stomach and duodenum). This thickening narrows (obstructs) the opening causing delayed emptying of food from the stomach into the intestine.

Hypoesthesia, skin – Sensory dysfunction in an area of the skin, characterized by decreased or absent sensation to stimuli including thermal, mechanical, electrical and vibration. The dysfunction may vary (i.e. ability to feel heat but not cold, sharp but not dull) and can be transient or permanent.

Hypospadias – Abnormal placement of the male urinary meatus (opening of the urethra) from its normal opening at the end of the penis.

Hypospadias, balanic – In balanic (glanular, coronal, first degree) hypospadias, the opening of the urethra is near the tip but on the underside of the glans penis (penile head).

Hypospadias, penile – Penile (second degree) hypospadias has an opening of the urethra anywhere along the underside of the penile shaft.

Hypospadias, penoscrotal – Third degree hypospadias where the urethral opening is located at the junction of the penile shaft and the scrotum.

Hypospadias, perineal – Third degree hypospadias where the urethral opening is along the perineum between the scrotum and the anus.

Immunotherapy (biologic therapy, biotherapy) – Treatment that utilizes the body's immune system to help fight diseases such as cancer. Immunotherapy may work by stimulating the immune system in general or by training it to attack cancer cells specifically.

Iniencephaly – Severe neural tube defect, characterized by an occipital bone defect, spinal bifida (myelomeningocele) at the level of the cervical vertebrae, and retroflexion (backward bend) of the head at the cervical spine. The condition can be further defined as having an encephalocele present (iniencephaly apertus) or absent (iniencephaly clausus).

Irritable bowel syndrome – Common, non-inflammatory functional bowel disorder that affects the colon (large intestine), with symptoms that include diarrhea and constipation (often alternating), abdominal pain or cramping, gas and bloating.

Irritant contact dermatitis – Inflammation of the skin caused by chemicals or other substances coming in direct with the skin characterized by redness, swelling and itching; may also include blisters/lesions with fluid drainage/oozing. The chemical or other substance is the cause of the inflammation as opposed to an allergic response causing the inflammation.

Isoimmunization – Isoimmunization is the development of antibodies in response to the exposure of isoantigens from foreign tissue or cells.

Jaundice, neonatal – Also called hyperbilirubinemia or neonatal icterus, newborn jaundice is characterized by a yellow discoloration of the sclera (eye) and skin, caused by elevated levels of unconjugated bilirubin.

Kyphosis – Pathological over curvature of the thoracic spine, characterized by a rounded or "humpback" appearance in the upper back.

Left anterior fascicular block – Conduction disorder of the heart that involves the electrical conduction of impulses from the atrioventricular node with the anterior half of the left bundle branch being defective causing the impulse to pass first to the posterior area of the ventricle and delaying activation of the anterior and upper ventricle. Also called left anterior hemiblock, it is the most common partial block of the left bundle branch.

Left posterior fascicular block – Conduction disorder of the heart that involves the electrical conduction of impulses from the atrioventricular node with the posterior half of the left bundle branch being defective causing the impulse to pass first to the anterior and upper ventricle and delaying activation of the posterior ventricle. Also called left posterior hemiblock.

Listeriosis – Infection caused by the bacterium Listeria monocytogenes.

Lordosis – Excessive inward curvature in the lumbar region of the spine, characterized by a swayback or saddle back appearance in the lower back.

Lumbago – Non-specific pain in the lower back region.

Lymphadenitis (lymphadenopathy) – Infection/inflammation of the lymph nodes (glands) which are small structures containing white blood cells (WBCs) that filter lymph fluid.

Lymphangitis – Infection/inflammation of the lymphatic channels that usually results from an infection distal to the channel. The condition is characterized by redness, swelling and warmth often in a "streaking" pattern from the site of the infection.

Malignant immunoproliferative disease – Disorders of the immune system involving abnormal proliferation of primary cells including B-cells, T-cells, Natural Killer (NK) cells and/or excessive production of immunoglobulins (antibodies).

Meckel's diverticulum – Congenital anomaly of the gastrointestinal tract, characterized by a small pouch located in the distal ileum that contains embryonic tissue remnants of the jejunum, duodenum, stomach or pancreas.

Meningococcemia – Infection of the blood caused by the bacteria Neisseria meningitides

Methicillin Resistant Staphylococcus Aureus (MRSA) – Strain of the Staphylococcus aureus bacterium that is resistant to first line antibiotics including penicillins and cephalosporins.

Methicillin Susceptible Staphylococcus Aureus (MSSA) – Strain of the Staphylococcus aureus bacterium sensitive to first line antibiotics including penicillins and cephalosporins.

Migraine – Common neurological disorder that often manifests as a headache that is usually unilateral and pulsating in nature. Caused by abnormal brain activity along nerve pathways and brain chemical (neurotransmitter) changes which affect blood flow in the brain.

Mitral valve – Heart valve located between the left atrium and left ventricle of the heart that is formed by 2 leaflets.

Mittelschmerz – Mid-cycle lower abdominal or pelvic pain usually associated with female ovulation. The pain may be unilateral or bilateral.

Mixed hearing loss – Conductive hearing loss in combination with sensorineural hearing loss.

Monoplegia – Paralysis of a single limb, muscle or muscle group.

Monteggia's fracture – Fracture of the proximal third of the ulna with dislocation of the radial head.

Morbid obesity – A large amount of excess body fat with a BMI>40 or body weight 50-100% greater than normal for height.

Multiple gestation – Pregnancy with more than one fetus.

Multiple Organ Dysfunction Syndrome (MODS) – Physiologic state in which body organs are incapable of maintaining homeostasis. Primary MODS is a direct result of a well-defined insult. Secondary MODS develops as a consequence of the host response within the context of Systemic Inflammatory Response Syndrome (SIRS).

Muscle spasm – Sudden, involuntary contraction of a single muscle or a muscle group.

Mycoplasma pneumoniae – Very small bacterium that lacks a peptidoglycan cell wall, instead having a cell membrane that incorporates a sterol compound. Causes an atypical pneumonia that is resistant to many antibiotics.

Myelodysplastic syndrome (MDS) – Diverse group of blood disorders involving poorly formed or dysfunctional myeloid stem cells.

Myocardial Infarction – Interruption of blood flow to an area of the heart muscle leading to cell damage or death, usually a result of occlusion (blockage) in the coronary arteries.

Myoclonus – Quick, involuntary muscle jerks.

Nephritic syndrome – Clinical disorder of the kidneys characterized by swelling and/or inflammation of the glomeruli which allows protein and red blood cells (RBCs) to filter into the urine. Hypertension and uremia may also be part of the syndrome.

Neutropenia – Low level of neutrophils, a type of white blood cell (WBC), in the circulating blood.

Obesity – Large amounts of excess fat in the body with a BMI of 30-39.9 or body weight at least 20% greater than normal for height.

Oligohydramnios – Decreased level of amniotic fluid during pregnancy.

Oligomenorrhea – Infrequent menstruation (cycle >35 days or 4-9 periods per year) in a woman with previously regular periods.

Oligospermia – Low level of sperm (<15 million sperm/ml) present in semen (ejaculate) and is associated with male infertility.

Omphalitis – Infection of the umbilical cord stump.

Oophoritis – Infection/inflammation of the ovary which can be unilateral or bilateral, and acute or chronic.

Osteoarthritis – Degenerative disease of the joints including articular cartilage and subchondral bone, characterized by pain, stiffness, immobility and swelling (effusion, fluid accumulation).

Osteomalacia – Softening of bone tissue due to inadequate intake or absorption of vitamin D, calcium and/or phosphorus (phosphate).

Osteoporosis – Disease that affects previously constructed bone tissue, characterized by decreased density, weakness and brittleness, making the bone more susceptible to fracture.

Otitis externa – Inflammation of the outer ear and ear canal.

Otitis media – Inflammation of the middle ear, between the tympanic membrane and inner ear and including the Eustachian tube.

Overweight – Excess body fat that can impair health. A BMI of 25-29.9 is considered overweight for most individuals.

Pancreatitis – Inflammation of the pancreas.

Pancytopenia – Reduced number of red blood cells (RBCs), white blood cells (WBCs) and platelets.

Paresthesia, skin – Sensory dysfunction affecting any area of the skin and characterized by a feeling of burning, numbness, tickling or tingling without any long term adverse effect.

Paraphimosis – Retraction of the prepuce (foreskin) behind the glans penis (head of the penis) that decreases blood flow to the glans causing a tight edematous (swollen) band of tissue to form. The swelling makes it difficult, sometimes impossible to move the foreskin back over the glans.

Parkinson's disease – Degenerative disorder of the brain and central nervous system caused by a loss of dopamine generating cells in the midbrain and an accumulation of the protein alpha-synuclein in structures called Lewy bodies also located in the brain.

Paroxysmal tachycardia – Heart rhythm disorder characterized by recurrent episodes of rapid heartbeats, usually with an abrupt onset and a spontaneous return to a normal. The condition is caused by an abnormal electrical focus that can originate in the atrium, atrioventricular node or ventricle.

Pathologic fracture associated with malignancy (cancer) – Fracture that results from primary or metastatic malignant (cancerous) lesions that invade and destroy normal bone tissue causing the bone to weaken and break.

Penile chordee, congenital – An abnormal upward or downward curvature of the penile head (glans penis) at the junction to the shaft that is present at birth.

Persistent vegetative state – Disorder of consciousness usually associated with severe brain damage, characterized by a state of partial arousal (wakeful unconsciousness) but not true awareness of the environment.

Persistent cloaca – Rare, complex, malformation of the female anorectal and genitourinary tracts, characterized by fusion of the rectum, vagina and urethra creating a single channel (cloaca).

Phimosis – Inability of the prepuce (foreskin) to be retracted behind the glans penis (head of the penis) in an uncircumcised male.

Phlebitis – Inflammation of a vein.

Pica – Patterned eating of non-nutritive substance, such as dirt or paper, for a duration of >1 month at an age when it is developmentally inappropriate.

Placenta previa – Obstetrical condition in which the placenta attaches low in the uterus, partially or totally obstructing the cervix, which may cause severe bleeding during pregnancy and/or delivery.

Placental insufficiency – Complication of pregnancy in which the fetus fails to receive adequate nutrition and/or oxygen because the placenta does not develop properly or becomes damaged during the pregnancy.

Placentitis – Inflammation of the placenta which is the organ that secretes hormones and provides nutrition, waste elimination and gas exchange (oxygen) to the developing fetus.

Pneumonia – Inflammatory condition of the lungs, primarily in the alveoli (terminal air sacs) which may be caused by infection (bacteria, virus, other pathogens), chemicals or drugs and certain autoimmune disorders.

Pneumonia, newborn/congenital – Inflammatory condition of the respiratory tract that is acquired in utero or during the birth process. Symptoms can be present at birth or occur in the neonatal period (up to 28 days following delivery).

Polyhydramnios – Increased level of amniotic fluid during pregnancy.

Post-term (postmature) newborn – Newborn with a gestational period (pregnancy) that has exceeded 42 weeks.

Pre-eclampsia – Obstetrical complication that typically occurs after the 20th week of gestation but may also occur as late as 6 weeks postpartum with the following symptoms: hypertension (BP >140/90 mmHg) with proteinuria (protein present in urine). Pre-eclampsia may be considered severe with a BP >160/110 and additional symptoms such as edema (swelling) and epigastric pain. The hypertension may be pre-existing or pregnancy induced.

Premenstrual dysphoric disorder (PMDD) – Severe form of premenstrual syndrome (PMS), PMDD is characterized by depression, anxiety, tension and irritability that typically begins after release of the ovum, as the follicle forms the corpus luteum and secretes progesterone (luteal phase).

Premenstrual syndrome (PMS) – Condition associated with the menstrual cycle that is characterized by a consistent pattern of physical and/or emotional symptoms, including irritability, tension, unhappiness (dysphoria), anxiety, insomnia, fatigue, breast tenderness, bloating, abdominal discomfort (cramps), muscle and joint pain.

Pre-term (premature) newborn – Neonate with a gestational period (pregnancy) less than 37 weeks.

Prune belly syndrome (Eagle-Barret syndrome, Triad syndrome) – Rare genetic condition characterized by three factors, a partial or total lack of abdominal muscles (giving skin a wrinkled appearance), undescended testis (cryptorchidism)and urinary tract problems (large ureters, distended bladder).

Pruritus – Itching.

Psoriasis – Chronic, noncontagious, immune mediated skin disorder characterized by thick silvery scales and dry, red, itchy patches that may be painful.

Psychogenic appetite loss – An aversion to food or eating without a pathologic/physiologic explanation for the condition.

Pterygium – Benign growth of tissue on the conjunctiva, that typically presents near the cornea as a painless, raised, white lesion that contains blood vessels.

Pulmonary valve – Heart valve located between the right ventricle of the heart and the pulmonary artery and is formed by 3 leaflets.

Pyosalpinx – Accumulation of pus in the fallopian tube leading to blockage and dilation of the tube.

Radiation proctitis – Inflammation and tissue damage of the lower colon following exposure to x-ray or ionizing radiation to treat certain cancers (cervical, prostate, colon).

Radiation therapy – The medical use of ionizing radiation to control or kill malignant (cancer) cells by damaging cell DNA.

Regional enteritis (Crohn's disease) – Chronic inflammatory bowel disease that can occur anywhere from the mouth to the anus but typically affects the intestines.

Renal agenesis (dysgenesis) (hypoplasia) – Failure of one (unilateral) or both (bilateral) kidneys to develop normally during gestation.

Restless leg syndrome (RLS) – An irresistible need to move the legs due to unpleasant sensations such as creeping, crawling, tingling or bubbling. The sensations are most often felt in the lower leg between the knee and ankle but can also be located in the upper leg or arms. Movement does not relieve the sensations.

Right fascicular block – Defect in the heart's electrical conduction system in which the right ventricle is not activated by an impulse from the right bundle branch but does depolarize when impulses from the left bundle branch travel through the myocardium.

Rolando's fracture – Comminuted intra-articular fracture through the base of the first metacarpal bone, usually in three fragments forming a T or Y shape.

Salpingitis – Infection/inflammation of the fallopian tube that may be unilateral or bilateral and acute or chronic.

Sciatica – Pain, paresthesia, and/or weakness in the low back, buttocks or lower extremities resulting from compression of one or more spinal nerves that form the sciatic nerves.

Scoliosis – Abnormal sideways curvature in the spine. The condition may be present at birth or develop later in life, usually around the time of puberty.

Scrotal varices (varicocele) – Enlarged veins along the spermatic cord.

Seborrheic dermatitis – Inflammatory skin disorder caused by over production of sebum, from oil producing sebaceous glands found in the scalp, face and torso. The condition is characterized by scaly or flaky skin, itching and redness.

Secondary hypertension – Abnormally elevated blood pressure levels due to an underlying condition or cause such as kidney disease, adrenal gland tumors, or medication.

Secondary parkinsonism – Parkinson's-like symptoms that are due to an identifiable underlying illness, injury or disease process, such as chemical or environmental toxins, drugs, encephalitis or meningitis and cerebral vascular disease.

Septicemia (bacteremia) – Presence of pathogens such as bacteria, virus, fungi or parasites in the blood. The condition may lead to sepsis.

Sialoadenitis – Inflammation and/or infection of one or more of the salivary glands.

Smith's fracture – Also referred to as a reverse Colles' fracture, this type of fracture occurs just above the radiocarpal junction with the radius displaced ventrally (volarly). It can present with multiple fragments and may or may not involve the articular surface of the wrist joint.

Somnolence – State of drowsiness that normally precedes sleep, but can occur outside of normal sleep patterns when there is a disruption or dysfunction in circadian rhythm, when fatigue causes periods of microsleep and when illness or infection are present and the body naturally rests to conserve energy.

Spermatocele – Fluid filled cyst that may contain spermatozoa and is located in a tubule at the head of the epididymis.

Spondylolisthesis – Anterior or posterior displacement of one or more vertebra(e).

Staphylococcus aureus – Bacterium that commonly colonizes in the human respiratory tract and on the skin and may lead to acute infections.

Stevens-Johnson syndrome – Mild form of toxic epidermal necrolysis (TEN), a complex hypersensitivity response that affects skin and mucus membranes causing cell death due to separation of the epidermis from the dermis.

Stress fracture – Small crack or break in a bone caused by unusual or repeated force/overuse in an area of the body, most commonly the lower legs and feet.

Stupor – Disorder of consciousness characterized by unresponsiveness except to noxious stimuli (pain). An individual in a state of stupor will usually have muscle rigidity, muteness, but eyes may open and appear to track surroundings.

Thrombophlebitis – Inflammation of a vein with formation of a blood clot within the vessel.

Tics – Tics or tic disorders involve a discrete group of muscles and are characterized by sudden, repetitive motor movement or phonic utterances.

Torus fracture – Fracture that occurs on one side of a long bone causing it to overlap (buckle) onto itself without disrupting the integrity of the bone on the opposite side.

Tracheoesophageal fistula, congenital – Abnormal connection between the trachea and the esophagus. The condition occurs when the tracheoesophageal ridges fail to fuse during early embryonic development.

Transient cerebral ischemia (transient ischemic attack, TIA) – Temporary disruption of cerebral blood flow without acute infarction or tissue death.

Transient global amnesia – Sudden, temporary loss of short term memory.

Tremor – Involuntary, often rhythmic contraction and relaxation of one or more muscles.

Tricuspid valve – Heart valve located between the right atrium and right ventricle of the heart and formed by 3 leaflets.

Ulcerative colitis – Chronic inflammatory bowel disease that affects the large intestine including the rectum. The condition is usually intermittent with exacerbation of symptoms (diarrhea with/without blood and/or mucus) and then extended periods without symptoms.

Undescended testis (cryptorchidism) – Failure of one or both testicles to descend from the groin (or abdomen) into the scrotum prior to birth.

Urethral stricture – Abnormal narrowing of the urethra, a channel through which urine passes from the bladder to the outside of the body.

Vaginismus – Sudden tension or spasm of vaginal muscles making vaginal penetration during intercourse painful or impossible.

Vaginitis – Inflammation of the female vagina usually due to irritation or infection (e.g., bacterial vaginosis, candidiasis, trichomoniasis) that may be acute or chronic.

Varicose veins – Enlarged, tortuous (twisted) and painful vein caused by incompetence of the valves in the vein and backflow of blood.

Ventricular fibrillation (V-fib) – Serious, life threatening heart rhythm disorder characterized by uncontrolled twitching or quivering of the heart muscle fibers and failure of the heart to effectively pump blood.

Vertigo – Sensation that one's body (subjective vertigo) or surroundings (objective vertigo) are in motion.

Vesicoureteral reflux (VUR) – Backflow of urine from the bladder to the ureters and sometimes into the kidneys.

Vulvovaginitis – Inflammation of the female vagina and vulva (labia, clitoris and vestibule of the vagina) that may be acute or chronic.